Biomechanics in Orthopedics

Biomechanics in Orthopedics

Editor: Jack Burrell

FOSTER
ACADEMICS

www.fosteracademics.com

www.fosteracademics.com

FOSTER ACADEMICS

Cataloging-in-Publication Data

Biomechanics in orthopedics / edited by Jack Burrell.
p. cm.
Includes bibliographical references and index.
ISBN 978-1-63242-528-7
1. Orthopedics. 2. Biomechanics. I. Burrell, Jack.
RD731 .B56 2018
617--dc23

Foster Academics,
118-35 Queens Blvd., Suite 400,
Forest Hills, NY 11375, USA

ISBN 978-1-63242-528-7 (Hardback)

Printed and bound in China.

Contents

Preface IX

Chapter 1 **A Replication Study for Genome-Wide Gene Expression Levels in Two Layer Lines Elucidates Differentially Expressed Genes of Pathways Involved in Bone Remodeling and Immune Responsiveness** 1
Christin Habig, Robert Geffers, Ottmar Distl

Chapter 2 **Surgical Membranes as Directional Delivery Devices to Generate Tissue: Testing in an Ovine Critical Sized Defect Model** 9
Melissa L. Knothe Tate, Hana Chang, Shannon R. Moore, Ulf R. Knothe

Chapter 3 **Glutamine Repeat Variants in Human RUNX2 Associated with Decreased Femoral Neck BMD, Broadband Ultrasound Attenuation and Target Gene Transactivation** 18
Nigel A. Morrison, Alexandre A. Stephens, Motomi Osato, Patsie Polly, Timothy C. Tan, Namiko Yamashita, James D. Doecke, Julie Pasco, Nicolette Fozzard, Graeme Jones, Stuart H. Ralston, Philip N. Sambrook, Richard L. Prince, Geoff C. Nicholson

Chapter 4 **Trabecular Reorganization in Consecutive Iliac Crest Biopsies when Switching from Bisphosphonate to Strontium Ranelate Treatment** 29
Björn Jobke, Andrew J. Burghardt, Burkhard Muche, Michael Hahn, Jutta Semler, Michael Amling, Sharmila Majumdar, Björn Busse

Chapter 5 **Common Genetic Variants are Associated with Accelerated Bone Mineral Density Loss after Hematopoietic Cell Transplantation** 39
Song Yao, Lara E. Sucheston, Shannon L. Smiley, Warren Davis, Jeffrey M. Conroy, Norma J. Nowak, Christine B. Ambrosone, Philip L. McCarthy Jr., Theresa Hahn

Chapter 6 **Cortical Bone Mechanical Properties are Altered in an Animal Model of Progressive Chronic Kidney Disease** 47
Christopher L. Newman, Sharon M. Moe, Neal X. Chen, Max A. Hammond, Joseph M. Wallace, Jeffry S. Nyman, Matthew R. Allen

Chapter 7 **Neovascular Niche for Human Myeloma Cells in Immunodeficient Mouse Bone** 55
Hirono Iriuchishima, Keiyo Takubo, Yoshitaka Miyakawa, Ayako Nakamura-Ishizu, Yoshiteru Miyauchi, Nobuyuki Fujita, Kana Miyamoto, Takeshi Miyamoto, Eiji Ikeda, Masahiro Kizaki, Yoshihisa Nojima, Toshio Suda

Chapter 8 ***Erk1* Positively Regulates Osteoclast Differentiation and Bone Resorptive Activity** 67
Yongzheng He, Karl Staser, Steven D. Rhodes, Yaling Liu, Xiaohua Wu, Su-Jung Park, Jin Yuan, Xianlin Yang, Xiaohong Li, Li Jiang, Shi Chen, Feng-Chun Yang

Chapter 9 **Targeting Bone Alleviates Osteoarthritis in Osteopenic Mice and Modulates Cartilage Catabolism** 77
Thomas Funck-Brentano, Hilène Lin, Eric Hay, Marie-Dominique Ah Kioon, Corinne Schiltz, Didier Hannouche, Rémy Nizard, Frédéric Lioté, Philippe Orcel, Marie-Christine de Vernejoul, Martine Esther Cohen-Solal

Chapter 10 **Cthrc1 is a Positive Regulator of Osteoblastic Bone Formation** 85
Hiroaki Kimura, Kin Ming Kwan, Zhaoping Zhang, Jian Min Deng, Bryant G. Darnay, Richard R. Behringer, Takashi Nakamura, Benoit de Crombrugghe, Haruhiko Akiyama

Chapter 11 **Accelerated Postero-Lateral Spinal Fusion by Collagen Scaffolds Modified with Engineered Collagen-Binding Human Bone Morphogenetic Protein-2 in Rats** 94
Xinglong Han, Wen Zhang, Jun Gu, Huan Zhao, Li Ni, Jiajun Han, Yun Zhou, Yannan Gu, Xuesong Zhu, Jie Sun, Xianglin Hou, Huilin Yang, Jianwu Dai, Qin Shi

Chapter 12 **Growth Hormone Improves Growth Retardation Induced by Rapamycin without Blocking its Antiproliferative and Antiangiogenic Effects on Rat Growth Plate** 103
Óscar Álvarez-García, Enrique García-López, Vanessa Loredo, Helena Gil-Peña, Natalia Mejía-Gaviria, Julián Rodríguez-Suárez, Flor Á. Ordóñez, Fernando Santos

Chapter 13 **Phase II Open Label Study of Valproic Acid in Spinal Muscular Atrophy** 112
Kathryn J. Swoboda, Charles B. Scott, Sandra P. Reyna, Thomas W. Prior, Bernard LaSalle, Susan L. Sorenson, Janine Wood, Gyula Acsadi, Thomas O. Crawford, John T. Kissel, Kristin J. Krosschell, Guy D'Anjou, Mark B. Bromberg, Mary K. Schroth, Gary M. Chan, Bakri Elsheikh, Louise R. Simard

Chapter 14 **Mechanical Behaviour of Umbrella-Shaped, Ni-Ti Memory Alloy Femoral Head Support Device during Implant Operation: A Finite Element Analysis Study** 121
Wei Yi, Qing Tian, Zhipeng Dai, Xiaohu Liu

Chapter 15 **Control of Bone Resorption by Semaphorin 4D is Dependent on Ovarian Function** 130
Romain Dacquin, Chantal Domenget, Atsushi Kumanogoh, Hitoshi Kikutani, Pierre Jurdic, Irma Machuca-Gayet

Chapter 16 **The Effect of HIV-Hepatitis C Co-Infection on Bone Mineral Density and Fracture** 141
Tyler J. O'Neill, Laura Rivera, Vladi Struchkov, Ahmad Zaheen, Hla-Hla Thein

Chapter 17 **Isolation and Characterization of Novel Murine Epiphysis Derived Mesenchymal Stem Cells** 152
Chun-Chun Cheng, Wei-Shiung Lian, Felix Shih-Hsiang Hsiao, I-Hsuan Liu, Shau-Ping Lin, Yen-Hua Lee, Chia-Chun Chang, Guan-Yu Xiao, Hsin-Yi Huang, Ching-Feng Cheng, Winston Teng-Kuei Cheng, Shinn-Chih Wu

Chapter 18 **Protection by Salidroside against Bone Loss via Inhibition of Oxidative Stress and Bone-Resorbing Mediators**......167
Jin-Kang Zhang, Liu Yang, Guo-Lin Meng, Zhi Yuan, Jing Fan, Dan Li, Jian-Zong Chen, Tian-Yao Shi, Hui-Min Hu, Bo-Yuan Wei, Zhuo-Jing Luo, Jian Liu

Chapter 19 **Time of Progression to Osteopenia /Osteoporosis in Chronically HIV-Infected Patients: Screening DXA Scan**......177
Eugenia Negredo, Anna Bonjoch, Moisés Gómez-Mateu, Carla Estany, Jordi Puig, Nuria Perez-Alvarez, Joaquin Rosales, Silvana di Gregorio, Luis del Rio, Guadalupe Gómez, Bonaventura Clotet

Chapter 20 **Coating with a Modular Bone Morphogenetic Peptide Promotes Healing of a Bone-Implant Gap in an Ovine Model**......186
Yan Lu, Jae Sung Lee, Brett Nemke, Ben K. Graf, Kevin Royalty, Richard Illgen III, Ray Vanderby Jr., Mark D. Markel, William L. Murphy

Chapter 21 **Determinants of Microdamage in Elderly Human Vertebral Trabecular Bone**......193
Hélène Follet, Delphine Farlay, Yohann Bala, Stéphanie Viguet-Carrin, Evelyne Gineyts, Brigitte Burt-Pichat, Julien Wegrzyn, Pierre Delmas, Georges Boivin, Roland Chapurlat

Chapter 22 **Generic Rules of Mechano-Regulation Combined with Subject Specific Loading Conditions can Explain Bone Adaptation after THA**......203
Tomasz D. Szwedowski, William R. Taylor, Markus O. Heller, Carsten Perka, Michael Müller, Georg N. Duda

Chapter 23 **Impaired Angiogenesis during Fracture Healing in GPCR Kinase 2 Interacting Protein-1 (GIT1) Knock Out Mice**......210
Guoyong Yin, Tzong-Jen Sheu, Prashanthi Menon, Jinjiang Pang, Hsin-Chiu Ho, Shanshan Shi, Chao Xie, Elaine Smolock, Chen Yan, Michael J. Zuscik, Bradford C. Berk

Permissions

List of Contributors

Index

Preface

This book has been a concerted effort by a group of academicians, researchers and scientists, who have contributed their research works for the realization of the book. This book has materialized in the wake of emerging advancements and innovations in this field. Therefore, the need of the hour was to compile all the required researches and disseminate the knowledge to a broad spectrum of people comprising of students, researchers and specialists of the field.

Bone is the most significant organ of our bodies. The skeletal system provides support and structure to the body and our organs. Bones are also crucial because they store minerals. Orthopedics deals with topics related to bone surgery, dislocation of bones, treatment and cure of tumors and cancers affecting bones and our musculoskeletal system. This book presents this complex subject in the most comprehensible and easy to understand language. It strives to provide a fair idea about this discipline and to help develop a better understanding of the latest advances within this field. It will serve as a valuable source of reference for graduate and post-graduate students.

At the end of the preface, I would like to thank the authors for their brilliant chapters and the publisher for guiding us all-through the making of the book till its final stage. Also, I would like to thank my family for providing the support and encouragement throughout my academic career and research projects.

Editor

1

A Replication Study for Genome-Wide Gene Expression Levels in Two Layer Lines Elucidates Differentially Expressed Genes of Pathways Involved in Bone Remodeling and Immune Responsiveness

Christin Habig[1], Robert Geffers[2], Ottmar Distl[1]*

1 Institute for Animal Breeding and Genetics, University of Veterinary Medicine Hannover (Foundation), Hannover, Germany, **2** Department of Cell Biology, Helmholtz Centre for Infection Research, Braunschweig, Germany

Abstract

The current replication study confirmed significant differences in gene expression profiles of the cerebrum among the two commercial layer lines Lohmann Selected Leghorn (LSL) and Lohmann Brown (LB). Microarray analyses were performed for 30 LSL and another 30 LB laying hens kept in the small group housing system Eurovent German. A total of 14,103 microarray probe sets using customized Affymetrix ChiGene-1_0-st Arrays with 20,399 probe sets were differentially expressed among the two layer lines LSL and LB (FDR adjusted P-value <0.05). An at least 2-fold change in expression levels could be observed for 388 of these probe sets. In LSL, 214 of the 388 probe sets were down- and 174 were up-regulated and vice versa for the LB layer line. Among the 174 up-regulated probe sets in LSL, we identified 51 significantly enriched Gene ontology (GO) terms of the biological process category. A total of 63 enriched GO-terms could be identified for the 214 down-regulated probe sets of the layer line LSL. We identified nine genes significantly differentially expressed between the two layer lines in both microarray experiments. These genes play a crucial role in protection of neuronal cells from oxidative stress, bone mineral density and immune response among the two layer lines LSL and LB. Thus, the different regulation of these genes may significantly contribute to phenotypic trait differences among these layer lines. In conclusion, these novel findings provide a basis for further research to improve animal welfare in laying hens and these layer lines may be of general interest as an animal model.

Editor: Ioannis P Androulakis, Rutgers University, United States of America

Funding: This project and CH have been supported by funds of the Federal Ministry of Food, Agriculture and Consumer Protection (BMELV) via the Federal Office for Agriculture and Food (BLE), Bonn, Germany, under the innovation support program (PGI 06.01 28 1-36.004-07). The funders had no role in study design, data collection and analysis, decision to publish, or preparation of the manuscript.

Competing Interests: The authors have declared that no competing interests exist.

* E-mail: ottmar.distl@tiho-hannover.de

Introduction

Whether and to what extent cellular development, differentiation, function and physiology occur does essentially depend on the repertoire, level and time point of expressed genes [1]. Therefore, experimental tools for direct and simultaneous monitoring of the expression levels of large numbers of genes in parallel are of great importance [1]. Affymetrix was the first company that developed a method to analyse large fragments and even entire genomes, called DNA microarrays [2]. Currently, the Affymetrix GeneChip microarrays are the most frequently used high-throughput technology to measure gene expression [3]. Microarrays are now available for a variety of different species, including agriculturally important species [4] like the chicken. Since the completion of the chicken genome sequence, assembly and annotation, as well as the availability of new high-throughput tools for the exploration of functional elements of the genome, the chicken became an important model organism [5,6] for evolutionary and developmental biology, immunology, genetics and agricultural science [7].

Microarray technologies enable the examination of expression levels of thousands of genes in a single hybridization experiment. Microarray analyses can permit the understanding of biological pathways important in various physiological processes [4] and may therefore contribute to improvements in important economic parameters in poultry, like egg production and reproduction traits in ducks or feed efficiency and growth in broilers [8–10]. Furthermore, behavioural disorders, like feather pecking, a serious animal welfare and economically important problem, especially in the laying hen husbandry has been examined by using microarray analyses in several studies [11–13]. Labouriau et al. [11] used 20K chicken oligonucleotide microarrays (ARK-Genomics) to compare gene transcription profiles of a high feather pecking White Leghorn line, selected for eight generations, with another group of birds performing feather pecking. Among a total of 14,077 investigated genes they identified 456 genes to be differentially expressed between these two groups of laying hens, supporting their evidence of the presence of a major dominant allele affecting feather pecking behaviour. Differences in feather pecking behaviour between the two widespread commercial layer lines Lohmann Selected Leghorn (LSL) and Lohmann Brown (LB) are also confessed from several studies [12–13]. Due to these behavioural differences, as well as further differences in phenotypic traits, LSL and LB laying hens are not equally suitable for different housing systems. In a previous study, we identified 6,276 microarray probe sets to be significant differentially expressed (FDR adjusted P-value <0.05) between the two layer lines LSL and LB [14]. Among these probe sets, 151 had a 2-fold change or greater in gene expression and could be assigned to immune system processes and phosphorus metabolic processes. In order to confirm the conclusions drawn from this microarray experiment, a replication study was performed to validate the reliability of the results, as well as to improve the sensitivity and specificity of our previous analyses.

Therefore, the aim of the present study was to replicate the previous study under the very similar conditions and determine which genes are differentially expressed in both experiments.

Results

Phenotypic traits

For the phenotypic traits the least square means (LSM) with their standard errors (SE) and the P-values for differences between the two layer lines LSL and LB in the present experiment are given in Table 1. Although the egg weights were approximately equal in both layer lines, LSL hens laid eggs with significantly higher albumen heights and Haugh units, heavier yolks and eggshells, but at the same time thinner eggshells. At each time of examination, LSL layers were scored significantly worse for the plumage condition of the different body regions, resulting in a worse total plumage score compared to LB. The body weights, bone weights, as well as the bone lengths were significantly higher in LB than in LSL. Furthermore, LB hens had significantly higher tibia and humerus bone breaking strengths than LSL. The calculated heterophil to lymphocyte ratio (H/L-ratio) of LB layers was approximately 3-times higher than the average H/L-ratio determined for LSL.

Gene expression analysis

A total of 388 probe sets with at least a 2-fold change in expression could be assigned among the 14,103 probe sets. In LSL, 214 of the 388 probe sets were down- and 174 were up-regulated (Table S1). By contrast, the 214 down-regulated probe sets were enriched and the 174 highly expressed probe sets were down-regulated in the LB layer line (Figure S1). GO annotation of biological process was only given for 45 of the 388 significant probe sets. Among the 174 up-regulated probe sets in LSL, we identified 51 significantly enriched GO-terms of the biological process category (Table S2). Figure S2 shows a tree graph, representing the hierarchical relationships of these enriched GO-terms. A total of 63 enriched GO-terms could be identified for the 214 down-regulated probe sets of the layer line LSL. Relationships between these GO-terms are represented in Figure S3.

We compared the outcomes for the differentially expressed probe sets among the two layer lines of the present study with our previous microarray analysis for the same layer lines. A 2-fold or greater change in gene expression was identified on 151 probe sets in the previous experiment [14]. These 151 probe sets could be assigned to 79 different genes. The 388 significant probe sets of the present experiment could be assigned to 264 different genes. A comparison of all genes (n = 14,338) assigned to the probe sets of both microarray experiments revealed that 66% of the genes were in common. A total of 2343 genes of the previous microarray experiment were not represented in the present experiment, whereas 2605 genes of the present experiment were missing in the previous experiment. Among the differentially expressed genes from both experiments (n = 334), there were 301/334 genes (90%) on both microarray platforms represented. We found nine genes to be differentially expressed between the two layer lines in both experiments (Table 2). Assuming the same rate of differentially expressed genes (9/301 = 0.03) for the genes not present on both microarray platforms, we assume that we may have missed $0.03 \times 65 = 1.95$ genes potentially significantly differentially expressed. The probability for observing nine differentially expressed genes in the two experiments was $P<0.0001$.

Discussion

The present study confirmed the layer lines as the most important factor influencing gene expression levels. While for the group size and tier of the housing system no significant differentially expressed genes could be found, we identified a great number of genes with different expression among the layer lines LSL and LB. Although the type of microarray chip was not identical in the two microarray experiments, we identified a total of nine genes to be significant differentially expressed in the same direction of regulation between the two layer lines in both experiments. Identification of these nine genes among the huge number of several ten thousands of probe sets indicates a crucial role of their gene products within processes that are different between the two layer lines.

The *aldo-keto reductase family 7, member A2* (*AKR7A2*) was one of these genes with higher expression in LSL in both experiments. AKR7A2 is one of the aldo-keto reductase enzymes that are necessary for detoxication and reduction of endogenous and exogenous aldehydes in mammals [15,16]. AKR7A2 plays a significant role in protecting the brain from oxidative stress, because of its protective function of cells against the cytotoxicity of products arised from lipid peroxidation and correspondingly DNA damage, as well as its contribution to lowering reactive oxygen species [16]. Furthermore, this succinic semialdehyde reductase is catalyzing the biosynthesis of the neuromodulator γ-hydroxybutyrate [15].

The expression of *catechol-O-methyltransferase domain containing 1* (*COMTD1*) was down-regulated in LSL in the first as well as in the second experiment. Its gene product the catechol O methyltransferase 1 is responsible for the O-methylation of catechol estrogens, physiologically important catecholamines and many other catechols [17]. A common genetic polymorphism in the orthologous human *COMT* gene is a functional G>A polymorphism, resulting in an amino acid substitution of valine to methionine at codon 158 [18–20]. In comparison to the valine variant, the methionine variant has a 3- to 4-fold lower enzymatic activity [19–21] and is also associated with individual thermolability of the enzyme [20–22]. A lower bone mineral density has been found in men being homozygous for the low-activity *COMT* allele [19]. The *COMT* genotype can be used as an independent predictor of areal bone mineral density in the total body and in all femur locations, but not in the spine [19]. An increase in sympathetic activity due to a decreased degradation of catecholamines in individuals has been associated with the low-activity *COMT* genotype [19]. This increased activity of the sympathetic nervous system has a catabolic effect on bone formation [23]. Therefore, these findings may explain the increased risk for osteoporotic fractures and for fragility fractures in human male carriers of the Met^{158} low-activity allele [18]. The low expression of the *COMTD1* gene in LSL in the current study may have resulted in low expression levels of the catechol-O-methyltransferase, and correspondingly a decrease in substrate conversion. Consequently, the LSL layers had a higher sympathetic activity, which might explain the significantly lower humerus and tibia bone breaking strengths

Table 1. Least-square means (LSM), their standard errors (SE) and P-values for the phenotypic traits analysed in the two layer lines Lohmann Selected Leghorn (LSL) and Lohmann Brown (LB).

Trait	LB		LSL		LB - LSL
	LSM	SE	LSM	SE	P-value
Egg quality traits					
Egg weight (g)	63.99	0.23	64.40	0.23	0.210
Eggshell weight (g)	6.51	0.04	6.79	0.04	<0.001
Eggshell breaking strength (N)	41.29	0.46	40.00	0.46	0.058
Albumen height (mm)	8.45	0.07	9.23	0.07	<0.001
Haugh units	90.29	0.41	94.41	0.41	<0.001
Yolk weight (g)	16.07	0.07	16.99	0.07	<0.001
Eggshell thickness (µm)	343.14	1.12	338.48	1.11	0.007
Plumage condition (1–4)					
-Neck	2.74	0.05	2.45	0.05	<0.001
-Back	3.63	0.12	2.56	0.12	<0.001
-Wings	2.53	0.07	2.43	0.07	0.321
-Tail	2.48	0.05	1.85	0.05	<0.001
-Breast	2.32	0.04	1.62	0.04	<0.001
-Belly	3.38	0.07	1.99	0.07	<0.001
-Total	17.09	0.34	12.91	0.34	<0.001
Body weight (kg)	1.91	0.01	1.58	0.01	<0.001
Bone length (cm)					
-Tibia (cm)	11.85	0.03	11.58	0.02	<0.001
-Humerus (cm)	7.90	0.02	7.60	0.01	<0.001
Bone weight (g)					
-Tibia (g)	11.59	0.09	8.81	0.08	<0.001
-Humerus (g)	4.52	0.05	3.43	0.05	<0.001
Bone breaking strength (N)					
-Tibia (N)	146.78	3.15	137.29	3.13	0.044
-Humerus (N)	237.83	3.57	185.68	3.52	<0.001
H/L-ratio	0.84	0.05	0.29	0.05	<0.001

measured in LSL compared to LB. Furthermore, the increase in sympathetic activity might be a reason for the significant differences of plumage condition between LSL and LB laying hens. The major reason for the observed damage of plumage up to bare regions, especially in LSL, could be found in feather pecking. This term describes a behaviour that involves hens destroying the plumage of their flock mates, in some cases even pulling out feathers and eating them [24]. Significantly higher plasma noradrenaline levels and a faster heart rate during manual restraint, both indicative for a high sympathetic reactivity, in high feather peckers have been reported for a White Leghorn line compared to low feather peckers of the same layer line [25,26].

The up-regulation of *EXT2* in LSL may also be contributed to their lower bone breaking strengths. *EXT2* encodes for exostosin 2, an enzyme that synthesizes heparan sulfate proteoglycans [27]. In human, a genetic mutation in exostosin 2 is associated with skeletal syndromes or predispositions to certain skeletal diseases [28].

Another gene with different expression between the two layer lines in both studies was *IGJ*, encoding the immunoglobulin J polypeptide, linker protein for immunoglobulin alpha and mu polypeptides. Beside the monomer IGM, IGJ is one of the components that mediate the B-cell-specific expression of IGM antibodies [29], and therefore plays an important role in the immune response. In LB, lower expression could be found for one transcript variant of IGJ in the first and even three transcript variants in the second experiment. In agreement with previous results, we attribute this down-regulation of immune system components to the elevated stress levels seen in LB [14]. Layers of the LB line showed almost 3-fold higher heterophil to lymphocyte (H/L) ratios than LSL hens. The measurement of the H/L-ratio is a common method to detect mild to moderate avian stress [30], which causes a heterophilia and a corresponding raised H/L-ratio [31]. Following a scale suggested by Gross and Siegel [32], LB layers of the present study have been exposed to long-term and high levels of stress, while LSL hens showed mean H/L-ratios of 0.29, indicative for low levels of stress. It is well known that the influence of stress causes a down-regulation of immune responsiveness [33–38]. The high stress levels measured for LB may therefore have suppressed the gene expression of *IGJ*.

In conclusion, the results of the two microarray studies in layer lines have shown *COMTD1*, *AKR7A2* and *IGJ* as strong candidates causing phenotypic differences in bone breaking strength, stress levels and immune responsiveness among layer lines. These findings have large implications for improving animal welfare and

Table 2. List of genes that were significant differentially expressed between the two layer lines Lohmann Selected Leghorn (LSL) and Lohmann Brown (LB) in both microarray experiments.

Gene symbol	Gene	Chr	Chromosome start index	Chromosome stop index	Regulation in LSL versus LB	Number of transcripts	Fold change
AKR7A2	*Aldo-keto reductase family 7,*	21	4669151	4673134	Up	2	2.24
	member A2 (aflatoxin aldehyde reductase)						2.17
C20ORF177	*chromosome 20 open reading frame*	20	7219219	7222018	Up	1	7.39
COMTD1	*Catechol-O-methyltransferase domain containing 1*	6	14390582	14396766	Down	1	-2.53
IGJ	*Immunoglobulin J polypeptide, linker protein for immunoglobulin*	4	49429222	49434990	Up	3	2.23
	alpha and mu polypeptides						2.42
							2.88
PTPN5	*Protein tyrosine phosphatise, non-receptor type 5 (striatum-enriched)*	5	12065964	12145215	Up	4	2.09
							3.15
					Down		−2.01
							−3.29
RNF207	*Ring finger protein 207*	21	634031	638889	Down	1	−2.53
RPL21	*Ribosomal protein L21*	1	175570306	175577122	Up	1	2.46
SYT1	*Synaptotagmin 1*	1	39261286	39381655	Down	1	−2.14
UPK1B	*Uroplakin 1B*	1	80215467	80223594	Up	2	2.55
							2.83

Given are the gene symbols and names, their chromosomal positions in base pairs and the chromosomes (Chr), up- or downregulation in LSL versus LB layers, the number of transcripts per gene with their fold changes.

demonstrate the chicken as a useful animal model for explaining these metabolic processes.

Material and Methods

Ethics statement

All animal work has been conducted according to the national and international guidelines for animal welfare. The Lower Saxony state veterinary office, Niedersächsisches Landesamt für Verbraucherschutz und Lebensmittelsicherheit, Oldenburg, Germany, was the responsible Institutional Animal Care and Use Committee (IACUC) for this specific study. Exsanguination of laying hens at the University of Veterinary Medicine Hannover was under the supervision of the Lower Saxony state veterinary office, Niedersächsisches Landesamt für Verbraucherschutz und Lebensmittelsicherheit, Oldenburg, Germany. The experiments for the present study have been approved by the Lower Saxony state veterinary office, Niedersächsisches Landesamt für Verbraucherschutz und Lebensmittelsicherheit, Oldenburg, as a notifiable experiment with the registration number 33.9-42502-05-11A154.

Layer lines and housing system

The investigated flock of laying hens was kept in the small group housing system Eurovent German provided by Big Dutchman (Vechta, Germany). The housing system was installed at the farm for education and research of the University of Veterinary Medicine Hannover (Foundation) in Ruthe. Investigations have been carried out on the duration of one laying period, starting in October 27, 2010 and ending in October, 14, 2011. The housing system comprised three tiers with ten compartments each. The two commercial layer lines, Lohmann Selected Leghorn (LSL) and Lohmann Brown (LB) were kept in group sizes of 36 and 54 hens per compartment. Each tier consisted of five successive compartments of LSL and another five of LB, which were arranged in alternate order. The layer lines were equally distributed among the two group sizes, but not mixed within a single compartment. All compartments had an equal height and depth of 60 cm and 135 cm, respectively. According to the different group sizes, the compartments were 240 and 362 cm wide, respectively. Hence, the available floor space per hen was 890 cm^2. The total flock size was 1350 laying hens, with 684 LB and 666 LSL hens. After a rearing period of 18 weeks in cages the birds were moved to the small group housing system. The equipment of each compartment comprised dust baths, nest boxes with flexible curtains, claw abrasion devices, perches and a manure belt ventilator. Per compartment, two white plastic and another two metal perches, as well as the central tube for the automatic distribution of dust bathing substrate cold be used for perching by the hens. The four perches were installed in a stepped position at two different heights of 9 cm and 28 cm. The perch length per hen was 15 cm. The distribution of the layer lines and group sizes within the housing system and the structure of a single compartment in cross section and top view are shown in Figure S4. The lighting period was gradually stepped up until reaching 14 hours of light at the fifth week of the laying period. Both layer lines had an approximately equal egg production per hen housed (78%), with an average egg mass per hen housed of around 19 kg. Even the egg production (83%) and egg mass (21 kg) per average hen were similar in LSL and LB. With 3.91%, dirty eggs were more common in LSL hens than in LB (2.56%). In LSL, as well as in LB almost 4% of the eggs were cracked. While the overall mortality was approximately 4% for LB, almost 6% of the LSL laying hens died or had to be culled during the laying period.

Management and feeding

All hens had identical feeding and management conditions throughout the whole laying period. A three-phase feeding program was provided to cover the amounts needed of calcium, phosphor and energy. Feed and water were provided ad libitum. A standard vaccination program for laying hens was applied during the rearing and laying period.

Phenotypic traits

A total of 480 eggs each were randomly sampled in the 3rd, 9th and 12th laying month and recorded for the following internal and external egg quality traits including egg weight, eggshell breaking strength, albumen height, Haugh units, yolk weight, eggshell thickness and eggshell weight.

In the 2nd, 8th and 13th laying month the plumage condition of 480 laying hens each was scored using an evaluation scheme comprising four scores. A massive damage of the plumage and bare regions was assessed with Score 1. Score 2 was given when an explicit damage of feathers and/or bare areas could be observed. Completely or nearly complete feathered birds, with only a few damaged feathers were scored with 3 and score 4 was given for a very good plumage condition with nearly no damaged feathers. The six body regions neck, breast, belly, back, wings and tail were scored separately and added to a total plumage score. Furthermore, all hens were weighed using a digital table scale.

Approximately 0.5 ml of blood was drawn from a wing vein of 360 hens out of the 480 birds investigated in the 13th laying month. Blood samples were used for preparing two methanol-fixed and one native blood smear within 30 minutes after sampling. After staining according to a modified Wright-Giemsa protocol, at least 400 leucocytes, including heterophils, lymphocytes, monocytes, basophils and eosinophils were counted on one slide per hen. The H/L-ratios were calculated by dividing the relative numbers of heterophils by the relative numbers of lymphocytes.

The 360 laying hens were subsequently transported to the Clinic for Poultry of the University of Veterinary Medicine Hannover (Foundation), where they were sacrificed by exsanguination after stunning them by rabbit punch. For further analyses of bone breaking strengths alternately the intact right or left *humeri* and *tibiae* were dissected and removed from the tissue surrounding the bones. Initially all bones were frozen at $-20°C$ and examined after thawing within the next four weeks. After determination of the bone lengths and weights (in cm and g, respectively), the bone breaking strengths were measured in Newton (N) using a three-point-bending machine (Zwick/Z2.5/TNIS, Zwick-Roell, Ulm, Germany), which was controlled and calibrated by the technical service of Zwick-Roell in regular intervals. The punching tool exerts a constant, perpendicular force on the midshaft of the bone until its fracture.

Statistical analysis of the phenotypic traits

Statistical analyses were performed using SAS, version 9.3 (Statistical Analysis System Institute Inc., Cary, North Carolina, USA). Egg quality traits, plumage condition, blood parameters and bone traits were analysed employing the procedure MIXED. Analysis of variance was applied after normal distribution of the logarithmically transformed white blood cell numbers and H/L-ratios, as well as the residuals of bone traits were confirmed using the Shapiro-Wilk and Kolmogorov-Smirnov tests of the UNIVARIATE procedure of SAS. The group size, tier, layer line and the interactions between layer line and group size, layer line and tier were regarded as fixed effects in the statistical model for the blood parameters and bone traits. The statistical model for the egg quality traits and the plumage condition additionally comprised the laying month as a fixed effect, as well as its interaction with the layer line. The individual compartments within layer line and trial were treated as randomly distributed effects. F-tests were conducted to examine whether an effect in the statistical model was significant or not, with a level of significance of $P<0.05$. A normal distribution was given for the residuals of all traits examined.

Statistical model for the blood parameters and bone traits:

$$(\log -) Y_{ijklm} = \mu + GR_i + TI_j + LL_k + LL * GR_{ik} + LL * TI_{jk} + comp(LL * TR)_{kl} + e_{ijklm},$$

where Y_{ijklm} = white blood cell numbers, H/L-ratios and bone traits, μ = model constant, GR_i = fixed effect of group size (i = 1 to 2), TI_j = fixed effect of tier (j = 1 to 3), LL_k = fixed effect of layer line (k = 1 to 2), $LL*GR_{ik}$ = fixed effect of interaction between layer line and group size, $LL*TI_{jk}$ = fixed effect of interaction between layer line and tier, $comp(LL*TR)_{kl}$ = randomly distributed effect of compartment within layer line (LL) and trial (TR), e_{ijklm} = random error variation.

Statistical model for the egg quality traits and the plumage condition:

$$(\log -) Y_{ijklmn} = \mu + GR_i + TI_j + LL_k + LM_l + LL * GR_{ik} + LL * TI_{jk} + LL * LM_{kl} + comp(LL * TR)_{km} + e_{ijklmn},$$

where LM_l = fixed effect of laying month, $LL*LM_{kl}$ = fixed effect of interaction between layer line and laying month.

Sampling and RNA isolation

When choosing hens for microarray analysis we selected between stressed and unstressed birds based on their behaviour during handling, their plumage condition and the number of skin lesions. In consideration of the group sizes, the tiers and the layer lines two to three hens per compartment were chosen for sampling, giving a total of 70 layers. After the hens were stunned and sacrificed by exsanguination, samples of four different regions of the cerebrum were taken from each hen at necropsy; one from the anterior left, one from the anterior right and another two from the posterior left and right side, respectively. All samples were extracted without meninges and immediately stored in 1.5 ml RNAlater stabilization solution (Qiagen, Hilden, Germany). As substitute sample of the remained cerebrum was stuck into cryogenic tubes and snap frozen in liquid nitrogen. The time from slaughtering to storing the samples was less then 15 minutes. RNAlater-samples were kept at +4°C for 24 hours and afterwards stored with the supplementary samples at −80°C. After thawing, approximately 50 mg tissue per sample were removed from RNAlater and transferred into microcentrifuge tubes (2 ml) containing 1 ml of QIAzol Lysis Reagent (Qiagen). Samples were disrupted and homogenized using 5 mm stainless steel beads (Qiagen) on a Tissue Lyser (Qiagen). The extraction of total RNA from the tissues was performed using the RNeasy Lipid Tissue Mini Kit (Qiagen) as described by the manufacturer, including the additional step of DNA-digestion. The total RNA concentration was measured using a NanoDrop 1000 spectralphotometer (Peqlab Biotechnologie, Erlangen, Germany).

Synthesis of cDNA and microarray hybridization

Microarray analyses of 60 samples from the posterior left and right site of the cerebrum were performed by Helmholtz Centre for Infection Research (HZI), Braunschweig, Germany. In a first step quality and integrity of total RNA was assessed using the Agilent Technologies 2100 Bioanalyzer (Agilent Technologies, Waldbronn, Germany). Target preparation for RNA microarray processing was carried out according to the Ambion WT Expression Kit. A total of 500 ng RNA were used for biotin labelling according the Ambion WT Expression Kit (Ambion, Austin, TX). 5.5 µg of fragmented biotinylated cRNA were placed in a hybridization cocktail containing four biotinylated hybridization controls (BioB, BioC, BioD and Cre) as recommended by the manufacturer. Samples were hybridized to an identical lot of Affymetrix ChiGene-1_0-st Arrays (Affymetrix) for 17 hours at + 45°C. After hybridization the microarrays were washed and stained with Streptavidin Phycoerythrin on the Fluidics Station 450 using the FS450-0002 protocol (Affymetrix). Finally, microarrays were scanned by the Affymetrix GCS3000 Scanner (Affymetrix) and the scanned images were analyzed with GCOS1.2 Software Suite (Affymetrix).

Analysis of microarray data

Each Affymetrix microarray contained 20,399 probe sets. The GeneSpring GX 11 Software (Agilent Technologies, Santa Clara, California, USA) was used for statistatical analysis. Raw microarray data were normalized using the Robust Multi-array Average method (RMA). After background correction data were transformed and quantile global normalized at probe level to the median using a non-linear algorithm. To sort out all the unexpressed genes, raw data were filtered according to expression levels by cut off the 20th percentile. Analyses for the effects layer line, group size and tier were performed using an unpaired T-test with multiple testing of Benjamini and Hochberg. The accepted level of significance was $P<0.05$. Genes with a 2-fold change or greater in gene expression were considered differentially expressed. We used the Gene Ontology (GO) Enrichment Analysis Toolkit (GOEAST, http://omicslab.genetics.ac.cn/GOEAST) to identify significantly enriched GO-terms among the lists of differentially expressed genes. The hypergeometric test method with Benjamini and Hochberg as multi-test adjustment method and $FDR<0.1$ as significance level of enrichment were selected for analyses. A GO-term was considered significantly enriched, if it could be assigned to at least two or more genes. The GO comprises three categories, named biological process, molecular function and cellular component. Within each of these categories the specific terms are considered children of more broad terms (child-parent relationships) [39]. For the current study the analyses only were made for terms belonging to the biological process of gene ontology. All significantly expressed probe sets were cross-checked against the data of the National Center for Biotechnology Information (National Center for Biotechnology Information (NCBI), http://www.ncbi.nlm.nih.gov/) and the chicken genome assembly (AmiGo, http://amigo.geneontology.org/cgi-bin/amigo/go.cgi).

NCBI GEO submission

The normalized data from the present microarray gene expression experiment has been submitted to NCBI's Gene Expression Omnibus (GEO, http://www.ncbi.nlm.nih.gov/geo/) and can be queried via GEO series accession number GSE55570 (http://www.ncbi.nlm.nih.gov/geo/query/acc.cgi?acc = GSE55570). The previous data set can be read via the GEO accession number GSE40802.

Supporting Information

Figure S1 Heat map of differentially expressed probe sets among the two layer lines. Heat map of the probe sets with absolute fold changes of 2-fold or greater detected in the comparison between the layer lines Lohmann Brown (LB) and Lohmann Selected Leghorn (LSL). The range of relative expression levels from lowest to highest is represented by the blue and red dyeing, respectively.

Figure S2 Tree graph of the enriched Gene ontology (GO) terms of the biological process category among the list of probe sets with higher expression in LSL (GOEAST, http://omicslab.genetics.ac.cn/GOEAST). The tree graph displays the hirachial relationships of biological processes identified to be enriched among the list of probe sets with given gene symbol that were significantly up-regulated in the layer line LSL. Significantly enriched GO terms are marked yellow. GO terms without significance are either shown as white boxes or drawn as points. Relationship between two enriched GO terms are marked with red edges, black solid edges stand for relationship between enriched and unenriched terms, black dashed edges stand for relationship between two unenriched GO terms. Each box represents a GO term, labeled by its GOID, the term definition, the P-value and detail informations.

Figure S3 Tree graph of the enriched Gene ontology (GO) terms of the biological process category among the list of down-regulated probe sets in LSL (GOEAST, http://omicslab.genetics.ac.cn/GOEAST). The tree graph displays the hirachial relationships of biological processes identified to be enriched among the list of probe sets with given gene symbol that were significantly up-regulated in the layer line LSL. Significantly enriched GO terms are marked yellow. GO terms without significance are either shown as white boxes or drawn as points. Relationship between two enriched GO terms are marked with red edges, black solid edges stand for relationship between enriched and unenriched terms, black dashed edges stand for relationship between two unenriched GO terms. Each box represents a GO term, labeled by its GO-ID, the term definition, the P-value and detail informations.

Figure S4 Arrangement and dimensions of the compartments of the small group housing system. A Cross section drawing of a single compartment. **B** Individual compartment for group sizes of 54 laying hens in a top view drawing. **C** Arrangement drawing of the tiers (A: first tier; B: second tier; C: third tier), layer lines (LB: Lohmann Brown; LSL: Lohmann Selected Leghorn) and group sizes (36 and 54 hens) of the small group housing system Eurovent German.

Table S1 Differentially expressed probe sets between the Lohmann Selected Leghorn (LSL) and Lohmann Brown (LB) laying hens.

Table S2 Enriched biological processes of probe sets with different expression in comparison between LSL and LB.

Acknowledgments

Thanks to Dr. Christian Sürie and Carolin Salitzky from the Farm for Education and Research of the University of Veterinary Medicine Hannover (Foundation) in Ruthe for supporting us during the investigations in the housing system. The authors wish to acknowledge Prof. Dr. Silke Rautenschlein from the Clinic for Poultry, University of Veterinary Medicine Hannover (Foundation), for her support in post-mortem examinations. We are grateful to Vanessa Sabrina Kaser for her expert technical assistance.

Author Contributions

Conceived and designed the experiments: CH OD. Performed the experiments: CH RG OD. Analyzed the data: CH OD RG. Contributed reagents/materials/analysis tools: RG OD. Wrote the paper: CH OD.

References

1. Lockhart DJ, Dong H, Byrne MC, Follettie MT, Gallo MV, et al. (1996) Expression monitoring by hybridization to high-density oligonucleotide arrays. Nature Biotechnol 14: 1675–1680.
2. Kamiński S (2002) DNA microarrays – a methodological breakthrough in genetics. J Appl Genet 43: 123–130.
3. McCall MN, Almudevar A (2012) Affymetrix GeneChip microarray preprocessing for multivariate analyses. Brief Bioinform 13: 536–546.
4. Yao J, Ren X, Ireland JJ, Coussens PM, Smith TPL, et al. (2004) Generation of a bovine oocyte cDNA library and microarray: resources for identification of genes important for follicular development and early embryogenesis. Physiol Genomics 19: 84–92.
5. Burt DW (2007) Emergence of the Chicken as a Model Organism: Implications for Agriculture and Biology. Poult Sci 86: 1460–1471.
6. Cogburn LA, Porter TE, Duclos MJ, Simon J, Burgess SC, et al. (2007) Functional Genomics of the Chicken- A Model Organism. Poult Sci 86: 2059–2094.
7. Nie H, Crooijmans RPMA, Lammers A, van Schothorst EM, Keijer J, et al. (2010) Gene expression in chicken reveals correlation with structural genomic features and conserved patterns of transcription in the terrestrial vertebrates. PLoS ONE 5(8): e11990.
8. Chang M-T, Cheng Y-S, Huang M-C (2013) Novel genetic markers of the carbonic anhydrase II gene associated with egg production and reproduction traits in Tsaiya ducks. Reprod Dom Anim 48: 98–104.
9. Bottje WG, Kong W-B, Song JJ, Lee JY, Hargis BM, et al. (2012) Gene expression in breast muscle associated with feed efficiency in a single male broiler line using a chicken 44K microarray. II. Differentially expressed focus genes. Poult Sci 91: 2576–2587.
10. Li CL, Wang XL, Li N, Wu CX (2012) Microarray analysis revealed that immunity-associated genes are primarily regulated by roxarsone in promoting broiler chicken (*Gallus gallus domesticus*) growth. Poult Sci 91: 3184–3190.
11. Labouriau R, Kjaer JB, Abreu GCG, Hedegaard J, Buitenhuis AJ (2009) Analysis of severe feather pecking behavior in a high feather pecking selection line. Poult Sci 88: 2052–2062.
12. Kjaer JB, Sørensen P (1997) Feather pecking behaviour in White Leghorns, a genetic study. Br Poult Sci 38: 333–341.
13. Kjaer JB (2000) Diurnal rhythm of feather pecking behaviour and condition of integument in four strains of loose housed laying hens. Appl Anim Behav Sci 65: 331–347.
14. Habig C, Geffers R, Distl O (2012) Differential gene expression from genome-wide microarray analyses distinguishes Lohmann Selected Leghorn and Lohmann Brown layers. PLoS ONE 7(10): e46787.
15. Picklo MJ Sr, Olson SJ, Hayes JD, Markesbery WR, Montine TJ (2001) Elevation of AKR7A2 (succinic semialdehyde reductase) in neurodegenerative disease. Brain Res 916: 229–238.
16. Li D, Ferrari M, Ellis EM (2012) Human aldo-keto reductase AKR7A2 protects against the cytotoxicity and mutagenicity of reactive aldehydes and lowers intracellular reactive oxygen species in hamster V79-4 cells. Chem Biol Interact 195: 25–34.
17. Zhu BT, Conney AH (1998) Functional role of estrogen metabolism in target cells: review and perspectives. Carcinogenesis 19: 1–27.
18. Stolk L, van Meurs JBJ, Jhamai M, Arp PP, van Leeuwen JPT, et al. (2007) The catechol-O-methyltransferase Met[158] low-activity allele and association with nonvertebral fracture risk in elderly men. J Clin Endocrinol Metab 92: 3206–3212.
19. Lorentzon M, Eriksson A-L, Mellström D, Ohlsson C (2004) The COMT val158met polymorphism is associated with peak BMD in men. J Bone Miner Res 19: 2005–2011.
20. Lachman HM, Papolos DF, Saito T, Yu YM, Szumlanski CL, et al. (1996) Human catechol-O-methyltransferase pharmacogenetics: description of a functional polymorphism and its potential application to neuropsychiatric disorders. Pharmacogenetics 6: 243–250.

21. Chen J, Lipska BK, Halim N, Ma QD, Matsumoto M, et al. (2004) Functional analysis of genetic variation in catechol-O-methyltransferase (COMT): effects on mRNA, protein, and enzyme activity in postmortem human brain. Am J Hum Genet 75: 807–821.
22. Scanlon PD, Raymond FA, Weinshilboum RM (1997) Catechol-O-methyl-transferase: thermolabile enzyme in erythrocytes of subjects homozygous for allele for low activity. Science 203: 63–65.
23. Takeda S, Elefteriou F, Levasseur R, Liu X, Zhao L, et al. (2002) Leptin regulates bone formation via the sympathetic nervous system. Cell 111: 305–317.
24. Hocking PM, D'Eath RB, Kjaer JB (2011) Genetic selection: Behavioural Problems: Feather pecking, removal and cannibalism in laying hens. In: Appleby MC, Mench JA, Olsson IAS, Hughes BO, editors. Animal Welfare 2011. Wallingford, Oxon, UK: CAB International. pp. 270–272.
25. Korte SM, Beuving G, Ruesink W, Blokhuis HJ (1997) Plasma catecholamine and corticosterone levels during manual restraint in chicks from a high and low feather pecking line of laying hens. Physiol Behav 62: 437–41.
26. Korte SM, Ruesink W, Blokhuis HJ (1999) Heart rate variability during manual restraint in chicks from high- and low-feather pecking lines in laying hens. Physiol Behav 65: 649–52.
27. Rubin JB, Choi Y, Segal RA (2002) Cerebellar proteoglycans regulate sonic hedgehog responses during development. Development 129: 2223–2232.
28. Shum L, Nuckolls G (2002) The life cycle of chondrocytes in the developing skeleton. Arthritis Res 4: 94–106.
29. Niles MJ, Matsuuchi L, Koshland ME (1995) Polymer IgM assembly and secretion in lymphoid and nonlymphoid cell lines: Evidence that J chain is required for pentamer IgM synthesis. Proc Natl Acad Sci USA 92: 2884–2888.
30. Gross WB, Siegel HS (1983) Evaluation of heterophil/lymphocyte ratio as a measure of stress in chickens. Avian Dis 27: 972–979.
31. Maxwell MH (1993) Avian blood leucocyte responses to stress. Worlds Poult Sci J 49: 34–43.
32. Gross WB, Siegel PB (1993) General principles of stress and welfare. In: Grandin T, editor. Livestock Handling and Transport. Wallingford, Oxon, UK: CAB International. pp. 21–34.
33. Berczi I (1998) The stress concept and neuroimmunoregulation in modern biology. Ann N Y Acad Sci 851: 3–12.
34. Dantzer R (1997) Stress and immunity: what have we learned from psychoneuroimmunology? Acta Physiol Scand Suppl 640: 43–46.
35. Dohms JE, Metz A (1991) Stress-mechanisms of immunosuppression. Vet Immunol Immunopathol 30: 89–109.
36. Glaser R, Kiecolt-Glaser JK, Malarkey WB, Sheridan JF (1998) The influence of psychological stress on the immune response to vaccines. Ann N Y Acad Sci 840: 649–655.
37. Magnusson U, Wattrang E, Tsuma V, Fossum C (1998) Effects of stress resulting from short-term restraint on in vitro functional capacity of leukocytes obtained from pigs. Am J Vet Res 59: 421–425.
38. Sheridan JF, Dobbs C, Jung J, Chu X, Konstantinos A, et al. (1998) Stress-induced neuroendocrine modulation of viral pathogenesis and immunity. Ann N Y Acad Sci 840: 803–808.
39. Dwight SS, Harris MA, Dolinski K, Ball CA, Binkley G, et al. (2002) Saccharomyces genome database (SGD) provides secondary gene annotation using the gene ontology (GO). Nucleic Acids Res 30: 69–72.

2

Surgical Membranes as Directional Delivery Devices to Generate Tissue: Testing in an Ovine Critical Sized Defect Model

Melissa L. Knothe Tate[1,2]*, Hana Chang[1], Shannon R. Moore[1], Ulf R. Knothe[3]

1 Department of Biomedical Engineering, Case Western Reserve University, Cleveland, Ohio, United States of America, **2** Department of Mechanical & Aerospace Engineering, Case Western Reserve University, Cleveland, Ohio, United States of America, **3** Department of Orthopaedic Surgery, Cleveland Clinic, Cleveland, Ohio, United States of America

Abstract

Purpose: Pluripotent cells residing in the periosteum, a bi-layered membrane enveloping all bones, exhibit a remarkable regenerative capacity to fill in critical sized defects of the ovine femur within two weeks of treatment. Harnessing the regenerative power of the periosteum appears to be limited only by the amount of healthy periosteum available. Here we use a substitute periosteum, a delivery device *cum* implant, to test the hypothesis that directional delivery of endogenous periosteal factors enhances bone defect healing.

Methods: Newly adapted surgical protocols were used to create critical sized, middiaphyseal femur defects in four groups of five skeletally mature Swiss alpine sheep. Each group was treated using a periosteum substitute for the controlled addition of periosteal factors including the presence of collagen in the periosteum (Group 1), periosteum derived cells (Group 2), and autogenic periosteal strips (Group 3). Control group animals were treated with an isotropic elastomer membrane alone. We hypothesized that periosteal substitute membranes incorporating the most periosteal factors would show superior defect infilling compared to substitute membranes integrating fewer factors (i.e. Group 3>Group 2>Group 1>Control).

Results: Based on micro-computed tomography data, bone defects enveloped by substitute periosteum enabling directional delivery of periosteal factors exhibit superior bony bridging compared to those sheathed with isotropic membrane controls (Group 3>Group 2>Group 1, Control). Quantitative histological analysis shows significantly increased *de novo* tissue generation with delivery of periosteal factors, compared to the substitute periosteum containing a collagen membrane alone (Group 1) as well as compared to the isotropic control membrane. Greatest tissue generation and maximal defect bridging was observed when autologous periosteal transplant strips were included in the periosteum substitute.

Conclusion: Periosteum-derived cells as well as other factors intrinsic to periosteum play a key role for infilling of critical sized defects.

Editor: Mário A. Barbosa, Instituto de Engenharia Biomédica, University of Porto, Portugal

Funding: The surgical study was supported by the Case-Coulter Translational Research Partnership. Hana Chang was supported through a Medtronic Fellowship. Shannon Moore was supported in part through a grant from the AO Foundation (F-07-99K) and the Whitaker International Fellows and Scholars Program. Melissa Knothe Tate was supported in part through the Alexander von Humboldt Foundation's Fellowship for Senior Researchers. The funders had no role in study design, data collection and analysis, decision to publish, or preparation of the manuscript.

Competing Interests: MLKT has a patent pending for flow directing materials and systems [23: Knothe Tate ML, Anderson EJ (2009) Flow Directing Materials and Systems. U.S. Patent and Trademark Office Appl. No. US 2009/0053109.]; MLKT and URK have a provisional patent pending for the biologics-enhanced mechanoactive reconstruction sheet technology used in this study [24: Knothe Tate ML, Knothe U (2010) MechanoActive Sheets for Surgical Reconstruction Procedures, IDA, U.S. Patent and Trademark Office Provisional Patent Application No. 61311056] and a patent issued in the arena of composition and method to induce bone healing and repair [35: Knothe Tate ML,Knothe UR (February 1, 2011) Composition and method for inducing bone growth and healing. U.S. Patent No.: US 7,879,107 B2.].

* E-mail: knothetate@case.edu

Introduction

Critical sized defects do not heal spontaneously without surgical intervention. Numerous surgical techniques have been employed to treat these defects with limited success and a large number of complications [1]. Distraction osteogenesis has become a standard of care for the treatment of large diaphyseal bone defects due to superior union rates achieved with it in comparison with other surgical techniques [1–19]. Nonetheless, distraction osteogenesis has several disadvantages including long and labor-intensive treatment times, significant demands on patient compliance, discomfort, and high rates of complications with associated requirements for multiple surgical procedures following the index procedure. In addition, the technique requires significant technical expertise, which limits the number of orthopaedic surgeons with the training and experience necessary to perform the procedure. Even when implemented by surgeons with significant expertise, the relatively high rate of complications and subsequent need for reoperations associated with the technique persists [11,13,17].

These and other factors provided the impetus for the development of a one stage bone transport procedure that harnesses the regenerative power of the periosteum to fill in critical sized defects without the need for adjuvant bone graft (**Fig. 1**) [20–22]. Histology and quantitative micro-computed tomography (μ-CT) studies indicate that the cells and blood supply within the periosteum are key to success of the one stage procedure [21,22]. Interestingly, filling of the periosteum enveloped defect with autologous bone graft from the iliac crest retards the infilling of the defect due to the need for prior osteoclastic resorption [22]. Based on experimental and several clinical cases, implementation of the one stage bone transport procedure appears to be limited only by the amount of healthy periosteum available [20–22]. The current study addresses that limitation.

In the current study we implement a newly developed surgical reconstruction membrane as a substitute for the periosteum to treat a critical sized (2.54 cm) defect in a previously developed adult ovine femur model with intramedullary nailing for mechanical stabilization [21]. Our goal was to design a periosteum substitute that mimics the structure-function properties inherent to native periosteum. As a bi-layered membrane, native periosteum exhibits anisotropic, composite structure conferring unique functional properties [23]. The periosteum's outer layer comprises mostly collagens, aligned with the longitudinal axis, and elastin; this outer layer is hypothesized to control bone shape/length during growth [24], to contribute to bone toughness, and to limit displacement of fracture fragments to stabilize bones after bone failure [25]. The cambium, or periosteum's innermost layer, comprises mostly cells that appose the underlying bone [26]. The progenitor cells within the inner cambial layer are responsible for continual periosteal bone apposition during life and confer regenerative properties to the periosteum [21,22,27–30].

Hence, we designed our periosteum substitute to serve as a delivery device *cum* implant exhibiting a modular design with pockets to allow for directional (outside→in), spatial (via anterior, posterior, medial and lateral pockets), and temporal control of factor delivery (**Fig. 2A**). The periosteum substitute design *per se* mimics the structure of native periosteum, the outer layer of which is made up of the structural proteins elastin and collagen. In this study, we used the periosteum substitute for the controlled addition of periosteal factors including the presence of collagen, the predominant structural protein of the extracellular matrix that is present in the outer sheath of the periosteum [26] (Group 1, **Fig. 2B**), cells residing within the periosteum (Group 2, **Fig. 2C**), and autologous periosteal strips (Group 3, **Fig. 2D**). Animals of the Control group were treated with an isotropic membrane alone. We hypothesized that periosteal substitute membranes incorporating the most periosteal factors would show superior defect infilling compared to substitute membranes integrating fewer factors (*i.e.* Group 3>Group 2>Group 1>Control).

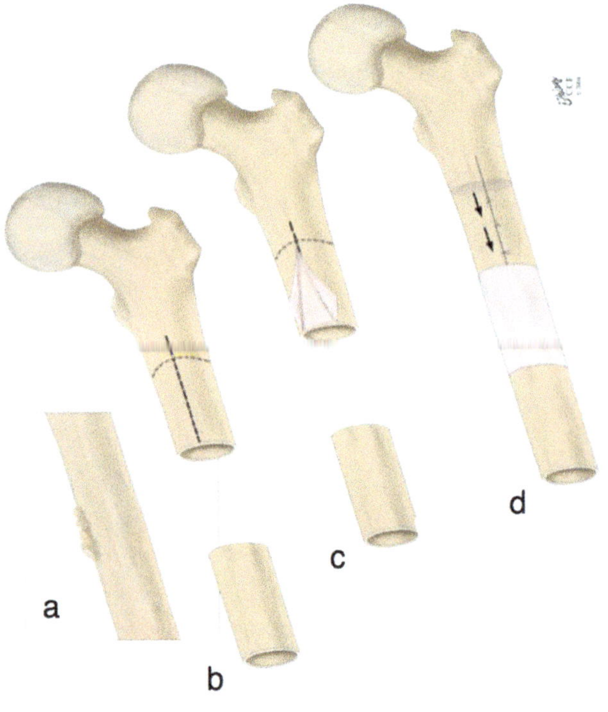

Figure 1. The one-stage bone-transport procedure [20–22] harnesses the regenerative potential of the periosteum and cells therein, *e.g.* for treatment of a critical sized long bone defect after tumor resection. (**a**) The tumor is first identified and (**b**) then resected *in toto*, leaving a critical sized defect. The periosteum is scored (dashed line, **b**) and (**c**) gently peeled back off the proximal bone, leaving denuded bone below. (**d**) The denuded bone is osteotomized and transported distally to fill the defect zone. It is docked to the distal, healthy femur using ligament sutures. A limiting factor in implementation of this technique is the availability of periosteum in areas easily accessible to the surgical site. This is particularly problematic in high impact trauma injuries such as blast wounds or high speed sports or traffic injuries. Images used with permission [21].

Methods

Ethics Statement

All work was conducted according to relevant national and international guidelines; full details of the study were approved by the Amt für Lebensmittelsicherheit und Tiergesundheit Graubünden (Institutional Review Board of the Canton of Grisons, Switzerland), Tierversuchsbewilligung (Animal Experiment Permission) No. 15/2008.

Overview

Previously described surgical protocols were used to create critical sized, middiaphyseal femur defects [21], first in one short term (3 week) pilot group treated with periosteum substitute implants incorporating collagen membranes (Group 1). Thereafter, we treated four groups of five skeletally mature Swiss alpine sheep for sixteen weeks, a period over which defects surrounded by periosteum *in situ* heal completely and untreated defects do not heal (providing proof of critical size) [21,22].

Each group was treated using a substitute periosteal membrane designed and manufactured according to our protocols [31,32] to deliver specific factors to the defect zone (**Fig. 2**, Table 1). The substitute periosteum implants comprised combinations of FDA-approved materials and/or autologous materials including periosteum derived cells and periosteal strips from the bone removed to create the defect. The FDA approved materials used to make the implants included medical grade silicone elastomer sheeting, absorbable collagen membrane derived from bovine achilles tendon, and nonresorbable sutures (**Fig. 2**). The periosteum substitutes were designed to be easily manufactured, modular (the pocket design allows for substitution as well as precise localization and timing for release of specific factors or combinations of factors), fully sterilizable with other surgical armamentaria, and easy to use by surgeons with varying degrees of expertise.

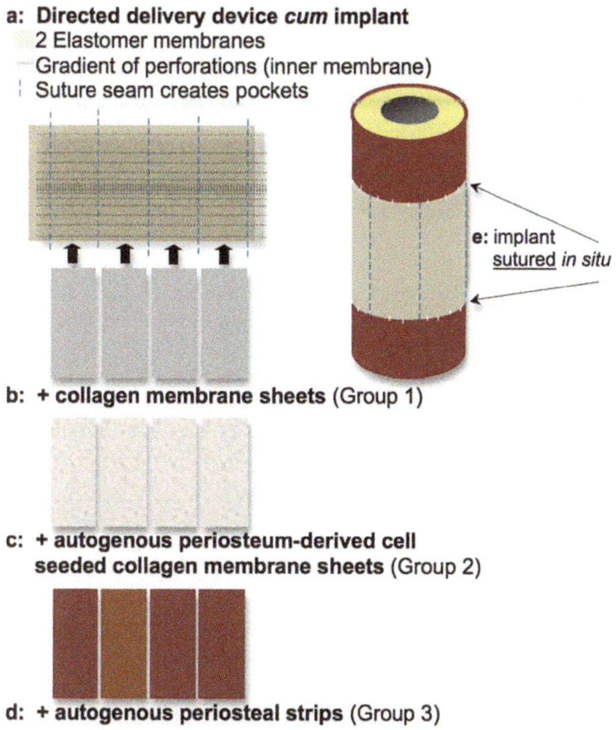

Figure 2. A periosteal substitute, novel directed delivery device *cum* implant was developed and implemented to mimic structure-function relationships intrinisic to the periosteum and to enable vectorial delivery, *i.e.* control of delivery direction and magnitude or concentration, of periosteal factors. In the current study we tested the efficacy of directional delivery of periosteal factors to enhance defect healing. (**A**) The implant comprises an outer elastomeric membrane (FDA approved material), an inner elastomeric membrane with a gradient of perforations of highest concentration furthest from the proximal and distal edges of the defect zone. The layers are sewn together with suture material, creating four pockets into which periosteal factors can be tucked. (**B**) Collagen membranes (FDA approved) were cut and tucked into the pockets of Group 1 implants. (**c**) Cells were isolated from periosteum of the bone removed to create the defect, seeded on the collagen membranes (FDA approved), and tucked into the pockets of Group 2 implants. (**D**) Strips of periosteum were resected from bone removed to create the defect and tucked into the pockets of Group 3 implants. Bony bridging of defects sheathed by each respective periosteum substitute was compared between groups and with a Control group implementing an isotropic, simple elastomeric membrane (FDA approved). (**E**) The periosteum substitute implant was then sutured to the proximal and distal edges of periosteum lifted along the edges of the defect and sutured close along the longitudinal axis of the lateral aspect. Refer to **Fig. 3** for intraoperative photo.

To create the modular design, an inner membrane was first perforated with a gradient of holes along its entire length, with the highest concentration of holes near the center of the defect region, decreasing toward the edges that are sutured to the periosteum of healthy bone proximal and distal to the defect zone. The pattern of holes was achieved using a double (parallel) sewing machine needle (without thread) and setting the sewing machine stitch length to achieve equidistance at the center of the defect between rows of double holes. The inner membrane was then sewn, using the suture material, to the outer membrane, which was devoid of perforations, creating a long sleeve (3.5×10 cm) with four, 2 cm wide pockets (**Fig. 2A**). The whole construct was then placed on surgical dressing gauze and encapsulated within a sterilization

Table 1. Defect bridging was scaled to assess objectively defect bridging without the ability to measure volume of bone generated quantitatively due to the presence of the intramedullary nail.

GROUPS	0–25%	25–50%	50–75%	75–100%
EMPTY	7/7			
Control Membrane	4/5	1/5		
1: Membrane + Collagen	5/5			
2: Membrane + Collagen + Cells	1/5	2/5	1/5	1/5
3: Membrane + Periosteal Strips		2/5	1/5	2/5
INTACT PERIOSTEUM				7/7

For comparative purposes, images from a previous study using the same animal model were assessed using the same scaling method, comparing to the empty defect zone (see **Fig. 7A**), which was left without treatment and which never healed, indicative of a true critical sized defect [21]. Also, the use of intact periosteum with adherent cortical bone chips on the inner surface, from the previous study, is compared as the "best observed outcome" which provides target specifications for the periosteum substitute implant [21].

sleeve for steam sterilization in an autoclave with other surgical instruments.

Shortly before surgical implantation (in the sterile surgical operating theatre), the substitute periosteum implant was removed from the sterile packaging and experimental (periosteal) factors were placed in the implant pockets (collagen membrane - Group 1, collagen membrane seeded with autogenous periosteum derived cells - Group 2, or strips of autogenous periosteum transplants from bone removed to create defect - Group 3, Table 1). The implant was then sutured to periosteum lifted along the edge of the remaining bone proximal and distal to the defect (**Fig. 2D, Fig. 3**). The control group was treated with a simple, isotropic silicone elastomer membrane (without flow directing architecture) around the critical sized defect. Group 1 was treated with a membrane and collagen sheets, incorporating flow directing architecture, which allows for directional transport, *i.e.* from the proximal and distal edges axially toward the center, and from the membrane

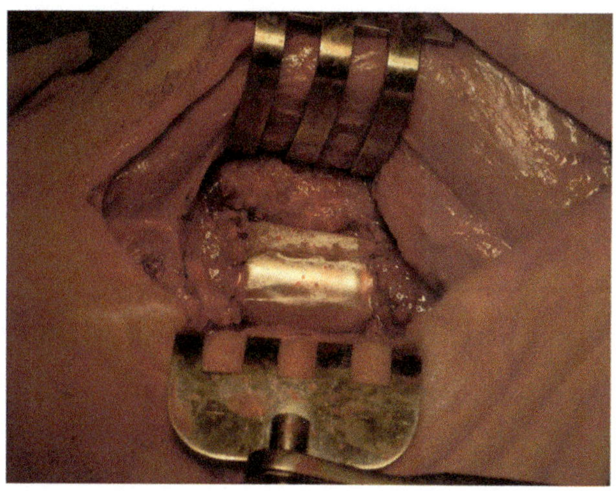

Figure 3. Intraoperative photo showing a periosteal substitute *in situ*, enveloping a critical sized defect in the middiaphysis of the ovine femur.

radially toward the intramedullary nail. Group 2 received the membrane as in Group 1, but the collagen sheet within the membrane was pre-seeded with cells isolated from periosteum of the autologous defect bone and incubated at 37°C overnight. After careful aspiration and washing, the cell-seeded membrane was then placed into the four pockets of the substitute periosteum. Finally, Group 3 received the membrane in combination with autologous periosteal transplant strips (isolated from the bone removed to create the defect zone) in place of the collagen sheets.

Animals were euthanized at 3 (pilot group) and 16 weeks after surgery. Femoral tissue blocks including surrounding musculature were scanned with the intramedullary (IM) nail *in situ* using high resolution μ-CT to determine efficacy of the periosteal substitutes for defect bridging. Due to the retention of the steel IM nail (which can cause imaging artifacts due to beam hardening), it was not possible to obtain volumetric data from the μ-CT images. For this reason, bridging of the defect was ranked, by a blinded observer, on a quartile scale (**Table 1**, 0–25%, 25–50%, 50–75%, 75–100%), indicating degree of defect coverage for each treated sample in each experimental group.

Finally, quantitative histomorphometry was carried out to measure bone generation in the defect zone and to compare the mean bone regenerated between groups.

Detailed Methods

Sheep and surgical procedures. The experimental protocol was carried out, using skeletally mature Swiss alpine sheep ($n = 5$ per group, 3 experimental and one control group), at the AO Research Institute in Davos, Switzerland, with the approval of the animal care and use commission of the Canton of Grisons.

All surgeries were performed by URK. Surgery was performed with sheep in the right lateral position. After general anaesthesia with intubation and spinal anaesthesia, the left hindlimb was shaved and prepped with Hibiscrub solution and draped. The right hind limb was strapped with a belt extending around the operating table and the abdomen. The sheep was then transported into the operating room and the left hind limb was prepped and draped in the usual sterile fashion. A lateral parapatellar approach was performed to enter the knee joint to prepare for retrograde IM nailing. The patella was dislocated medially. A 4 mm entry hole was then placed in the midline of the trochlea, approximately 8 mm anterior to the intracondylar notch. Sequential reaming of the intramedullary canal was performed with increasing sized cutting reamers, starting at 7 mm, going up to 14 mm. The flexible Synthes reamer system was then used to ream 15 mm, up to 16 mm, in 0.5 mm increments.

Attention was then turned lateral to the femur and a second, approximately 12.5 cm incision was made lateral over the femur. The *vastus lateralis fasciae* and the intramuscular plane were developed to expose the lateral aspect of the femur. Meticulous hemostasis and ligation of larger vessels was performed, distal third of the femur. The *vastus lateralis* was then detached from the bone with a scalpel to expose the distal femur with a 1–2 mm layer of muscle attached. A 2.54 cm critical sized defect was then created 8 cm proximal to the knee joint line with an oscillating saw using small amplitude and preserving the soft tissue with rounded custom retractors.

The periosteum was then lifted circumferentially, approximately 5 mm from the proximal and distal defect/osteotomy edges, with a periosteal elevator. Thereafter, the intramedullary nail was inserted retrograde and care was taken to maintain the 2.5 cm critical defect size. Two proximal and two distal 4.9 mm interlocking bolts were then placed.

The 3.5 cm periosteum substitute membrane was then introduced around the defect using a custom S-shaped retractor to maintain space medial to the femur-nail. The membrane was placed from anterolateral side and brought posterior around the defect. The membrane was designed to overlap 0.5 cm distal and proximal to the defect. In the case of the experimental membrane, the outer layer overlapped the elevated periosteum by 5 mm and the inner layer was placed so that the periosteum was sandwiched between and sutured carefully in place with Dermalon 4.0 sutures, while applying inner and outer rotation of the hind limb as needed to reach regions behind the IM nail. In the case of the simple control membrane, the membrane was placed overlapping the elevated periosteum by 5 mm and sutured in place. The edges of the membrane were connected laterally using Dermalon 4.0 sutures and trimmed to fit the circumference of the defect.

The knee and lateral femoral incisions were then closed in layers with no suction tube trains, using vicryl #1 for fascia, 2.0 for subcutaneous, and Moncryl 3.0 for subcuticular running sutures.

Periosteum substitute implant manufacture. Substitute periosteal membrane were designed and manufactured by MKT as sterilizable, modular units to deliver specific factors to the defect zone. Delivery devices (modular implant with pockets) were manufactured from FDA approved materials, including medical grade silicone sheeting (Bioplexus, 0.005″ thick medium durometer silicone elastomer, Ventura, CA), and nonresorbable sutures (Dermalon 4-0, monofilament nylon, Syneture, Covidien Surgical, Dublin, Ireland). Absorbable collagen membranes (Biomend®, derived from bovine achilles tendon, Zimmer Dental, Carlsbad, CA), designed for periodontal use, were cut to size and placed in implant pockets in Groups 1 (collagen membrane alone) and 2 (collagen membrane seeded with cells isolated from autologous periosteum). Autologous periosteal strips were placed in the pockets of implants from Group 3, retaining the anatomic orientation of the inner and outer surfaces. Cut to size but otherwise unaltered, isotropic medical grade silicone sheets were used in the control group. Bone growth within implants incorporating increasing numbers of periosteal factors were compared with control implants as well as with the baseline critical sized defect control (untreated) and "gold standard" *in situ* periosteum treated defects studied previously [21].

Cell culture methods - isolation and proliferation of periosteum derived cells. Cell culture was carried out by HC. Ovine periosteum explants resected from the bone removed to create the defect were immediately placed in TBSS with 1% Penicillin/Streptomycin (P/S). The explants were then minced and placed in spinner flasks with high glucose DMEM (GIBCO, Grand Island, NY) with 1% P/S and 0.3% Collagenase II (Worthington Biochemical Corporation, Lakewood, NJ). This was incubated for 3 hours in a 37°C incubator in 95% humidified air and 5% CO_2. The cells were filtered through a 40 mm vacuum filter to remove fibrous tissue, centrifuged to remove the collagenase solution, and resuspended in high glucose DMEM with 10% FBS and 1% P/S. The cells were then seeded on precut collagen membranes, which were sized to fit into the periosteal implant pockets. The seeded membranes were then incubated overnight at 37°C, in 95% humidified air with 5% CO_2. The next morning, after careful aspiration and rinsing in TBSS to remove any cell culture chemicals, the seeded membranes were then placed into the four pockets of the substitute periosteum implant, under sterile conditions, in the surgical theater.

Prior to the surgical study we characterized growth rates of the ovine periosteum derived cells. Adherent periosteum derived cells were plated at 34,000 cells/cm^2 high sets of 8 in 96-well plates in high glucose DMEM with 10% FBS and 1% P/S. Cell culture media was changed every 2–3 days. Cell numbers were analyzed for 7 days using WST-1 reagent (Roche Applied Science, Indianapolis, IN) and incubated for 4 hours before measuring absorbance.

Undecalcified histological preparation and measurements of tissue generation. Histological sectioning and analysis was carried out by SM and MKT. Following resection and μ-CT imaging, the femur and surrounding tissue were fixed and embedded in poly(methyl methacrylate) (PMMA) for undecalcified histology processing. A diamond wire saw was used to produce three transverse sections through the tissue block with intramedullary nail *in situ;* sections were taken at intervals of approximately 6.5 mm to span the entire defect (Well Precision Diamond Wire Saw 6234, Norcross, GA), and polished with a variable speed Grinder-Polisher (Buehler EcoMet 4000, Lake Bluff, IL). Both sides of each section were imaged, and full collages of the cross-sections were created first, at 1.6× magnification to establish a qualitative perspective on *de novo* bone generation and healing trends between and across groups. Thereafter, cut surfaces were stained with Giemsa and Eosin to quantify new tissue area and distribution. The stain colors cell nuclei and connective tissue dark blue, and mineralized tissue (bone) pink. Collages were made of the proximal and distal side of all slices at 5× magnification using an inverted epifluorescent microscope with automated, computerized stage, (Leica DMIRE2, Wetzlar, Germany) and using broad spectrum UV excitation to quantify *de novo* bone generation and compare areas of new bone generated between groups. Whole collages were processed using a custom designed algorithm to identify and segment out mineralized (pink) and cartilage (blue) tissue (Adobe Photoshop CS5, Adobe Systems Incorporated, San Jose, CA). Thereafter, total areas of regenerates for mineralized and cartilage tissue were calculated using a pixel-to-area scaling factor (Image J version 10.2, NIH, Bethesda, MD).

To summarize the sample size for histological measures, three sections were made through the mid-diaphyseal region of each defect site, resulting in a total of six surfaces (both proximal and distal) for each animal. With five animals in each group, this resulted in a total of 30 high-resolution collages for each group (Control, Group 1, Group 2 and Group 3), *i.e.* 120 collages in total. Three collages were excluded because due to their near proximity to the proximal or distal bone outside of the defect zone. This resulted in an $n \geq 27$ collages for all groups.

Results

Histomorphometric and μ-CT data showed that membranes incorporating periosteal factors significantly improved bone generation in the critical sized defect compared to isotropic, unstructured control membranes made of the same material (Group 3>Group 2>Control, Table 1, **Fig. 4, Fig. 5, Fig. S1, S2, S3, S4**). Bone generation in defects treated with isotropic control membranes appeared to emanate from the proximal and distal periosteal edges of the defect zone, tapering along the surface of the intramedullary nail, from the intact bone toward the center of the defect (**Fig. S1**); more new bone was observed in the proximal half of the defect than the distal half and limited contact was observed between the two areas of bone ingression. In addition, limited proliferative woven bone was observed to radiate inward from the isotropic membrane in only one specimen treated with the isotropic control membrane (9047, **Fig. S1**).

At three weeks after treatment with periosteum substitute implants incorporating collagen sheets (Group 1), intramembranous, woven bone was observed emanating from the implant toward the intramedullary nail in four of five defects studied

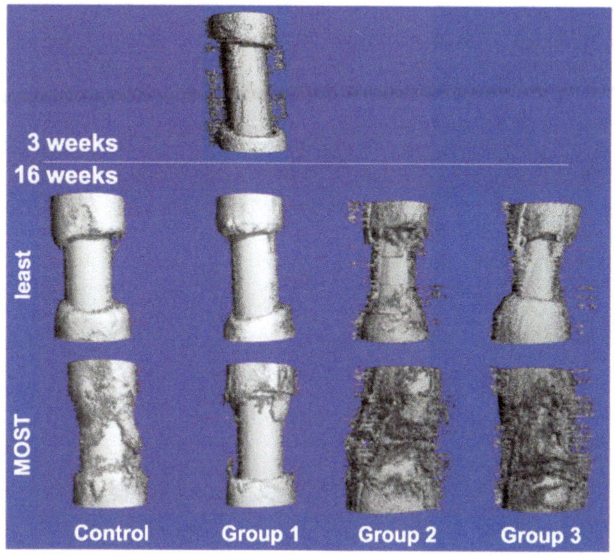

Figure 4. High resolution micro-computed tomography (μ-CT) of bone regenerate in Group 1 at 3 weeks and in all groups at 16 weeks after surgery. The intramedullary nail is present along the longitudinal axis of all specimens. Each group comprised five sheep and the sample images showing the least and most amount of new bone are depicted for each group.

(**Fig. 4, Fig. S2A**). At three weeks after surgery, almost no ingression of bone was observed from the intact periosteum of the proximal and distal edges. The intramembranous bone observed at three weeks was no longer evident in μ-CT images at sixteen weeks (**Fig. S2B**). In fact, at 16 weeks, Group 1 did not show evidence of improved defect filling compared to the isotropic control membrane, and the best case of the Control membrane showed more infilling than the best case of the implants incorporating collagen sheets alone. Furthermore, in contrast to the control group, less ingression of bone was observed from the proximal and distal edges of the defect. Bone that did ingress proximally and distally appeared to exhibit less tapering toward the intramedullary nail than in the Control group.

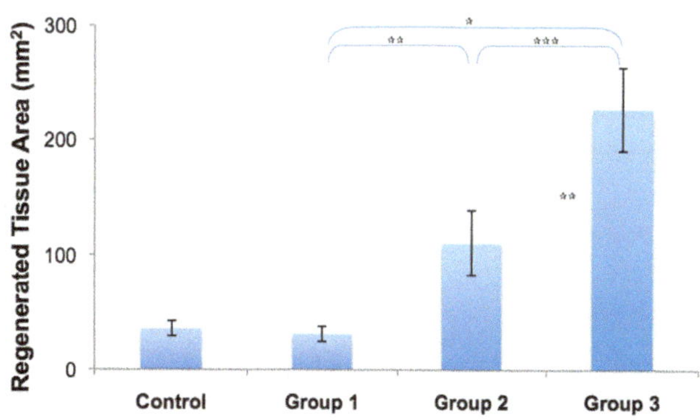

Figure 5. Mean area of *de novo* bone regenerate in defect zone, measured in histological sections through the defect zone. Error bars represent standard error of the mean. Statistical significance of differences between groups was tested using the Mann-Whitney (Wilcoxon) test, with significance defined as $p<0.05$. $^{*}p=0.0003$, $^{**}p=0.0459$, $^{***}p=0.037$.

Insertion of collagen sheets seeded with periosteal derived cells (Group 2) within the periosteum substitute implant resulted in significantly increased bone generation (**Fig. 5, Fig. 6**) and defect bridging (**Fig. 4, Fig. S3**) compared to the isotropic control membrane (Control) as well as compared to the periosteum substitute with collagen sheets alone (Group 1). In contrast to both the Control and Group 1 at 16 weeks, woven intramembranous bone was evident in μ-CT images from Group 2 at 16 weeks. In addition, bone infilling appeared to have ingressed from the proximal and distal edges of the defect, in nearest proximity to healthy bone (with a tendency toward more bone in the proximal than the distal half of the defect). In one specimen exhibiting the most robust infilling/healing response of all in Group 2, the inwardly radiating intramembranous bone also coalesced most with proximally and distally ingressing bone, compared to other specimens within the group (9046, **Fig. S3**).

Maximal bone infilling of the defect was observed in Group 3, where autologous strips of periosteum were tucked into the pockets of the modular periosteum substitute (**Fig. 4**, **Fig. 5, Fig. 6, Fig. S4**). Two specimens exhibited coalescence of intramembranous bone emanating from the membrane and bone ingressing from the proximal and distal edges of the defect (9049, 9050, **Fig. S4**). Two specimens exhibited a weaker intramembranous proliferative bone response and ingression from the proximal, respectively distal, edges (9048, 9051, **Fig. S4**) and one exhibited an intermediate response (9052, **Fig. S4**).

Periosteum-derived cells proliferate exponentially during the first seven days of seeding; linear regression gives the following equation to predict cell number (y) as a function of days (x):

$$y = 0.0045e^{1.1382x}$$

Although the cell proliferation studies could not be conducted on the collagen membrane due to the colorimetric measurements needed for the proliferation assay, proliferation data shows that the isolated cells are viable and proliferate steadily over the course of 7 days (**Fig. 7**).

Discussion

The current set of experiments indicate a key role for directional delivery of periosteum-derived cells as well as other factors intrinsic to periosteal transplants for infilling of critical sized defects. Based on quantitive histomorphometry measurements as well as micro-computed tomography data, bone defects enveloped by substitute periosteum enabling directional delivery of periosteal factors show significantly more bone generation as well as superior bony bridging compared to those sheathed with isotropic elastomer membrane controls. Maximal bridging was observed when autologous periosteal transplant strips were included in the periosteum substitute, followed by the group in which the periosteum substitute delivered cells (derived from the periosteum), radially, to the defect. Whereas the periosteum substitute incorporating collagen membranes showed evidence for woven bone generation, radially inward from the inner surface of the implant, at three weeks after surgery, the radial woven bone generation was not evident at sixteen weeks after surgery. Similar to the isotropic control membrane, bone generation in the defect zone at sixteen weeks after surgery occurred mainly via bone ingression from proximal and distal edges of intact bone and periosteum.

To place the results of the current study in context with our previous work on treatment of criticial sized bone defects in the same ovine model, we compared our current results with the those of the baseline, untreated control as well as those of the "best outcomes group" where the periosteum (with adherent cortical bone on its inner surface) was left *in situ* around the defect (**Fig. 7**) [21]. Due to the necessity to retain the intramedullary nail in the femoral blocks of the current study, μ-CT observations were compared using a defect coverage scale. Thereafter we used histomorphometric measures to compare quantitatively bone

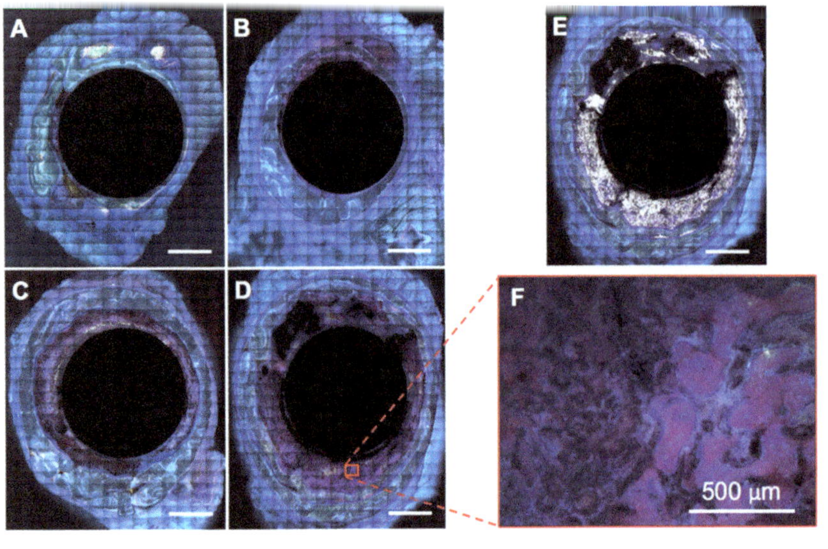

Figure 6. Histological cross-sections for Giemsa and eosin-stained specimens showing representative areas of tissue regeneration for each control and experimental group. (**A**) Stained and unprocessed specimen for the Control Group. (**B**) Stained and unprocessed specimen for Group 1 incorporating collagen sheets. (**C**) Stained and unprocessed specimen for Group 2 incorporating periosteum derived cells seeded on collagen sheets. (**D**) Stained and unprocessed specimen for Group 3 incorporating periosteal strips. (**E**) Segmented image from Group 3 (**D**) highlighting mineralized tissue. (**F**) Demonstration of collage resolution, as shown in a single field-of-view (acquired from **D**). Scale bar for (**A**–**E**) is 5 mm.

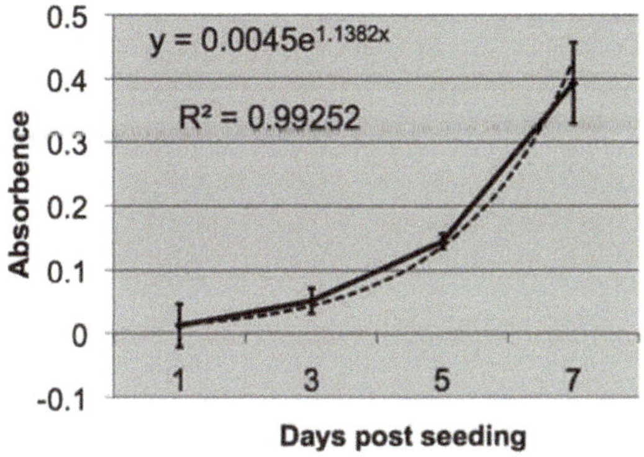

Figure 7. Proliferation of seeded cells derived from ovine periosteum. Error bars depict standard deviations.

generated *de novo* in the defect zone. In the previous study, the baseline control specimens were left empty; the lack of infilling and bridging of the defect in all five specimens of this group provided evidence for the defect's critical size (**Fig. 8A**). Both the Control group and Group 1 of the current study showed similar results, with no bridging of the defect at 16 weeks after surgery. Thus, neither implementation of the isotropic control membrane nor use of the directional delivery membrane incorporating a collagen sheet showed improvement in healing compared to the untreated defect of the previous study. In contrast, Groups 2 and 3 of the current study, which implemented the directional delivery membrane in conjunction with periosteum-derived cells seeded on the collagen sheet and strips of endogenous periosteum, respectively, showed superior defect bridging and bone generation in the defect zone compared to the untreated control of the previous study. Accounting for all five specimens of each respective group, healing was not as robust as that observed in the best outcomes group of the previous study, where five of five defects completely bridged (**Fig. 8B**) [21].

Given our explicit goal to mimic structure-function relationships in the design of our periosteum substitute membrane, we were surprised that inclusion of collagen sheets within the elastomeric modular pockets showed no significant improvement in bone generated within or bridging of the defect zone, compared to isotropic membrane controls. At 16 weeks after surgery, previous studies showed all critical sized defects to have healed completely when surrounded by periosteum *in situ* [21]. Hence, based on quantitative histomorphometric and qualitative μ-CT data of the current study, it appears the delivery of cells (seeded on collagen sheets), or in combination with periosteum intrinsic factors, provides a much more potent stimulus for tissue building than delivery of collagen alone. Using this previously tested ovine defect model with mechanical stabilization via a solid intramedullary nail, the medullary niche and its resident, multipotent marrow stromal cells are removed at the time of surgery. In native periosteum, collagen and elastin form the outer, fibrous sheath, encompassing the cambium (cellular) layer. When left *in situ* around the defect, periosteum derived cells egress from the cambium layer, inwards, to fill the defect with intramembranous bone [21,22]. Of particular note, proliferation of periosteum derived cells cultured on tissue culture styrene does not appear to be contact inhibited, in contrast to other pluripotent cell lines [33]. Surprisingly little reference data exists with regard to characterization of periosteum derived multipotent cells in sheep, likely due to the paucity of ovine surface markers (for FACS) or rtPCR primers. In future studies it will be interesting to better mimic molecular and cellular interactions to further functionalize the periosteum substitute membrane.

From a clinical perspective, it would be expected that, in surgical cases where insufficient periosteum is available to suture *in situ* around tissue defects, use of the directional delivery implant in conjunction with periosteum strips harvested from other areas would provide a superior alternative to treatment with a simple isotropic membrane sleeve. However, harvesting of periosteum strips from elsewhere (*e.g.* proximal or distal to the area of tumor resection or trauma) was not tested directly in the current study and potentially could be associated with other complications when implemented in patients. In the current study, periosteal strips were resected from the bone to create the defect. Inclusion of autologous periosteal strips would be expected to yield superior results to inclusion of autologous periosteum-derived cells for similar reasons, given the necessity of harvesting tissue and subjecting the patient to a two stage procedure in order to harvest and proliferate autologous cells on collagen membranes for implantation in the directional delivery device. However, another potential scenario would be to pre-seed collagen membranes with pluripotent cells from a stem cell bank (*e.g.* [34,35]) prior to surgery and then to incorporate the pre-seeded collagen sheets into the directional delivery membrane at the time of surgery. This clinical scenario would not only avoid the necessity of a two stage procedure, but it would also not involve additional harvesting of tissue (and potential additional complications associated with more extensive surgical approaches) from the patient.

The current study implicates different spatiotemporal patterns of bone formation via bone induction and bone conduction that are modulated differently, depending on the surgical membrane used. Whereas use of the directional delivery membrane appeared to enable (rapid) early bone induction, radially inward from the implant to the surface of the intramedullary nail, both the isotropic and directional delivery membranes appeared to serve as an osteoconductive sleeve as well, allowing for ingression of bone from the proximal and distal edges of the defect, axially into the defect zone. Albrektsson and Johansson differentiate osteo*induction*, "the recruitment of immature cells and stimulation of these cells to develop into preosteoblasts", from osteo*conduction* or surface mediated bone growth [36]. Albrektsson and Johansson's

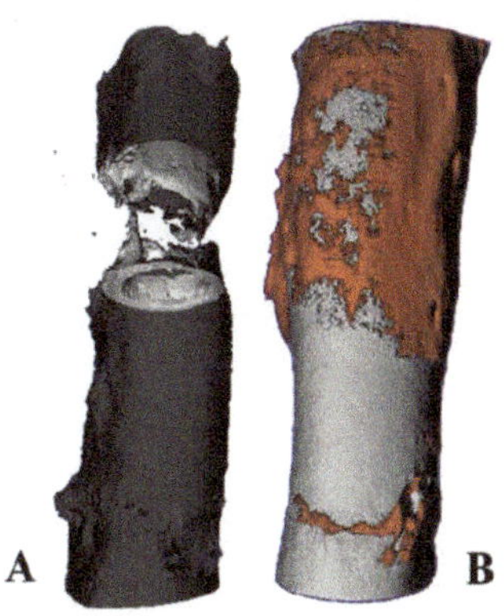

Figure 8. High resolution micro-computed tomograph (μ-CT) images of healing 16 weeks after critical sized defect from the previous study [21] (used with permission). (A) Baseline, untreated control defect, confirming critical size of defects (does not heal without treatment). Defect is completely healed in experimental groups, e.g. (B) including group treated with periosteum, left *in situ* with small cortical bone chips adherent to inner surface, around defect.

definition somewhat contrasts with earlier descriptions of osteoinduction via demineralized bone which initiates a biological cascade resulting in endochondral ossification [37,38]. In the current and previous studies, we describe the observed early, woven bone proliferation as intramembranous rather than endochondral [21,22,39], which better fits with Albrektsson and Johansson's definition. Taken one step further, we consider the relative barrier properties of the membrane sleeve, in conjunction with the impermeable surface of the intramedullary nail, to provide a conduit that guides bone regeneration inwards radially, similar (but in an opposite direction) to that suggested by Gogolewski and colleagues [40]. Finally, a gradient of cells and osteogenic factors is expected to develop between the inner surface of the directional delivery membrane and the outer surface of the IM nail, as well as between the edges and center of the defect zone; cellular and biochemical gradients can further facilitate osteogenesis via osteoinduction and osteoconduction.

Histomorphological studies are underway to elucidate quantitatively the time course of defect infilling via osteoinductive and osteoconductive mechanisms. In the previous study, in groups where periosteum, with small cortical bone chips adherent to the inner surface, was left *in situ* around critical sized defects, rapid proliferative woven bone was shown to infill the defect zone within two weeks of surgery (as evidenced by fluorochrome labeling during this time period) [21,22]. In that study, by sixteen weeks after surgery, bone consolidated and its density and volume were shown to be highly modulated by the loading history to which the bone generated within the defect zone was subjected. Namely, in areas along the bone axis most able to resist bending loads (along the major centroidal axis), regenerate bone volume was higher and regenerate bone density was lower than in areas along the bone axis least able to resist bending (along the minor centroidal axis). Furthermore, at the conclusion of the previous study, it was impossible to assess wither bone induction or conduction had played a more important role in healing, although the rapid proliferative woven bone laid down in defects not packed with morcellized bone graft appeared to favor a more rapid maturation and remodeling of regenerate bone in the sixteen weeks of the experimental study [21,22]. Of note, in the current study, the axial ingression (osteoconduction) was more apparent in the proximal half of the defect and was observed in the specimens examined at 16 weeks after surgery but not in those examined 3 weeks after surgery (where osteoinduction **was** observed radially from the implant toward the IM nail surface). An ongoing quantitative histomorphological analysis of the specimens from the current study should allow us to elucidate the spatiotemporal mechanisms of bone generation occurring radially via periosteum derived cells and axially via bone and periosteum of the proximal and distal bone segments.

Previously published studies have underscored the need to engineer periosteum substitutes [41] but have met with limited success [42,43] in bridging critical sized defects and few have been tested in large animal models where scale up of cell mediated tissue generation is expected to be a major limitation. The approach employed in the current study capitalizes on osteoinductive and osteoconductive properties of periosteum substitutes, while providing a means for directional delivery of cells and osteoinductive factors inherent to the periosteum as well as modulation of the concentration of factors through tuning of the pore gradient on the inner membrane surface. In effect, this allows for vectorial delivery (a *vector* being defined by its magnitude and direction) of cells and osteoinductive factors, filling in the defect from the outside in, much like the mechanism by which osteoblasts infill resorption cavities during bone remodeling [32,44].

There are several limitations inherent to the design, as well as to financial constraints, associated with *in vivo* studies in large animal models. First and foremost, we decided to retain the custom, stainless steel IM nail in the femoral tissue blocks at the conclusion of the study in order to retain the precise spatial organization of the biological samples. This was not necessary in our previous study using periosteal sleeves around the defect, because all defects were bridged and thus mechanically stable at the conclusion of the study. Retention of the nail had a further implication of not allowing for quantitative μ-CT analysis due to beam hardening and due to artifacts in imaging attributable to the presence of metallic implants [45]. However, histomorphometric study of femoral blocks that are fixed, embedded in PMMA, and sectioned serially *in toto* allowed for quantitation of tissue generation and comparison between groups. Ongoing histological analysis will allow for maximally precise reconstruction of spatial and temporal (though analysis of chelating fluorochromes administered at defined timepoints in the study) bone apposition in the sixteen weeks after surgery. Furthermore, given unlimited resources, it would have been desirable to include more experimental groups in the study to better elucidate effects of independent variables. Nonetheless, the current study provides a foundation that will help us to prioritize follow on studies, including *in silico* (virtual) models that allow for prediction of outcomes through variation of model parameters [46].

In trauma patients, as well as in surgical reconstruction patients, the amount of remaining healthy periosteum represents a limit to the use of the endogenous engineering approach demonstrated to bridge critical sized defects in the ovine femur (one-stage bone-transport procedure) [21,22]. The current studies, implementing the newly developed periosteal substitutes, augmented through addition of periosteal transplant from other bone sites, test the use of the technology as a delivery vehicle for the patient's endogenous bone healing factors, expanding the indications for surgical reconstruction sheets in treatment of long bone defects. In addition, the periosteal substitutes, enhanced through seeding with auto- or allogenic stem cells, further expand the use of the technology for a range of tissue defects. The technology, which is based on a modular platform combining FDA approved materials, is poised for translation from the lab bench to the surgical patient.

Supporting Information

Figure S1 Sixteen weeks after surgery. High resolution micro-computed tomography (μ-CT) images from the five femora making up the Control group, which was treated with an isotropic surgical membrane. Infilling occurs mainly through axial osteoconduction from proximal and distal edges toward the center of the defect zone.

Figure S2 **A.** Three weeks after surgery. High resolution micro-computed tomography (μ-CT) images from the five femora making up Group 1, which was treated with the directional delivery membrane incorporating collagen sheets. Infilling occurs mainly radially, via inward intramembranous bone formation, from the inner surface of the surgical membrane towards the outer surface of the intramedullary nail. **B.** Sixteen weeks after surgery. High resolution micro-computed tomography (μ-CT) images from the five femora making up Group 1 of the current study, which was treated with the directional delivery membrane incorporating collagen sheets. Radial intramembranous bone formation observed at three weeks is no longer evident. Small amounts of infilling occur via axial osteoconduction from proximal and distal edges of the defect zone.

Figure S3 Sixteen weeks after the two stage surgery with a directional delivery membrane incorporating collagen sheets seeded with autogenous periosteum-derived cells. High resolution micro-computed tomography (μ-CT) images of the femoral defect zones in the five femora making up Group 2. Infilling occurs radially via osteoinduction and axially via osteoconduction. Best infilling is observed in cases where the two coalesce.

Figure S4 Sixteen weeks after the two stage surgery with a directional delivery membrane incorporating strips of autogenous periosteum from the bone removed to create the defect. High resolution micro-computed tomography (μ-CT) images of the femoral defect zones in the five femora making up Group 3. Infilling occurs radially via osteoinduction and axially via osteoconduction. Best infilling is observed in cases where the two coalesce.

Acknowledgments

We thank U. Lanker and his team (AO Research Institute, Davos, Switzerland) for their expert and compassionate care of experimental animals.

Author Contributions

Conceived and designed the experiments: MLKT URK. Performed the experiments: MLKT HC SRM URK. Analyzed the data: MLKT HC SRM URK. Wrote the paper: MLKT URK. Customized software used in anlysis: HC.

References

1. Tucker HL, Kendra, Kinnebrew T (1990) Reconstruction using the method of Ilizarov as an alternative. Orthopedic Clinics of North America 21: 629–637.
2. Alonso J, Regazzoni P (1997) Bridging bone gaps with the Ilizarov technique. Clinics in Plastic Surgery 18: 497–504.
3. Watson JT, Anders M, Moed BR (1995) Management strategies for bone loss in tibial shaft fractures. Clinical Orthopaedics and Related Research 315: 138–152.
4. Aronson J (1997) Limb-lengthening, skeletal reconstruction, and bone transport with the Ilizarov Method. Journal of Bone and Joint Surgery American 79: 1243–1258.
5. Prokuski L, Marsh J (1994) Segmental bone deficiency after acute trauma. Orthopedic Clinics of North America 25: 753–763.
6. Atesalp AS, Basbozkurt M, Erler E, Sehirlioglu A, Tunay S, et al. (1998) Treatment of tibial bone defects with the Ilizarov circular external fixator in high-velocity gunshot wounds. International Orthopaedics 22: 343–347,1998.
7. Smrke D, Arnez Z (2000) Treatment of extensive bone and soft tissue defects of the lower limb by traction and free flap transfer. Injury 31: 153–162.
8. Paley D, Maar D (2000) Ilizarov bone transport for tibial defects. Journal of Orthopaedic Trauma 14: 76–85.
9. Polyzois D, Papachristou G, Kotsiopoulos K, Plessas S (1997) Treatment of tibial and femoral bone loss by distraction osteogenesis. Experience in 28 infected and 14 clean cases. Acta Orthopaedica Scandinavica Supplement 275: 84–88.
10. DeCoster TA, Gehlert RJ, Mikola EA, Pirela-Cruz MA (2004) Management of Posttraumatic Segmental Bone Defects. Journal of the American Academy of Orthopaedic Surgeons 12: 28–38.
11. Paley D (1990) Problems, obstacles, and complications of limb lengthening by the Ilizarov technique. Clinical Orthopaedics and Related Research 250: 81–104.
12. Dagher F, Roukoz SR (1991) Compound tibial fractures with bone loss treated by the Ilizarov technique. Journal of Bone and Joint Surgery British 73: 316–321.
13. DeCoster TA, Gehlert RJ, Garcia-Cimbrelo E, Olsen B, Ruiz-Yague M, et al. (1992) Ilizarov Technique: results and difficulties. Clinical Orthopaedics and Related Research 283: 116–123.
14. Marsh DR, Shah S, Elliott J, Kurdy N (1997) The Ilizarov method in nonunion, malunion, and infection of fractures. Journal of Bone and Joint Surgery British 79: 273–279.
15. Gugenheim J (1998) The Ilizarov Method: orthopedic and soft tissue applications. Clinics in Plastic Surgery 25: 567–578.
16. Saleh M, Yang L, Sims M (1999) Limb reconstruction after high energy trauma. British Medical Bulletin 55: 870–884.
17. Slomka R. Complications of ring fixators in the foot and ankle. Clinical Orthopaedics and Related Research 391: 115–122.
18. Pavolini B, Maritato M, Turelli L, D'Arienzo M (2000) The Ilizarov fixator in trauma: a 10-year experience. Journal of Orthopaedic Science 5: 108–113.
19. Polak WG, Pawlowski S, Skora J, Morasiewicz L, Janczak D, et al. (2001) Vascular complications after the treatment with Ilizarov external fixators. Vasa 30: 138–140.
20. Knothe U, Springfield DS (2005) A novel surgical procedure for bridging of massive bone defects. World Journal of Surgical Oncology 3: 5.
21. Knothe Tate ML, Ritzman TF, Schneider E, Knothe U (2007) Testing of a new one-stage bone-transport surgical procedure exploiting the periosteum for the repair of long-bone defects. Journal of Bone and Joint Surgery American 89: 307–316.
22. Knothe U, Dolejs S, Miller RM, Knothe Tate ML (2010) Effects of mechanical loading patterns, bone graft, and proximity to periosteum on bone defect healing. Journal of Biomechanics 43: 2728–37.
23. McBride SH, Evans S, Knothe Tate ML (2011) Anisotropic mechanical properties of ovine femoral periosteum and the effects of cryopreservation. Journal of Biomechanics 44: 1954–1959.
24. Taylor J (1992) The periosteum and bone growth. In: Bone: Bone Growth v.6 BK. Hall, ed. Boca Raton, FL: CDC Press. pp 21–52.
25. Yiannakopoulos CK, Kanellopoulos AD, Trovas GP, Dontas IA, Lyritis GP (2008) The biomechanical capacity of the periosteum in intact long bones. Arch Orthop Trauma Surg 128: 117–20.
26. Allen MR, Hock JM, Burr DB (2004) Periosteum: biology, regulation, and response to osteoporosis therapies. Bone 35: 1003–1012.
27. Colnot C (2009) Skeletal cell fate decisions within periosteum and bone marrow during bone regeneration. J Bone Miner Res 24: 274–82.
28. Ozaki A, Tsunoda M, Kinoshita S, Saura R (2000) Role of fracture hematoma and periosteum during fracture healing in rats: interaction of fracture hematoma and the periosteum in the initial step of the healing process. J Orthop Sci 5: 64–70.
29. Zhang X, Xie C, Lin AS, Ito H, Awad H, et al. (2005) Periosteal progenitor cell fate in segmental cortical bone graft transplantations: implications for functional tissue engineering. J Bone Miner Res 20: 2124–2137.
30. Arnsdorf EJ, Jones LM, Carter DR, Jacobs CR (2009) The periosteum as a cellular source for functional tissue engineering. Tissue Eng A 15: 2637–2642.
31. Knothe Tate ML, Anderson EJ Flow Directing Materials and Systems. U.S. Patent and Trademark Office Appl. No. US 2009/0053109.
32. Knothe Tate ML, Knothe U (2011) Multilayer Surgical Membrane. PCT International Publication Number WO 2011/109817 A2.
33. Evans MJ, Kaufman MH (1981) Establishment in culture of pluripotent cells from mouse embryos. Nature 292: 154–156.
34. National Stem Cell Bank (NCSB) website. Available: http://www.nationalstemcellbank.org/. Accessed 2011 Nov 15.
35. United Kingdom Stem Cell Bank website. http://www.ukstemcellbank.org.uk/. Accessed 2011 Nov 15.
36. Albrektsson T, Johansson C (2001) Osteoinduction, osteoconduction and osteointegration. European Spine Journal 10: S96–101.
37. Glowacki J, Mulliken JB (1985) Demineralized bone implants. Clinics in Plastic Surgery 12: 233–41.
38. Urist MR (1972) Osteoinduction in undermineralized bone implants modified by chemical inhibitors of endogenous matrix enzymes. A preliminary report. Clinical Orthopaedics and Related Research 87: 132–7.
39. Knothe Tate ML, Falls TD, McBride SH, Atit R, Knothe UR (2008) Mechanical modulation of osteochondroprogenitor cell fate. International Journal of Biochemistry and Cell Biology 40: 2720–38.
40. Faro Nielsen F, Karring T, Gogolewski S (1992) Biodegradable guide for bone regeneration. Polyurethane membranes tested in rabbit radius defects. Acta Orthopaedica Scandinavica 63: 66–9.
41. Zhang X, Awad HA, O'Keefe RJ, Guldberg RE, Schwarz EM (2008) A perspective: engineering periosteum for structural bone graft healing. Clinical Orthopaedics and Related Research 466: 17777–87.
42. Yamamiya K, Okuda K, Kawase T, Hata K, Wolff LF, et al. (2008) Tissue-engineered cultured periosteum used with platelet-rich plasma and hydroxyapatite in treating human osseous defects. Journal of Periodontology 79: 811–8.
43. Zhao L, Zhao JL, Wan L, Wang SK (2008) The study of the feasibility of segmental bone defect repair with tissue-engineered bone membrane: a qualitative observation. Strategies in Trauma and Limb Reconstruction 3: 57–64.
44. Knothe Tate ML, Knothe UR (2011) Composition and method for inducing bone growth and healing. U.S. Patent No.: US 7,879,107 B2.
45. Meganck JA, Kozloff KM, Thornton MM, Broski SM, Goldstein SA (2009) Beam hardening artifacts in micro-computed tomography scanning can be reduced by X-ray beam filtration and the resulting images can be used to accurately measure BMD. Bone 45: 1104–16.
46. Miller RM, McBride SH, Dolejs S, Knothe U, Knothe Tate ML (2011) Modeling the Mechanobiology of the Periosteum to Predict & Harness its Regenerative Capacity. Transactions of the Orthopaedic Research Society 36: 2213.

3

Glutamine Repeat Variants in Human RUNX2 Associated with Decreased Femoral Neck BMD, Broadband Ultrasound Attenuation and Target Gene Transactivation

Nigel A. Morrison[1*], Alexandre A. Stephens[1], Motomi Osato[2], Patsie Polly[3], Timothy C. Tan[3], Namiko Yamashita[4], James D. Doecke[1], Julie Pasco[5], Nicolette Fozzard[1], Graeme Jones[6], Stuart H. Ralston[7], Philip N. Sambrook[8†], Richard L. Prince[9], Geoff C. Nicholson[10]

1 School of Medical Sciences, Griffith University, Southport, Australia, **2** Institute of Molecular and Cell Biology, Singapore, Singapore, **3** Department of Pathology and Inflammation and Infection Research Centre, School of Medical Sciences, University of New South Wales, Sydney, Australia, **4** Cancer Science Institute of Singapore, National University of Singapore, Singapore, Singapore, **5** School of Medicine, Deakin University, Geelong, Australia, **6** The Menzies Institute, Hobart, Australia, **7** Centre for Molecular Medicine, The University of Edinburgh, Edinburgh, Scotland, **8** Royal North Shore Hospital, The University of Sydney, Sydney, Australia, **9** Western Australian Institute of Medical Research and the Department of Endocrinology and Diabetes, Sir Charles Gairdner Hospital, Perth, Australia, **10** Rural Clinical School, School of Medicine, The University of Queensland, Toowoomba, Australia

Abstract

RUNX2 is an essential transcription factor required for skeletal development and cartilage formation. Haploinsufficiency of RUNX2 leads to cleidocranial displaysia (CCD) a skeletal disorder characterised by gross dysgenesis of bones particularly those derived from intramembranous bone formation. A notable feature of the RUNX2 protein is the polyglutamine and polyalanine (23Q/17A) domain coded by a repeat sequence. Since none of the known mutations causing CCD characterised to date map in the glutamine repeat region, we hypothesised that Q-repeat mutations may be related to a more subtle bone phenotype. We screened subjects derived from four normal populations for Q-repeat variants. A total of 22 subjects were identified who were heterozygous for a wild type allele and a Q-repeat variant allele: (15Q, 16Q, 18Q and 30Q). Although not every subject had data for all measures, Q-repeat variants had a significant deficit in BMD with an average decrease of 0.7SD measured over 12 BMD-related parameters ($p = 0.005$). Femoral neck BMD was measured in all subjects (-0.6SD, $p = 0.0007$). The transactivation function of RUNX2 was determined for 16Q and 30Q alleles using a reporter gene assay. 16Q and 30Q alleles displayed significantly lower transactivation function compared to wild type (23Q). Our analysis has identified novel Q-repeat mutations that occur at a collective frequency of about 0.4%. These mutations significantly alter BMD and display impaired transactivation function, introducing a new class of functionally relevant RUNX2 mutants.

Editor: Elizabeth G. Laird, University of Liverpool, United Kingdom

Funding: Alex Stephens and James Doecke were supported by Griffith University postgraduate scholarships. The funders had no role in study design, data collection and analysis, decision to publish, or preparation of the manuscript.

Competing Interests: The authors have declared that no competing interests exist.

* E-mail: N.Morrison@mailbox.gu.edu.au

† Deceased.

Introduction

Osteoporosis is the major metabolic bone disease among developed nations. The disease is characterized by low bone density and reduced bone quality through the deterioration of bone micro architecture. As a consequence, sufferers have impaired skeletal strength and an increased susceptibility to osteoporotic fractures. Bone mineral density (BMD) is a complex trait and is controlled by environmental and genetic factors [1]. BMD is a primary predictor of osteoporotic fractures; it is however a continuous trait related to age and weight. Osteoporosis as a category is a truncation of this continuous normally distributed trait, defined by a BMD value less than 2.5 SD from the population mean of young adults [2]. The proportion of fractures attributable to osteoporosis ranges from 10%–44% [3].

RUNX2 is a key regulator of skeletogenesis, bone and cartilage formation [4–8] and has been genetically associated with BMD [9–15]. RUNX2 transactivates genes such as osteocalcin, type 1 collagen and osteopontin and is initially expressed in mesenchymal condensations where it plays an essential role in osteoblast differentiation and in chondrocyte maturation [16]. RUNX2 deficient mice have un-mineralized skeletons with few immature osteoblasts and an absence of vascular and mesenchymal cell invasion in the cartilaginous templates. Heterozygous mutations in coding and promoter sequences of RUNX2 cause the dominantly inherited skeletal syndrome cleidocranial dysplasia (CCD). The disorder is characterised by persistently open or delayed closure of sutures, hypoplasia/aplasia of clavicles, Wormian bones, supernumerary teeth, short stature and other skeletal abnormalities [17,18]. A spectrum of severity of CCD symptoms is correlated with the extent of transcriptional activity remaining in the cognate mutant RUNX2 with severest symptoms associated with complete loss of RUNX2 function [19] and milder symptoms correlated with some residual RUNX2 transactivation function [20].

RUNX2 has consecutive polyglutamine and polyalanine repeats (Q/A repeat) in the protein sequence. Such repeat regions have the capacity to mutate via strand slippage during DNA replication. Glutamine repeat sequence expansion has been the cause of some diseases that show genetic anticipation, where severity increases in subsequent generations as repeat length increases due to errors in replication [21]. Wild type human RUNX2 contains a 23Q/17A repeat; 23 consecutive glutamine followed by 17 alanine residues. An insertion of the polyalanine tract (23Q/27A) was observed in one patient with CCD [7] although no further polyalanine-related CCD patients have been reported and no evidence currently associates the Q-repeat region with CCD. We previously identified Q-variants (15Q, 16Q, 24Q and 30Q) in an Australian fracture cohort [9] and two 16Q variants as well as a single alanine expansion variant (23Q/23A) in a randomly selected population from Aberdeen [10]. Pineda et al. [22] observed three Q-variants (16Q, 18Q and 30Q) in a Spanish population. Evidence exists that the RUNX2 Q-repeat is a site of functional variation; in carnivores the length of the Q repeat is significantly associated with mid-face length and nose curvature [23], indicating an effect on bone growth rates. Sears et al. [24] confirmed the functional nature of carnivore related Q/A repeat alterations, showing correlation of transcriptional variation with facial length in carnivores. These lines of evidence suggest that RUNX2 repeat variation may be functionally different in the human population. We hypothesised that glutamine repeat variants would exist in normal populations and may influence adult BMD and/or risk of fracture.

Materials and Methods

Study Subjects

The study subjects were obtained from four different epidemiological studies of bone density and are summarised in Table 1. All subjects were female. Voting in elections in Australia is compulsory and each region maintains an electoral roll. The West Australian study [25] consisted of females between the ages of 70 and 85 years who were randomly ascertained from the electoral role and approached by letter. The Geelong Osteoporosis study comprised a cohort recruited at random from the electoral role (GOS random) [26] and a specific fracture study (GOS fracture), where all fracture cases over the age of 35 years presenting at the only two radiology practices in the region were invited to join, as described [27]. Genotype was obtained on 834 subjects with no history of fracture from the random sample of GOS and 578 of the GOS fracture cases. The Sydney study comprised monozygotic and dizygotic twins who volunteered for studies of general medical issues through the Australian twin registry, as described [28]. Self reported history of fracture was available among a series of questionnaires completed by volunteers. Data were obtained on 980 participants. In the Tasmanian older adult cohort (TASOAC) study, 388 DNA of females were available of which 385 yielded genotype data. In this study, subjects ranged from 50 to 80 and were recruited by random ascertainment from the electoral roll [29]. For the Aberdeen study, subjects were postmenopausal women aged between 45 and 55 years who were approached at random using Community Health Index records of Aberdeen, Scotland as previously described [30]. Data were obtained on 991 study participants. In addition, 101 elderly female clinic patients with established osteoporosis and at least one osteoporotic fracture were available from the Geelong endocrine clinic. A similar cohort of 200 clinical patients with established osteoporosis defined by recurrent vertebral fracture was available from a New Zealand study, as described [31,32]. BMD data were not available for clinic patients. Individuals in all studies were female Caucasians and no subjects were excluded. Appropriate written consent was obtained from subjects under procedures in accordance with the Declaration of Helsinki approved by the relevant human research ethics committees (HREC) as previously described [25–32]. The committees are as follows: Sir Charles Gairdner Hospital HREC, Barwon Health HREC, Northern Sydney Local Health District HREC, Southern Tasmanian Health and Medical HREC and University of Otago HREC.

Bone measures

Bone density was measured by dual energy X-ray absorptiometry (DEXA). In the Aberdeen study a Norland XR26 or XR36 was used (Norland Corporation, Fort Atkinson, WI, USA). A Lunar DPX-L machine was used for the GOS. The Western Australian study used a Hologic 4500A fan beam densitometer to measure total BMD of the hip region. A Lunar Achilles ultrasound machine was used to measure the left calcaneus bone. Measures of speed of sound (SOS), broadband ultrasound attenuation (BUA) and bone stiffness were available. In the Sydney study, a Hologic 4500A fan beam densitometer was used to measure BMD at the lumbar spine, total hip, femoral neck and whole body. Western Australian, TASOAC and Sydney studies used the same type of densitometer and were calibrated with the same standard phantoms.

Detection of Q-variants

PCR was used to amplify RUNX2 exon 1 fragments harboring the Q/A repeat using the primers forward 5′-CCGGCAAAATGAGCGACG-3′ and reverse 5′-GGGCGGTGTAGCCTCTTACCTT-3′. The PCRs were carried out in 20 µl reactions containing $5\times10{-}7$ M primers, PCR reaction buffer, 125 µM dNTPs, 80 ng genomic DNA, 0.5 units *Taq* polymerase in 20 µl as specified by the supplier (Promega, Sydney, Australia). The study populations were genotyped separately by differing means: testing 100 random DNA by all methods gave the same genotypes. For the GOS and TASOAC, the resulting 336 bp fragments were resolved via nondenaturing 10% polyacrylamide gel electrophoresis (PAGE). Heteroduplex analysis was used to determine the presence of Q-repeat variants. For the Aberdeen populations the PCR fragment was digested with MspA1I (New England Biolabs) and resolved on 3% agarose. For the Western Australian samples, all PCR products were initially analysed via dHPLC (Varian Prostar 430, Varian Industries, Sydney, Australia) and subsequently by heteroduplex PAGE. Genotyping was done twice for all samples and all variant genotypes confirmed by PAGE to reveal heteroduplexes. All PCR amplified DNA fragments that displayed unique mobility patterns on PAGE were sequenced using BigDye

Table 1. Characteristics of population studies.

Study	Age range	N genotyped	Recruitment via	Reference
Western Australian	70–82	1078	Electoral roll	25
GOS random	20–92	822	Electoral roll	26
GOS fracture	35–95	598	Present with fracture	27
Sydney	19–78	980	Twin registry	28
TASOAC	50–80	385	Electoral roll	29
Aberdeen	45–55	991	Health records	30

Terminator v1.1 ready mix according to the manufacturer's protocol (Applied Biosystems).

Plasmids, transfection and cell culture

Expression plasmids containing mutant Q/A domains were constructed by cloning the *XbaI-XbaI* fragment from full length RUNX2 expression plasmid pEF-αA [33] into pUC18 to create pUC18RUNX2 which served as a template to create glutamine variants via PCR cloning. PCR was used to amplify partial RUNX2 promoter and exon 1 fragments from DNA samples harboring Q/A mutations using the oligonucleotide primers 5′-TTCACCACCGGACTCCAACT-3′ for the 5′ side and 5′-CATCTGGTACCTCTCCGAGGGCTACCACCTTGAAGG-CCACGGGCAGGGTC-3′ for the 3′ side. The reverse primer contained an *EcoNI* tag facilitating the cloning of the PCR amplified product into the *BglII-EcoNI* site of pUC18RUNX2. Mutant Q/A regions were confirmed by DNA sequencing and the *XbaI-XbaI* fragments were cloned into the *XbaI-XbaI* site of the mammalian expression vector pEF-BOS [34]. Restriction digest analysis and DNA sequencing confirmed the orientations of RUNX2 inserts. pGL3-Basic served as a template to create the reporter constructs. *BglII* and *HindIII* sites were introduced by PCR amplification in the human osteocalcin gene using oligonucleotide primers 5′-CAGGAGATCTCTGACCGTCGAGCTG-3′ for the 5′ side and 5′-GGGCAAGCTTGGTGTCTCGGGTGG-C-3′ for the 3′ side. The resulting *BglII-HindIII* fragment was cloned into the corresponding sites of pGL3-Basic to create pOSLUC, which has 590 basepairs of the human osteocalcin promoter, including 70 base pairs of the untranslated message. Oligonucleotides containing a consensus mouse osteocalcin RUNX2 response element (RRE: 5′-GATCCGCTGCAATCACCAACCACAGCA, with RUNX2 consensus binding site underlined) were cloned into the *BglII* site of pOSLUC to create pRRE, which had three copies of the RRE inserted as direct repeats. Transfections were performed using FuGENE (Roche) as the manufacturer's protocols. Antibody immuno-staining was performed as described in Yoshida et al. [35]. 1,25 dihydroxyvitamin D_3 (1,25$(OH)_2D_3$) was kept in the dark under argon in isopropanol and added with appropriate vehicle controls after dilution in ethanol. No more than 0.1 μl ethanol per ml medium was present in cell culture. Western blots of transfected cells were done by standard methods using anti-RUNX2 antibody (D130-3, MBL International) according to the manufacturer's instructions.

Luciferase Assay

NIH3T3 cells and HEK293 cells were maintained in DMEM (Gibco) supplemented with 10% FBS (v/v) (Gibco), 1% Penicillin-Streptomycin (v/v) (Gibco) in a 5% CO_2 humidified atmosphere at 37°C. For the luciferase assay NIH3T3 cells were seeded into 6-well plates at a density of 1×10^5 cells/well 24 hours prior to transfection. HEK293 cells were seeded into 12-well plates at a density of 1×10^5 cells/well 24 hours prior to transfection. NIH3T3 and HEK293 cells were transfected using FuGENE6 transfection reagent according to the manufacturer's instructions (Promega). Cells were harvested 48 hours post-transfection. Luciferase activities were determined using the dual luciferase assay system described by Dyer et al. 2000 [36]. pRL-CMV (Promega) was used as an internal control to normalize results.

Gel shift assays, *in vitro* protein translation and GST pull-down assays

Gel shift assays were done by standard methods as previously described, using 5% PAGE and *in vitro* translated proteins [37]. DNA probes representing RUNX2 binding sites were end labelled using a fill in reaction of 5′ overhangs using DNA polymerase 1 Klenow fragment and fragments purified by PAGE. *In vitro* translated human RUNX2 variant proteins 23Q wild type, 16Q-variant, and 30Q-variant were generated from DNA fragments representing 23Q, 16Q, or 30Q variants recloned into a T7 promoter containing hRUNX2 vector by using T7 RNA polymerase (TNT® Promega, USA) and coupled transcription-translation reactions containing [^{35}S]-methionine. Protein products were visualised and quantified by [^{35}S]-methionine incorporation. Bacterial over-expression of glutathione-S-transferase coupled human VDR (GSThVDR) fusion protein was performed by induction with isopropyl-β-D-thio-galactopyranoside (IPTG, 1.25 mM) for 3 h at 30°C in the JM109 *E.coli* strain as described previously [37]. GST pull-down assays were performed by incubation of GSThVDR with either [^{35}S]-23Q RUNX2 wild type, [^{35}S]-16Q variant, [^{35}S]-30Q variant RUNX2. As a binding agent, a GSThVDR-Sepharose bead slurry (50% w/v of beads) in PPI buffer (20 mM HEPES, pH 7.9; 200 mM KCl; 1 mM EDTA, 4 mM MgCl2, 1 mM dithiothreitol, 0.1% Nonidet P-40 and 10% glycerol) was used. GST fusion-Sepharose slurries were pre-blocked in PPI buffer containing bovine serum albumin (1 μg/μl) prior to use in pull-down assays. Unbound [^{35}S]-23Q RUNX2 wild type, [^{35}S]-16Q variant or [^{35}S]-30Q variant RUNX2 labelled proteins were washed away with PPI buffer. *In vitro* translated [^{35}S] 23Q, [^{35}S] 16Q or [^{35}S] 30Q that had bound to GSThVDR-Sepharose was released from the Sepharose, electrophoresed through a 12% SDS-PAGE, and detected by autoradiography using either phosphor screens (BioRad) or X-ray film. Densitometric analysis on resolved bands was performed using the ChemicDoc system (BioRad).

Statistical methods

Within studies, Q-variants were analysed using analysis of variance (ANOVA) and Student's T-test. Genotype status (Q-variant carrier or not) was coded as one and zero, respectively, and used as a variable in ANCOVA analysis to test the effect of covariates such as age and weight. Age, age-weight and age-weight^{-1} adjusted values of bone density parameters were produced using linear regression. Stiffness was $\log_e$ transformed to comply with equality of variance assumptions in ANOVA. These adjustments had no material influence on the conclusions and Z scores of age-weight^{-1} regression are presented. Incident fracture during five years of observation was available for the Western Australian study. Incident fracture was categorised as zero and one for absence and presence of fracture, respectively, for analysis by logistic regression and the number of such fracture events also examined in genotype groups using contingency tables. Results of logistic regression are presented as p values and odds ratios (OR) with 95% confidence intervals (CI). Genotypes were examined pooled (all variants) and separately as either deletions or insertions. The only measure in common across all studies was femoral neck BMD. In order to pool all studies, each individual was expressed within a study as a Z-score of residual femoral neck BMD from the age-weight^{-1} regression specific for that study. Under the null hypothesis of no effect at this locus on BMD, the Z scores should be distributed randomly around a mean of zero. Population simulations were constructed in excel, using the Monte Carlo simulation plugin, PopTools [38], and the correlated variable tool to simulate bone density parameters as a series of correlated normal distributions, based on the correlations observed in the populations studied. Results of transfections were analysed using ANOVA with Fisher's least significant difference test for pair wise comparisons. Counts of cells were analysed using contingency tables and Chi-square. Analysis of covariance was used to analyse categorical and continuous covariates.

Results

Q-variants identified

From the 1078 individuals genotyped in the Western Australian study, there were five 16Q alleles, one 18Q allele and two 30Q alleles. In the GOS random population sample three Q-variants were identified in 822 subjects: these were one 15Q and two 16Q variants. In the GOS fracture study, where recruitment was based on any fracture at any age, four Q-variants were identified in 598 subjects: these were two 16Q and two 30Q variants. In a prior publication [9], three of these variants were reported (two 16Q and one 30Q): in this study more samples from the GOS fracture cohort were genotyped and an additional variant identified. In the Sydney population of 980, five individuals with Q-variants were identified: carrying 16Q, 18Q and 30Q. The 16Q and 18Q variants were found in two pairs of monozygotic twins. The 30Q variant was in one individual of a dizygotic twin pair. For analysis, the average bone density values of the monozygotic twin pairs were taken and the pair considered as a single genetically unique individual. In the Tasmanian study (TASOAC) no Q-variants were found in 385 genotyped. In the Aberdeen study, two 16Q variants were identified previously from 991 subjects [10]; in this study their bone parameters are reported. In order to estimate the frequency of the Q-variants without bias, only those populations where the recruitment strategy involved volunteers were considered (Western Australia, Geelong, Tasmania and Aberdeen). In this case, 13 Q-variants were observed within 3276 subjects, yielding a population frequency estimate of 0.004 (95%CI, 0.002 to 0.007). Using the binomial theorem and the observed frequency of Q-variants, it is estimated that 95% of repeat studies of a similar size (approximately 3000 subjects) will detect between 6 and 19 such Q-variant carriers, if allele frequency is similar in other populations. In 103 female post-menopausal clinic patients with established osteoporosis with fracture, 16Q and 30Q variants were found. In a similar population of vertebral fracture cases from New Zealand [31,32], two 30Q variants were found in 200 patients genotyped. Therefore, in clinic patients with osteoporosis, four Q-variants were found in 303 patients genotyped. Apart from those Q-variants described above, three examples of 24Q alleles were detected overall. These 24Q subjects were not considered in this analysis. All Q-repeat variants were heterozygous carriers with the other chromosome containing a 23Q/17A wild type allele.

Bone density in Q-variants

Characteristics of Q-variant carriers with respect to femoral neck (FN) Z scores are presented in Table 2. Figure 1 shows the mean Z score of Q-variants for each measured parameter in each study cohort. The Q-variant carriers in Western Australian were compared to non carriers ($N=1021$) for differences in the ultrasound measures of bone density: broadband ultrasound attenuation (BUA) and speed of sound (SOS). Q-variants had significantly lower BUA measures ($n=8$, BUA, $p=0.025$) at the calcaneus, with a difference of -0.80 standard deviations (SD, or Z score) and significantly lower SOS ($p=0.05$) and log stiffness ($p=0.013$). Weight, height and age were not significantly different in Q-variants. For all BMD values, age and age-weight^{-1} adjustment was done using regression and adjusted values produced. Individual values were then expressed as Z scores around the relevant population mean. While the particulars of reported measures change depending on such adjustment, the general outcomes reported here are not dependent on this mathematical adjustment. Measures of bone density using DEXA were similarly lower in Q-variants (Fig. 1A) although only nominally significant with the total hip BMD measure ($p=0.028$). At other sites there was a trend for Q-variants to have lower BMD compared with all others in the study: femoral neck ($p=0.22$), trochanter ($p=0.065$), and intertrochanteric region ($p=0.06$). Of the seven Q-variants identified from GOS there was a trend for negative Z scores (BMD below the population mean value, Fig. 1A) with 6 of 7 sites having negative average BMD. The Q-variant subjects from the Aberdeen study had negative Z-scores for both femoral neck and lumbar spine BMD (averaging -1.39SD and -1.36SD, $p=0.01$ and $p=0.11$ respectively, Fig. 1A). In the Sydney study, the data from each monozygotic twin pair were averaged and thus three were available with BMD data. The Q-variants had negative BMD Z-scores for the femoral neck with an average effect of -0.62SD. There was a trend for negative Z scores for all bone measures (Table 3).

Combining BMD data using Monte Carlo simulation

Bone density measures at different anatomical sites are correlated: additional measures in individuals therefore contribute useful information to explore the bone phenotype of Q-variants. All these data from skeletal sites can be used collectively to explore the genotype-phenotype relationship. Empirical p values based on Monte Carlo modelling make use of the additional data available in bone studies, where the scanning methods provide BMD measures of multiple sites. Considering only Z scores derived from within each study eliminates the effect of using different DEXA devices. A simulation was made based on the likelihood of sampling such individuals with measurements of correlated bone related variables. Correlated variables were simulated based on the measured correlations of bone parameters in the various populations, and a simulation of sampling was done in order to determine how many such samples met or exceeded the observed data. This approach was first taken with the Western Australian study, considering just deletion variants. There were six deletion variants, identified in a population sample of 1078 subjects, each with seven measured parameters related to bone. In this case, of 100,000 simulations of sampling six individuals measured for seven correlated bone parameters, only 252 such samples had an overall group mean equal to or more negative than the observed mean of -0.74 Z scores for all variables. This yields an empirical multivariate p value of 0.0025. The GOS study came from a similar population via similar recruitment with seven bone related parameters measured; although the bone parameters were measured using different equipment. The three deletions observed in GOS study were combined with those from Western Australia and a simulation done based on the idea of sampling from the combined population: in this case the observed mean was -0.63 Z scores and 235 samples from 100,000 trials met or exceeded the observed mean, giving an empirical p value of 0.0024. When 30Q variants were combined with all other variants from the two Australian studies the Monte Carlo based multivariate p value was: 0.0007. Of the 75 bone related measures from the Q variants identified in Aberdeen, Western Australia and Geelong studies, 59 measures had negative Z score values. Combining data from the three studies for Monte Carlo simulation resulted in 9 samples in 100,000 trials; giving an empirical probability of $p=0.0009$. These simulations suggest that the additional measures provide useful data supporting the hypothesis that Q-variant carriers have lower bone density and that the average deficit is of the order of 0.7 Z scores of age, weight^{-1} adjusted BMD.

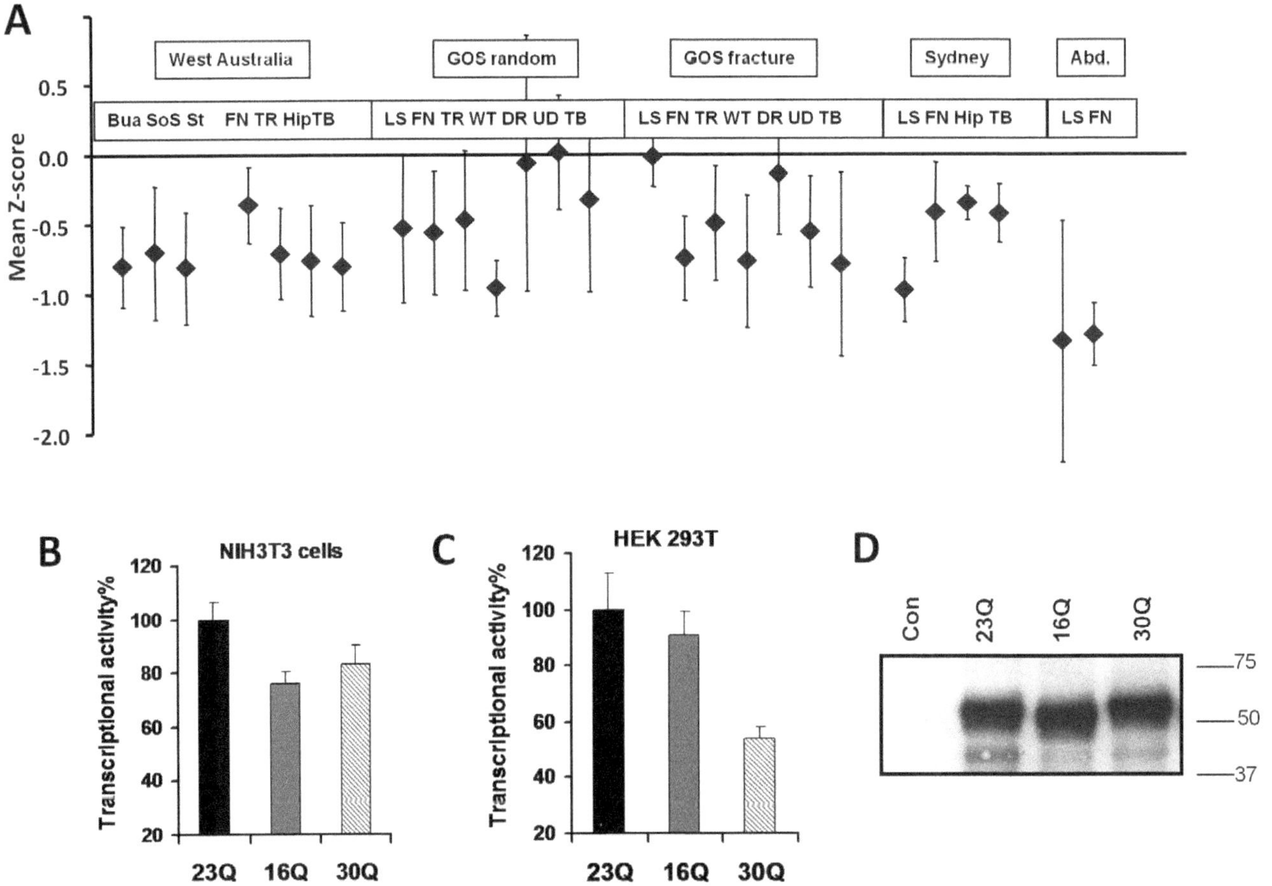

Figure 1. Characterization of RUNX2 Q variants with respect to clinical measures of bone density and *in vitro* transactivation. A. RUNX2 Q-variant carriers from Western Australia, Geelong (GOS random sample and GOS fracture), Sydney and Aberdeen studies have lower mean bone density parameters. Q-variants have lower mean Z-scores of bone density measured by calcaneal ultrasound (BUA, SOS, Stiff) and by DEXA at various skeletal sites. Abbreviations: Abd., Aberdeen; BUA, broadband ultrasound attenuation; SOS, speed of sound; Stiff, bone stiffness; FN, femoral neck BMD; TR, trochanteric region BMD; Hip, Hip BMD; TB, total body BMD; LS, lumbar spine BMD; WT, Ward's triangle BMD; DR, distal radius BMD; UD, ultradistal radius BMD. Error bars are standard error. Z scores presented are the within study age weight^{-1} adjusted Z score derived from within that cohort. **B** and **C**. Q-variant expression vectors have diminished capacity to transactivate target promoters in NIH3T3 mouse fibroblasts (**B**) and human embryonic kidney cell (HEK293) (**C**). Cells were transfected as described in the methods. In **B** the target was pRRE which is the human osteocalcin promoter with three additional synthetic mouse RUNX2 target sites added upstream, and in **C** the target promoter construct was 590 bp of the authentic human osteocalcin promoter driving luciferase (pOSLUC). **D.** Transfected cells show appropriate sizes of expressed product and exhibit equivalent amount of protein. NIH3T3 cells were transfected with empty vector (Con) or expression constructs as indicated. Cellular extracts were Western blotted after electrophoresis on SDS-PAGE. Numbers indicate molecular weight markers in kilodaltons. In **B** and **C** transactivation is expressed as percentage relative to the 23Q variant in order to normalise scales of NIH3T3 and HEK293 cells.

Using BMD data from the Q-variants derived from the GOS fracture cohort is not necessary, since a significant p value was already obtained using data from studies with no apparent recruitment bias. However, if the GOS fracture and Sydney cohort data were used in the Monte Carlo simulations the result was still significant. Addition of all subjects for whom BMD data were available to the Monte Carlo simulation supported the hypothesis that Q-variant carriers have significantly lower BMD (3 samples in one million trials with mean values equal to or more extreme than the observed means).

Femoral neck BMD was the only measure in common between the GOS random sample, GOS fracture, Aberdeen, Sydney and Western Australian studies. In order to combine the effects of these studies, age-weight^{-1} adjusted Z-scores for each study were taken giving a mean Z score of -0.60. Simply combining all populations, as if there were one global population from which the samples were drawn, gave a p value of 0.0007. The conclusions were not altered appreciably by taking the average of those who were twins.

Relationship to fracture

In the GOS study, the random sample that was genotyped excluded any with history of fracture, whereas in the Western Australian study, although recruitment was essentially random, fracture was not a reason for exclusion. Of the eight Q-variants found in the Western Australian study, four had prior osteoporosis related fractures (hip, spine and arm fractures). Data on incident fracture during a five year observation period were available for those who had completed the follow-up. Incident fracture during the study period was coded as 0 or 1 for absence and presence of fracture and the type of fracture was ignored. Four of 8 Q-variant carriers sustained incident fracture whereas the fracture rate was 17.8% in 1036 subjects with the normal 23Q RUNX2 allele. Q-variant carriers were significantly more likely (Fisher's exact test,

Table 2. Characteristics of Q-variant allele carriers.

Allele	Age	Weight	Height	Z-FN
15Q	41	69	159	−0.33
16Q	30	79	171	−1.42
16Q	45	56	166	0.07
16Q	47	68	174	−1.52
16Q	49	66	161	−1.07
16Q*	69	71	165	−0.15
16Q	70	56	152	−0.34
16Q	72	80	168	0.89
16Q	75	71	165	−1.69
16Q	76	52	156	−0.91
16Q	78	61	152	−0.70
16Q	79	65	167	−0.31
16Q	85	70	147	−0.13
18Q*	65	66	161	−0.21
18Q	74	69	156	−0.24
30Q	39	97	161	−1.34
30Q	48	62	160	−1.37
30Q	72	57	161	0.07
30Q	74	54	162	−0.02
30Q	87	50	155	−1.18

Age (years), weight (kg), height (cm) and Z-score of femoral neck BMD are presented. Subjects are ranked by allele length and then age.
*indicates average of identical twin pair. In addition, a 16Q and three 30Q variants were observed in clinic patients.

Table 3. Bone parameters in standardized Z scores averaged over all Q-variants carriers.

Site	Mean Z	N	P value
Z_Spine	−0.709	14*	0.0032
Z_FN	−0.601	22*	0.0006
Z_WT	−0.484	6	0.1449
Z_TR	−0.774	14*	0.0022
Z_UD	−0.102	5	0.8358
Z_MI	−0.271	5	0.4149
Z_TB	−0.531	10*	0.0844
Z_INT	−0.760	7	0.0206
Z_HIP	−0.653	11*	0.0146
BUA	−0.798	8	0.0254
SOS	−0.700	8	0.0505
STIFF	−0.809	8	0.0130

N is the number of observations available.
*Asterisk indicates sites with data from more than one study combined using Z scores. P value is the test of the hypothesis that the mean Z score is zero. Key: Z_ indicates a Z score adjusted by age weight^{-1} regression, FN is femoral neck, WT is Ward's triangle, TR is trochanteric region, UD is ultra distal radius, MI is Mid shaft of the radius, TB is total body, INT is intertrochanteric region, HIP is total hip, BUA is broadband ultrasound attenuation measured at the calcaneus, SOS is speed of sound, STIFF is stiffness and p value refers to $\log_e$ transformed stiffness.

p = 0.036) to be in the fracture category (OR 4.7 with 95% CI 1.2 to 19.2). Overall, 6 of 8 Q-variants from the Western Australian study had prior or incident fractures. If the Geelong fracture study (n = 598) is combined with Western Australian study subjects who had ever fractured (n = 426), 1024 Australian subjects are available who had sustained fracture. Combining Western Australian [25] and GOS [39] subjects who had not reported fracture gave 1478 Australian non-fracture subjects. Despite the fact that no age matching was done, there was a significant increase (p = 0.036) in Q-variants within the fracture category in this comparison. Overall, of 22 Q-repeat variants identified, 12 had sustained some form of bone fracture, including the clinically important sites of femur, hip, spine and arm. Within the 30Q variants, three of five had fractured.

Reduced capacity to transactivate RUNX2 target genes

Expression vectors were constructed to express 23Q, 16Q and 30Q variants of RUNX2. Significantly lower transactivation of target gene promoters occurred after transfection for 16Q and 30Q compared to the wild type 23Q was observed using a semi-synthetic RUNX2 reporter construct (pRRE) in mouse fibroblastic NIH3T3 cells (p = 0.002 and 0.016, for 16Q and 30Q, respectively, Fig. 1B). Similar data was obtained using the human osteocalcin promoter driving luciferase (pOSLUC) in HEK293 cells (Fig. 1C). Western blot of total protein from transfected NIH3T3 cells demonstrated the expected differences in apparent molecular weight in PAGE while there was no evidence a difference in relative abundance of Q-variants compared to 23Q wild type. Control cells transfected with empty vector showed no immunoreactivity (Fig. 1D).

Comparison with CCD-related RUNX2 mutants

CCD is a disease where severe inactivating mutations of *RUNX2* exist. Some CCD-related RUNX2 mutants have no transactivation capacity while others, related to milder phenotypes, have a residual activity. CBFB is a heterodimer binding partner of RUNX2, known to increase DNA binding. The ability of RUNX2 variants to co-localise with endogenous CBFB in either nuclear, and/or cytoplasmic compartments was assessed by confocal immunomicroscopy with simultaneous staining with RUNX2 and CBFB with different fluorophores (Fig. 2 A–C). Cells were counted with exclusively nuclear staining, nuclear plus cytoplasmic and cytoplasmic only staining. The data were expressed as percentages of cells counted with a particular type of staining. For RUNX2, more cells with cytoplasmic staining were observed in transfected cells with 16Q and 30Q variants than expected compared with wild type 23Q (p = 0.007), with the 30Q having the stronger effect (p = 0.01). The majority (90%) of cells transfected with wild type 23Q RUNX2 also showed nuclear localization of CBFB: the other 10% represented cells with both nuclear and cytoplasmic staining. For transfected 16Q variant, 75% of positive cells showed nuclear RUNX2 while only 45% showed nuclear CBFB ($p = 7.5 \times 10^{-5}$) with the difference appearing in the combined nuclear and cytoplasmic compartment (Fig. 2C). For transfected 30Q, the difference in CBFB binding was not as great: 64% showed nuclear RUNX2 while 54% of cells were also being positive for nuclear CBFB (p = 0.002) with a 10% increase in the nuclear and cytoplasmic compartment for CBFB.

The transactivation functions of the Q-variants were analysed using a third RUNX2 target gene reporter assay and activity compared to RUNX2 mutants known to cause CCD. Using the mouse osteocalcin reporter (p147) in NIH3T3 mouse fibroblastic cells: 16Q and 30Q variants had reduced capacity to transactivate

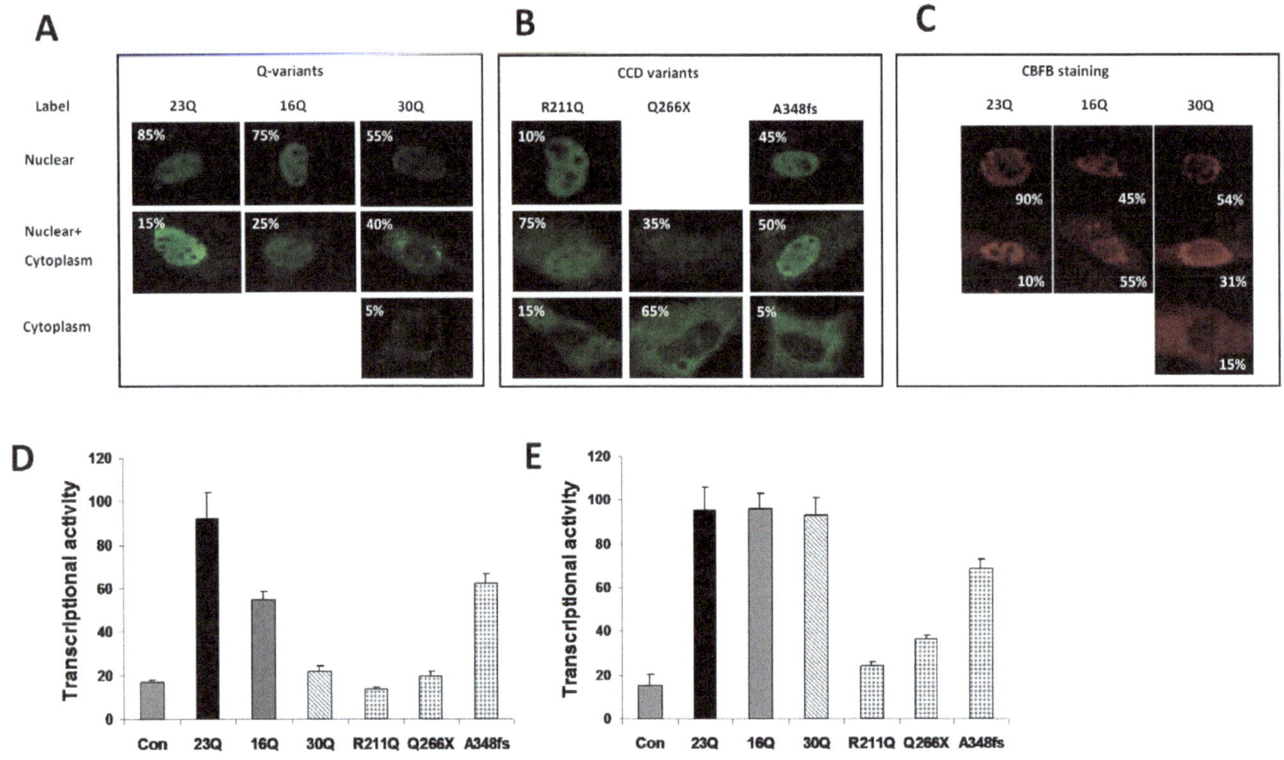

Figure 2. RUNX2 Q-variants have reduced nuclear localization and transactivation activity. A. Expression constructs were transfected into NIH3T3 cells and RUNX2 detected using confocal immunofluorescence, counts were then made of the number of cells with staining in the nuclear or cytoplasmic compartment, or both. The figures show representative cells and the insert percentage numbers indicates the proportion of cells that show that particular staining location. Panel **A** shows Q-variant forms of RUNX2 and panel **B** shows RUNX2 mutants that are associated with the condition cleidocranial dysplasia (CCD). **C.** Nuclear or cytoplasmic localization of CBFB in cells transfected with RUNX2 Q-variant constructs. **D.** RUNX2 Q-variants compared with CCD-associated RUNX2 mutants, tested against the p147 mouse osteocalcin construct. In this assay Q-variants 16Q and 30Q have a deficit of transcriptional activity that overlaps that of CCD-associated variants. **E.** Co-transfection of CBFB expression vector with RUNX2 Q-variants completely overcomes the defect in transcriptional activity detected by the p147 promoter. In contrast, the transcriptional activity of CCD-associated RUNX2 mutants on the p147 construct is not rescued by CBFB co-transfection. The transcriptional activities of 16Q and 30Q alleles were compared to wild type 23Q RUNX2 and known CCD-related mutants using an *in vitro* target gene reporter assay consisting of the proximal mouse osteocalcin promoter (p147) driving luciferase target gene construct and transfected with expression vector for RUNX2 variants in mouse NIH3T3 fibroblast-like cells. In **D** and **E**, transactivation data are not percentages relative to 23Q wild type, but arbitrary units related to the ratio of firefly luciferase to Renilla luciferase. Key to symbols: Con, control cells with target gene promoter p147 but transfected with empty expression vector; 23Q, wild type; 16Q and 30Q, Q variants; R211Q, missense mutation at residue 211; Q266X, early termination at residue 266; A348fs, frames shift mutation at alanine residue 348.

and this was a stronger effect than had been observed in the prior reporter-cell line combinations (Fig. 2D). The depressed transactivation ability of the 30Q variant was approximately the same as that observed in the Q266X CCD mutant, whereas the 16Q variant was similar to that seen in the A348fs mutant. Exogenous transfected CBFB enhanced wild type RUNX2 activity and rescued, to a large extent, the transactivation activity on the p147 target promoters when Q-variants were considered (Fig. 2E). Under the same conditions, the activity of CCD-related RUNX2 mutants was not rescued fully by co-transfection of CBFB partner (Fig. 2E).

Endogenous CBFB nuclear translocation was significantly related to RUNX2 Q-variants when observed using confocal microscopy (Fig. 2 A–C). Despite the fact that endogenous CBFB localization might be altered in RUNX2 variants, we reasoned that transfection of CBFB expression vector, may alter the phenotype of the Q-variants by augmenting endogenous CBFB levels. Expression vector for CBFB was transfected with Q-variants and activity on the p147 target in NIH3T3 cells examined.

Vitamin D receptor (VDR) and Q variants

In order to test the interaction of VDR with RUNX2 Q-variants in cells, the human osteocalcin promoter luciferase construct (pOSLUC) was transfected into NIH3T3 fibroblasts, with or without VDR expression vector and with or without $1,25(OH)_2D_3$ and RUNX2 expression vector (Fig. 3A). Differences in target promoter activity were once again observed, as described above, with 16Q and 30Q showing significantly lower activity compared to wildtype 23Q (Fig. 3A). As expected, transfection of VDR resulted in induction of pOSLUC. In the presence of 45 ng RUNX2 vector, 10 ng VDR vector and $1,25(OH)_2D_3$ (at 10^{-8} M) approximately 63 fold induction of the target vector occurred compared to empty vector vehicle treated cells (Fig. 3A). In the absence of $1,25(OH)_2D_3$, transfected VDR had no significant effect on promoter activity. Treatment of cells with $1,25(OH)_2D_3$, in the absence of transfected VDR, resulted in some induction of pOSLUC, consistent with activation of endogenous VDR. Induction by $1,25(OH)_2D_3$ was increased in the presence of transfected VDR ($p = 1.7 \times 10^{-10}$). In the absence of $1,25(OH)_2D_3$, both 16Q and 30Q variants had significantly lower target gene promoter activity compared to 23Q wild type construct (23Q versus 16Q, $p = 1.1 \times 10^{-5}$; 23Q versus 30Q, $p = 4.0 \times 10^{-6}$), regardless of the presence or not of transfected VDR. In contrast, in the presence of $1,25(OH)_2D_3$ and transfected VDR the difference between 23Q and other Q-variant constructs measured by osteocalcin promoter activity was eliminated or reduced (23Q versus 16Q, $p = 0.95$; 23Q versus 30Q, $p = 0.08$).

VDR is a RUNX2 partner protein that can be activated by ligand, $1,25(OH)_2D_3$. To examine the interaction of VDR and RUNX2 variants, *in vitro* translated proteins were made and tested in glutathione-S transferase (GST) pull down reactions for differences in protein-protein interaction. Unlabelled GST-VDR fusion construct was used to pull down ^{35}S labelled Q variant RUNX2 proteins (Fig. 3B). Under these conditions, GST-VDR demonstrated a strong interaction with RUNX2 (approximately 25% of label being recovered in pull down) but no significant difference in capacity to pull down RUNX2 Q-variants ($p = 0.08$), suggesting that protein-protein interactions of RUNX2 and VDR are unaffected by either variation in the glutamine repeat or the GST moiety added to VDR. There was no difference in the

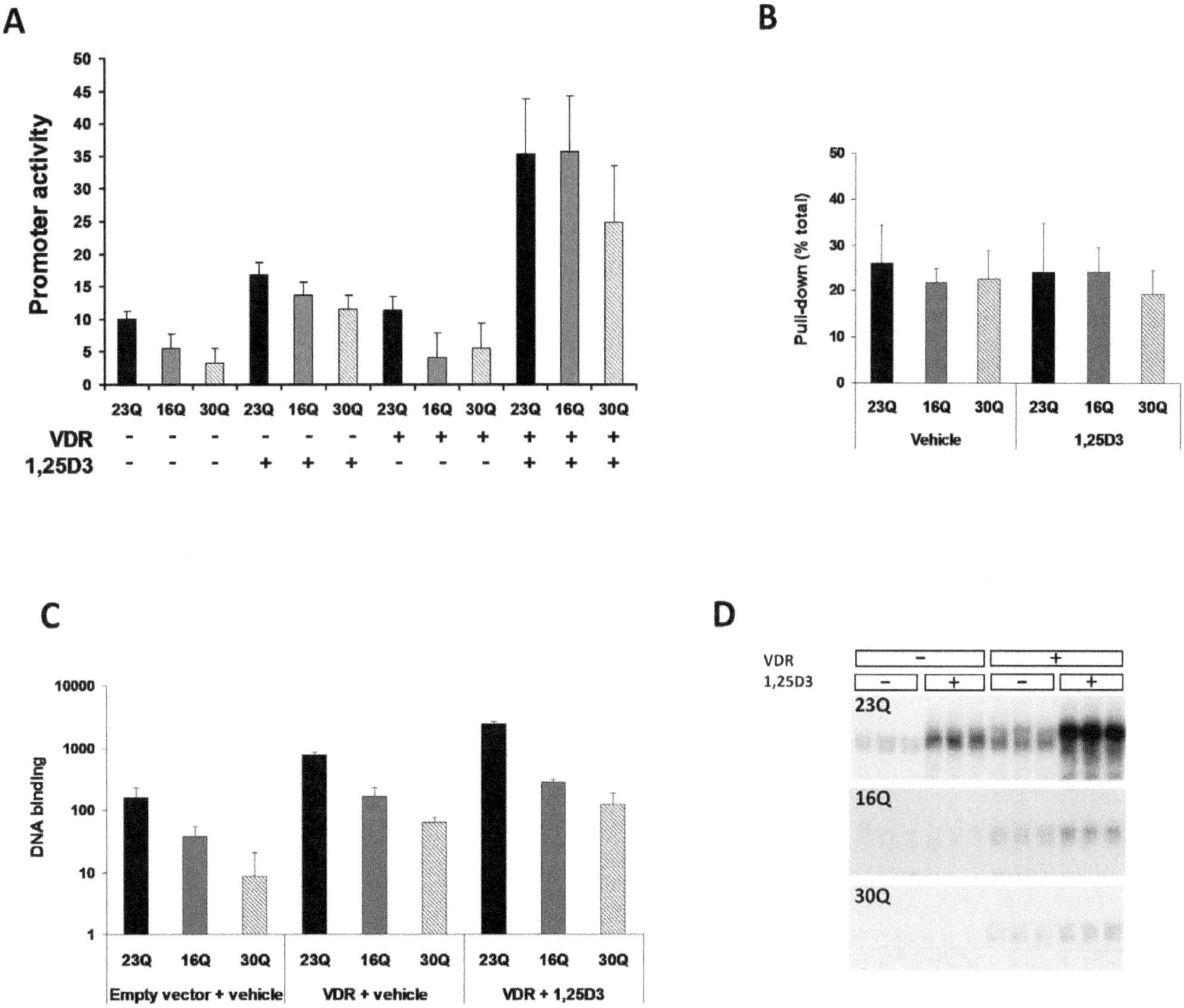

Figure 3. RUNX2 Q-variant interaction with the vitamin receptor (VDR). A. Transfected VDR, activated by $1,25(OH)_2D_3$, can overcome the deficit in Q-variant transcriptional activity on a target human osteocalcin promoter. Although 16Q and 30Q variants show significantly reduced transactivation in NIH3T3 cells, as seen previously, transfected VDR alone does not alter the significant defect, however activation of VDR by the natural ligand $1,25(OH)_2D_3$, results in essentially no difference in activation on the target gene promoter between the Q-variants. Promoter activity refers to human osteocalcin promoter construct driving fire fly luciferase (pOSLUC). Transactivation units are arbitrary based on the ratio of fire fly to Renilla luciferase. Empty vector controls are not shown but had activity of about one half unit on this graph. **B.** There was no detectable difference in the affinity of [^{35}S] RUNX2 Q-variants for binding labelled VDR protein in *in vitro* pull-down assays where VDR was used to pull down ^{35}S labelled RUNX2 protein via an affinity column. **C.** The ability of *in vitro* translated RUNX2 Q-variants to bind a RUNX2 DNA element from the mouse osteocalcin promoter (known as ORE) is enhanced by VDR in a ligand dependant manner. DNA binding was measured by phosphor analysis of labelled bands in gel shift assays after 5% PAGE. A difference in binding capacity existed on this element. Although addition of VDR or VDR and $1,25(OH)_2D_3$, resulted in a increased total binding, in a ligand dependent manner, there was still a difference in Q-variants relative to 23Q. **D.** Images show gel shift data, with triplicates, RUNX2 variants indicated on the image and above the additional proteins added. Data suggest a difference in DNA binding and interaction with VDR. 1,25D3 in figure indicates $1,25(OH)_2D_3$.

amount of GST-pull down signal in the presence or absence of $1,25(OH)_2D_3$ ligand.

Quantitative gel-shift assays were done using *in vitro* translated RUNX2 variants and a synthetic RUNX2 element from the mouse osteocalcin gene. These data showed a significant difference in the binding capacity of the Q-variants to the response element, suggesting that variation in the Q repeat can influence DNA binding, at least on some elements. *In vitro* conditions for ligand ($1,25(OH)_2D_3$) dependent VDR binding to DNA were previously described [36]. Under these conditions, the RUNX2 response element binding activity was increased by addition of *in vitro* translated VDR protein and further enhanced by addition of $1,25(OH)_2D_3$. Despite increased DNA affinity in the presence of VDR and $1,25(OH)_2D_3$ a significant difference in the *in vitro* DNA binding activity of Q-variants persisted such that 16Q and 30Q variants were less active than 23Q wild type (Fig. 3 C, D).

Discussion

Various lines of evidence suggest that the RUNX2 Q/A repeat region has functional polymorphism. We screened samples from various studies for Q-repeat mutations in RUNX2. A total of 26 Q-variant carriers were identified, involving 24 genetically unique individuals. The Q-variants did not present with cleidocranial dysplasia (CCD) and thus we hypothesized that the Q-variants may alter another skeletal phenotype such as BMD. Overall, Q-variants were significantly lower for BMD measures including bone ultrasound attenuation of the calcaneus, and DEXA measures of BMD at several sites. After pooling BMD measures from all studies, using Z scores, an overall estimate of the effect of Q-variant status was obtained. The genetic effect of Q-variants was around 0.7 Z-score (SD) reduction in bone density whether measured by DEXA or ultrasound. These data confirm that the Q-tract of RUNX2 has a reasonably high rate of population variation and furthermore, suggest that this variation manifests in the phenotype of lower BMD. Q-variant heterozygotes were detected at around 0.4%, or around 40,000 per ten million inhabitants. Q-variant homozygotes are expected to be infrequent; but such homozygotes may have a more severe phenotype with a mean effect of −1.4 Z-scores, if the genetic effect is additive. Whether Q-insertions have a more extreme phenotype than deletions, as suggested by the BMD data, remains to be determined in larger populations.

New repeat variants can occur through strand slippage during replication of repeat sequences such as that encoding the RUNX2 Q-repeat. Expansion of Q-repeats is known in other diseases such as Kennedy's disease where expanded androgen receptor repeats result in motor neuron disease [40] and, incidentally, the length of the repeat has been related to transcriptional function [41]. Long Q-repeats are thought to adopt β-sheet structures [42] that coil into a nanotube by forming a super helix with a critical point of increased stability at a length of 30Q [43]. This might suggest that the super structure of the Q-repeat, rather than the length, is important for altered function. Although the Q-variants observed in this study were either 30Q or less, it seems possible that longer repeat expansion of RUNX2 may be observed and may be associated with some other pathology. Interestingly, the most frequent variants observed are 16Q and 30Q, each being 7 amino acids difference from the standard wild type 23Q allele. This represents a deletion or expansion of 21 base pairs in the DNA helix, being exactly two turns of the helix increase or decrease, given the accepted value of 10.5 base pairs per helical turn in DNA.

The transcriptional activities of the 16Q and 30Q mutants were analysed using three different luciferase reporter gene assays. The variants exhibited transactivation function, however at significantly reduced levels compared to wild type (23Q). The effect was of greater magnitude using a truncated mouse osteocalcin promoter, p147, where 16Q and 30Q variant activity overlapped that of some RUNX2 mutations that are associated with cleidocranial dysplasia. The reduction in transactivation function is consistent with the decrease in BMD observed. In the case of a heterozygote with a normal wild-type allele, the net effect would be expected to reflect the activity of individual alleles. The significant effect of Q-variant RUNX2 on transactivation activity in transfection assays could result from effects on DNA binding, nuclear residence and interactions with partner proteins. Nuclear residence of Q-variants was decreased significantly in transfected cells while quantitative gel shift assays suggested a difference in binding to consensus DNA elements. We cannot distinguish between the nuclear import effects and direct effects on transcriptional machinery, since we did not examine *in vitro* transcription. Regardless of the mechanism, it seems plausible that the quantitative reduction in the transactivation capacity of RUNX2 is associated with overall decrease in BMD seen in human carriers. Accumulated over a lifetime, this may be enough to explain the observed effects on bone density. On the other hand, only one semi-synthetic and two natural target genes were tested, so the effect of Q-variants on other genes is not known. The vitamin D receptor (VDR) is ligand activated, is known to bind RUNX2 by interaction on the osteocalcin promoter [44], and has potent direct effects on bone cells. In the human, but not in mouse, VDR activates osteocalcin through a vitamin D response element. In this case, partial recovery of the transactivation potential of the RUNX2 Q-variants on the human osteocalcin promoter was observed on co-transfection and activation of VDR with the ligand $1,25(OH)_2D_3$.

Are the Q-variants related to fracture? While it is suggestive that a significant effect on incident fracture was observed within the Western Australian study, this outcome should be viewed with caution due to the small numbers of Q variants. In addition, the apparent enrichment of Q-variants in post-menopausal clinic fracture cases (four variants in 303 cases genotyped) should also be considered with caution. Given the rare nature of these Q-variants, much larger studies are required to determine the relationship with fracture with precision. A frequently quoted proposition is that for every one standard deviation decrease in BMD, a person increases two fold in liability for fracture. If the effect on BMD of Q-variants is similar to the measured amount (0.7SD deficit), we can expect an increase in liability to fracture of slightly less than two-fold, if the effect of a gene such as RUNX2 on fracture acts solely via BMD. Based on the observed allele frequency, very large studies indeed (10,000 cases and controls) would be required for reasonable power test the hypothesis of association with fracture at 99% confidence for an odds ratio of around 2. If the hypothetical effect on fracture is greater than that suggested by BMD differences, then it may be possible to detect an effect in smaller numbers.

Severe RUNX2 mutations that cause CCD have a more profound effect in transfection assays, usually abolishing transactivation [6,7,19,20]. Milder phenotypes are associated with RUNX2 mutants that have some transactivation function. In some transactivation assays, notably using the p147 mouse osteocalcin promoter, the 30Q RUNX2 variant resulted in transactivation in a manner similar to CCD mutant RUNX2 forms (Q266X), suggesting a phenotype similar to CCD in terms of transfection. The subjects that carry Q-repeat mutations do not present with CCD, thus the Q-variant proteins transactivate target promoters at levels that are high enough to avoid the manifestations of CCD but at levels that reduce bone density within the normal range. Alternatively, some other mechanism may keep the phenotype out of the range of CCD, such as the CBFB or VDR interactions that were investigated in this study. The transfection data are consistent with this hypothesis. Our constructs were based on the RUNX2 protein that starts MRIPV, an isoform that is expressed off the second promoter of RUNX2. At least in mouse, and possibly in human, an isoform beginning MASNS is expressed off the first promoter. We have not tested the effect of Q-variants within the context of the isoform RUNX2-II, expressed off the first promoter. In addition, recent evidence suggests that Q-repeat regions contain an activity similar to a trans-activation domain [45,46]. Furthermore, RUNX2 Q/A repeat variation is related to skull shape in carnivores [25,26] suggesting that functional polymorphism is associated with this repeat: unfortunately no data on facial characteristics or skull shape was taken from the subjects presented in this study. It is also notable that the RUNX2 locus shows evidence of intense evolutionary selection in the comparison between Neanderthal and modern human DNA sequences [47]. How this relates to functional change remains to be established. Our data support a role for the Q-repeat in contributing to transactivation activity, although we have no data on a biochemical mechanism. It seems reasonable to conclude that a number of activities are altered to arrive at a change in target gene transactivation: including nuclear localization, DNA binding and possibly the activity of the Q-repeat as a transactivation function. The data suggests lower transcriptional activity of RUNX2, contributing to lower bone density and possibly flow-on increased risk of fracture, through reduced transcriptional activity in osteoblasts.

There are several limitations of this study. No subjects were rejected from the collections for any reason prior to genotyping although some DNA failed to amplify for technical reasons. Recruitment bias was minimised as far as could be done in such clinical collections and there is no reason to suspect that genetic stratification might have influenced the outcome, although this was not formally tested. Similar results were observed in different locations, although all populations were essentially Caucasian. Bone phenotype data were derived from different commercial devices in each population and were compared through the use of standardized Z scores or Monte Carlo modelling; which should remove device-related differences. The study was limited to female Caucasians. The statistical outcome observed was not dependent on modelling covariates, although adjusted standardized values are presented. While statistically significant, these outcomes do not extend to the whole genome level of significance used in genome scans, although this study was not designed as a genome scan. The Q-variants observed in this study may be new mutations, although intergenerational studies are needed to verify this. If these are new mutants such a mutable locus may not be detected in a whole genome association study, as new mutations would be sporadically associated with genetic markers used in genome scans studies such as haplotype blocks. We have not formally established that these variants are new mutations, although the range of alleles (15Q, 16Q, 18Q and 30Q) suggests new mutations and these are compatible with strand slippage models of DNA replication through repeated sequences. Furthermore, the biochemical data based on transfections for Q-variants were tested only in 16Q and 30Q types and only within the context of RUNX2-I isoform. Biochemical effects of Q-variants may be different in the RUNX2-II isoform, which is more osteoblast specific [48] and has a differential interaction with CBFB [49] compared to RUNX2-I. Three different target constructs were tested, with similar results, although other target promoters may give different results. Finally, interactions of VDR and RUNX2 were tested in artificial constructs with a GST moiety, and tested on a single DNA element, so differences observed may not relate to the situation in the human and on other promoters.

In conclusion, the lines of evidence presented here suggest that variation in the glutamine repeat of RUNX2 has functional consequence. Significantly different phenotypic values for bone density parameters were observed in individuals heterozygous for the Q-variants. Significant functional differences were observed in assays of transcription factor activity on different target gene promoters. Furthermore, an alteration in both *in vitro* DNA binding activity and nuclear residence was observed, suggesting a number of different cumulative effects might occur with these variants. A partial correction of the defect in Q-variant transcriptional activity was observed in studies of interaction with two nuclear partners, CBFB and VDR, which are candidates for increasing residence of the RUNX2 variant on DNA. In addition, due to the large number of potential carriers, this genetic marker may be of some interest in the clinical setting. Intriguingly, transfection of the VDR, in the presence of active $1,25(OH)_2D_3$ overcame some of the *in vivo* defect in RUNX2 Q-variant, suggesting a possible route for clinical studies of Q-variant carriers or at least future studies of the bone phenotype of Q-variants relative to vitamin D status.

Acknowledgments

Investigators for clinical collections are as follows: Western Australia, RLP; Sydney PNS, Geelong, GCN; TASOAC, GJ; Aberdeen, SHR. Alex S. Stephens and James D. Doecke were supported by Griffith University postgraduate scholarships. With sadness we announce that our respected colleague, Professor Philip Sambrook, passed away just prior to submission of this manuscript.

Author Contributions

Conceived and designed the experiments: NAM ASS JDD MO GCN PP. Performed the experiments: NAM ASS MO PP TCT NY JDD NF. Analyzed the data: NAM ASS JDD. Contributed reagents/materials/analysis tools: GJ SHR PNS RLP JAP GCN. Wrote the paper: NAM.

References

1. McGuigan FE, Murray L, Gallagher A, Davey-Smith G, Neville CE, et al. (2002) Genetic and environmental determinants of peak bone mass in young men and women. J Bone Miner Res 17:1273–1279.
2. Kanis JA, Melton III LJ, Christiansen J, Johnston CC, Khaltaev N (1994) The diagnosis of osteoporosis. J Bone Miner Res 9:1137–1141.
3. Chan MY, Nguyen ND, Center JR, Eisman JA, Nguyen TV (2012) Absolute fracture-risk prediction by a combination of calcaneal quantitative ultrasound and bone mineral density. Calcif Tissue Int 90:128–136.
4. Ducy P, Zhang R, Geoffroy V, Ridall AL, Karsenty G (1997) Osf2/Cbfa1: a transcriptional activator of osteoblast differentiation. Cell 89:747–754.
5. Komori T, Yagi H, Nomura S, Yamaguchi A, et al. (1997) Targeted disruption of Cbfa1 results in a complete lack of bone formation owing to maturational arrest of osteoblasts. Cell 89:755–764.
6. Otto F, Thornell AP, Crompton T, Denzel A, Gilmour KC, et al. (1997) Cbfa1, a candidate gene for cleidocranial dysplasia syndrome, is essential for osteoblast differentiation and bone development. Cell 89:765–771.
7. Mundlos S, Otto F, Mundlos C, Mulliken JB, Aylsworth AS, et al. (1997) Mutations involving the transcription factor CBFA1 cause cleidocranial dysplasia. Cell 89:773–779.
8. Enomoto H, Enomoto-Iwamoto M, Iwamoto M, Nomura S, Himeno M, et al. (2000) Cbfa1 is a positive regulatory factor in chondrocyte maturation. J Biol Chem 275:8695–8702.

9. Vaughan T, Pasco JA, Kotowicz MA, Nicholson GC, Morrison NA (2002) Alleles of RUNX2/CBFA1 gene are associated with differences in bone mineral density and risk of fracture. J Bone Miner Res 17:1527–1534.
10. Vaughan T, Reid DM, Morrison NA, Ralston SH (2004). RUNX2 alleles associated with BMD in Scottish women; interaction of RUNX2 alleles with menopausal status and body mass index. Bone 34:1029–1036.
11. Napierala D, Garcia-Rojas X, Sam K, Wakui K, Chen C, et al. (2005) Mutations and promoter SNPs in RUNX2, a transcriptional regulator of bone formation. Mol Genet Metab 86:257–268.
12. Doecke JD, Day CJ, Stephens AS, Carter SL, van Daal A, et al. (2006) Association of functionally different RUNX2 P2 promoter alleles with BMD. J Bone Miner Res 21:265–273.
13. Bustamante M, Nogués X, Agueda L, Jurado S, Wesselius A, et al. (2007) Promoter 2 -1025 T/C polymorphism in the RUNX2 gene is associated with femoral neck BMD in Spanish postmenopausal women. Calcif Tissue Int 81:327–332.
14. Ermakov S, Malkin I, Keter M, Kobyliansky E, Livshits G (2008) Family based association study of polymorphisms in the RUNX2 locus with hand bone length and hand BMD. Ann Hum Genet 72:510–518.
15. Lee HJ, Koh JM, Hwang JY, Choi KY, Lee SH, et al. (2009) Association of a RUNX2 promoter polymorphism with bone mineral density in postmenopausal Korean women. Calcif Tissue Int 84:439–445.
16. Long F (2011) Building strong bones: molecular regulation of the osteoblast lineage. Nat Rev Mol Cell Biol 13:27–38.
17. Online Mendelian Inheritance in Man, OMIM®. McKusick-Nathans Institute of Genetic Medicine, Johns Hopkins University (Baltimore, MD) (2012) World Wide Web URL: http://omim.org/#119600, CLEIDOCRANIAL DYSPLASIA; **CCD**
18. Cohen MM Jr (2009) Perspectives on *RUNX* genes: an update. Am J Med Genet 149: 2629–2646.
19. Yoshida T, Kanegane H, Osato M, Yanagida M, et al. (2002) Functional analysis of RUNX2 mutations in Japanese patients with cleidocranial dysplasia demonstrates novel genotype-phenotype correlations. Am J Hum Genet 71:724–738.
20. Zhang YW, Yasui N, Kakazu N, Abe T, Takada K, et al. (2000) PEBP2alphaA/CBFA1 mutations in Japanese cleidocranial dysplasia patients. Gene 244:21–28.
21. McMurray CT (2010) Mechanisms of trinucleotide repeat instability during human development. Nat Rev Genet 11:786–799.
22. Pineda B, Hermenegildo C, Laporta P, Tarín JJ, Cano A, et al. (2010) Common polymorphisms rather than rare genetic variants of the Runx2 gene are associated with femoral neck BMD in Spanish women. J Bone Miner Metab 28:696–705.
23. Fondon JW 3rd, Garner HR (2004) Molecular origins of rapid and continuous morphological evolution. Proc Natl Acad Sci USA. 101:18058–18063.
24. Sears KE, Goswami A, Flynn JJ, Niswander LA (2007) The correlated evolution of Runx2 tandem repeats, transcriptional activity, and facial length in carnivora. Evol Dev 9:555–565.
25. Prince RL, Devine A, Dhaliwal SS, Dick IM (2006) Effects of calcium supplementation on clinical fracture and bone structure: results of a 5-year, double-blind, placebo-controlled trial in elderly women. Arch Intern Med 166:869–875.
26. Henry MJ, Pasco JA, Nicholson GC, Seeman E, Kotowicz MA (2000) Prevalence of osteoporosis in Australian women: Geelong Osteoporosis Study. J Clin Densitom 3:261–268.
27. Sanders KM, Seeman E, Ugoni AM, Pasco JA, Martin TJ, et al. (1999) The age- and gender-specific rate of fractures in Australia: a population based study. Osteoporosis Int 10: 240–247.
28. Makovey J, Nguyen TV, Naganathan V, Wark JD, Sambrook PN (2007) Genetic effects on bone loss in peri- and postmenopausal women: a longitudinal twin study. J Bone Miner Res 22:1773–1780.
29. Ding C, Parameswaran V, Cicuttini F, Burgess J, Zhai G, et al. (2008) Association between leptin, body composition, sex and knee cartilage morphology in older adults: the Tasmanian older adult cohort (TASOAC) study. Ann Rheum Dis 67:1256–1261.
30. MacDonald HM, McGuigan FA, New SA, Campbell MK, Golden MHN, et al. (2001) COL1A1 Sp1 polymorphism predicts perimenopausal and early postmenopausal spinal bone loss. J Bone Miner Res 16:1634–1641.
31. Tilyard MW, Spears GF, Thomson J, Dovey S (1992) Treatment of postmenopausal osteoporosis with calcitriol or calcium. N Engl J Med. 326:357–362.
32. Morrison NA, George PM, Vaughan T, Tilyard MW, Frampton CM, et al. (2005) Vitamin D receptor genotypes influence the success of calcitriol therapy for recurrent vertebral fracture in osteoporosis. Pharmacogenet Genomics 15:127–135.
33. Zhang YW, Yasui N, Ito K, Huang G, Fujii M, et al. (2000) A RUNX2/PEBP2alpha A/CBFA1 mutation displaying impaired transactivation and Smad interaction in cleidocranial dysplasia. Proc Natl Acad Sci USA 97:10549–10554.
34. Mizushima S, Nagata S (1990) pEF-BOS, a powerful mammalian expression vector. Nucleic Acids Res 18: 5322.
35. Yoshida T, Kanegane H, Osato M, Yanagida M, Miyawaki T, et al. (2002) Functional analysis of RUNX2 mutations in Japanese patients with cleidocranial dysplasia demonstrates novel genotype-phenotype correlations. Am J Hum Genet 71:724–738.
36. Dyer BW, Ferrer FA, Klinedinst DK, Rodriguez R (2000) A noncommercial dual luciferase enzyme assay system for reporter gene analysis. Anal Biochem 282:158–161.
37. Polly P, Herdick M, Moehren U, Baniahmad A, Heinzel T, et al. (2000) VDR-Alien: a novel, DNA-selective vitamin D(3) receptor-corepressor partnership. FASEB J 14:1455–1463.
38. Hood GM (2010) PopTools version 3.2.3 (CSIRO Canberra, Australia). Available on the internet. URL http://www.poptools.org
39. Pasco JA, Seeman E, Henry MJ, Merriman EN, Nicholson GC, et al. (2006) The population burden of fractures originates in women with osteopenia, not osteoporosis. Osteoporos Int 17:1404–1409.
40. Finsterer J (2010) Perspectives of Kennedy's disease. J Neurol Sci 298:1–10.
41. Chamberlain NL, Driver ED, Miesfeld RL (1994) The length and location of CAG trinucleotide repeats in the androgen receptor N-terminal domain affect transactivation function. Nucleic Acids Res 22:3181–3186.
42. Perutz MF, Finch JT, Berriman J, Lesk A (2002) Amyloid fibers are water-filled nanotubes. Proc Natl Acad Sci USA 99:5591–5595.
43. Ogawa H, Nakano M, Watanabe H, Starikov EB, Rothstein SM, et al. (2008) Molecular dynamics simulation study on the structural stabilities of polyglutamine peptides. Comput Biol Chem 32:102–110.
44. Paredes R, Arriagada G, Cruzat F, Villagra A, Olate J, et al. (2004) Bone-specific transcription factor Runx2 interacts with the 1alpha,25-dihydroxyvitamin D_3 receptor to up-regulate rat osteocalcin gene expression in osteoblastic cells. Mol Cell Biol 24:8847–8861.
45. Atanesyan L, Nther V, Dichtl B, Georgiev O, Schaffner W (2012) Polyglutamine tracts as modulators of transcriptional activation from yeast to mammals. Biol Chem 393:63–70.
46. Whan V, Hobbs M, McWilliam S, Lynn DJ, Lutzow YS, et al. (2010) Bovine proteins containing poly-glutamine repeats are often polymorphic and enriched for components of transcriptional regulatory complexes. BMC Genomics 11:654–665.
47. Green RE, Krause J, Briggs AW, Maricic T, Stenzel U, et al. (2010) A draft sequence of the Neandertal genome. Science 328:710–722.
48. Kanatani N, Fujita T, Fukuyama R, Liu W, Yoshida CA, et al. (2006) Cbf beta regulates Runx2 function isoform-dependently in postnatal bone development. Dev Biol 296:48–61.
49. Xiao Z, Awad HA, Liu S, Mahlios J, Zhang S, et al. (2005) Selective Runx2-II deficiency leads to low-turnover osteopenia in adult mice. Dev Biol 283:345–356.

4

Trabecular Reorganization in Consecutive Iliac Crest Biopsies when Switching from Bisphosphonate to Strontium Ranelate Treatment

Björn Jobke[1,2], Andrew J. Burghardt[1], Burkhard Muche[3], Michael Hahn[4], Jutta Semler[3], Michael Amling[4], Sharmila Majumdar[1], Björn Busse[4,5]*

1 Musculoskeletal Quantitative Imaging Research Group, Department of Radiology, University of California San Francisco, San Francisco, California, United States of America, **2** Institute of Radiology, Helios Klinikum Berlin-Buch, Berlin, Germany, **3** Department of Bone Metabolism and Osteology, Immanuel Hospital Berlin-Wannsee, Berlin, Germany, **4** Department of Osteology & Biomechanics, University Medical Center Hamburg-Eppendorf, Hamburg, Germany, **5** Materials Sciences Division, Lawrence Berkeley National Laboratory, University of California, Berkeley, California, United States of America

Abstract

Background: Several agents are available to treat osteoporosis while addressing patient-specific medical needs. Individuals' residual risk to severe fracture may require changes in treatment strategy. Data at osseous cellular and microstructural levels due to a therapy switch between agents with different modes of action are rare. Our study on a series of five consecutively taken bone biopsies from an osteoporotic individual over a six-year period analyzes changes in cellular characteristics, bone microstructure and mineralization caused by a therapy switch from an antiresorptive (bisphosphonate) to a dual action bone agent (strontium ranelate).

Methodology/Principal Findings: Biopsies were progressively taken from the iliac crest of a female patient. Four biopsies were taken during bisphosphonate therapy and one biopsy was taken after one year of strontium ranelate (SR) treatment. Furthermore, serum bone markers and dual x-ray absorptiometry measurements were acquired. Undecalcified histology was used to assess osteoid parameters and bone turnover. Structural indices and degree of mineralization were determined using microcomputed tomography, quantitative backscattered electron imaging, and combined energy dispersive x-ray/μ-x-ray-fluorescence microanalysis.

Conclusions/Significance: Microstructural data revealed a notable increase in bone volume fraction after one year of SR treatment compared to the bisphosphonate treatment period. Indices of connectivity density, structure model index and trabecular bone pattern factor were predominantly enhanced indicating that the architectural transformation from trabecular rods to plates was responsible for the bone volume increase and less due to changes in trabecular thickness and number. Administration of SR following bisphosphonates led to a maintained mineralization profile with an uptake of strontium on the bone surface level. Reactivated osteoclasts designed tunneling, hook-like intratrabecular resorption sites. The appearance of tunneling resorption lacunae and the formation of both mini-modeling units and osteon-like structures within increased plate-like cancellous bone mass provides additional information on the mechanisms of strontium ranelate following bisphosphonate treatment, which may deserve special attention when monitoring a treatment switch.

Editor: Wei-Chun Chin, University of California Merced, United States of America

Funding: The authors have no support or funding to report.

Competing Interests: The authors have declared that no competing interests exist.

* E-mail: b.busse@uke.uni-hamburg.de

Introduction

Currently, several agents are available to address patients' specific medical needs when treating osteoporosis. Anti-resorptive drugs with various modes of action (e.g., bisphosphonates (BP), hormone replacement therapy, selective estrogen-receptor modulators and RANK ligand (RANKL) inhibitors slow the progression of bone loss [1,2,3,4], whereas other agents stimulate bone formation (e.g., parathyroid hormone fragments) to support increases in bone mass [4,5,6]. Strontium Ranelate (SR) is promoted as a treatment for postmenopausal osteoporosis with a dual mechanism on bone remodeling: inhibition of osteoclastic resorption and activation of osteoblastic apposition. Its antifracture efficacy in the treatment of postmenopausal osteoporosis has been shown in previous clinical trials [7,8,9,10], where Bone Mineral Density (BMD) increases under SR treatment were measured with Dual X-Ray Absorptiometry (DXA). The observed BMD gain is partially due to SR deposition in bone [9,10,11]. To what extent this mechanism occurs in humans as well as how it has to be considered during long-term treatment is mostly based on theoretical models and is still under investigation [12,13,14]. It has been shown that SR is incorporated in a dose-dependent manner into new bone (and less into pre-existing old bone) without detrimental effects on bone mineralization [11,15,16]. Only a few *in vivo* microstructural studies or human (histological) data have been reported about the desired effect of a positively influenced uncoupling of bone formation and bone resorption on cohorts following long-term BP treatment [11,17]. Focusing on the previously mentioned issues, this study presents the time-associated development of cellular characteristics, serum markers, bone microstructure and mineralization caused by a therapy switch from an antiresorptive (bisphosphonate) to a dual action bone agent (strontium ranelate) in five progressively taken bone biopsies from an osteoporotic individual over a six-year period.

Materials and Methods

Bone biopsies were obtained from the Hamburg Bone Register at the University Medical Center Hamburg-Eppendorf. The Hamburg Bone Register is a collection of diseased human bone samples representing patients covering various bone pathologies; the samples are prepared and archived in an undecalcified state. Documentation is available for each biopsy regarding the details of the patients, including their history, treatment course, and clinical complications. This resource enabled tracking and analysis of the following case of osteoporosis in a female patient over a six-year time period. The patient characteristics for this study are as follows. The patient was postmenopausal, 75 years old and had multiple vertebral fractures (Th 6–8; LS 2–4) before initiating the BP treatment. During the BP treatment, new or progressive vertebral fractures were detected with an additional reduction in height accompanied by an unchanged low BMD; thus, treatment was switched from BP to SR. The study was approved by the institutional review boards of the University of California, Berkeley & San Francisco and IDG Immanuel Diakonie Group Berlin/Brandenburg. Informed written consent was given by the patient for the study and publication of the data. Five consecutive iliac crest biopsies were obtained from the patient over a period of six years; at the same time as the biopsies, the associated hip T-Scores (comparison of the patient's BMD value to the mean BMD of the young adult healthy population) [11] and serum biomarkers were determined. Both the presence and concentration of type I collagen's crosslink peptide sequence were measured by the biomarker for carboxy-terminal collagen crosslinks (CTX). The portion of this peptide sequence that is cleaved by osteoclasts during bone resorption provides bone turnover information, where its serum levels are a proportional measure of osteoclastic activity [18]. Serum bone-specific alkaline phosphatase (bAP) was measured as a biochemical indicator of bone turnover. The bone-specific isoform of alkaline phosphatase is a tetrameric glycoprotein found on the surface of osteoblasts and can be used as an index of active bone formation [19]. Calcium and phosphorus blood samples were analyzed to differentiate between osteoporosis and other diseases associated with fracture risk and low bone mineral density [20].

All of the bone biopsies were performed at the same clinic by one of the authors (JS, Immanuel-Hospital Berlin-Wannsee, Berlin, Germany), who has experience with over 5000 iliac crest biopsies. All of the biopsies were taken during the BP and SR treatment periods (Fig. 1), see the timeline in figure 1. The side of the pelvis that the biopsy was extracted from was alternated at each visit; biopsies taken from the same side were extracted at a similar site but at a different biopsy angle. Therefore, biopsies 1,3,5 and biopsies 2,4 were taken in an alternating caudocranial or craniocaudal direction to avoid regional overlaps and possible interference from regional acceleratory phenomenon (RAP) or other bone healing effects [6,21]. JS used an 8-gauge Jamshidi needle with an inner diameter of 3 mm to obtain the biopsies. The biopsies meet the standard required for histomorphometry because the length of the biopsies averages 2 cm (0.79 in.). Thus, the bone volume of Jamshidi biopsies for histomorphometry equates to the bone volume of transiliacal Bordier biopsies without the limiting factor of bilateral subcortical bone heterogeneity [6,11].

Micro-computed Tomography (µCT)

Undecalcified and polymethylmethacrylate (PMMA) embedded biopsies were scanned with a micro-computed tomography system (µCT 40, Scanco Medical AG, Basserdorf, Switzerland) with a 12-µm isotropic nominal resolution. Application of the threshold algorithm is based on previous studies and has been described in detail [22,23]. The bone volume fraction (BV/TV), trabecular thickness (Tb.Th.), trabecular separation (Tb.Sp.), trabecular number (Tb.N.), connectivity density (Conn.D), structure model index (SMI) and trabecular bone pattern factor (TBPf) were measured from the segmented images as described elsewhere [24].

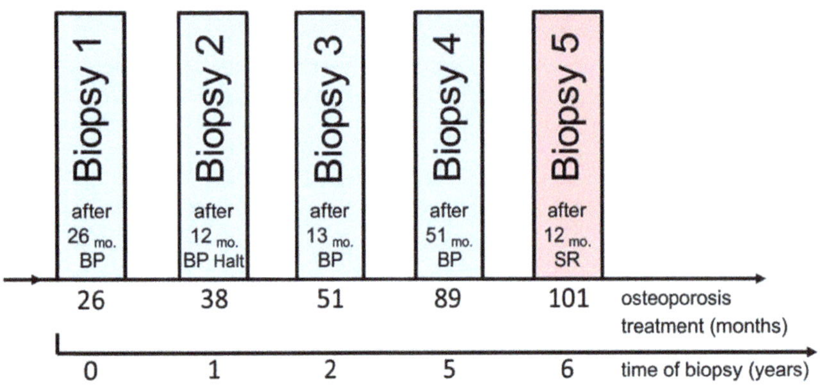

Figure 1. Timeline of treatment and biopsy obtainment. We investigated 5 serial iliac crest biopsies from a 75-year-old female patient over a period of 6 years. The patient was diagnosed with osteoporosis with multiple vertebral fractures and was first treated with bisphosphonates (BP) for 26 months (biopsy 1). The BP treatment was halted for 12 months until a second biopsy was obtained (biopsy 2). The BP treatment was then continued and another biopsy was taken after 13 months (biopsy 3). The antiresorptive therapy was stopped after an additional 51 months of treatment and another biopsy was taken (biopsy 4). Next, strontium ranelate was administered for 12 months (2g/d) in total before another iliac crest biopsy was conducted. BP and SR were administered according to the manufacturer's instructions and the patient additionally received a Vitamin D3 metabolite during osteoporosis treatment.

Conn.D, SMI and TBPf are closely related to each other and provide information about the characteristics of the cancellous bone structure. Calculation of the Euler characteristics can be applied to networks to provide information regarding the number of connected entities within the structure [25,26]. In networks of cancellous bone, the connectivity density (Conn.D) can be calculated by dividing the connectivity estimate by the volume of the sample. Basically, Conn.D provides an estimation of the number of trabecular connections per unit volume [25,26]. The structure model index (SMI) determines the geometry of the intertrabecular network. It is based on the change in surface area with an infinitesimal increase in volume. Quantification of the SMI gives an impression of whether the trabecular structure consists of a plate-like (SMI $\approx$ 0) or rod-like (SMI $\approx$ 3) configuration [26,27]. In cortical bone, the SMI may shift towards negative values if many concave surfaces are present [27]. The TBPf describes the ratio of intertrabecular connectivity, which was first developed to analyze histological sections in 2D [28]. The concept of TBPf is based on varying values for the convexity and/or concavity of a structure. Due to dilation, there will always be increases in bone area but increases in bone perimeter only occur with convex surfaces. Trabecular bone with many concave structures has a negative TBPf, whereas many convex structures results in a positive value (osteopenia/osteoporosis) [28]. A low TBPf value reflects a cancellous morphology that has adapted from a rod-like configuration to a plate-like configuration. Excellent correlation has been reported between the SMI and 2D-TBPf [28,29]. The bone tissue density was determined from the original µCT grayscale images. The binary image map from the segmentation step was eroded by two voxels to remove partial volume components and to mask the grayscale data. The mean linear attenuation was calculated as the sum of the masked image divided by the number of bone voxels in the eroded mask. This value was converted to mineral density (MD) in mg HA/cm^3 based on a phantom-derived linear calibration [22,30].

Undecalcified histology

Bone biopsies were sectioned to a 4-µm thickness and stained with Goldner-Masson, Giemsa and Tartrate Resistant Acid Phosphatase (TRAP). Osseous cells and osteoid indices were assessed quantitatively in accordance with the guidelines of the American Society of Bone and Mineral Research [31,32] using histomorphometry software OSTEO II (Bioquant, Nashville, TN, USA). The ratio of the osteoid surface to the bone surface (OS/BS,%), the ratio of the osteoblast surface to the bone surface (Ob.S/BS,%), the ratio of the number of osteoblasts to the bone surface (N.Ob/BS, #/mm) and the ratio of the number of osteoclasts to the bone surface (N.Oc/BS, #/mm) were determined. Bone turnover was classified by analyzing serum markers (bAP and CTX) [33,34,35,36,37,38,39] and osteoid indices [40,41,42,43,44], which were compared to reference values from the literature for naïve and treated patients. Furthermore, visible bone remodeling units were evaluated [45] as an additional supportive measurement indicating bone turnover information and were based on the following histological criteria. The total number of osteoblasts and osteoclasts were counted at individual bone remodeling units (magnification 40x) and divided by the total number of assessed fields of view (approx. 4–6). *'Low turnover'* is attributed to bone tissue under low endosteal remodeling showing <1 bone remodeling unit with cubic-shaped osteoblasts and a maximum of one osteoclast per field of view (magnification 40x) in the underlying histological section. *'Normal turnover'* is attributed to bone tissue with maintained endosteal remodeling showing 1–2 bone remodeling units with cubic-shaped osteoblasts and 2–4 single osteoclasts per field of view (magnification 40x). *'High turnover'* is attributed to bone tissue with both increased endosteal remodeling and osteoclastic resorption showing >2 bone remodeling units with prominent seams of osteoblasts and >4 groups of osteoclasts per field of view (magnification 40x) in the underlying histological section. Polarized light was used to observe collagen birefringence and lamellar orientation [46,47].

Bone mineral density distribution and microanalysis

The bone mineral density distribution was measured on plastic-embedded cross-sections of iliac crest biopsies with coplanar, polished and carbon-coated surfaces using quantitative backscattered electron imaging (qBEI) [11,48,49,50]. The scanning electron microscope (LEO 435 VP, LEO Electron Microscopy Ltd., Cambridge, England) was operated at 15 kV and 665 pA at a constant working distance (BSE Detector, Type 202, K.E. Developments Ltd., Cambridge, England). The pixel size was 3 ìm, as recommended by Roschger et al. [50]. Synthetic hydroxyapatite (HA) samples were used to create a calibration curve. These HA samples (DOT Medical Solutions, Rostock, Germany) contained different Ca/P ratios, which were determined with energy dispersive X-ray analysis (DX-4, EDAX, Mahwah, NJ) and qBEI. A highly linear relationship between the gray values of backscattered signal intensities and the calcium content of each sample has been reported previously by other authors [49,51], enabling calibration of the method. The generated mineralization profile (gray value histogram) reflects the degree of mineralization in the cross-sectioned bone.

Strontium deposition in mineralized bone tissue was measured using µXRF (Micro-X-ray Fluorescence Analysis; IMOXS, IFG, Germany) in combination with EDX (Energy Dispersive X-ray Analysis); EDAX DX-4, USA). An XRF-module with capillary zoom optics enables x-ray fluorescence analysis in the SEM with a high sensitivity. The advantage of this method is the high spatial resolution [11,52]. The detection limit ranges between 1 and 0.01 weight percent (wt%) due to electron-induced Bremsstrahlung background. The strontium (Sr) content in the bone biopsies was evaluated in wt% via software that enabled combined EDX/µXRF quantification (IMOXS Quant 2.10, IFG, Berlin, Germany).

Results

Clinical data

C-terminal cross-linking telopeptides of type I collagen (CTX) were consistently at very low levels (43–95 pg/ml) under antiresorptive therapy (Fig. 2A) in comparison to the range of mean CTX values (331–562 pg/ml) in the literature for naïve postmenopausal women [33,38]; after antiresorptive treatment, the CTX values may range at approx. a quarter of the baseline [34,35]. CTX rose to moderate levels (255 pg/ml) [33,38] after the SR treatment was initiated (Fig. 2A). At the same time, the bone specific alkaline phosphatase (bAP) level rose from 13.5 to 21.7 µg/l (Fig. 2B) in comparison to the range of mean bAP values (13.6–17.3 µg/l) from the literature for naïve postmenopausal woman [33,36], which may decrease by approx. 45% during bisphosphonate treatment [37,39]. Calcium/phosphorus levels were in the normal range [53]. During BP treatment, new or progressive vertebral fractures (Th 7, 8, 12; LS 2, 3) were determined with an additional 6-cm reduction in height. DXA measurements showed only minor changes in the BMD at the femoral neck following BP treatment and following SR treatment (Fig. 2C). The T-score at the lumbar spine increased by 0.3 T-score points to −3.5, but its interpretation was very limited due to

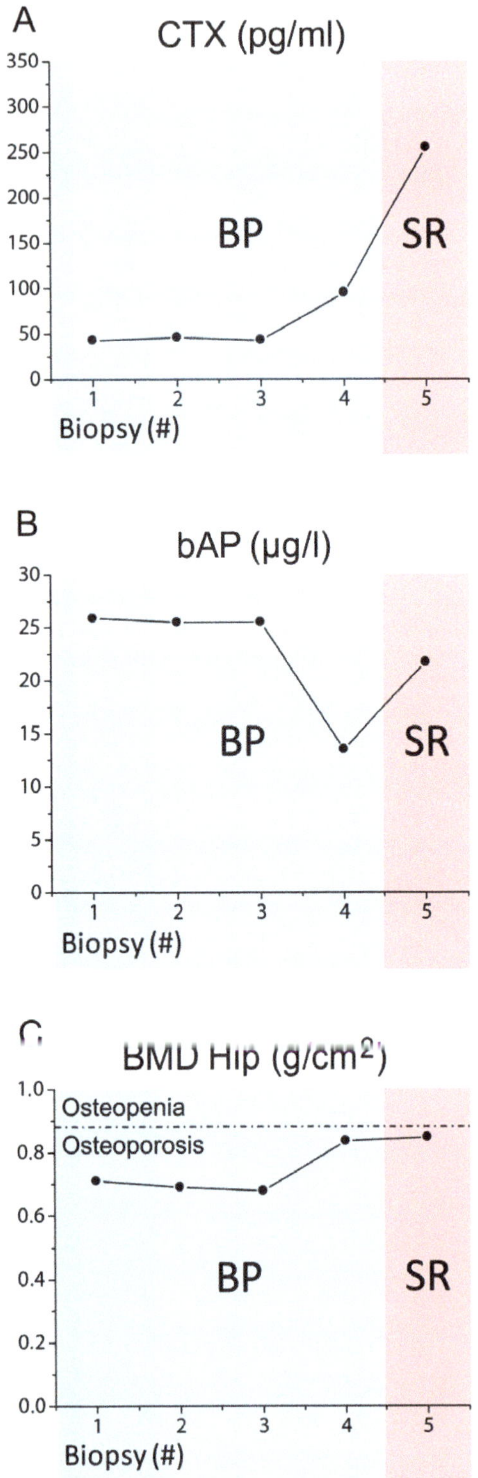

Figure 2. Clinical data. A) C-terminal cross-linking telopeptides of type I collagen (CTX) showed very low levels under antiresorptive therapy and rose to normal levels after SR treatment was initiated. **B**) The bone specific alkaline phosphatase (bAP) level varied under BP treatment from 25.9 to 13.5 µg/l. After the treatment was switched to SR, the bAP level rose again to 21.7 µg/l. **C**) DXA measurements showed only marginal changes in bone mineral density at the femoral neck following both the BP and SR treatments.

multiple fractures. No DXA density correction factor related to the period of strontium ranelate treatment was applied.

µCT tomography

The bone volume fraction, structural parameters and bone tissue density data from all five biopsies collected by µCT are shown in figure 3. In comparison with all biopsies after BP treatment (Biopsy 1, 2, 3 and 4), the trabecular architecture after SR administration (Biopsy 5) changed notably (Fig. 3A–E). The trabecular architecture in biopsies 1–4 (Fig. 3A–D) consisted mainly of thin rod-like structures or plates connected by very thin rods. In biopsy 5 (Fig. 3E), a high increase in BV/TV (22% vs. 6%) along with an increase in Tb.Th. (0.2 vs. 0.17) was observed (Fig. 3F,G). The 3D reconstruction shows thick, plate-like structures that seemed to be connected mainly by plates and a small number of rods, which represents a small reduction in trabecular number and a very high connectivity density (Conn.D.: 8.2) (Fig. 3H–J). The SMI (Structural Model Index) and trabecular bone pattern factor (TBPf) presented had improved values (SMI; −0,81 vs. 5,49 and TBPf; −1,15 vs. 2,27) (Fig. 3K,L). Reconstruction of biopsies 1,4 and 5 showed small microcallus formations as a result of biomechanical instability and thus trabecular fracture (Fig. 3A,D,E). The mean density measured by µCT in milligrams of hydroxyapatite per bone tissue volume had already reached a high value of 1126 mg HA/cm^3 after 26 months of BP treatment (Biopsy 1), dropped after cessation of antiresorptive treatment to 1085 mgHA/cm^3 (Biopsy 2) and increased again to 1144 mgHA/cm^3 under a status of reduced bone turnover (Biopsy 4). The mean density after 12 months SR remained almost unchanged at 1133 mg HA/cm^3 (Biopsy 5) during a normal bone turnover situation (Fig. 3M).

In contrast to flat, reticulate, perforating resorption cavities in biopsies during BP treatment (Fig. 3A–D), multiple deep, hook-like [15] resorption patterns were visible on the surface and on sections of biopsy 5 (Fig. 3E,4A). Small humps of endosteal bone (peritrabecular surfaces) were detected in µCT reconstructions and histology (Fig. 4B–E). Peak densities measured in the cancellous bone ranged between 1200–1300 mg HA/cm^3 (Fig. 4D). A maximum value of 1400–1500 mg HA/cm^3 was detected in a microcallus formation in biopsy 5 (Fig. 3E). The lowest values in recently mineralized modeling sites ranged between 650 to 850 mg HA/cm^3 (Fig. 4D).

Undecalcified histology

Following 12 months of SR administration, individual trabeculae were thicker as expected in healthy women of that age group [54,55] and presented a somewhat irregular connectivity (Fig. 4B,E). Woven bone was not observed in any of the biopsies. However, following strontium ranelate treatment, several thick trabeculae had deep intratrabecular resorption cavities filled with fibrovascular tissue (Fig. 4B). Osteon-like structures in the trabecular bone were seen frequently (Fig. 4B). Seams of osteoid only partially covered with osteoblasts were occasionally present in the form of endosteal humps (Fig. 4C,E) on top of straight cement lines, which suggests that endosteal apposition took place without prior resorption (modeling). A genuine fibro-osteoclasia was not visible. Remodeling indices (Fig. 4G–J) determined by 2D histomorphometry (Fig. 5A) provide histological bone turnover information. Normal mean values for OS/BS have been reported between 9.51% and 35% for female cohorts [40,41,42], whereas a bisphosphonate treatment regime is known to decrease OS/BS mean values to within a range of 1.02% to 3%, in accordance with low bone turnover [43,44] (Fig 4G).

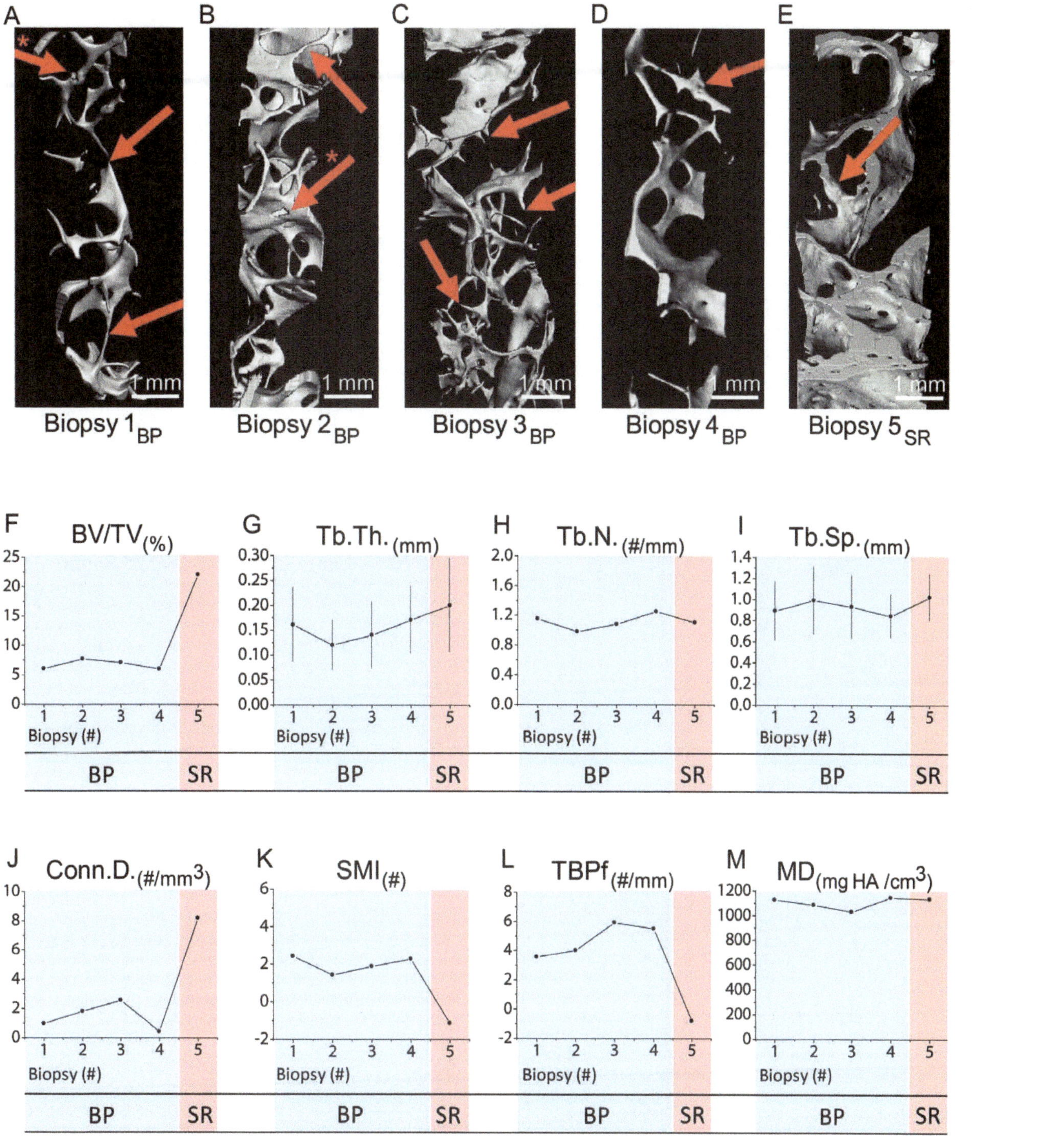

Figure 3. μCT reconstructions of biopsies and structural indices. A) μCT-3D reconstruction of the complete bone core (biopsy 1). Rod-like structures with a microcallus formation (*→) are evident in the trabecular architecture. Some rods are likely to be perforated (→). **B)** μCT reconstruction of biopsy 2. Bone core with a combination of plate- and rod-like architecture. Note the thinning of the connecting rods (→) and reticulate perforation sites on a plate (*→). **C)** μCT reconstruction of biopsy 3. The trabecular architecture of this bone core presents an irregular composition of fine rod-like elements with some small plates. Several dead-ending rods are visible (→). **D)** μCT reconstruction of biopsy 4. The trabecular architecture in this iliac crest sample is almost completely deteriorated. Another trabecular fracture of a rod leading to microcallus formation is visible (→). Microcallus formations are bulky nodes with an irregular oftentimes clefted structure. **E)** μCT reconstruction of the biopsy after one year of SR treatment showing thick plate-like structures containing multiple intratrabecular 'tunnels'. Although a very dense architecture is evident in the structure, big gaps of lost connectivity are also visible. Bulky microcallus formation (→). **F–L)** Changes in the trabecular network emphasized by structural indices evaluated through assessment of 3D μCT reconstructions. The dots represent mean values, and the error bars represent standard deviations of the mean. **M)** Mean density measured by μCT showed already high values during BP treatment that can be traced back to low bone turnover. The mean density after 12 months of SR remained almost unchanged suggesting maintained mineralization during a normal bone turnover situation.

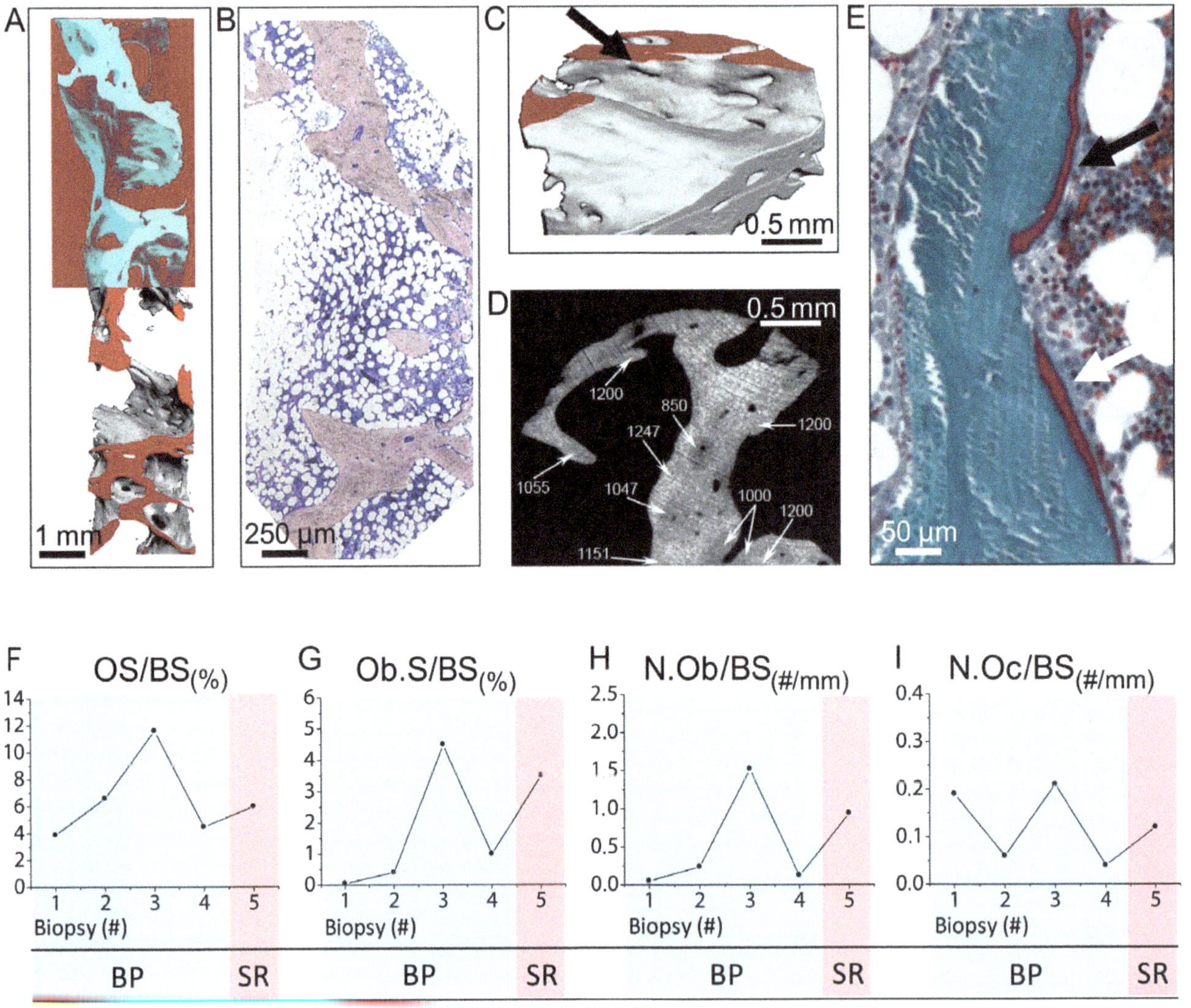

Figure 4. Reorganization pattern, µCT mean density and 2D histomorphometry. A) µCT reconstruction of biopsy 5. Note the coarse structure with surface irregularities and the occurrence of an intratrabecular 'tunnel'. The area with the dark-colored background demonstrates the 2D section plane as it can be seen on the histology section in panel B. **B**) Congruent histology section following the µCT slice in panel A. Note the irregular trabecular structure with varying trabecular diameter. The thickened trabecular architecture indicates intratrabecular resorption sites filled with fibrovascular tissue (mineralized bone = light purple; Giemsa, 40x). **C**) A high magnification of the µCT reconstruction of biopsy 5 indicates the irregular trabecular surface with multiple hook-like, tunneling and sometimes perforating resorption lacunae. Virtual serial sections can show that all intratrabecular 'tunnels' are connected at some point and have openings to the trabecular surface. Small humps due to bone formation (mini-modeling) arise from the trabecular surface (→). **D**) Axial µCT section of biopsy 5: Distribution of local mineral densities (mg HA/cm^3) represented by different gray levels. Due to bone formation, a low mineral content is detected in the proximity of new osteons, whereas the interstitial regions show a higher mineral content due to an older tissue age. **E**) Two (re-)modeling sites with distinct osteoid seems are visible. The osteoid seam on the trabecular surface at the bottom (white arrow) is covered with some cubic-shaped osteoblasts that become flattened to the lower image border. Non-active endosteal appostion is evident on the top of the image (black arrow) without prior resorption (modeling) as flat osteoblasts or lining cells cover osteoid (mineralized bone = green, osteoid = red; Goldner-Masson, 400x). **F–I**) Osteoid and cellular indices determined by 2D histomorphometry point to a low bone turnover situation at the time of biopsies 1, 2 and 4. Normal bone turnover, leading to an increase in osteoid apposition and thus increasing osteoid surface and volume appeared only after 50 months of BP treatment and after the treatment was switched to strontium ranelate. Osteoid indices did not indicate any signs of hyperosteoidosis considering the reference ranges reported by Lips et al. [73].

Bone mineral density distribution and microanalysis

Backscattered signal intensities reflected a maintained mean hard tissue mineralization (Fig. 5B). Combined EDX/µXRF microanalysis revealed a deposition of 1.63 Wt% strontium in the mineralized tissue after SR treatment (Fig. 5C,D). Lower mineralized regions (dark gray values) showed increased strontium content and appeared more commonly around osteon-like structures (Fig. 5B,C) but were also present in modeling sites on endosteal surfaces (peritrabecular surfaces) (Fig. 5C). Before treatment, the strontium content ranged at the detection limit of the method.

Discussion

One year of SR administration following long-term bisphosphonate treatment revealed a notable increase in bone volume fraction. This structural change reflected more of a transformation of trabecular rods to plates than an increase in trabecular thickness

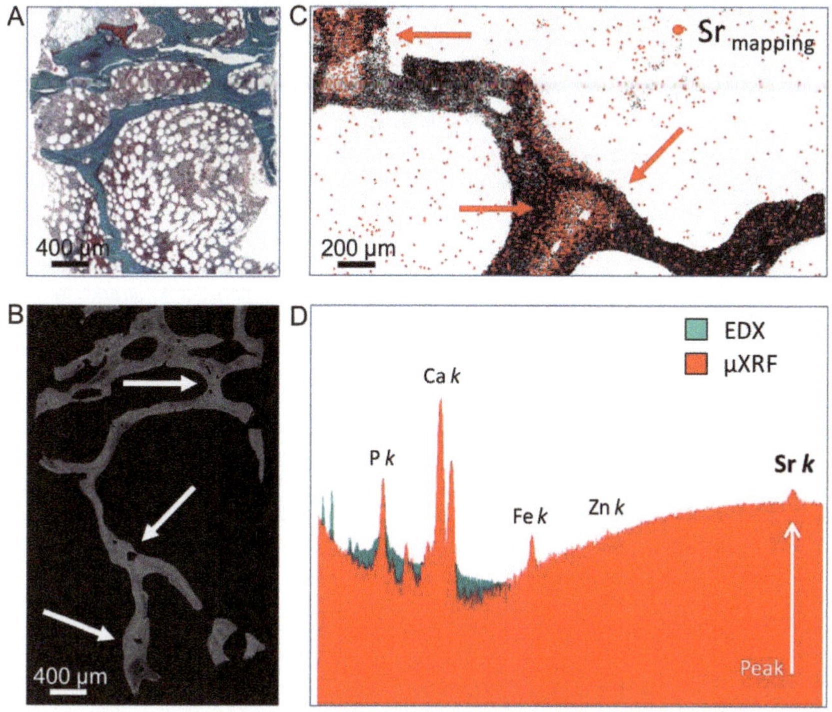

Figure 5. Bone mineral density distribution and microanalysis. A) Histology of the cancellous bone area after strontium ranelate treatment. Intratrabecular cavities and thin osteoid seams are visible (mineralized bone = green, Goldner-Masson, 40x). **B**) Quantitative backscattered image of the selected area in panel A. Intratrabecular resoption sites showed osteon-like structures (→). The gray level distribution reflects the mineralization density, which varied between new and old bone. Newly formed osteon-like structures showed dark-gray pixels in comparison to older bright-gray bone packets. **C**) Microanalysis mapping showed that increased strontium deposition (red dots) appeared predominantly around newly formed osteon-like structures (→) as well as in modeling sites on endosteal surfaces (→). **D**) Combined EDX/µXRF microanalysis spectra demonstrated a deposition of 1.63 Wt% strontium (peak) in the mineralized tissue after SR treatment.

and number because indices of connectivity density, structure model index and trabecular bone pattern factor were predominantly enhanced. The degree of mineralization was maintained although strontium deposition occurred on the bone surface level. No mineralization defects (e.g. entrapped osteoid) or accumulation of osteoid were detected. The appearance of tunneling resorption lacunae, the new formation of osteon-like entities and mini-modeling of endosteal humps in trabecular structures reflected a novel particularity after treatment switch accompanied by an increase in cancellous bone mass.

The enhancement in bone volume fraction following SR treatment, which was evaluated by micro-tomography, was not equally represented by increases in trabecular thickness or trabecular number. The characteristics of the trabecular architecture changed to a partly disorganized and somewhat compact network without separated trabeculae; thus, the number of individual trabeculae decreased but the connectivity density increased. The structure model index (SMI) and trabecular bone pattern factor (TBPf) were both negative, which may indicate the formation of very dense, plate-like structures or many concave structures created by tunneling resorption [29,56]. The discovered reorganization mechanism also raises the question of whether this could eventually lead to an increase in 'new' trabeculae. Compared to normal trabecular thickness values obtained from histomorphometric studies [54,55], an unusual thickness of 300–400 µm was measured for many plate-like structures. Many of these thick trabeculae included newly formed osteon-like structures, which are characteristically found in the cortex around Haversian canals [57]. µCT observations revealed that a majority of these canals or tunnels create a complex, interconnected system as can be seen in the cortex between Haversian and Volkmann canals. The relevancy of its development in cancellous bone remains uncertain. It can only be speculated whether this new intratrabecular canal system that has developed outside of the cortex maintains blood supply to the osteocyte network in the inner regions of unusually thick trabeculae [58]. Inta-trabecular osteons may act to ensure adequate diffusion of nutrients to, and waste products from, osteocytes by limiting the maximum distance between the osteocytes and the bone surface [59]. In particular, thin nonmineralized pericellular zones between osteocytes and their surrounding bone allow a strain-derived flow of interstitial fluid over the osteocytes' surfaces that is important for the osteocytes' health because it facilitates the exchange of nutrients and waste products between the haversian channel and the osteocyte network [60,61]. Although not investigated in this study, a dramatic change in the cancellous structure from a plate-like to rod-like shape with aging and osteoporosis has been reported and results in a decrease in mechanical competence [62,63]. The measured reversal of the bone structure due to changes in treatment may therefore improve the bone's elastic modulus [64]. There are several possible factors that may account for the dramatic increase in bone volume. Because the trabecular thickness only slightly increased by a mean of 0.03 mm, which only explains about one third of the gain in bone volume, a possible explanation was found in the reorganization pattern. Endosteal appostion on the trabecular surfaces without prior resorption (modeling) was found in the biopsy after SR treatment. These small modeling sites, which are also known as *mini-modeling*

[65,66], thicken and rearrange the remaining trabeculae to best adapt to functional demands. Multiple long and deep, hook-like resorption cavities, which are frequently seen and reported in renal osteopathies (e.g. ROD type IIIb) [67], were observed. Similar resorption sites were first described by Woods (1972) and later quantified by Sato (1981) under conditions of osteoidosis and increased PTH serum levels [68,69]. The cause was suspected to be multifactorial, including maintenance of calcium homeostasis through a compensatory increase in resorption depth in osteomalacic situations and PTH-induced overstimulation of osteoclasts. Low calcium or abnormal PTH serum levels were not found in our patient but could have played a role in the early stages of SR-induced bone formation that created a temporary calcium deficit and a need for increased bone resorption. The SR treatment stimulated bone turnover, which was demonstrated by moderate serum bone markers (bAP, CTX), and indicated increased bone formation (endosteal humps with osteoblast coverage and newly formed bone packets with an accumulation of strontium). An uncoupling with a pronounced suppression of osteoclastic resorption was not present histologically or biochemically after 12 months of SR administration. However, a complete uncoupling was not expected because it is known that an osteoclast-derived stimulus is required for normal bone remodeling involving bone formation. In this connection, osteoclastic resorption re-activated by strontium ranelate's mode of action may account not only for the improvement in bone mass and structural integrity but also for the maintenance of calcium metabolism.

Previous reports have shown that strontium is predominantly incorporated into new, and to a lesser degree, old bone in a dose-dependent matter without altering the degree of bone mineralization [11,15,16]. Based on theoretical models, other groups report that calcium substitution by strontium at the crystal level and its higher attenuation of x-rays could account for up to 10% of the total bone mineral density as measured by DXA, depending on the time of SR administration [12,14,70]. Clinical BMD scores acquired from the hip with DXA did not change significantly in our patient. The only assumption the authors could make from these results was that newly formed bone with a low mineral content was not able to offset the deterioration of the trabecular architecture in the femoral neck that may have irreversibly progressed before SR treatment was initiated. μCT uses a similar X-ray (fan beam) technique and is potentially influenced by the degree of attenuation. The strontium content in the bone after 12 months of treatment in the investigated patient clearly rose significantly to 1.63 Wt%. Despite the fact that we observed some areas with an unusually high degree of mineralization (>1200 mg HA/cm^3), the average mean tissue density (μCT) after SR administration did not change significantly. This finding might be due to the fact that the tissue density in biopsy 4 (1133 mg HA/cm^3) was already high and had reached a maximum saturation point. Therefore, tissue mineralization would not have a major impact on bone mineral density measurements.

This study has several limitations. First, the heterogeneity of the trabecular microstructure in different sites of the skeleton may have an effect on the accuracy of the measured structural indices [48,71,72]. Second, because more than one biopsy was obtained on each side of the Ilium, there remains the possibility that a later biopsy will overlap in parts with the location of a prior biopsy and include regions of the Ilium that healed following the earlier biopsy. Third, the study of five biopsies is limited to only one individual.

In this study, analyses of progressively obtained iliac crest bone biopsies over six years of osteoporosis treatment highlight remarkable changes in cancellous architecture, which are reinforced by a switch from an antiresorptive agent to a dual action bone agent. The clinical and microstructural information gained by an unusually high number of bone biopsies demonstrated treatment-associated responses in a novel case. These insights may support the understanding of reorganization mechanisms due to alternating osteoporosis treatments. Clinical bone markers showed that strontium ranelate stimulated bone formation and simultaneously bone resorption despite prior long-term antiresorptive treatment. In this case, administration of strontium ranelate for one year led to remarkable changes in trabecular structure with an impressive gain in bone volume fraction at the iliac crest, which may contribute to changes in bone quality.

Acknowledgments

The authors would like to thank Benjamin Boudignon from the Dept. of Endocrinology at the Veterans Hospital in San Francisco for his assistance with the use of the image analysis system OSTEO II, Bioquant, and Elizabeth A. Zimmermann who provided helpful comments and research support on the manuscript.

Author Contributions

Conceived and designed the experiments: BJ BB. Performed the experiments: BJ AJB BB. Analyzed the data: BJ AJB MH MA SM BB. Contributed reagents/materials/analysis tools: BJ AJB BM JS BB. Wrote the paper: BJ BB.

References

1. Torgerson DJ, Bell-Syer SE (2001) Hormone replacement therapy and prevention of nonvertebral fractures: a meta-analysis of randomized trials. JAMA 285: 2891–2897.
2. Bilezikian JP (2009) Efficacy of bisphosphonates in reducing fracture risk in postmenopausal osteoporosis. Am J Med 122: S14–21.
3. Ensrud KE, Stock JL, Barrett-Connor E, Grady D, Mosca L, et al. (2008) Effects of raloxifene on fracture risk in postmenopausal women: the Raloxifene Use for the Heart Trial. J Bone Miner Res 23: 112–120.
4. Rachner TD, Khosla S, Hofbauer LC (2011) Osteoporosis: now and the future. Lancet 377: 1276–1287.
5. Neer RM, Arnaud CD, Zanchetta JR, Prince R, Gaich GA, et al. (2001) Effect of parathyroid hormone (1-34) on fractures and bone mineral density in postmenopausal women with osteoporosis. N Engl J Med 344: 1434–1441.
6. Jobke B, Muche B, Burghardt A, Semler J, Link T, et al. (2011) Teriparatide in Bisphosphonate-Resistant Osteoporosis: Microarchitectural Changes and Clinical Results After 6 and 18 months. Calcified Tissue International. pp 1–10.
7. Meunier PJ, Roux C, Ortolani S, Diaz-Curiel M, Compston J, et al. (2009) Effects of long-term strontium ranelate treatment on vertebral fracture risk in postmenopausal women with osteoporosis. Osteoporos Int 20: 1663–1673.
8. Meunier PJ, Roux C, Seeman E, Ortolani S, Badurski JE, et al. (2004) The effects of strontium ranelate on the risk of vertebral fracture in women with postmenopausal osteoporosis. N Engl J Med 350: 459–468.
9. Reginster JY, Felsenberg D, Boonen S, Diez-Perez A, Rizzoli R, et al. (2008) Effects of long-term strontium ranelate treatment on the risk of nonvertebral and vertebral fractures in postmenopausal osteoporosis: Results of a five-year, randomized, placebo-controlled trial. Arthritis Rheum 58: 1687–1695.
10. Reginster JY, Seeman E, De Vernejoul MC, Adami S, Compston J, et al. (2005) Strontium ranelate reduces the risk of nonvertebral fractures in postmenopausal women with osteoporosis: Treatment of Peripheral Osteoporosis (TROPOS) study. J Clin Endocrinol Metab 90: 2816–2822.
11. Busse B, Jobke B, Hahn M, Priemel M, Niecke M, et al. (2010) Effects of strontium ranelate administration on bisphosphonate-altered hydroxyapatite: Matrix incorporation of strontium is accompanied by changes in mineralization and microstructure. Acta Biomater 6: 4513–4521.
12. Blake GM, Fogelman I (2007) Effect of bone strontium on BMD measurements. J Clin Densitom 10: 34–38.
13. Liao J, Blake GM, McGregor AH, Patel R (2010) The effect of bone strontium on BMD is different for different manufacturers' DXA Systems. Bone 47: 882–887.
14. Nielsen SP, Slosman D, Sorensen OH, Basse-Cathalinat B, De Cassin P, et al. (1999) Influence of strontium on bone mineral density and bone mineral content measurements by dual X-ray absorptiometry. J Clin Densitom 2: 371–379.
15. Boivin G, Farlay D, Khebbab MT, Jaurand X, Delmas PD, et al. (2010) In osteoporotic women treated with strontium ranelate, strontium is located in bone

formed during treatment with a maintained degree of mineralization. Osteoporos Int 21: 667–677.
16. Li C, Paris O, Siegel S, Roschger P, Paschalis EP, et al. (2010) Strontium is incorporated into mineral crystals only in newly formed bone during strontium ranelate treatment. J Bone Miner Res 25: 968–975.
17. Middleton ET, Steel SA, Aye M, Doherty SM (2010) The effect of prior bisphosphonate therapy on the subsequent BMD and bone turnover response to strontium ranelate. J Bone Miner Res 25: 455–462.
18. Marx RE, Cillo JE, Jr., Ulloa JJ (2007) Oral bisphosphonate-induced osteonecrosis: risk factors, prediction of risk using serum CTX testing, prevention, and treatment. J Oral Maxillofac Surg 65: 2397–2410.
19. Gomez B, Jr., Ardakani S, Ju J, Jenkins D, Cerelli MJ, et al. (1995) Monoclonal antibody assay for measuring bone-specific alkaline phosphatase activity in serum. Clin Chem 41: 1560–1566.
20. DVO (2011) Guideline 2009 for Prevention, Diagnosis and Therapy of Osteoporosis in Adults Osteologie 20: 55–74.
21. Frost HM (1983) The regional acceleratory phenomenon: a review. Henry Ford Hosp Med J 31: 3–9.
22. Burghardt AJ, Kazakia GJ, Laib A, Majumdar S (2008) Quantitative assessment of bone tissue mineralization with polychromatic micro-computed tomography. Calcif Tissue Int 83: 129–138.
23. Burghardt AJ, Kazakia GJ, Majumdar S (2007) A local adaptive threshold strategy for high resolution peripheral quantitative computed tomography of trabecular bone. Ann Biomed Eng 35: 1678–1686.
24. Patel V, Issever AS, Burghardt A, Laib A, Ries M, et al. (2003) MicroCT evaluation of normal and osteoarthritic bone structure in human knee specimens. J Orthop Res 21: 6–13.
25. Odgaard A, Gundersen HJ (1993) Quantification of connectivity in cancellous bone, with special emphasis on 3-D reconstructions. Bone 14: 173–182.
26. Doube M, Klosowski MM, Arganda-Carreras I, Cordelières FP, Dougherty RP, et al. (2010) BoneJ: Free and extensible bone image analysis in ImageJ. Bone 47: 1076–1079.
27. Hildebrand T, Rüegsegger P (1997) Quantification of Bone Microarchitecture with the Structure Model Index. Computer Methods in Biomechanics and Biomedical Engineering 1: 15–23.
28. Hahn M, Vogel M, Pompesius-Kempa M, Delling G (1992) Trabecular bone pattern factor–a new parameter for simple quantification of bone microarchitecture. Bone 13: 327–330.
29. Thomsen JS, Laib A, Koller B, Prohaska S, Mosekilde L, et al. (2005) Stereological measures of trabecular bone structure: comparison of 3D micro computed tomography with 2D histological sections in human proximal tibial bone biopsies. J Microsc 218: 171–179.
30. Mulder L, Koolstra JH, Van Eijden TM (2004) Accuracy of microCT in the quantitative determination of the degree and distribution of mineralization in developing bone. Acta Radiol 45: 769–777.
31. Parfitt AM (1988) Bone histomorphometry: proposed system for standardization of nomenclature, symbols, and units. Calcif Tissue Int 42: 284–286.
32. Parfitt AM, Drezner MK, Glorieux FH, Kanis JA, Malluche H, et al. (1987) Bone histomorphometry: standardization of nomenclature, symbols, and units. Report of the ASBMR Histomorphometry Nomenclature Committee. J Bone Miner Res 2: 595–610.
33. Iki M, Akiba T, Matsumoto T, Nishino H, Kagamimori S, et al. (2004) Reference database of biochemical markers of bone turnover for the Japanese female population. Japanese Population-based Osteoporosis (JPOS) Study. Osteoporos Int 15: 981–991.
34. Zikan V, Stepan JJ (2009) Marked reduction of bone turnover by alendronate attenuates the acute response of bone resorption marker to endogenous parathyroid hormone. Bone 44: 634–638.
35. Sebba AI, Bonnick SL, Kagan R, Thompson DE, Skalky CS, et al. (2004) Response to therapy with once-weekly alendronate 70 mg compared to once-weekly risedronate 35 mg in the treatment of postmenopausal osteoporosis. Current Medical Research and Opinion 20: 2031–2041.
36. Schafer A, Vittinghoff E, Ramachandran R, Mahmoudi N, Bauer D (2010) Laboratory reproducibility of biochemical markers of bone turnover in clinical practice. Osteoporosis International 21: 439–445.
37. Garnero P, Darte C, Delmas PD (1999) A model to monitor the efficacy of alendronate treatment in women with osteoporosis using a biochemical marker of bone turnover. Bone 24: 603–609.
38. Garnero P, Borel O, Delmas PD (2001) Evaluation of a Fully Automated Serum Assay for C-Terminal Cross-Linking Telopeptide of Type I Collagen in Osteoporosis. Clin Chem 47: 694–702.
39. Watts NB, Jenkins DK, Visor JM, Casal DC, Geusens P (2001) Comparison of Bone and Total Alkaline Phosphatase and Bone Mineral Density in Postmenopausal Osteoporotic Women Treated with Alendronate. Osteoporosis International 12: 279–288.
40. Dos Reis LM, Batalha JR, Muñoz DR, Borelli A, Correa PHS, et al. (2007) Brazilian normal static bone histomorphometry: effects of age, sex, and race. Journal of Bone and Mineral Metabolism 25: 400–406.
41. Vedi S, Compston JE, Webb A, Tighe JR (1982) Histomorphometric analysis of bone biopsies from the iliac crest of normal British subjects. Metabolic Bone Disease and Related Research 4: 231–236.
42. Schnitzler CM, Pettifor JM, Mesquita JM, Bird MDT, Schnaid E, et al. (1990) Histomorphometry of iliac crest bone in 346 normal black and white South African adults. Bone and Mineral 10: 183–199.
43. Chavassieux PM, Arlot ME, Reda C, Wei L, Yates AJ, et al. (1997) Histomorphometric assessment of the long-term effects of alendronate on bone quality and remodeling in patients with osteoporosis. The Journal of clinical investigation 100: 1475–1480.
44. Eriksen EF, Melsen F, Sod E, Barton I, Chines A (2002) Effects of long-term risedronate on bone quality and bone turnover in women with postmenopausal osteoporosis. Bone 31: 620–625.
45. Jobke B (2006) Bisphosphonat-Therapie bei Osteoporosepatienten: Veränderung der dreidimensionalen Spongiosastruktur und Entwicklung des endostalen Umbaus [Dissertation]: University Medical Center Hamburg-Eppendorf .
46. Hahn M, Vogel M, Delling G (1991) Undecalcified preparation of bone tissue: report of technical experience and development of new methods. Virchows Arch A Pathol Anat Histopathol 418: 1–7.
47. Bromage TG, Goldman HM, McFarlin SC, Warshaw J, Boyde A, et al. (2003) Circularly polarized light standards for investigations of collagen fiber orientation in bone. Anat Rec B New Anat 274: 157–168.
48. Busse B, Hahn M, Soltau M, Zustin J, Puschel K, et al. (2009) Increased calcium content and inhomogeneity of mineralization render bone toughness in osteoporosis: mineralization, morphology and biomechanics of human single trabeculae. Bone 45: 1034–1043.
49. Roschger P, Fratzl P, Eschberger J, Klaushofer K (1998) Validation of quantitative backscattered electron imaging for the measurement of mineral density distribution in human bone biopsies. Bone 23: 319–326.
50. Roschger P, Paschalis EP, Fratzl P, Klaushofer K (2008) Bone mineralization density distribution in health and disease. Bone 42: 456–466.
51. Skedros JG, Bloebaum RD, Bachus KN, Boyce TM, Constantz B (1993) Influence of mineral content and composition on graylevels in backscattered electron images of bone. J Biomed Mater Res 27: 57–64.
52. Bjeoumikhov A, Arkadiev V, Eggert F, Hodoroaba VD, Langhoff N, et al. (2005) A new microfocus x-ray source, iMOXS, for highly sensitive XRF analysis in scanning electron microscopes. X-Ray Spectrometry 34: 493–497.
53. Seitz S, Schnabel C, Busse B, Schmidt HU, Beil FT, et al. (2010) High bone turnover and accumulation of osteoid in patients with neurofibromatosis 1. Osteoporos Int 21: 119–127.
54. Glorieux FH, Travers R, Taylor A, Bowen JR, Rauch F, et al. (2000) Normative data for iliac bone histomorphometry in growing children. Bone 26: 103–109.
55. Won YY, Chung YS, Park YK, Yoo VY (2003) Correlations between microcomputed tomography and bone histomorphometry in Korean young females. Yonsei Med J 44: 811–815.
56. Stauber M, Muller R (2006) Volumetric spatial decomposition of trabecular bone into rods and plates–a new method for local bone morphometry. Bone 38: 475–484.
57. Busse B, Hahn M, Schinke T, Puschel K, Duda GN, et al. (2010) Reorganization of the femoral cortex due to age-, sex-, and endoprosthetic-related effects emphasized by osteonal dimensions and remodeling. J Biomed Mater Res A 92: 1440–1451.
58. Eriksen EF, Eghbali-Fatourechi GZ, Khosla S (2007) Remodeling and vascular spaces in bone. J Bone Miner Res 22: 1–6.
59. Doube M, Kłosowski MM, Wiktorowicz-Conroy AM, Hutchinson JR, Shefelbine SJ (2011) Trabecular bone scales allometrically in mammals and birds. Proceedings of the Royal Society B: Biological Sciences.
60. Busse B, Djonic D, Milovanovic P, Hahn M, Puschel K, et al. (2010) Decrease in the osteocyte lacunar density accompanied by hypermineralized lacunar occlusion reveals failure and delay of remodeling in aged human bone. Aging Cell 9: 1065–1075.
61. Kufahl RH, Saha S (1990) A theoretical model for stress-generated fluid flow in the canaliculi-lacunae network in bone tissue. J Biomech 23: 171–180.
62. Ding M, Hvid I (2000) Quantification of age-related changes in the structure model type and trabecular thickness of human tibial cancellous bone. Bone 26: 291–295.
63. Laib A, Kumer JL, Majumdar S, Lane NE (2001) The Temporal Changes of Trabecular Architecture in Ovariectomized Rats Assessed by MicroCT. Osteoporosis International 12: 936–941.
64. Liu XS, Sajda P, Saha PK, Wehrli FW, Guo XE (2006) Quantification of the Roles of Trabecular Microarchitecture and Trabecular Type in Determining the Elastic Modulus of Human Trabecular Bone. Journal of Bone and Mineral Research 21: 1608–1617.
65. Ma YL, Zeng Q, Donley DW, Ste-Marie LG, Gallagher JC, et al. (2006) Teriparatide increases bone formation in modeling and remodeling osteons and enhances IGF-II immunoreactivity in postmenopausal women with osteoporosis. J Bone Miner Res 21: 855–864.
66. Jee WS, Tian XY, Setterberg RB (2007) Cancellous bone minimodeling-based formation: a Frost, Takahashi legacy. J Musculoskelet Neuronal Interact 7: 232–239.
67. Amling M, Grote HJ, Vogel M, Hahn M, Delling G (1994) Three-dimensional analysis of the spine in autopsy cases with renal osteodystrophy. Kidney Int 46: 733–743.
68. Woods CG, Bishop MC, Nicholson GD (1972) Bone histological changes occurring after haemodialysis treatment for chronic renal failure. J Pathol 107: 137–143.
69. Sato K, Byers PD (1981) Quantitative study of tunneling and hook resorption in metabolic bone disease. Calcif Tissue Int 33: 459–466.
70. Blake GM, Fogelman I (2005) Long-term effect of strontium ranelate treatment on BMD. J Bone Miner Res 20: 1901–1904.

71. Amling M, Herden S, Pösl M, Hahn M, Ritzel H, et al. (1996) Heterogeneity of the skeleton: Comparison of the trabecular microarchitecture of the spine, the iliac crest, the femur, and the calcaneus. Journal of Bone and Mineral Research 11: 36–45.
72. Hauge EM, Mosekilde L, Melsen F, Frydenberg M (2001) How many patients are needed? Variation and design considerations in bone histomorphometry. Bone 28: 556–562.
73. Lips P (2001) Vitamin D Deficiency and Secondary Hyperparathyroidism in the Elderly: Consequences for Bone Loss and Fractures and Therapeutic Implications. Endocrine Reviews 22: 477–501.

5

Common Genetic Variants Are Associated with Accelerated Bone Mineral Density Loss after Hematopoietic Cell Transplantation

Song Yao[1], Lara E. Sucheston[1], Shannon L. Smiley[2], Warren Davis[1], Jeffrey M. Conroy[3], Norma J. Nowak[3,4], Christine B. Ambrosone[1], Philip L. McCarthy Jr.[2]⁹, Theresa Hahn[2]*⁹

1 Department of Cancer Prevention and Control, Roswell Park Cancer Institute, Buffalo, New York, United States of America, **2** Department of Medicine, Roswell Park Cancer Institute, Buffalo, New York, United States of America, **3** Department of Cancer Genetics, Roswell Park Cancer Institute, Buffalo, New York, United States of America, **4** Department of Biochemistry, University at Buffalo, Buffalo, New York, United States of America

Abstract

Background: Bone mineral density (BMD) loss commonly occurs after hematopoietic cell transplantation (HCT). Hypothesizing that genetic variants may influence post-HCT BMD loss, we conducted a prospective study to examine the associations of single nucleotide polymorphisms (SNP) in bone metabolism pathways and acute BMD loss after HCT.

Methods and Findings: We genotyped 122 SNPs in 45 genes in bone metabolism pathways among 121 autologous and allogeneic HCT patients. BMD changes from pre-HCT to day +100 post-HCT were analyzed in relation to these SNPs in linear regression models. After controlling for clinical risk factors, we identified 16 SNPs associated with spinal or femoral BMD loss following HCT, three of which have been previously implicated in genome-wide association studies of bone phenotypes, including rs2075555 in *COL1A1*, rs9594738 in *RANKL*, and rs4870044 in *ESR1*. When multiple SNPs were considered simultaneously, they explained 5–35% of the variance in post-HCT BMD loss. There was a significant trend between the number of risk alleles and the magnitude of BMD loss, with patients carrying the most risk alleles having the greatest loss.

Conclusion: Our data provide the first evidence that common genetic variants play an important role in BMD loss among HCT patients similar to age-related BMD loss in the general population. This infers that the mechanism for post-HCT bone loss is a normal aging process that is accelerated during HCT. A limitation of our study comes from its small patient population; hence future larger studies are warranted to validate our findings.

Editor: Michael Hendricks, Harvard University, United States of America

Funding: This work was supported, in part, by a Cancer and Leukemia Group B (CALGB) Investigator Award for junior oncology faculty (S.L.S). The DataBank and BioRepository and the Genomics Shared Resource at Roswell Park Cancer Institute are Cancer Center Support Grant (CCSG) Shared Resources (NIH 5P30CA016056-34). The funding organizations played no roles during the conduct of the study or the preparation of the manuscript. The funders had no role in study design, data collection and analysis, decision to publish, or preparation of the manuscript.

Competing Interests: The authors have declared that no competing interests exist.

* E-mail: Theresa.hahn@roswellpark.org

⁹ These authors contributed equally to this work.

Introduction

After the second decade of life, bone mineral density (BMD) gradually declines as a result of normal aging [1]. This process is accelerated in patients undergoing hematopoietic cell transplantation (HCT) [2,3]. Rapid bone loss weakens bone strength and may permanently impair bone remodeling capability [4,5], putting HCT survivors at high risk of premature fracture. We previously demonstrated that BMD loss within 4 months after HCT is equivalent to 7 to 17 years of normal bone aging [6]. Moreover, this loss occurs following autologous and allogeneic HCT with a similar incidence and severity.

In the general population, the inherited genetic background accounts for a large proportion of phenotypic variation in BMD loss and fracture risk [7,8]. In numerous candidate gene association studies, a variety of genetic variants, mostly in the form of single nucleotide polymorphisms (SNP), have been associated with regulation of BMD and risk of fracture [9], with less than a handful of them confirmed in a recent large-scale meta-analysis performed by the Genetic Factors for Osteoporosis (GEFOS) Consortium [10]. A genome-wide association (GWA) approach has also been used to search for loci associated with various bone phenotypes, which identified a number of novel SNPs [11,12,13,14,15]. These genetic markers may have clinical significance in predicting risk of BMD loss and/or osteoporosis. Moreover, some may also be predictive for response to therapies targeting related molecules or pathways, such as a human monoclonal antibody against receptor activator of nuclear factor κB ligand (RANKL) (denosumab), which was recently approved by the FDA for postmenopausal women at risk for fracture [16].

Among HCT recipients, rapid BMD loss may be due to an accelerated bone aging process after exposure to high doses of corticosteroids, chemotherapy and/or total body irradiation. Indeed, we have previously demonstrated that bone loss occurs within three months of HCT in both allogeneic and autologous HCT patients [6]. Therefore, predisposing genetic variants for low BMD and osteoporosis in the general population may also predispose carriers to risk of severe post-HCT BMD loss. Recently, McClune and colleagues proposed comprehensive guidelines for the screening, prevention and treatment of osteoporosis after HCT. They recommend dual-energy X-ray absorptiometry (DXA) scans for all adult patients 1 year post-HCT or earlier for patients at high risk of bone loss [17]. Bisphosphonates are effective in reducing or reversing HCT-related bone loss in several small randomized studies; however, they rarely resolve bone loss to pre-HCT levels and have a significant side-effect, osteonecrosis of the jaw. We hypothesized that genetic variants are associated with BMD loss in HCT patients, and sought to identify a panel of genetic biomarkers that can be incorporated into the above guidelines to personalize prevention and treatment strategy.

Methods

Ethics statement: Stem cell transplant patients at the Blood and Marrow Transplantation Program included in this study are part of an institution-level Data Bank and Biorepository (DBBR) at Roswell Park Cancer Institute (RPCI). All participants have provided written consent for their data and biospecimens to be used for research purposes. This study has been reviewed and approved by RPCI Institutional Review Board.

Patients, BMD measurement, and DNA specimens

A detailed description of the patient population has been published previously [6]. Briefly, between 1/2006 and 1/2009, 206 consecutive adult (≥18 years) patients underwent their first HCT in the Blood and Marrow Transplantation Program at Roswell Park Cancer Institute (RPCI). As part of routine clinical care, the average BMD at lumbar spine (L2–L4) and dual femurs were measured by DXA scans at baseline (pre-HCT) and day +100 post-HCT. The median time for 197 patients (96%) who had a baseline DXA scan was 20 days before HCT and 98 days for 146 patients (74%) who had a second DXA scan after HCT. Reasons for not obtaining a follow-up DXA scan were unstable medical status (n = 14), or disease relapse/early death (n = 37). Before HCT, patients were invited to participate in the DataBank and BioRepository (DBBR), a comprehensive data and biospecimen core facility at RPCI [18]. Upon their consent to the DBBR, blood samples were drawn and genomic DNA was extracted and stored for multidisplinary research. For this study, 121 patients including 67 autologous and 54 allogeneic HCT patients, consented to the DBBR and had adequate DNA available for genotyping.

Candidate gene and SNP selection and genotyping

Candidate genes from bone metabolism pathways were selected based on the following criteria: (1) genes that have been well studied and established in association with osteoporosis or other bone phenotypes in the general population; (2) key genes in bone metabolism pathways, including osteoblast or osteoclast differentiation, proliferation and activation; calcitronic hormone metabolism and activation; and bone matrix formation and regulation. As listed in Table S1, a total of 45 candidate genes were clustered into 4 groups based on underlying biological function, including (1) RANKL-RANK-OPG central signaling axis and regulating cytokines, (2) bone matrix proteins and regulating factors, (3) vitamin D receptor and metabolizing enzymes, and (4) steroid hormones and receptors.

SNPs for each candidate gene were selected based on the following criteria: (1) minor allele frequency (MAF) ≥0.10 in the population of European ancestry; (2) SNPs that have been well studied and established in association with osteoporosis or other bone traits in the general population, including those identified in recent GWA studies and the large prospective study Genetic Factors for Osteoporosis (GEFOS) Consortium [10]; (3) coding SNPs and SNPs in the 3′ or 5′ untranslated region (UTR); and (4) tagSNPs selected by the Tagger program [19] from the HapMap Project data [20], if no functional SNPs or well studied SNPs were available. In all, 158 SNPs were initially selected from the 45 candidate genes. To remove redundant SNPs due to high linkage disequilibrium (LD), pair-wise r^2 was computed for SNPs in each gene and in genes clustered on the same chromosome by PLINK [21]; SNP_tools [22] was used for necessary data formatting. For SNP pairs in high LD ($r^2 \geq 0.90$), one SNP was randomly selected from each pair for further consideration. As a result, a total of 122 SNPs were included in the final analysis (see Table S1).

Genotyping of DNA extracted from peripheral blood was performed in the Genomics Shared Resource at RPCI utilizing the MassARRAY® technology and iPLEX Gold assay (Sequenom). Nine percent duplicate samples and in-house Coriell trio samples were included within plates and across plates for genotyping quality assurance. The average qualified call rate was 98.1% for each SNP and 98.3% for each DNA sample. There was no discordance among duplicate pairs, and no SNPs violated Mendelian inheritance or Hardy-Weinberg equilibrium.

Statistical analysis

All analyses were performed stratified by autologous and allogeneic HCTs since these two treatments, and the characteristics of the patients given these two treatments, are significantly different. Change in BMD was standardized to 100 days (BMD change divided by the number of days between the two DXA scans then times 100) and used as a continuous variable; thus, a negative value indicates BMD loss and a positive value indicates BMD gain. We used linear regression models to analyze the association of clinical factors and genetic variants with four separate outcomes: BMD changes at the spine and at the femur in autologous and allogeneic HCT patients. Assuming an additive genetic model, 54 patients in the small allogeneic HCT group and two-sided p-value of 0.05, we had 80% power to detect a minimum BMD change of 0.023–0.040 g/cm^2 for a SNP with a minor allele frequency between 0.10–0.50. In the autologous HCT group which had a larger sample size of 67, we had 80% power to detect effect sizes <0.023 g/cm^2.

Single SNP analysis. SNPs associated with HCT-induced BMD change were identified as follows. First, each SNP was tested individually in a simple linear regression model without controlling for covariates; SNPs with $p<0.10$ were then added to regression models previously built with clinical factors for each of the four outcomes, including the cumulative dose of corticosteroids (in prednisone equivalents) between the two DXA scans for BMD loss in allogeneic HCT patients [6]. We measured the proportion of variance explained by all the covariates retained in a model, R^2, and determined, ΔR^2, an estimate of the proportion of variance that can be explained by the SNP(s) added to the base model, with adjustment for the number of covariates in the model. A SNP with a ΔR^2 of 5% or higher was deemed significant. Effect size (i.e., absolute BMD change) per copy of the variant allele and 95% confidence intervals (CI) were calculated for each significant SNP, with and without adjustment for clinical risk factors. The rate of annualized BMD change between pre- and post-HCT DXA scans was compared and plotted by the genotypes of each significant

SNP. To explore potential functionality of the significant SNPs, the SNP and CNV Annotation Database (SCAN) [23] was surveyed to explore whether it is a potential expression quantitative trait loci (eQTL) that has been associated with altered gene expression.

Multiple-SNP analysis. We examined the combined effects of multiple variants using backward elimination. SNPs with a $p \leq 0.05$ were retained in the final models. Adjusted R^2 was calculated for the complete models with both clinical and genetic factors and compared to the base models with only clinical factors, to determine the overall contribution of genetic factors. For SNPs retained in the model, the number of risk alleles was summed for each patient, and the annualized rate of BMD change was compared across patients by number of risk alleles. Although we measured change in BMD between a set interval of approximately 100 days, we presented annualized BMD loss rates for comparisons to the general population. Prior reports of BMD loss post-HCT demonstrated that reversal of BMD loss takes several years after HCT [3]. Multiple-SNP analysis was not performed for spinal BMD loss after allogeneic HCT because only

Table 1. Characteristics of HCT patients with BMD measurement and genomic DNA samples.

Characteristics	Autologous HCT (n = 67)	Allogeneic HCT (n = 54)
Age at HCT in years	57 (25–74)	47 (18–71)
Spine BMD at baseline, median (range), g/cm^2	1.23 (0.71–1.65)	1.20 (0.86–1.83)
Femur BMD at baseline, median (range), g/cm^2	1.04 (0.60–1.41)	1.09 (0.71–1.45)
Gender		
Male	42 (63%)	30 (56%)
Female	25 (37%)	24 (44%)
Race		
White	59 (88%)	52 (96%)
Other	8 (12%)	2 (4%)
Diagnosis		
Acute leukemia	3 (4%)	34 (63%)
Lymphoma	37 (55%)	9 (17%)
Myeloma	27 (40%)	0
Other	0	11 (20%)
Disease status at HCT		
CR1/untreated MDS	29 (43%)	38 (70%)
CR2+/PIF/Relapse	38 (57%)	16 (30%)
Graft source		
Bone marrow ± PBSC	6 (9%)	8 (15%)
PBSC	61 (91%)	46 (85%)
Conditioning regimen		
Myeloblative	67 (100%)	19 (35%)
Reduced Intensity	0	32 (59%)
Non-myeloblative	0	3 (6%)
GvHD prophylaxis regimen		
CsMt/FKMt	-	19 (35%)
FK/FKMMF	-	15 (28%)
FKMtMMF		20 (37%)
Donor relation		
Unrelated	-	36 (67%)
Related	-	18 (33%)
HLA match		
Matched	-	45 (83%)
Mismatched	-	9 (17%)
Acute GvHD		
Grade 0–I	-	26 (48%)
Grade II–IV	-	28 (52%)

Abbreviations: BMD, bone mineral density; CR, complete remission; Cs, cyclosporine; FK, tacrolimus; GvHD, graft-versus-host disease; HCT, hematopoietic cell transplantation; HLA, human leukocyte antigen; MDS, myelodysplastic syndrome; MMF, mycophenolate mofetil; Mt, methotrexate; PIF, primary induction failure; PBSC, peripheral blood stem cell.

one SNP was retained in the final comprehensive model. All analyses were two-tailed and were performed with SAS 9.2 (SAS Institute, Cary, NC).

Results

Individual SNP analysis

Table 1 summarizes the demographic and clinical characteristics of the study population separately by auto- and allo-HCT groups, which were statistically similar to the overall patient population described in our prior report [6]. Unadjusted p-values for associations between individual SNPs and BMD change between pre- and post-HCT are shown in Figure S1. After controlling for clinical risk factors, at least one SNP remained significant for each of the four outcomes, with a total of 16 significant SNPs for all four outcomes. SNP rs2075555 in the *COL1A1* gene remained significant after Bonferroni correction for multiple comparisons ($p = 0.037$).

Table 2 summarizes the unadjusted and adjusted BMD change associated with each of the 16 SNPs significant in individual SNP tests. Annualized rate of BMD change by genotype are shown in Figure 1. There was a significant dose-response trend between rate of BMD loss and number of risk alleles at the spine and the femur in autologous HCT and at the femur in allogeneic HCT. The functions of these genes, SNPs and published literature are summarized in Table S2. Among these, three SNPs, including rs2075555 in *COL1A1* gene [11,24], rs9594738 in *RANKL* gene [13] and rs4870044 in *ESR1* gene [13], were significantly associated with bone phenotypes in GWA studies of the general population. Moreover, rs2075555 and rs9594738 were associated with altered gene expression in the SCAN ($p<0.0001$). Another 9 significant SNPs in our analysis were previously linked to bone phenotypes in candidate gene association studies, including rs4588 in *GC*, rs6256 in *PTH*, rs419598 in *IL1RN*, rs1801131 in *MTHFR*, rs1800896 in *IL10*, and rs1061624 in *TNFRSF1B*, rs1042358 in *ALOX12*, rs759330 in *BGLAP*, and rs2235579 in *CLCN7*. Four of these SNPs (rs759330, rs2235579, rs1800896 and rs1061624) were also associated with altered gene expression in the SCAN. The other 4 SNPs, including rs3787557 and rs2296241 in *CYP24A1*, rs25645 in *CSF3*, and rs1321080 in *RUNX2*, were selected as tagSNPs or SNPs in functional genomic regions, with no known associations with bone phenotypes. Two of these SNPs (rs2296241 and rs25645) were associated with altered gene expression in the SCAN.

Multiple-SNP analysis

The multiple-SNP models are shown in Table 3. For the spinal BMD change after autologous HCT, three SNPs (rs759330 in

Table 2. Change in bone mineral density per copy of the variant allele for individual SNPs which were significant in the multivariable models including clinical risk factors[1].

Gene	SNP	Unadjusted BMD change per copy of variant allele (95% CI), g/cm^2	Unadjusted P-value	Adjusted BMD change per copy of variant allele (95% CI), g/cm^2	Adjusted P-value
Spinal bone mineral density change after autologous hematopoietic cell transplantation					
BGLAP	rs759330	−0.024 (−0.045−0.002)	0.03	−0.026 (−0.047−0.006)	0.01
CLCN7	rs2235579	0.016 (−0.001-0.034)	0.07	0.019 (0.002-0.036)	0.03
GC	rs4588	−0.031 (−0.051−0.011)	0.003	−0.024 (−0.045−0.003)	0.02
CYP24A1	rs3787557	−0.055 (−0.095−0.016)	0.007	−0.049 (−0.087−0.010)	0.01
PTH	rs6256	0.036 (0.004-0.067)	0.03	0.032 (0.002-0.063)	0.04
Femoral bone mineral density change after autologous hematopoietic cell transplantation					
IL1RN	rs419598	−0.014 (−0.026−0.003)	0.01	−0.014 (−0.025−0.004)	0.009
CSF3	rs25645	0.011 (0.002-0.021)	0.02	0.011 (0.002-0.020)	0.02
MTHFR	rs1801131	0.022 (0.009-0.036)	0.001	0.020 (0.08-0.033)	0.008
ALOX12	rs1042357	−0.016 (−0.027−0.005)	0.004	−0.014 (−0.025−0.003)	0.01
CYP24A1	rs2296241	0.014 (0.004-0.024)	0.01	0.014 (0.004-0.024)	0.01
ESR1	rs4870044	−0.011 (−0.023−0.000)	0.06	−0.015 (−0.025−0.004)	0.008
Spinal bone mineral density change after allogeneic hematopoietic cell transplantation					
RANKL	rs9594738	−0.029 (−0.052−0.007)	0.01	−0.020 (−0.039−0.001)	0.04
Femoral bone mineral density change after allogeneic hematopoietic cell transplantation					
RANKL	rs9594738	−0.022 (−0.042−0.003)	0.02	−0.018 (−0.036−0.001)	0.05
IL10	rs1800896	−0.016 (−0.035−0.002)	0.08	−0.022 (−0.039−0.005)	0.01
TNFRSF1B	rs1061624	−0.023 (−0.041−0.004)	0.02	−0.021 (−0.039−0.003)	0.02
COL1A1	rs2075555	−0.052 (−0.080−0.024)	0.0003	−0.050 (−0.077−0.023)	0.0006
RUNX2	rs1321080	−0.028 (−0.051−0.006)	0.02	−0.024 (−0.047−0.002)	0.03

Footnote:

[1]The clinical risk factors included in the multivariable models are: (1) Spinal BMD change after autologous HCT: spinal BMD at baseline and diagnosis (lymphoma vs others); (2) Femoral BMD change after autologous HCT: age at HCT and diagnosis (lymphoma vs others); (3) Spinal BMD change after allogeneic HCT: spinal BMD at baseline, weight at baseline, and steroid dose; (4) Femoral BMD change after allogeneic HCT: femoral BMD at baseline, weight at baseline, and steroid dose. Please refer to Table S2 for description of functions of these genes and SNPs. *Abbreviation:* BMD, bone mineral density; CI, confidence interval; HCT, hematopoietic cell transplantation; SNP, single nucleotide polymorphism.

A. Annualized spinal BMD loss rate in autologous HCT patients

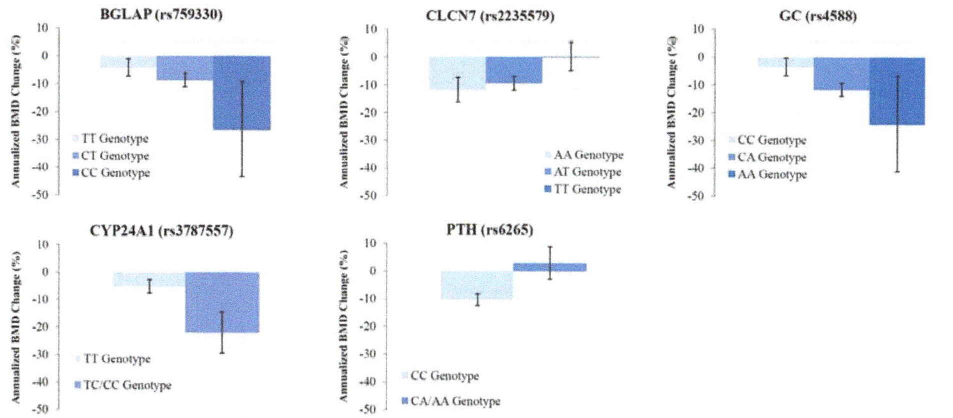

B. Annualized femoral BMD loss rate in autologous HCT patients

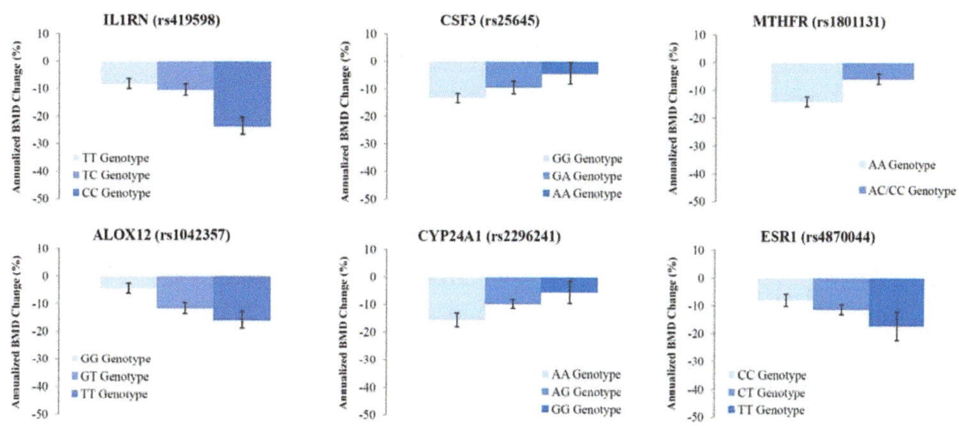

C. Annualized spinal BMD loss rate in allogeneic HCT patients

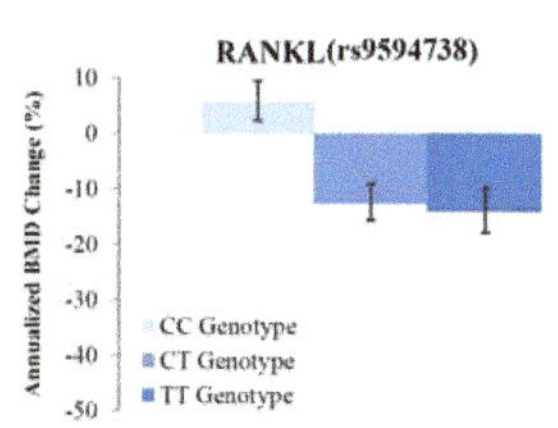

D. Annualized femoral BMD loss rate in allogeneic HCT patients

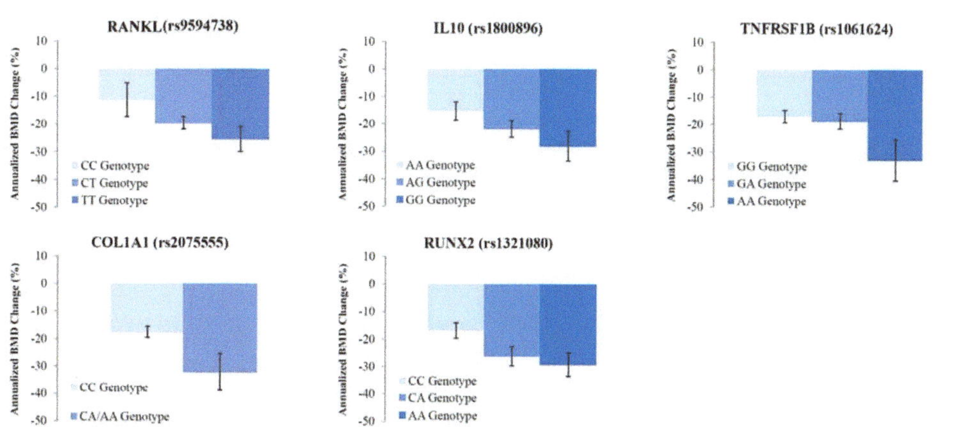

Figure 1. Annualized rate of bone mineral density change after hematopoietic cell transplantation by genotype for SNPs significant in the multivariable models including clinical risk factors. Mean and standard error of the annualized rate of BMD change is plotted by genotype for significant SNPs in the multivariable models including clinical risk factors. If the frequency of the homozygous variant genotype was ≤5%, it was combined with the heterozygous genotype (includes rs3787557 [*CYP24A1*], rs6265 [*PTH*], rs1801131 [*MTHFR*] and rs2075555 [*COL1A1*]). Please refer to Table S2 for a description of functions of these genes and SNPs. *Abbreviation:* BMD, bone mineral density; HCT, hematopoietic cell transplantation; SNP, single nucleotide polymorphism.

BGLAP, rs4588 in *GC*, and rs3787557 in *CYP24A1*) remained in the final model and explained 16% of the variance in BMD loss, in addition to the 10% determined by the clinical risk factors. Similarly, SNPs retained in the final models explained an additional 35%, 5% and 29% of the variance in femoral BMD loss after autologous HCT, spinal BMD loss after allogeneic HCT, and femoral BMD loss after allogeneic HCT, respectively.

When the annualized rate of BMD loss was compared by the number of risk alleles, there was a significant association between higher number of risk alleles and higher BMD loss (Figure 2). In addition, the multiple-SNP models identified patients at the highest risk of BMD loss. Patients carrying the highest number of risk alleles had the most severe BMD loss.

Discussion

Our analysis identified a number of SNPs in bone metabolism pathways predictive for acute BMD loss following HCT. Because our candidate genes and SNPs have been previously implicated in age-related bone loss, osteoporosis and/or bone phenotypes in the general population, our findings support the hypothesis that HCT-related BMD loss is an acceleration of the normal bone aging process. Moreover, SNPs showed greater effects in HCT patients in our study than those identified in the general population for bone phenotypes. Four SNPs accounted for 35% of variance in femoral BMD change after autologous HCT, whereas the 12 most significant loci in a GWA study accounted for only about 3% of variance in hip and spine BMD in a healthy Icelandic population [13]. The stronger effect may be driven by potent exposures during HCT.

Among the 16 SNPs significant in our analysis, only rs9594738 in *RANKL* gene was related to BMD loss at both the spine and the femur in allogeneic patients. This marginal overlap could be attributed to differences in exposures related to allogeneic versus autologous transplant procedures, as well as to differences in susceptibility to HCT-induced BMD loss at these two anatomic sites. The trabecular interconnection of the lumbar spine is much higher than that of the femur [25]. Thus, the difference in bone microarchitecture may explain the lack of overlap of SNPs associated with BMD and risk of fracture at the two sites in previous studies in the general populations [10] and the observations that femoral bone was more susceptible to HCT-induced bone loss than spinal bone [6,26].

A limitation of our study comes from the relatively small sample size and the large number of tests performed: 122 SNPs in relation to 4 quantitative outcomes in 121 patients stratified by autologous and allogeneic HCT. The statistical power was thus limited. Instead of using a Bonferroni correction, which would be over conservative, we propose a hierarchy of evidence in our findings based on curated knowledge of the SNPs in the literature.

The first level of evidence includes three SNPs implicated in two GWA studies of bone phenotypes. We found that rs2075555 in the intronic region of *COL1A1* is associated with femoral BMD loss after allogeneic HCT. The gene encodes for type I collagen, a major matrix protein for bone formation and this SNP has been previously associated with femoral neck width in women and shaft width in men [11]. Two other SNPs, rs9594738 near *RANKL* and rs4870044 near *ESR1* from a GWA study of BMD in an Icelandic population [13], and a meta-analysis of GWA studies of BMD[14], were also significant in our study. *RANKL* plays a central role in coupling the activities of osteoblasts and osteoclasts; and *ESR1* encodes for estrogen receptor alpha, which is key in estrogen-regulated activities.

The second level of evidence includes 9 SNPs, which have been previously studied in relation to various bone phenotypes using a candidate gene approach: rs4588 in *GC*, rs6256 in *PTH*, rs419598 in *IL1RN*, rs1801131 in *MTHFR*, rs1800896 in *IL10*, and rs1061624 in *TNFRSF1B*, and rs1042358 in *ALOX12*, rs759330 in *BGLAP*, and rs2235579 in *CLCN7* (Table S2). The first 5 SNPs are among the most widely studied candidates for osteoporosis and/or other bone phenotypes.

Table 3. Multiple SNP models of bone mineral density change after hematopoietic cell transplantation.

Outcome	Base model of clinical factors	Adjusted R^2	SNP (Gene)	Adjusted R^2	ΔR^2
Spinal BMD change after autologous HCT	Spinal BMD at baseline; lymphoma vs others	0.10	rs759330 (*BGALP*); rs4588 (*GC*); rs3787557 (*CYP24A1*)	0.26	0.16
Femoral BMD change after autologous HCT	Age at HCT; lymphoma vs others	0.12	rs419598 (*IL1RN*); rs1801131(*MTHFR*); rs1042357 (*ALOX12*); rs4870044 (*ESR1*)	0.46	0.35
Spinal BMD change after allogeneic HCT	Weight at HCT; spinal BMD at baseline; cortico-steroid dose	0.35	rs9594738 (*RANKL*)	0.40	0.05
Femoral BMD change after allogeneic HCT	Weight at HCT; femoral BMD at baseline; cortico-steroid dose	0.14	rs9594738 (*RANKL*); rs1061624 (*TNFRSF1B*); rs2075555(*COL1A1*); rs1321080 (*RUNX2*)	0.45	0.29

Footnote: R^2, coefficient of determination, provides an estimate of the proportion of BMD change that can be accounted for by all covariates in the model. ΔR^2 denotes the increase in model accountability by adding SNP(s) to the base clinical risk factor model. All R^2 are adjusted by the number of covariates in the model. A higher ΔR^2 suggests an important role of genetics in addition to clinical risk factors for HCT-inducted BMD loss. Please refer to Table S2 for a description of the functions of these genes and SNPs. *Abbreviation:* BMD, bone mineral density; HCT, hematopoietic cell transplantation; SNP, single nucleotide polymorphism.
single nucleotide polymorphism.

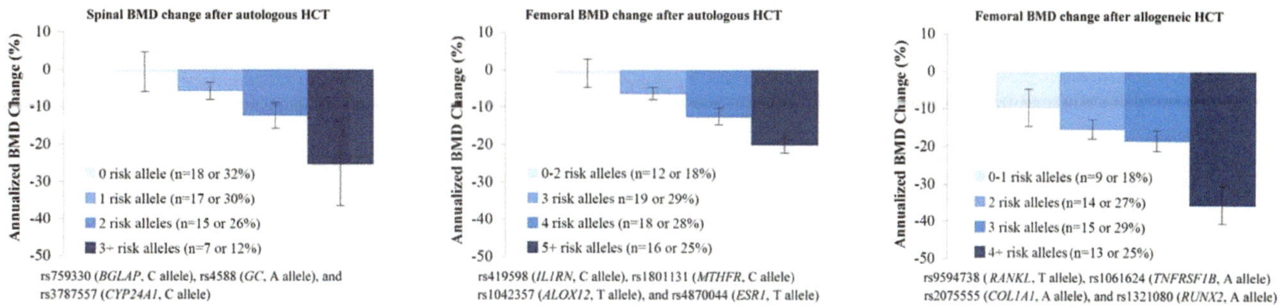

Figure 2. Annualized rate of bone mineral density change after hematopoietic cell transplantation by the number of risk alleles of the SNPs significant in the multiple SNP models. Mean and standard error of annualized rate of BMD change is plotted by the number of risk alleles in significant SNPs from the multiple SNP models as shown in Table 3. The p-values for a trend between the number of risk alleles and BMD change were ≤0.003 for all three outcomes. The proportion of HCT patients carrying the specified number of risk alleles is shown. The multiple SNP analysis was not performed for spinal BMD change after allogeneic HCT since only one SNP was significant in the multiple SNP model. Please refer to Table S2 for a description of these genes and SNPs. *Abbreviation:* BMD, bone mineral density; HCT, hematopoietic cell transplantation; SNP.

The third level of evidence includes 4 SNPs which have not been previously studied in relation to bone phenotypes: rs3787557 and rs2296241 in *CYP24A1*, rs25645 in *CSF3*, and rs1321080 in *RUNX2*. These SNPs are either tagSNPs or located in potentially functional regions, and these genes were selected for their importance in bone metabolism (Table S2).

As discussed above, we relied on *a priori* knowledge to rank our confidence in our results: those previously implicated in GWA studies were deemed most reliable, followed by those implicated in candidate gene studies, and lastly those without support from the literature. Although this knowledge-based hierarchy of evidence is not statistically stringent, and we cannot exclude the possibility of false positive (or negative) findings in our results, it aligns with our exploratory purpose and provides support that genetic variants contribute to post-HCT bone loss. Moreover, our findings may provide clues for future studies. Thus, in addition to rs2075555 in *COL1A1*, which remained significant in our analysis under the most stringent threshold of significance, we also reported other SNPs that may be interesting. Our study was designed to evaluate only one post-HCT BMD measurement (about +100 days); thus we do not know how the genetic variants described in our study affect long-term BMD post-HCT. We chose day +100 for post-HCT BMD measurement for three reasons. First, BMD loss occurs at the highest rate within the first 3–6 months after HCT [3], thus a true gene-exposure influence would be strongest in the time period closest to the exposure. Second, patients who were osteoporotic at their day +100 DXA scan were treated with a bisphosphonate soon afterwards which may distort the association between genotypes and BMD loss. Third, as an exploratory study, BMD loss at day +100 was an outcome immediately available, while we continue to follow-up patients with the plan to assess genotypes and long-term BMD loss.

It is of interest to investigate the association of donor genotype with BMD loss in allogeneic HCT recipients, considering their hematopoietic cells, and thus osteoclast precursors, are replaced by donors' hematopoietic cells once complete donor chimerism has been achieved. Unfortunately, donor DNA is not available from the allogeneic HCT patients in this study. However, given that the acute BMD loss we observed occurred quickly following transplantation, prior to complete donor chimerism, and that the acute BMD loss in our study was similar between autologous and allogeneic HCT recipients (ie., in the absence and presence of donor genomes), any effect of donor genotype may only be evidenced in chronic BMD loss with longer follow-up. This question warrants further investigation.

In summary, given the continuous bone loss due to normal aging, accelerated post-HCT bone loss may never recover without aggressive therapy, and HCT patients may be at much higher risk of fracture compared to their age-matched peers. Considering the well established relationship between low BMD and fracture risk in the general population, we support the routine post HCT surveillance guidelines developed by McClune et al [17]. Further studies are needed to determine the impact and timing of different prevention and/or intervention strategies.

Supporting Information

Figure S1 Log-transformed p-values for associations between bone mineral density change and individual SNPs without adjustment for clinical risk factors. Individual SNP (gene) remained significant in the multivariable models including clinical risk factors are labeled in circles. A number of other SNPs significant in univariate analysis but dropped out of multivariate analysis were not labeled. Please refer to Table S2 for description of functions of these genes and SNPs. *Abbreviation:* HCT, hematopoietic cell transplantation; SNP, single nucleotide polymorphism.

Table S1 Selected 122 single nucleotide polymorphisms from 46 candidate genes in bone metabolism pathways. [1]SNPs that have been previously studied in the large prospective study Genetic Markers for Osteoporosis (GENOMOS) Consortium were labeled as "GENOMOS SNPs". SNPs that have been identified in genome wide association (GWA) studies were labeled as "GWAS SNP". TagSNPs selected to represent genetic variations in genes that have not been previous studied and have no common SNPs in functional regions were labeled as "tagSNP". Functional regions include 3′ and 5′ untranslated region (UTR) and codon. For coding SNPs, amino acid changes are shown.

Table S2 Functions and summary of the published literature for genes and SNPs significant in the individual SNP models including clinical risk factors

Acknowledgments

The authors are grateful to the RPCI patients who agreed to participate in this study, the BMT nursing and laboratory staff, the nurse practitioners, physician assistants and the entire clinical team who cares for these patients, and the BMT data managers for assistance with data collection.

Author Contributions

Conceived and designed the experiments: SY LES SLS CBA PLM TH. Performed the experiments: SY WD JMC NJN. Analyzed the data: SY LES SLS CBA PLM TH. Contributed reagents/materials/analysis tools: WD JMC NJN CBA. Wrote the paper: SY LES SLS WD JMC NJN CBA PLM TH.

References

1. Benjamin RM (2010) Bone health: preventing osteoporosis. J Am Diet Assoc 110: 498.
2. Kelly PJ, Atkinson K, Ward RL, Sambrook PN, Biggs JC, et al. (1990) Reduced bone mineral density in men and women with allogeneic bone marrow transplantation. Transplantation 50: 881–883.
3. Schulte CM, Beelen DW (2004) Bone loss following hematopoietic stem cell transplantation: a long-term follow-up. Blood 103: 3635–3643.
4. Tauchmanova L, Serio B, Del Puente A, Risitano AM, Esposito A, et al. (2002) Long-lasting bone damage detected by dual-energy x-ray absorptiometry, phalangeal osteosonogrammetry, and in vitro growth of marrow stromal cells after allogeneic stem cell transplantation. J Clin Endocrinol Metab 87: 5058–5065.
5. Lee WY, Cho SW, Oh ES, Oh KW, Lee JM, et al. (2002) The effect of bone marrow transplantation on the osteoblastic differentiation of human bone marrow stromal cells. J Clin Endocrinol Metab 87: 329–335.
6. Yao S, Smiley SL, West K, Lamonica D, Battiwalla M, et al. (2010) Accelerated bone mineral density loss occurs with similar incidence and severity, but with different risk factors, after autologous versus allogeneic hematopoietic cell transplantation. Biol Blood Marrow Transplant 16: 1130–1137.
7. Peacock M, Turner CH, Econs MJ, Foroud T (2002) Genetics of osteoporosis. Endocr Rev 23: 303–326.
8. Eisman JA (1999) Genetics of osteoporosis. Endocr Rev 20: 788–804.
9. Liu YZ, Liu YJ, Recker RR, Deng HW (2003) Molecular studies of identification of genes for osteoporosis: the 2002 update. J Endocrinol 177: 147–196.
10. Richards JB, Kavvoura FK, Rivadeneira F, Styrkarsdottir U, Estrada K, et al. (2009) Collaborative meta-analysis: associations of 150 candidate genes with osteoporosis and osteoporotic fracture. Ann Intern Med 151: 528–537.
11. Kiel DP, Demissie S, Dupuis J, Lunetta KL, Murabito JM, et al. (2007) Genome-wide association with bone mass and geometry in the Framingham Heart Study. BMC Med Genet 8 Suppl 1: S14.
12. Richards JB, Rivadeneira F, Inouye M, Pastinen TM, Soranzo N, et al. (2008) Bone mineral density, osteoporosis, and osteoporotic fractures: a genome-wide association study. Lancet 371: 1505–1512.
13. Styrkarsdottir U, Halldorsson BV, Gretarsdottir S, Gudbjartsson DF, Walters GB, et al. (2008) Multiple genetic loci for bone mineral density and fractures. N Engl J Med 358: 2355–2365.
14. Rivadeneira F, Styrkarsdottir U, Estrada K, Halldorsson BV, Hsu YH, et al. (2009) Twenty bone-mineral-density loci identified by large-scale meta-analysis of genome-wide association studies. Nat Genet 41: 1199–1206.
15. Styrkarsdottir U, Halldorsson BV, Gretarsdottir S, Gudbjartsson DF, Walters GB, et al. (2009) New sequence variants associated with bone mineral density. Nat Genet 41: 15–17.
16. Perrone M (June 01, 2010) FDA clears Amgen's bone-strengthening drug Prolia. Available: http://www.biosciencetechnology.com/News/FeedsAP/2010/06/fda-clears-amgens-bone-strengthening-drug-prolia/ Accessed 2011 September 14.
17. McClune BL, Polgreen LE, Burmeister LA, Blaes AH, Mulrooney DA, et al. (2011) Screening, prevention and management of osteoporosis and bone loss in adult and pediatric hematopoietic cell transplant recipients. Bone Marrow Transplant 46: 1–9.
18. Ambrosone CB, Nesline MK, Davis W (2006) Establishing a cancer center data bank and biorepository for multidisciplinary research. Cancer Epidemiol Biomarkers Prev 15: 1575–1577.
19. de Bakker PI, Yelensky R, Pe'er I, Gabriel SB, Daly MJ, et al. (2005) Efficiency and power in genetic association studies. Nat Genet 37: 1217–1223.
20. The International HapMap Consortium (2003) The International HapMap Project. Nature 426: 789–796.
21. Purcell S, Neale B, Todd-Brown K, Thomas L, Ferreira MA, et al. (2007) PLINK: a tool set for whole-genome association and population-based linkage analyses. Am J Hum Genet 81: 559–575.
22. Chen B, Wilkening S, Drechsel M, Hemminki K (2009) SNP_tools: A compact tool package for analysis and conversion of genotype data for MS-Excel. BMC Res Notes 2: 214.
23. Gamazon ER, Zhang W, Konkashbaev A, Duan S, Kistner EO, et al. (2010) SCAN: SNP and copy number annotation. Bioinformatics 26: 259–262.
24. Murabito JM, Rosenberg CL, Finger D, Kreger BE, Levy D, et al. (2007) A genome-wide association study of breast and prostate cancer in the NHLBI's Framingham Heart Study. BMC Med Genet 8 Suppl 1: S6.
25. Amling M, Herden S, Posl M, Hahn M, Ritzel H, et al. (1996) Heterogeneity of the skeleton: comparison of the trabecular microarchitecture of the spine, the iliac crest, the femur, and the calcaneus. J Bone Miner Res 11: 36–45.
26. Yao S, McCarthy PL, Dunford LM, Roy DM, Brown K, et al. (2008) High prevalence of early-onset osteopenia/osteoporosis after allogeneic stem cell transplantation and improvement after bisphosphonate therapy. Bone Marrow Transplant 41: 393–398.

Cortical Bone Mechanical Properties Are Altered in an Animal Model of Progressive Chronic Kidney Disease

Christopher L. Newman[1], Sharon M. Moe[2,3], Neal X. Chen[2], Max A. Hammond[4], Joseph M. Wallace[4,5], Jeffry S. Nyman[6,7], Matthew R. Allen[1]*

1 Department of Anatomy and Cell Biology, Indiana University School of Medicine, Indianapolis, Indiana, United States of America, **2** Division of Nephrology, Department of Medicine, Indiana University School of Medicine, Indianapolis, Indiana, United States of America, **3** Roudebush VA Medical Center, Indianapolis, Indiana, United States of America, **4** Weldon School of Biomedical Engineering, Purdue University, West Lafayette, Indiana, United States of America, **5** Department of Biomedical Engineering, Indiana University—Purdue University, Indianapolis, Indiana, United States of America, **6** Department of Orthopaedic Surgery and Rehabilitation and Vanderbilt Center for Bone Biology, Vanderbilt University Medical Center, Nashville, Tennessee, United States of America, **7** Department of Veterans Affairs, Tennessee Valley Healthcare System, Nashville, Tennessee, United States of America

Abstract

Chronic kidney disease (CKD), which leads tocortical bone loss and increasedporosity,increases therisk of fracture. Animal models have confirmed that these changes compromise whole bone mechanical properties. Estimates from whole bone testing suggest that material properties are negatively affected, though tissue-level assessmentshavenot been conducted. Therefore, the goal of the present study was to examine changes in cortical bone at different length scales using a rat model with theprogressive development of CKD. At 30 weeks of age (~75% reduction in kidney function), skeletally mature male Cy/+ rats were compared to their normal littermates. Cortical bone material propertieswere assessed with reference point indentation (RPI), atomic force microscopy (AFM), Raman spectroscopy,and high performance liquid chromatography (HPLC). Bones from animals with CKD had higher (+18%) indentation distance increase and first cycle energy dissipation (+ 8%) as measured by RPI.AFM indentation revealed a broader distribution of elastic modulus values in CKD animals witha greater proportion of both higher and lower modulus values compared to normal controls. Yet, tissue composition, collagen morphology, and collagen cross-linking fail to account for these differences. Though the specific skeletal tissue alterations responsible for these mechanical differences remain unclear, these results indicate that cortical bone material properties are altered in these animals and may contribute to the increased fracture risk associated with CKD.

Editor: Damian Christopher Genetos, University of California Davis, United States of America

Funding: National Institutes of Health grants AR58005 (SM) and DL100093 (CN); Indiana Clinical Translational Science Institute grant TR000162 (CN). The funders had no role in study design, data collection and analysis, decision to publish, or preparation of the manuscript.

Competing Interests: The authors have declared that no competing interests exist.

* E-mail: matallen@iupui.edu

Introduction

Chronic kidney disease—mineral and bone disorder (CKD-MBD) is characterized by hyperphosphatemia, secondary hyperparathyroidism, and an increased risk offractures[1–3].Unlike osteoporosis, CKD-MBD appears to have a preferential impact on cortical bone, leading to reduced bone mass and increased porosity [4–6].These effects likely underlie the increased fracture risk observed in patients with CKD[7–9].

Whole bone (structural)mechanical properties are dependent upon a number of variables [10–11]. While bone mass is a major determinant, both the distribution of bone and its material properties (inherent physical and chemical properties) also play crucial roles. Most biomechanical studies in rodent models of CKD have focused on structural mechanical properties, employing three-point bending or dynamic mechanical analysis (DMA) [12–18]. These studies indicate that the bending and viscoelastic properties of bone are compromised in animals with CKD. Specifically, DMA indicates that diseased animals have lower storage modulus (a measure of stiffness) and tan delta (a measure of energy dissipation) [14–15], while three point bending studies indicate that ultimate load, stiffness, and energy to failure are lower in CKD animals [12].

While there is an increasing awareness of the importance of bone quality in CKD [19], few studies have explicitly examined material properties in animal models[14–15,20]. Material properties can be estimated from whole bone mechanical tests using standardengineering equations that account for whole bone structure and geometry.Because these estimates assume that skeletal tissue is homogeneous, isotropic, and linearly elastic, direct measures ofmaterial properties in bone would provide additionalinsight into how the disease is affecting fracture resistance. Therefore, the goal of the present study was to examine material-level changes in cortical bone at several length scales using a rat model with the progressive development of CKD. Specifically, we hypothesized that CKD adversely impacts cortical bone material properties as determined by material-level mechanical testing and assessments of bone composition and collagen morphology.

Materials And Methods

Animal Model

The current study utilized a slowly progressive animal model of CKD, the Cy/+ rat. Cy/+ ratsare characterized by autosomal dominant polycystic kidney disease [21]. These animals have a mutation (R823W) in *Anks6*, a gene that codes for the protein SamCystin. Currently, the function of this protein is unknown, and the specific role of this mutation in the development of polycystic kidney disease is unclear. Aside from its expression in the kidney, however, little is known about its role in the cell [22].Unlike most other PKD-related proteins, though, SamCystin does not localize to the primary cilia of kidney cells [23]. While there is no known human disease associated with this gene, thespontaneous onset of disease provides a helpful phenotypic model of human CKD [21].Unlike the more common surgical models[24], Cy/+ rats display a gradual onset of disease.And unlike most genetic models[25–26], they exhibit a slow enough progression that bone disease does not begin to occur until after skeletal maturity.

Skeletal tissuefrom animals in a previous study wasutilized [12]. All animals were fed a casein diet (Purina AIN-76A; 0.7% Pi) to increase phosphorus availability in order to produce a more consistent kidney disease phenotype.Fresh frozen tibiaefrom 30-week-old male Cy/+ ratsand their age-matched non-affected littermates were assessed mechanically, compositionally, and morphologically at several length scales.Fresh frozen femora were used for collagen cross-linking analyses. Blood was collected at the end of the experiment for biochemical analyses (previously reported in [12]).All procedures were conducted under the approval of Indiana University School of Medicine Institutional Animal Care and Use Committeeprotocol # 10479.

Reference Point Indentation

Tibiae were thawed to room temperature and soaked overnight in phosphate-buffered saline. The anteromedial surface of the proximal diaphysis of the tibia was assessed using reference point indentation (RPI) (Biodent Hfc, Active Life Scientific, Santa Barbara, CA). The reference probe, which housed a BP2 test probe, waslowered vertically, normal to the surface, until itrested on the surface of the bone.In order to stabilize the unit, a reference force of ~13 N was applied before each measurement was initiated.Each test included a series of 10 cycles at 2 Hz to a force of 10 N. Bones were maintained in a hydrated state throughout the test. Five locations per sample, each ~2 mm apart, were indented. Raw data from the RPI analysis software (version 2.0) were imported into a customized MATLAB code (Mathworks) designed to provide cycle-by-cycle data for each test [27], from which first cycle unloading slope, indentation distance increase, first cycle energy dissipation, creep indentation distance, first cycle indentation distance, total indentation distance, and total energy dissipation were calculated for each test. All five tests from each animal were averaged to produce a single value for each variable.

Tissue Composition

Raman spectroscopy was performed using a LabRAM HR 800 Raman Spectrometer (HORIBA JobinYvon, Edison, NJ) connected to a BX41 microscope (Olympus, Tokyo, Japan). A 660 nm laser was focused on the bone surface using a 50X objective to a spot size of ~10 μm. Five locations were imaged ~1 mm apart on the anteromedialmid-diaphysiswith five 20 second acquisitions at each location as previously published [28]. A five point linear baseline correction was applied in LabSpec 5 (HORIBA JobinYvon). Using OriginPro 8.6 (OriginLab, Northampton, MA), a single Gaussian peak was fit to the PO_4^{3-}ν1 peak, and the areas under the PO_4^{3-}ν1, CO_3^{2-}ν1, and Amide I peaks were calculated at each location. Type B carbonate substitution was found by the band area ratio of CO_3^{2-}ν1/PO_4^{3-}ν1. The degree of matrix mineralization was determined by the band area ratios of PO_4^{3-}ν1/Amide I. Mineral maturity (crystallinity) was determined by the inverse of the full width at half maximum (FWHM) of the PO_4^{3-}ν1 peak.

AFM Indentation

The anteromedial portion of the mid-diaphysis used above was polished with a 3 μm polycrystalline water-based diamond suspension in order to create a flat region for testing. Nanoindentation was performed using a BioScope Catalyst atomic force microscope (Bruker, Santa Barbara, CA), operating in peak force tapping mode using previously published methods [29]. Indentations were performed using a polycrystalline diamond probe (NaDia ND-DYC series; Advanced Diamond Technologies, Inc.) with a measured spring constant of 29.25 N/m. Four locations per sample were indented and, at each location (20 μm×20 μm grid), 49 indentationswere performed. Samples were loaded to 200 nN with force-separation curves acquired from each indentation. Within each location, indentations were spaced about 2 μm apart in order to avoid interactions from neighboring indentations. In total, 196 indentations were performed for each sample. The indentation elastic modulus was calculated from 5% to 95% of the withdrawal curve using the classic Hertz model of contact between a rigid sphere and an elastic half space because the indentation depth is much smaller than the radius of curvature of the probe [29]. The indentation elastic modulus was determined from the following equation: $E = 3F(1-v^2)/(4r^{1/2}\delta^{3/2})$ where E is the indentation elastic modulus, F is the indentation force, v is the Poisson's ratio of the sample (assumed to be 0.35), r is the tip radius (nominal radius of 50 nm, with the same probe used for all samples), and δ is the indentation depth. All of the individual indentations were averaged to produce a single value for each animal though individual tests were used for distribution comparisons among the groups.

Collagen Morphology

Following AFMindentation, the polished surface was partially decalcified by soaking the bones in 0.5 M EDTA for 25 minutes followed by five minutes of sonication in a water bath. This process was repeated five times for each sample. For imaging, RTESPA probes were used (Bruker; radius nominally 8 nm, spring constant = 40 N/m). The scan size was set at 3.5 μm with 512×512 pixels and a scan rate of 0.5 lines/s. For measurements of collagen morphology, four locations were imaged per sample, and 10 to 15 fibrils were measured at each location. 40 to 50 fibrils per sample were averaged to produce a single value for each animal, though the individual tests were used for distribution comparisons. Using SPIP 5.1.10 (Image Metrology, Hrsholm, Denmark),D-periodic spacing was calculated using2D Fast Fourier Transformations (2D FFTs) as previously described [28].

Collagen Cross-Linking

Segments of bone (~3 mm in length) from the proximal femoral diaphysis were fully demineralized in 20% EDTA (0.68 M, pH 7.4). Approximately 10 mg of demineralized bonewerehydrolyzedin6 N HCl (~10 μL per 1 mg) at 110°C for 20 to 24 hours. After evaporating the acidusing a SpeedVAC centrifuge with coldtrap, each hydrolysate was resuspended in ultrapure water, split into two equal portions, and dried. Half the residue was resuspended in ultrapure water with an internal standard

(5×10^{-6} g/L pyridoxine). The solution was filtered and diluted with 0.05% heptafluorobutyric acid in 10% acetonitrile, and 50 μL of each hydrolysate were assayed by a high performance liquid chromatography (HPLC) system (Beckman-Coulter System Gold 168) with a silica-based column (Waters Spherisorb). Standards with varying concentrations of pyridinoline (Pyd) (Quidel),deoxypyridinoline (Dpd) (Quidel),pentosidine(PE) (International Maillard Reaction Society), and a constant amount of pyridoxinewere also assayed. Using a Waters 2475 fluorescence detector (excitation/emission of295/400 nm for Pyd and Dpd and 328/378 nm for PE), chromatograms were recorded to determine the amount of each crosslink. These amounts were then normalized by collagen content, which was determined from the other half of each hydrolysate by another HPLC assay [30]. Briefly, withα-amino-butyric acid (α-ABA) included as an internal standard, the amino acids were subjected to derivatization withphenyl isothiocyanate (PITC). Along with standards of varying concentrations of hydroxyproline (Sigma) and proline (Sigma)and a constant amount of α-ABA, the derivatized samples were resuspendedin a buffer solution of 5% acetonitrile in 5 mM disodium phosphate. Upon injecting 50 μLof this sample, chromatograms were generated with a UV detector (Beckman-Coulter System Gold 168). The calculated mass of hydroxyproline was then multiplied by 7.5 (assuming 13–14% of type I collagen by mass) and divided by the molecular weight of collagen (30,000 Da) [31], thereby giving crosslink concentration as mol/mol of collagen.

Statistical Analysis

All analyses were performed using SPSS software. Comparisons between groups were made with Student's t-tests (assumptions validated by Shapiro-Wilk and Levene tests). When non-normal distributions or unequal variances were present, comparisons were made using Wilcoxon ranked-sum tests and unequal variance t-tests, respectively. Distributions included all measures from each individual, and comparisons were made using Kolmogorov-Smirnov tests. *A priori* α-levels were set at 0.05 to determine significance.

Results

Animal Model

Details about the phenotype of these animals have been previous published [12]. Briefly, measures of kidney function, including BUN (+116%) and the albumin-to-creatinine ratio (+301%), weresignificantly higher in Cy/+ animals compared to the normal controls. Similar to what is observed in humans with CKD, there were no differences between groups for phosphorus or calcium levels, but both serum PTH (+240%) and FGF23 (+195%) weredrastically higher(**FIGURE 1**).Cy/+ animals had higher numbers of osteoclasts and higher levels of bone remodeling. Using three-point bending, they exhibited lower ultimate load (−28%), stiffness(−17%), and energy to fracture (−46%). Estimates of material properties indicate that they had lower ultimate stress (−20%) and toughness (−47%) (**FIGURE 2**)[12].

Reference Point Indentation

Indentation distance increase (IDI)provides an assessment of the change in depth between the first cycle and the final cycle. Cy/+ animals had significantly higher IDI (+18%), indicating that the tissue ismore prone to damage under the same applied load (**FIGURE 3**). The amount of energy dissipated during the first cycle was also significantlyhigher in animals with CKD (+8%). While the first cycle creep indentation distance (+18%) was higher in Cy/+ animals, there was no difference in microstructural stiffness (first cycle unloading slope)between the two groups.No differences were noted in first cycle indentation distance, total indentation distance, or total energy dissipation (**Table 1**).

AFM-based indentation

There was no difference in the indentation elastic modulus between the groups (**FIGURE 4a**). However, when all indentations within each groupwere considered as a population, the distribution of elastic modulus values did differ between the two groups. Animals with CKD had a greater proportion of both high and low values of elastic modulus than their normal counterparts (**FIGURE 4b**).

Tissue Composition

Raman spectroscopy revealed no differences between animals with CKD and their normal counterparts with regard to overall compositionof the mineral and organic matrices (**Table 2**). Specifically, there were no differences between the groups in the phosphate-to-amide I ratio (the mineral-to-matrix ratio), mineral crystallinity, or the carbonate-to-phosphate ratio (a reflection of type B carbonate substitution).

Collagen Morphology and Cross-Linking

There were no mean differences in D-periodicity between the two groups (**Table 2**). There were also no differences in the distribution of D-periodicity when all fibrils were considered. In addition, both enzymatic and non-enzymatic cross-linksas assessed by HPLC were similar between groups (**Table 2**).

Discussion

The mechanical integrity of skeletal tissue is determined by the amount of tissue present, its distribution, and its quality. Compromises in any of these factors can lead to an increased fracture risk. The notable loss of cortical bone mass associated with CKD is assumed to be primarily responsible for the increased fracture risk seen in patients [5]. The current study advances our understanding of bone fragility in CKD by showing that microscale and nanoscale mechanical properties are alteredindependently of changes in bone mass and porosity.

Our lab has previously documented reductions in both structural and estimated materialproperties in Cy/+ rats, animals with progressive CKD [12,32]. But, whole bone testing only provides indirect estimates of material properties, which is why wedirectly assessedmicroscale mechanical propertiesusing reference point indentation (RPI).RPI data from the present study indicate that animals with CKD had higher IDI, higher first cycle creep indentation distance, and first cycle energy dissipation. Taken together, these results indicatethat the tissue in animals with CKD is less resistant to indentation and more prone to damage. Indentation distance increase was nearly 20% higher in CKD animals compared to their normal counterparts. Similar differences in IDI have been previously reported in diabetic rats[33]. These data have two important implications. First, they show that CKD negatively affects skeletal tissue independently of bone mass, which means that estimates of bone massalone likely underestimate the overall mechanical effects of CKD.These differences in bone quality may explain the conflicting data available on BMD and fracture risk in CKD patients[6,34–40]. Second, our data provide a basis for considering *in vivo* applications of RPI in the clinical setting of CKD. RPI has been used to successfully differentiate patients with and without hip fractures[41] as well as those with and without atypical femoral fractures [42]. A related

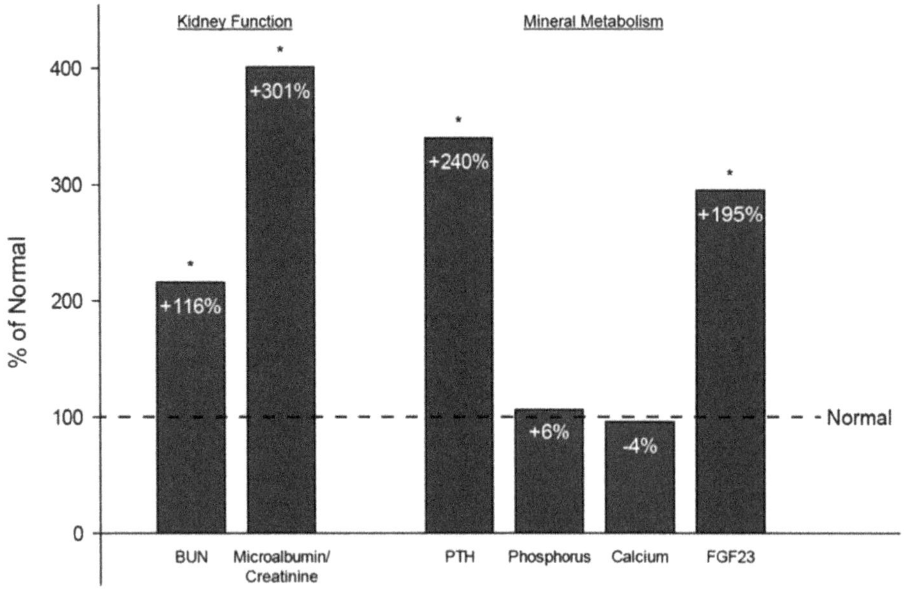

Figure 1. Biochemical assessment of kidney function and mineral metabolism. These previously published data (Allen *et al.*, 2013) show abnormalities in kidney function and mineral metabolism resulting from hyperparathyroidism in the animals utilized in the current work. Data are presented as a percentage of non-affected normal animals with (*) representing statistical significance.

indentation device has also been shown to discriminate patients with diabetes from their normal counterparts[43]. Assessment of tissue-level mechanical properties, combined with standard imaging modalities to measure bone mass, cortical geometry (especially porosity), and trabecular architecture, may prove to be an ideal combination by which to assess the overall mechanical integrity of bones in patients with CKD.

The current study also employed a hierarchical approach by examining nanoscale mechanical properties with atomic force microscopy. AFM indentation provides a direct assessment of the nanoscale stiffness produced by the collagen and mineral composite. Consistent with measurements of microscale stiffness (first cycle unloading slope), these results show that the average indentation elastic modulus was not significantly different between the two groups.Yet, the distribution of elastic modulus values was different. Animals with CKD displayed a greater degree of heterogeneity in nanoscale elasticity. Because increased material heterogeneity is often considered advantageous [44], these results may reflect an adaptive response to declining integrity at larger length scales. Alternatively, extreme variations in nanoscale properties maylead to localized stress concentrations that result in damage accumulation from lower forces[45]. Although heterogeneity is likely necessary for normal mechanical integrity, extreme heterogeneity may be problematic from a mechanical

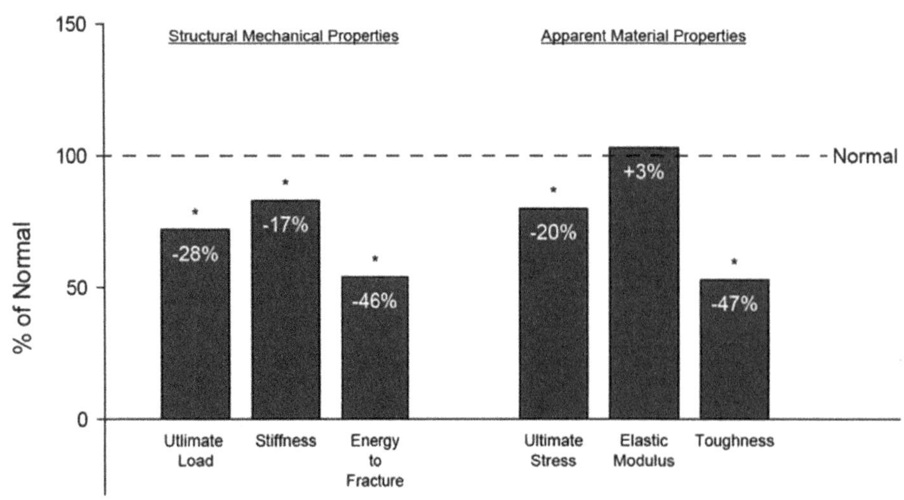

Figure 2. Structural mechanical properties and estimated material properties. These previously published data (Allen *et al.*, 2013) show compromised whole bone mechanical properties from femoral 3-point bending and apparent material-level mechanical properties derived from standard beam bending equations in the animals utilized in the current work. Data are presented as a percentage of non-affected normal animals with (*) representing statistical significance.

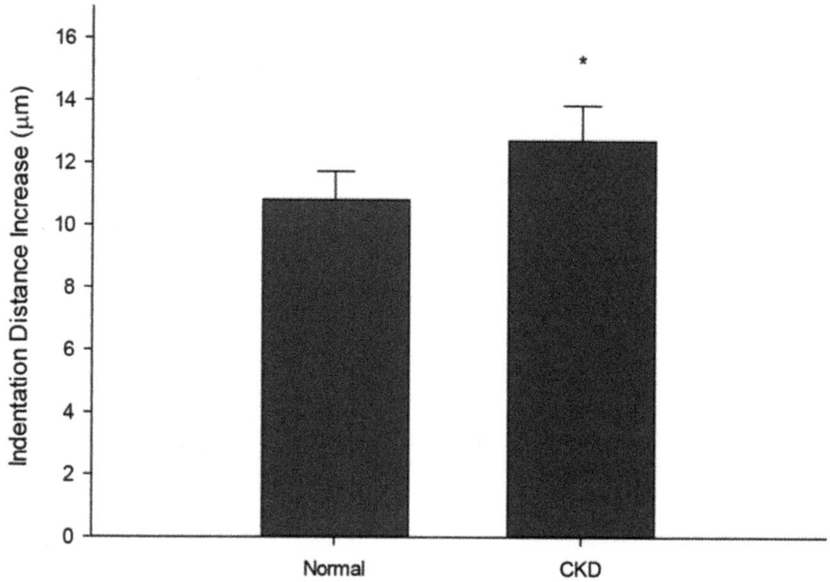

Figure 3. Microindentation reveals that CKD skeletal tissue is less able to resist damage. Using reference point indentation (RPI), the indentation distance increase (IDI) was found to be significantly higher in CKD animals compared to normal. These data indicate that the mechanical integrity of the bone is less able to resist microscale damage formation and propagation. Data are presented as mean and standard deviation. *$p < 0.05$ versus normal controls.

standpoint [46]. Future studies should attempt to better understand the role of material heterogeneity in CKD in order to specifythe contributionofmicroscale and nanoscalepropertiesto whole bone mechanical properties.

While whole bone, microscale, and nanoscale mechanical differences are present in animals with CKD, tissue composition, collagen morphology, and collagen cross-linking fail to account for the differences. These data conflict with studiesshowing higher mineral-to-matrix ratios, lower mineral crystallinity, increased advanced glycationendproducts (AGEs), and decreased gene expression of lysyl oxidase in alternative models of CKD [14–15,47]. One potential explanation for these disparate results is that these previous studies utilized younger animals that developed advanced CKD during skeletal growth. Teasing apart the interaction between growth and disease is difficult, which is why the present study employed the use of a model in which kidney disease occurs after skeletal maturity.

Previous studies have demonstrated that non-enzymatic cross-links (pentosidine, specifically) are increased in the circulation of patients with CKD[48–51]. These findings coincide with the accumulation of AGEs in soft tissues detected by fluorescence methods[52]. Because high levels in the circulation are associated with the deposition of AGEs in other tissues, this may be true of skeletal tissue as well. To date, this has only been confirmed in one small clinical study in patients on dialysis [53]. Currently, there are few data in animal models, and clinical trials examining predialysis patients are lacking. Using a low turnover 5/6 nephrectomy model, two studies have reported increased pentosidineusing

Table 1. Mechanical properties from microindentation and nanoindentation.

RPI	Normal (n = 6)	Cy/+ (n = 6)	p-values
First Cycle Indentation Distance (μm)	83.38±3.15	88.24±5.45	*0.088
First cycle Energy Dissipation (μJ)	275.53±14.00	297.94±19.35	***0.044**
First Cycle Unloading Slope (N/μm)	0.47±0.02	0.45±0.03	*0.113
First Cycle Creep Indentation Distance (μm)	6.08±0.43	7.17±0.95	***0.028**
Indentation Distance Increase (μm)	10.81±0.92	12.71±1.13	***0.009**
Total Indentation Distance (μm)	89.39±2.73	95.21±5.13	#0.080
Total Energy Dissipation (μJ)	663.06±43.53	712.30±89.19	*0.252
AFM	**Normal (n = 5)**	**Cy/+ (n = 4)**	**p-values**
Indentation Elastic Modulus (MPa)	962.99 345.98	996.73 588.99	0.920

Values are presented as mean ± standard deviation.
*equal variance t-test.
#Wilcoxon ranked-sum test.
p-values less than 0.05 are in bold.

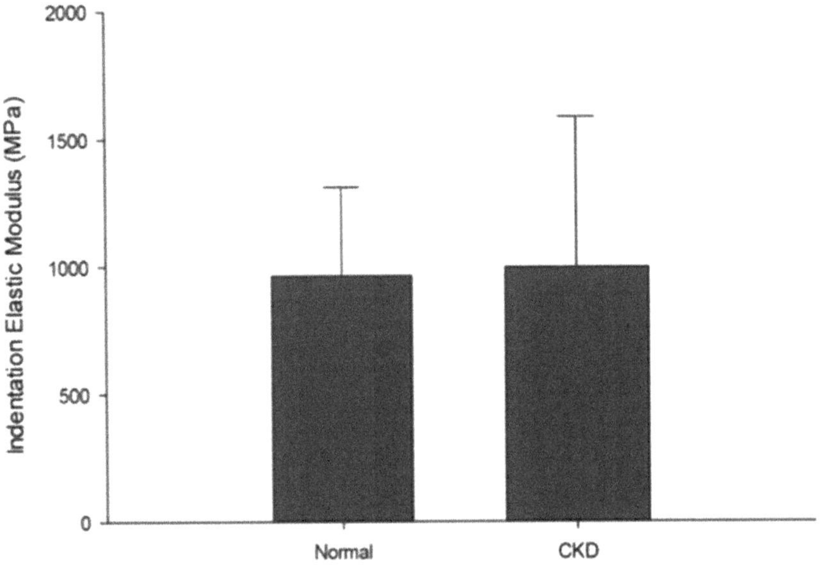

Figure 4b

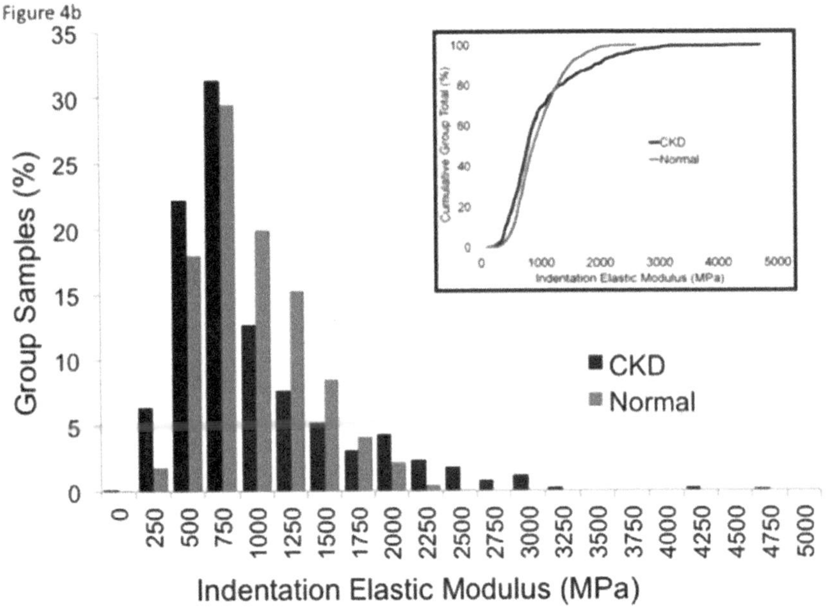

Figure 4. Nanoindenation reveals that CKD skeletal tissue has increased heterogeneity in the elastic modulus compared to normal bone. There was no significant difference in the average elastic modulus (A), but the distribution of elastic modulus values was significantly broader (B), with a greater proportion of both high and low values in CKD relative to normal ($p<0.0001$).

Raman spectroscopy[14–15]. While Raman spectroscopy has been utilized to detect AGEs in ocular tissue[54], its ability to detect changes in bone is unknown as HPLC is the standard method used to measure AGEs in skeletal tissue[53,55–58]. Here, having employed HPLC, thehypothesized increases in AGE content were not observed. While increases may occur with more advanced disease in theseanimals, the relationship between circulating pentosidineand its accumulation in bone collagen in CKDremains unresolved.

At present, clinical data on bone quality in CKD are minimal. Aside from the aforementioned dialysis study [53], CKD patients with high bone turnover had reduced stiffness and a decreased mineral-to-matrix ratio as assessed on iliac crest biopsies [59]. As these data are from cancellous bone, though, direct comparison with the current work on cortical bone is difficult. Connecting these dots by examining cortical bone properties in patients (which is possible with iliac crest biopsies) and cancellous properties in rats will be an essential step in moving forward.

Limitations to the current study should also be recognized. First, because tissue from a previous study was used, the sample sizes used here were small. Hence, any applications to other animal models or patients should occur with a measure of caution. Second, the mechanical assessments were localized to the periosteal surface, which may not be fully representative of the entire cortex. As such, the assessed parameters may differ at other cortical sites. Finally, this study assessed material properties in 30-week-old animals. As the disease progresses, differences in composition and morphologymay arise.Nevertheless, the advan-

Table 2. Tissue composition and collagen morphology.

Raman	Normal (n = 6)	Cy/+ (n = 6)	p-values
Crystallinity (1/FWHM PO_4^{3-}v1)	0.054±0.001	0.055±0.001	*0.4421
Carbonate Substitution (CO_3^{2-}v1/PO_4^{3-}v1)	0.618±0.037	0.608±0.019	#0.5375
Relative Mineralization (PO_4^{3-}v1/Amide I)	2.539±0.253	2.699±0.317	*0.9372
AFM	**Normal (n = 6)**	**Cy/+ (n = 5)**	**p-values**
D-Periodicity (nm)	65.641±0.646	65.864±0.838	*0.631
HPLC	**Normal (n = 8)**	**Cy/+ (n = 6)**	**p-values**
Pyridinoline per Collagen (mol/mol)	0.60±0.17	0.54±0.10	**0.252
Deoxypyridinoline per Collagen (mol/mol)	0.37±0.07	0.37±0.04	**0.974
Pentosidine per Collagen (mol/mol)	878± 153	921±148	*0.523

Values are presented as mean ± standard deviation.
*equal variances t-test.
**unequal variances t-test.
#Wilcoxon ranked-sum test.

tage of using 30-week-old animals is that these animals are skeletally mature but do not yet exhibit the rampant increase in cortical porosity present at 35 weeks [32].

In conclusion, these data show that both microscale and nanoscale cortical bone material properties are altered in an animal model of CKD. The specific skeletal tissue alterations responsible for these mechanical differences remain unclear. Nevertheless, in addition to bone loss and cortical porosity, defects in material-level mechanical properties may also contribute to the increased fracture risk associated with CKD.

Acknowledgments

We would like to thank Mr. Drew Brown for his assistance with analysis and tissue harvesting. We would also like to acknowledge the late Dr. Vincent H. Gattone II, who was instrumental in developing this animal model.

Author Contributions

Conceived and designed the experiments: CLN SMM JMW MRA. Performed the experiments: CLN NXC MAH JMW JSN. Analyzed the data: CLN MAH JMW JSN. Contributed to the writing of the manuscript: CLN SMM JMW JSN MRA.

References

1. Levey AS, Eckardt KU, Tsukamoto Y, Levin A, Coresh J, et al. (2005). Definition and classification of chronic kidney disease: a position statement from Kidney Disease Improving Global Outcomes (KDIGO). Kidney Int 67:2089–2100.
2. Levin A, Bakris GL, Molitch M, Smulders M, Tian J, et al. (2007) Prevalence of abnormal serum vitamin D, PTH, calcium, and phosphorus in patients with chronic kidney disease: results of the study to evaluate early kidney disease. Kidney Int 71:31–38.
3. KDIGO Working Group (2009) KDIGO clinical practice guideline for the diagnosis, evaluation, prevention, and treatment of Chronic Kidney Disease-Mineral and Bone Disorder (CKD-MBD). Kidney Int 76: S1–S130.
4. Cejka D, Patsch JM, Weber M, Diarra D, Riegersperger M, et al. (2011) Bone microarchitecture in hemodialysis patients assessed by HR-pQCT. Clin J Am Soc Nephrol 6:2264–71.
5. Nickolas TL, Stein E, Cohen A, Thomas V, Staron RB, et al. (2010) Bone mass and microarchitecture in CKD patients with fracture. J Am Soc Nephrol 21:1371–1380.
6. Nickolas TL, Cremers S, Zhang A, Thomas V, Stein E, et al. (2011) Discriminants of prevalent fractures in chronic kidney disease. J Am Soc Nephrol 22:1560–1572.
7. Fried LF, Biggs ML, Shlipak MG, Seliger S, Kestenbaum B, et al. (2007) Association of kidney function with incident hip fracture in older adults. J Am Soc Nephrol 18:282–286.
8. Nickolas TL, McMahon DJ, Shane E (2006) Relationship between moderate to severe kidney disease and hip fracture in the United States. J Am Soc Nephrol 17:3223–3232.
9. Nitsch D, Mylne A, Roderick PJ, Smeeth, Hubbard R, et al. (2009) Chronic kidney disease and hip-fracture-related mortality in older people in the UK. Nephrol Dial Transplant 24:1539–1544.
10. Cole JH, van der Muelen MCH (2011) Whole bone mechanics and bone quality. ClinOrthopRelat Res 469:2139–2149.
11. Seeman E, Delmas PD (2006) Bone quality: the material and structural basis of bone strength and fragility. N Engl J Med 354:2250–2261.
12. Allen MR, Chen NX, Gattone II VH, Chen X, Carr AJ, et al. (2013) Skeletal effects of zoledronic acid in an animal model of chronic kidney disease. OsteoporosInt 24:1471–1481.
13. Iwamoto J, Seki A, Sato Y, Matsumoto H (2012) Vitamin K2 improves renal function and increases femoral bone strength in rats with renal insufficiency. Calcif Tissue Int 90:50–59.
14. Iwasaki Y, Kazama JJ, Yamato H, Fukagawa M (2011) Changes in chemical composition of cortical bone associated with bone fragility in rat model with chronic kidney disease. Bone 48:1260–1267.
15. Iwasaki Y, Kazama JJ, Yamato H, Shimoda H, Fukagawa M (2013) Accumulated uremic toxins attenuate bone mechanical properties in rats with chronic kidney disease. Bone 57:477–483.
16. Jokihaara J, Porsti I, Pajamaki I, Vuohelainen T, Jolma P, et al. (2006) Paracalcitol [19-nor-1,25-(OH)2D2] in the treatment of experimental renal bone disease. J Bone Miner Res 21:745–751.
17. Moe SM, Radcliffe JS, White KE, Gattone VH II, Seifert MF, et al. (2011) The pathophysiology of early-stage chronic kidney disease–mineral bone disorder (CKD-MBD) and response to phosphate binders in the rat. J Bone Miner Res 26:2672–2681.
18. Sabbagh Y, Graciolli FG, O'Brien S, Tang W, dos Reis LM, et al. (2012) Repression of osteocyte Wnt/β-catenin signaling is an early event in the progression of renal osteodystrophy. J Bone Miner Res, 27:1757–1772.
19. Malluche HH, Porter DS, Pienkowski D (2013) Evaluating bone quality in patients with chronic kidney disease. Nat Rev Nephrol 9:671–680.
20. Kadokawa S, Matsumoto T, Naito H, Tanaka M (2011) Assessment of trabecular bone architecture and intrinsic properties of cortical bone tissue in a mouse model of chronic kidney disease. J Hard Tissue Biol 20: 79–86.
21. Moe SM, Chen NX, Seifert MF, Sinders RM, Duan D, et al. (2009) A rat model of chronic kidney disease-mineral bone disorder. Kidney Int 75:176–184.
22. Nagao S, Kugita M, Yoshihara D, Yamaguchi T (2012) Animal models for human polycystic kidney disease. Exp Anim Tokyo 61:477–488.
23. Stagner EE, Bouvrette DJ, Cheng J, Bryda EC (2009) The polycystic kidney disease-related proteins Bicc1 and SamCystin interact. BiochemBioph Res Co 383:16–21.
24. Shobeiri N, Adams MA, Holden RM (2010) Vascular calcification in animal models of CKD: a review. Am J Nephrol 31:471–481.
25. Gattone VH II, Tourkow BA, Trambaugh CM, Yu AC, Whelan S, et al. (2004)Development of multiorgan pathology in the *wpk* rat model of polycystic kidney disease. Anat Rec 277A:384–395.

26. Nagao S, Morita M, Kugita M, Yoshihara D, Yamaguchi T, et al. (2010) Polycystic kidney disease in Han:SPRD Cy rats is associated with elevated expression and mislocalizationof SamCystin. Am J Physiol Renal Physiol 299:F1078–F1086.
27. Aref M, Gallant MA, Organ JM, Wallace JM, Newman CL, et al. (2013) *In vivo* reference point indentation reveals positive effects of raloxifene on mechanical properties following 6 months of treatment in skeletally mature beagle dogs. Bone 56:449–53.
28. Hammond MA, Gallant MA, Burr DB, Wallace JM (2014) Nanoscale changes in collagen are reflected in physical and mechanical properties of bone at the microscale indiabetic rats. Bone 60:26–32.
29. Wallace JM (2012) Applications of atomic force microscopy for the assessment of nanoscale morphological and mechanical properties of bone. Bone 50:420–427.
30. Buckley A, Hill KE, Davidson JM (1988) Collagen metabolism. In:Colowick SP, Kaplan NO, Di SabatoG, editors. Methods in Enzymology: Immunochemical Techniques, Part M: Chemotaxis and inflammation. London: Academic Press. pp. 674–693.
31. Saito M, Marumo K, Fujii K, Ishioka N (1997) Single-column high-performance liquid chromatographic-fluorescence detection of immature, mature, and senescent cross-links of collagen. Anal Biochem 253:26–32
32. Moe SM, Chen NX, Newman CL, Gattone VH II, Organ JM, et al. (2014) A comparison of calcium to zoledronic acid for improvement of cortical bone in an animal model of CKD. J Bone Miner Res 29:902–910.
33. Gallant MA, Brown DM, Organ JM, Allen MR, Burr DB (2013) Reference-point indentation correlates with bone toughness assessed using whole-bone traditional mechanical testing. Bone 53:301–305.
34. Iimori S, Mori Y, Akita W, Kuyama T, Takada S, et al. (2012) Diagnostic usefulness of bone mineral density and biochemical markers of bone turnover in predicting fracture in CKD stage 5D patients—a single-center cohort study. Nephrol Dial Transplant 27:345–351.
35. Jamal SA, Hayden JA, Beyene J (2007) Low bone mineral density and fractures in long-term hemodialysis patients: a meta-analysis. Am J Kidney Dis 49:674–681.
36. Jamal SA, Cheung AM, West SL, Lok C (2012) Bone mineral density by DXA and HR pQCT can discriminate fracture status in men and women with stages 3 to 5 chronic kidney disease. OsteoporosInt 23:2805–2813.
37. Jassal SK, von Muhlen D, Barrett-Connor E (2007) Measures of renal function, BMD, bone loss, and osteoporotic fracture in older adults: the Rancho Bernardo study. J Bone Miner Res 22:203–210.
38. Klawansky S, Komaroff E, Cavanaugh PFJr, Mitchell DY, Gordon MJ, et al. (2003) Relationship between age, renal function and bone mineral density in the US population. OsteoporosInt 14:570–576.
39. Piraino B, Chen T, Cooperstein L, Segre G, Puschett J (1988) Fractures and vertebral bone mineral density in patients with renal osteodystrophy. ClinNephrol 30:57–62.
40. Yamaguchi T, Kanno E, TsubotaJ, Shiomi T, Nakai M, et al. (1996) Retrospective study on the usefulness of radius and lumbar bone density in the separation of hemodialysis patients with fractures from those without fractures. Bone 19:549–555.
41. Diez-Perez A, Güerri R, Nogues X, Caceres E, Pena MJ, et al. (2010)Micro-Microindentationfor in vivo measurement of bone tissue mechanical properties in humans. J Bone Miner Res 25:1877–1885.
42. Güerri-Fernández RC, Nogués X, Quesada Gómez JM, Torres Del Pliego E, Puig L, et al. (2013)Microindentation for in vivo measurement of bone tissue material properties in atypical femoral fracture patients and controls. J Bone Miner Res 28:162–168.
43. Farr JN, Drake MT, Amin S, Melton LJ III, McCready LK, et al. (2014) *In Vivo* assessment of bone quality in postmenopausal women with type 2 diabetes. J Bone Miner Res 29:787–795.
44. Tai K, Dao M, Suresh S, Palazoglu A, Ortiz C (2007) Nanoscale heterogeneity promotes energy dissipation in bone. Nat Mater 6:454–462.
45. Phelps JB, Hubbard GB, Wang X, Agrawal CM (2000) Microstructural heterogeneity and the fracture toughness of bone. J Biomed Mater Res 51:735–741.
46. Currey J (2005) Structural heterogeneity in bone: good or bad? J MusculoskeletNeuronal Interact 5:317.
47. Aoki C, Uto K, Honda K, Kato Y, Oda H(2013) Advanced glycation end products suppress lysyl oxidase and induce bone collagen degradation in a rat model of renal osteodystrophy. Lab Invest 93:1170–1183.
48. Galli F (2007) Protein damage and inflammation in uraemia and dialysis patients. Nephrol Dial Transplant 22 (Suppl 5):v20–36.
49. Miyata T, Ueda Y, Shinzato T, Iida Y, Tanaka S, et al. (1996) Accumulation of albumin-linked and free-form pentosidine in the circulation of uremic patients with end-stage renal failure: renal implications in the pathophysiology of pentosidine. J Am Soc Nephrol 7:1198–1206.
50. Sakata N, Noma A, Yamamoto Y, Okamoto K, Meng J, et al. (2003) Modification of elastin by pentosidine is associated with the calcification of aortic media in patients with end-stage renal disease. Nephrol Dial Transplant 18:1601–1609.
51. Zoccali C, Mallamaci F, Asahia K, Benedetto FA, Tripepi G, et al. (2001) Pentosidine, carotid atherosclerosis and alterations in left ventricular geometry in hemodialysis patients. J Nephrol 14:293–298.
52. Arsov S, Graaff R, van Oeveren W, Stegmayr B, Sikole A, et al. (2014) Advanced glycation end-products and skin autofluorescence in end-stage renal disease: a review. ClinChem Lab Med 52:11–20.
53. Mitome J, Yamamato H, Saito M, Yokoyama K, Marumo K, et al. (2011)Nonenzymaticcross-linking pentosidine increase in bone collagen and are associated with disorders of bone mineralization in dialysis patients. Calcif Tissue Int 88:521–529.
54. Glenn JV, Beattie JR, Barrett L, Frizzell N, Thorpe SR, et al. (2007) Confocal Raman microscopy can quantify advanced glycation end product (AGE) modifications in Bruch's membrane leading to accurate, nondestructive prediction of ocular aging. FASEB J 21:3542–52.
55. Nyman JS, Roy A, Acuna RL, Gayle HJ, Reyes MJ, et al. (2006). Age-related effect on the concentration of collagen crosslinks in human osteonal and interstitial bone tissue. Bone 39:1210–1217.
56. Odetti P, Rossi S, Monacelli F, Poggi A, Cirnigliaro M, et al. (2005) Advanced glycationend products and bone loss during aging. Ann NY AcadSci 1043:710–717.
57. Saito M, Fujii K, Mori Y, Marumo K (2006) Role of enzymatic and glycation induced cross-links as a determinant of bone quality in spontaneously diabetic WBN/Kob rats. Osteoporosis Int 17: 1514–1523.
58. Silva MJ, Brodt MD, Lynch MA, McKenzie JA, Tanouye KM, et al. (2009) Type 1 diabetes in young rats leads to progressive trabecular bone loss, cessation of cortical bone growth, and diminished whole bone strength and fatigue life. J Bone Miner Res 24: 1618–1627.
59. Malluche HH, Porter DS, Monier-Faugere M, Mawad H, Pienkowski D (2012)Differences in bone quality in low- and high-turnover renal osteodystrophy. J Am Soc Nephrol 23:525–532.

7

Neovascular Niche for Human Myeloma Cells in Immunodeficient Mouse Bone

Hirono Iriuchishima[1,6,❡], Keiyo Takubo[1*,❡], Yoshitaka Miyakawa[2], Ayako Nakamura-Ishizu[1], Yoshiteru Miyauchi[3], Nobuyuki Fujita[3], Kana Miyamoto[3], Takeshi Miyamoto[3], Eiji Ikeda[4], Masahiro Kizaki[2,5], Yoshihisa Nojima[6], Toshio Suda[1*]

1 Department of Cell Differentiation, The Sakaguchi Laboratory of Developmental Biology, Keio University School of Medicine, Tokyo, Japan, **2** Division of Hematology, Department of Internal Medicine, Keio University School of Medicine, Tokyo, Japan, **3** Department of Orthopedic Surgery, Keio University School of Medicine, Tokyo, Japan, **4** Department of Pathology, Yamaguchi University Graduate School of Medicine, Ube, Yamaguchi, Japan, **5** Department of Hematology, Saitama Medical Center, Saitama Medical University, Saitama, Japan, **6** Department of Medicine and Clinical Science, Gunma University Graduate School of Medicine, Maebashi, Gunma, Japan

Abstract

The interaction with bone marrow (BM) plays a crucial role in pathophysiological features of multiple myeloma (MM), including cell proliferation, chemoresistance, and bone lesion progression. To characterize the MM-BM interactions, we utilized an *in vivo* experimental model for human MM in which a GFP-expressing human MM cell line is transplanted into NOG mice (the NOG-hMM model). Transplanted MM cells preferentially engrafted at the metaphyseal region of the BM endosteum and formed a complex with osteoblasts and osteoclasts. A subpopulation of MM cells expressed VE-cadherin after transplantation and formed endothelial-like structures in the BM. $CD138^{+}$ myeloma cells in the BM were reduced by p53-dependent apoptosis following administration of the nitrogen mustard derivative bendamustine to mice in the NOG-hMM model. Bendamustine maintained the osteoblast lining on the bone surface and protected extracellular matrix structures. Furthermore, bendamustine suppressed the growth of osteoclasts and mesenchymal cells in the NOG-hMM model. Since VE-cadherin^{+} MM cells were chemoresistant, hypoxic, and HIF-2α-positive compared to the VE-cadherin^{-} population, VE-cadherin induction might depend on the oxygenation status. The NOG-hMM model described here is a useful system to analyze the dynamics of MM pathophysiology, interactions of MM cells with other cellular compartments, and the utility of novel anti-MM therapies.

Editor: Wolfgang Wagner, RWTH Aachen University Medical School, Germany

Funding: H.I. is a research fellow of Japan Society for the Promotion of Science. K.T. is supported by a MEXT Grant-in-Aid for Young Scientists (A). T.S. and K.T. were supported by MEXT a Grant-in-Aid for Scientific Research on Innovative Areas and a MEXT Grant-in-Aid for Scientific Research (A). The funders had no role in study design, data collection and analysis, decision to publish, or preparation of the manuscript.

Competing Interests: T.S. is a member of the scientific advisory board of Symbio Pharmaceuticals Ltd.

* E-mail: keiyot@gmail.com (KT); sudato@sc.itc.keio.ac.jp (TS)

❡ These authors contributed equally to this work.

Introduction

Multiple myeloma (MM) is a clonal disorder of late-stage B cells, in which transformed plasma cells expand and accumulate in the bone marrow (BM), leading to cytopenia, bone resorption and the production of the characteristic monoclonal immunoglobulin [1]. The bone marrow (BM) is believed to play a crucial role in the pathophysiological features of MM, including cell proliferation, chemoresistance and bone lesion progression. The "MM niche" is composed of osteoblasts, osteoclasts, vascular endothelial cells, stromal cells, adipocytes, and extracellular matrix (ECM) proteins [2]. MM cells are thought to be maintained by these various stromal cells [3], which regulate their survival, proliferation and apoptosis. However, the cellular and anatomical features of stromal cells have not been thoroughly examined in the MM. In this study, the MM niche was characterized in the BM of a mouse transplanted with human MM cells.

Recently, chemotherapeutic strategies for the treatment of MM have significantly advanced, including the development of anti-angiogenic drugs [4]. Using the MM mouse model, the suppressive effects of bendamustine, a bifunctional chemotherapeutic agent with a nitrogen mustard structure and a purine benzimidazole ring, were examined. Because of its unique structure, bendamustine exhibits only partial cross-resistance with other alkylators [5–7] and is widely used for the treatment of various hematological malignancies, including low-grade lymphoma and MM [8,9]. Although the clinical utility of bendamustine in the treatment of MM has been clearly demonstrated [10,11], the specific cellular and molecular effects of bendamustine on MM cells and the MM niche *in vivo* have not been determined. Therefore, this issue was investigated in a mouse model of human MM.

Results

Establishment of a human multiple myeloma in NOD/SCID/γ_c^{null} mice

When U266 cells, a human IgE-producing myeloma cell line, were transplanted into super-immunodeficient NOG mice [12], the cells engrafted and proliferated in the BM but not in any other organs. These mice exhibited various MM clinical symptoms, including the development of osteolytic bone lesions [13]. To analyze the myeloma niche more precisely, U266 cells stably expressing EGFP (U266-GFP) were transplanted into NOG mice (NOG-hMM model). 2×10^6 U266-GFP cells were intravenously inoculated into irradiated NOG mice (2.4 Gy), and recipient mice were sacrificed 2–6 weeks after transplantation to assess the establishment of the MM (Fig. 1A). After 4 weeks, the recipient NOG mice all developed bilateral paralysis and pathological fractures. Radiologic examination revealed severe scoliosis (Fig. 1B). Because GFP fluorescence in transplanted U266-GFP cells tended to decrease *in vivo* (data not shown), we used CD138, a pan-myeloma marker, to detect U266-GFP cells. Flow cytometric analysis of the BM revealed myeloma cells positive for human CD138 and negative for mouse CD45 (Fig. 1C). Furthermore, human IgE was detected in the sera of recipient mice at 5 days after transplantation and was drastically increased at day 35 post-transplantation (Fig. 1D).

The human MM niche in the BM of NOG mice

Engraftment of GFP-positive myeloma cells was detected in the BM but not in the spleen, liver, or any other organs (Fig. 1E). To characterize the myeloma niche *in vivo*, the recipient long bones, including the femur and tibia, were analyzed because their anatomical and histological structures in the hematopoietic niche have been well characterized. Within the BM of the long bone, myeloma cells were located mainly in the endosteal zone in the femur (Fig. 1E), indicating that the endosteal zone of the BM is the preferential location for myeloma engraftment. Next, the temporal distribution of myeloma cells in the BM was investigated. At the early stage (2–4 weeks after transplantation), myeloma cells were

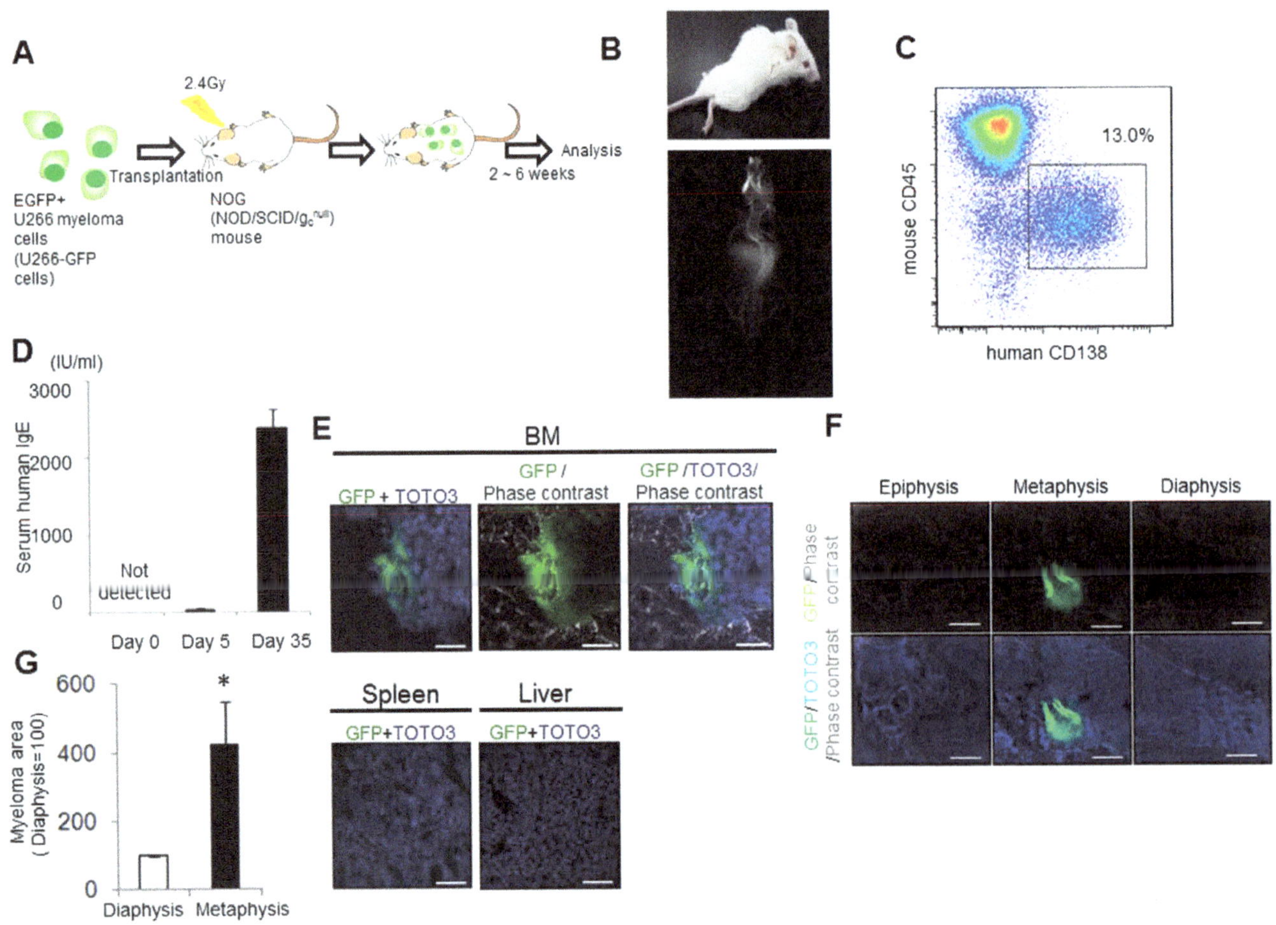

Figure 1. Interaction between multiple myeloma cells and the niche in an *in vivo* human myeloma model. A. Study design of the NOG-hMM model. Two million EGFP$^+$ U266 myeloma (U266-EGFP) cells were intravenously inoculated into 2.4 Gy irradiated NOG (NOD/SCID/g_c^{null}) mice. Two to six weeks after transplantation, mice were sacrificed for analysis. **B.** Representative clinical manifestation (upper panel) and radiologic examination (lower panel) of mice 4 weeks after transplantation. All mice showed hind leg paralyses (left) associated with spinal compression fractures (left; arrow). This clinical manifestation was observed in more than 20 mice. **C.** Representative FACS plot of U266-EGFP cell-transplanted NOG mice. Bone marrow of NOG mice was analyzed by FACS 4 weeks after U266-EGFP cell transplantation using anti-human CD138 antibody and anti-murine CD45 antibody. The experiment was performed in more than forty mice with similar results. **D.** Serum levels of human IgE. Human IgE levels in the serum of NOG mice at 0 (non-transplanted, non-irradiated mice), 5 or 35 days after transplantation with U266-EGFP cells were analyzed by ELISA ($n = 3$–5, mean $\pm$ SD). The experiment was performed twice with similar results. **E.** Double immunohistochemistry (IHC) of EGFP (green) and TOTO3 (blue) of the BM (upper panels), spleen or liver (lower panels) at 2 weeks after transplantation. U266-EGFP cells engrafted only in the BM. Representative data from 10 to 20 fields from the BM of two mice from three independent experiments are shown. Bars = 200 μm. **F.** Immunohistochemical (IHC) analysis of EGFP (green) and TOTO3 (blue) at the anatomical region of long bones at the early stage. Representative data from 10 to 20 fields from the BM of two mice from three independent experiments are shown. Bars = 200 μm. **G.** Quantification of U266-EGFP cells at the diaphysis and the metaphysis of the long bones. U266-EGFP at the metaphysis regions is represented relative to the diaphysis region (diaphysis = 100, $n = 3$, mean $\pm$ SEM). The experiment was performed twice with similar results.

primarily observed at the metaphyseal region (the wide portion of a long bone adjacent to the epiphyseal plate) but not in the epiphyseal region (the rounded end of a long bone) or the diaphyseal region (the mid-section of a long bone) of the BM (Fig. 1F). CD138$^+$ myeloma cells at the later stage (4–9 weeks after transplantation) were distributed mainly in the metaphyseal region and were relatively rare in the diaphyseal region in the femur (Fig. 1G).

Immunohistochemical analysis of the MM component at the early stage (2 weeks after transplantation) revealed that GFP-positive myeloma cells formed a complex with alkaline phosphatase (ALP)-positive osteoblasts and matrix metalloprotease (MMP) 9-positive osteoclasts in the femoral endosteum (Fig. 2A). Under normal conditions, NOG mice possess more tartrate-resistant acid phosphatase (TRAP)-positive osteoclasts in the metaphyseal region than in the diaphyseal region in the femur (Fig. 2B, left panels). At 4 weeks after transplantation, increased TRAP activity, which represents an increase in osteoclasts, was observed in the metaphyseal region but not in the femoral diaphyseal region (Fig. 2B, right panels). These data suggest that the myeloma niche is located in the metaphyseal endosteal zone of the longitudinal bone and is composed of osteoblasts and osteoclasts *in vivo*.

VE-cadherin expression and vascular mimicry of the MM cells

It is well known that increased vasculature accompanies active myeloma [14–16]. Therefore, the relationship between endothelial and myeloma cells was analyzed. Flow cytometric analysis revealed a VE-cadherin$^+$ subpopulation of human CD138$^+$ myeloma cells *in vivo* (Fig. 3A). Interestingly, these VE-cadherin$^+$ cells were not detected *in vitro* and were only observed after the transplantation of U266-GFP cells into NOG mice (Fig. 3A). These VE-cadherin$^+$ cells formed vascular-like structures in the femoral BM (Fig. 3B). To further characterize the VE-cadherin$^+$ cell population, VE-cadherin$^+$ cells and VE-cadherin$^-$ cells were sorted from the CD138$^+$ fraction and the expression of angiogenesis-related genes in each subpopulation was analyzed using human-specific primer sets. MM cells have been reported to secrete vascular endothelial growth factor (VEGF)-A into the BM microenvironment to induce angiogenesis [17]. Consistent with previous reports, human interleukin (IL)-6, VEGF-A, and fibroblast growth factor (FGF)-2 were expressed in both fractions (Fig. 3C–E). In particular, the expression of FGF-2 was significantly increased in the VE-cadherin$^+$ fraction (Fig. 3E). These data suggest that FGF-2 is involved in myeloma angiogenesis and may induce the formation of vascular endothelial-like structures by a subpopulation of VE-cadherin$^+$ cells. Although it is rare, human cancer cells are known to sometimes fuse with endothelial cells to form hybrid cells [18]. To address this possibility, fluorescence *in situ* hybridization (FISH) analysis was performed on the VE-cadherin$^+$ and VE-cadherin$^-$ CD138$^+$ cells from NOG-hMM mice. Cultured U266-GFP cells were used as a negative control. Fused cells were very rare ($<0.1\%$) and not specific to the VE-cadherin$^+$ subpopulation (Table S1). These data indicate that human VE-cadherin$^+$ CD138$^+$ cells were generated in the BM microenvironment *in vivo*.

In vivo effect of bendamustine

Using the NOG-hMM model, the antitumor effect of bendamustine was assessed *in vivo*. A single dose (Fig. 4A) or two doses over the course of a week (Fig. 4B) of bendamustine (20 mg/kg) were injected intraperitoneally into myeloma-inoculated NOG mice 5 days after transplantation, at which point MM cells had already engrafted into the BM. These mice were analyzed at 4–6 weeks after administration (Fig. 4A) or when the mice had developed symptoms (Fig. 4B). At the early stage after transplantation, myeloma cells were only observed at the metaphyseal region of the BM (Fig. 1F). However, in the later stage (Fig. 4C left), at which time the recipient mice were treated with bendamustine, myeloma cells had infiltrated the diaphyseal zone of the bone. In response to sequential bendamustine administration, femoral diaphyseal myeloma cells were largely depleted (Fig. 4C). In non-treated mice, myeloma cells accumulated in the metaphyseal region rather than in the diaphyseal region of the femur (Fig. 4D, left). Although bendamustine treatment largely depleted the MM cells (Fig. 4D, right), there were some instances of bendamustine-resistant myeloma cells which were positive for VE-cadherin (Fig. 4E).

Remaining VE-cadherin$^+$ MM cells express HIF-2α in response to hypoxia

The hypoxic status of the BM is an important niche characteristic [19]. The hypoxia-inducible transcription factor HIF-2α is known to induce VE-cadherin expression [20]. Therefore, levels of the hypoxic marker pimonidazole and levels of HIF-1α and HIF-2α were compared between the VE-cadherin$^+$ and VE-cadherin$^-$ MM fractions. The expression level of HIF-2α was higher in the VE-cadherin$^+$ cell fraction than in the VE-cadherin$^-$ cell fraction, and, interestingly, was induced after transplantation into NOG mice (Fig. 4F). VE-cadherin$^+$ MM cells showed higher levels of pimonidazole and HIF-1α protein than VE-cadherin$^-$ MM cells (Fig. 4G, H). These data indicate that the HIF-2α-VE-cadherin pathway is activated by hypoxia in a subset of MM cells.

The effect of bendamustine treatment on the paracrine loop of angiogenic factors was also examined *in vivo*. Human VEGFA and IL-6 transcript levels were significantly reduced after bendamustine treatment, but FGF-2 transcript levels remained unchanged (Fig. 4I). These results indicate that bendamustine could suppress myeloma cells and affect the myeloma niche by inhibiting VEGFA and IL-6 production.

Characterization of the extracellular matrix components and mesenchymal cells in the MM niche

To further characterize the myeloma niche, the expression and structure of the extracellular matrix (ECM) components of the BM, including fibronectin, type IV collagen (col IV) and α-laminin, were analyzed. Metaphyseal MM BM of the femur showed disruption of each of these ECM components (Fig. 5B, right; 5D, right; 5F, right). In addition, ECM structures in the non-MM diaphyseal areas of the femur were increased and disorganized compared to normal NOG mice (Fig. 5A–F). The presence of another component of the BM, nestin$^+$ mesenchymal cells [21], was also examined in myeloma. While nestin$^+$ cells were rare in the femoral BM of normal NOG mice (Fig. 5G, top), nestin$^+$ cells were drastically increased in the femoral BM of MM mice (Fig. 5G, middle). Interestingly, CD138$^+$ MM cells were located in close contact with nestin$^+$ cells (Fig. 5G, middle). Moreover, nestin$^+$ cells in NOG-hMM mice were increased in the non-MM areas of the femoral BM (Fig. 5G, bottom). Although nestin$^+$ cells are normally located adjacent to the vasculature [21], nestin$^+$ cells in NOG-hMM mice did not co-localize with endothelial cells (Fig. 5H). These data suggest that myeloma cells promote ECM reorganization and nestin$^+$ cell proliferation, which might create an abnormal microenvironment that promotes tumor progression and drug resistance in MM.

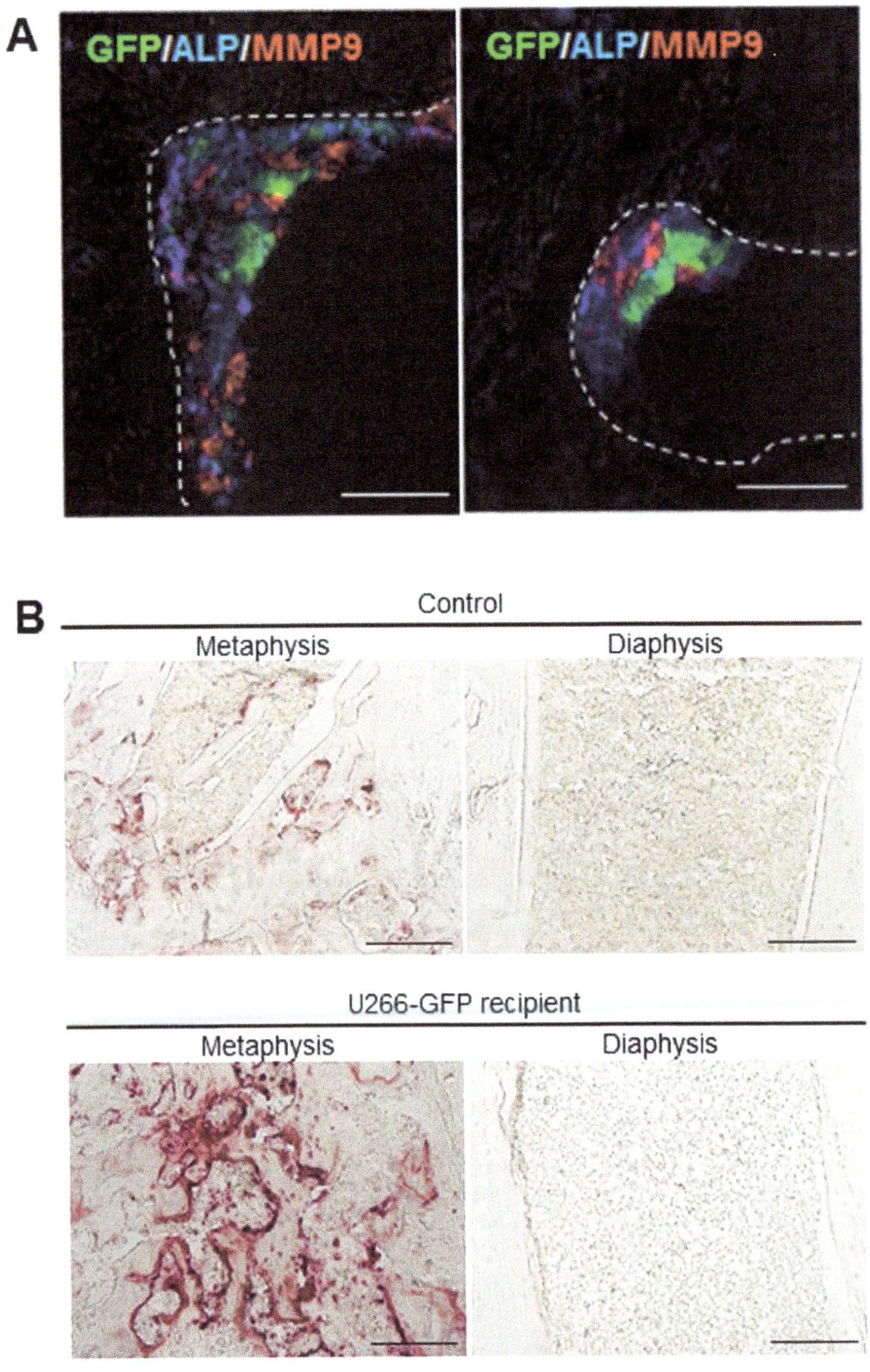

Figure 2. Dynamics of osteoblasts and osteoclasts at the MM niche. A. Triple IHC of GFP (green), ALP (blue) and MMP-9 (red) in the metaphyseal region at 2 weeks after U266-EGFP cell transplantation. Myeloma cells form a cellular complex with osteoblasts and osteoclasts *in vivo*. Representative data from 10 to 20 fields from the BM of two mice from three independent experiments are shown. Bars = 50 μm. **B.** Regional differences in TRAP-positive osteoclast cells in the long bones. Micrographs of TRAP staining of the metaphysis and the diaphysis at 4 weeks after U266-EGFP cell transplantation. Whereas the development of TRAP-positive osteoclast cells is barely discernable in the diaphysis region, a number of TRAP-positive osteoclast cells are evident in the metaphysis region. The experiment was performed three times with similar results. Bars = 200 μm.

Bendamustine maintains the normal BM niche and suppresses pathological myelofibrosis

After a single bendamustine treatment, the osteoblast lining on the femoral surface of the treated mice, which was disrupted without treatment, was observed to be intact (Fig. 6A). TRAP staining of single bendamustine-treated mice showed a decrease in the number and size of osteoclasts compared to PBS-treated (non-treated) mice (Fig. 6B), while bendamustine had no direct effect on osteoclast numbers (data not shown). ECM structures of the femoral BM, such as fibronectin, col IV and α-laminin, were maintained by single bendamustine treatment (Fig. 6C–E). Moreover, treatment with bendamustine also suppressed the

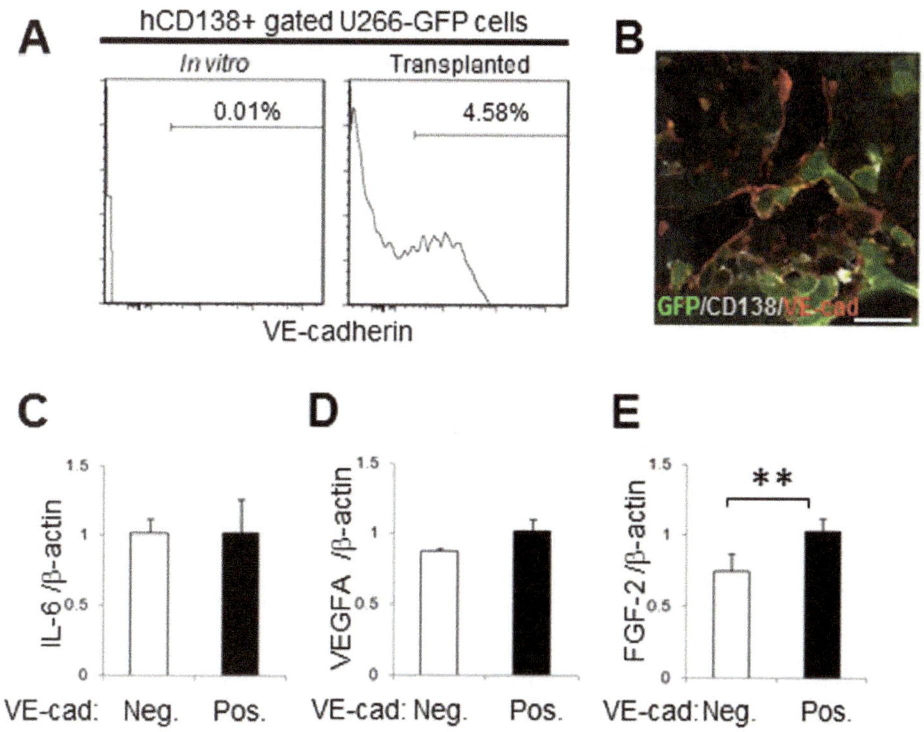

Figure 3. MM cells express VE-cadherin and form endothelial-like structures in the BM. A. Flow cytometric detection of VE-cadherin in U266-EGFP cells *in vitro* (left) or transplanted U266-EGFP cells (right) using anti-human VE-cadherin antibody. The experiment was performed with more than twenty mice with similar results. **B.** Triple IHC of GFP (green), human CD138 (gray) and VE-cadherin (red) within the diaphyseal region at 4 weeks after U266-EGFP cell transplantation. Representative data from four fields from the BM of three mice in two independent experiments are shown. Bars = 20 μm. **C–E.** Quantitative PCR analysis of IL-6 (**B**), VEGFA (**C**) or FGF-2 (**D**) transcripts in the VE-cadherin$^+$ or VE-cadherin$^-$ MM fractions five weeks after U266-EGFP cell transplantation. Each value was normalized to β-actin expression and is expressed as the fold induction compared to VE-cadherin$^+$ samples (mean ± SD, $^{**}P<0.01$, n = 4). The experiment was performed twice with similar results.

proliferation of nestin$^+$ cells (Fig. 6F). These data suggest that bendamustine treatment affects not only myeloma cells but also the surrounding niche cells.

Because myeloma often includes pathological myelofibrosis [22], the effect of bendamustine on myelofibrosis was examined. Moderate reticulin-positive fibrosis was noted in the non-treated BM of thoracic vertebrae (Fig. 6G, left); however, no fibrosis was observed in the BM of mice treated with a single dose of bendamustine (Fig. 6G, right). Masson trichrome staining, which detects collagen deposition, revealed several significant fibrotic regions in the non-treated BM of thoracic vertebrae (Fig. 6H, left). On the other hand, no collagen fibrosis was evident in the BM of mice treated with a single dose of bendamustine (Fig. 6H, right). These data indicate that bendamustine suppresses pathological myelofibrosis *in vivo*.

Hematological maintenance by bendamustine administration

Human IgE levels in the serum of mice receiving a single bendamustine administration were significantly suppressed compared to the non-treated group (Fig. 7A). In histological studies, massive infiltration of myeloma cells was observed in the thoracic vertebrae of non-treated mice, and normal hematopoiesis was minimal (Fig. 7B, left). However, a number of normal hematopoietic cells, including megakaryocytes, were observed in the BM of single bendamustine-administrated NOG mice (Fig. 7B, right). Flow cytometric analysis of non-treated and bendamustine-treated groups showed that the percentage of myeloma cells was decreased in bendamustine-treated mice (Fig. 7C).

Bendamustine induces p53-dependent apoptosis and suppresses myeloma cells *in vivo*

To clarify the molecular mechanism of bendamustine *in vivo*, apoptotic activity was analyzed by detection of cleaved caspase-3. In bendamustine-treated mice, the number of cleaved caspase-3$^+$ myeloma cells was significantly increased (Fig. 8A, B). Immunocytochemical analysis of apoptosis-related proteins showed that the levels of total and activated p53, a crucial participant in the apoptotic pathway, were drastically increased in bendamustine-treated myeloma cells (Fig. 8C–F). Although the level of Bax was unchanged by bendamustine treatment (Fig. 8G, H), p21, which induces cell cycle arrest preceding p53-dependent apoptosis, was significantly increased in bendamustine-treated MM cells (Fig. 8I, J).

Discussion

The present study contributes to the characterization of the MM niche in the BM, which is still incompletely elucidated *in vivo*. Here we show that MM cells preferentially engraft at the metaphyseal region of the BM endosteum and form a complex with osteoblasts and osteoclasts (Fig. 1F, G, 2A). The preferential engraftment of MM cells at the metaphyseal region is thought to be due to the abundance of vasculature in the metaphysis, which is composed of trabecular-rich cancellous bone and a dense vascular network made up of numerous sinusoid capillaries [23]. Similarly, transplanted hematopoietic stem and progenitor cells (HSPC) also engraft preferentially to the metaphysic [24,25], as do bone metastases of several hematological malignancies [26] and solid

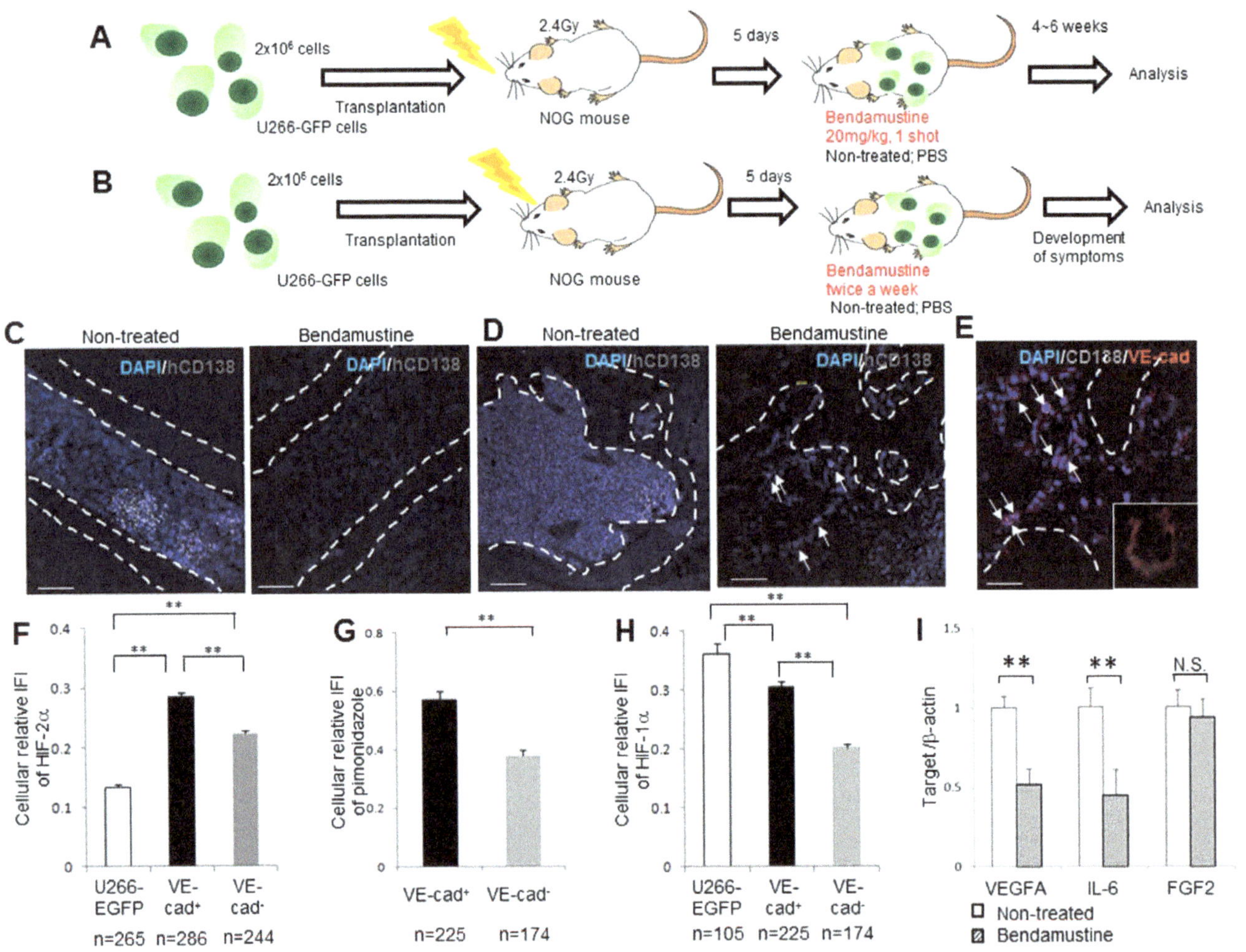

Figure 4. Bendamustine-treated MM cells remaining at the metaphyseal region express VE-cadherin and show hypoxic phenotypes. A. A single dose of bendamustine (20 mg/kg) or an equivalent amount of PBS was administered intraperitoneally to engrafted mice 5 days after U266-EGFP cell transplantation. Four to six weeks after administration, mice were sacrificed for analysis. **B.** Over the course of a week, two sequential doses of bendamustine (20 mg/kg) or equivalent amounts of PBS were administered intraperitoneally to engrafted mice 5 days after U266-EGFP cell transplantation. These mice were sacrificed for analysis when the mice had developed disease symptoms. **C, D.** IHC of human CD138 (gray) at the diaphyseal region (**C**) or the metaphyseal region (**D**) at 4 weeks after treatment in bendamustine-treated mice (right panel) or non-treated (PBS-treated) mice (left panel). Representative data from five fields of the BM of two mice per group in two independent experiments are shown. In A and B, the left bars = 200 μm, and in B, the right bar = 100 μm. **E.** Double IHC of human CD138 (gray) and VE-cadherin (red) at 4 weeks after treatment in bendamustine-treated mice. The arrows indicate human CD138-positive MM cells. Representative data from five fields of the BM of two mice in two independent experiments are shown. Bar = 50 μm. **F–H.** Quantification of HIF-2α (**F**) or HIF-1α (**H**) protein levels in cultured U266-EGFP cells, or VE-cadherin$^+$ or VE-cadherin$^-$ fractions, 6 weeks after U266-EGFP cell transplantation and quantification of pimonidazole retention (**G**) in VE-cadherin$^+$ or VE-cadherin$^-$ fractions at 6 weeks after transplantation. The experiment was performed twice with similar results. **I.** Human CD138$^+$ mouse CD45$^-$ MM cells were sorted from non-treated or bendamustine-treated mice, and VEGFA, IL-6 or FGF-2 transcripts were examined by qRT-PCR. Each value was normalized to β-actin expression (mean ± SD, $^{**}P<0.01$, n = 4). The experiment was performed twice with similar results.

tumors [23]. These observations suggest that the vasculature is important for the homing of transplanted HSPC or malignant cells to the bone marrow.

VE-cadherin is a cell adhesion molecule that is crucial for tube formation by endothelial cells [27]. Myeloma cells express various angiogenic factors and promote angiogenesis in the BM. In particular, VEGF [17], its receptors [28], and b-FGF [29] are reportedly produced by MM cells. In this paper, MM cells were also observed to express VE-cadherin, but only *in vivo* (Fig. 3A, B). Since we observed a small population of bendamustine-resistant myeloma cells that were positive for VE-cadherin (Fig. 4E), similar events might occur in the MM *in vivo*. Furthermore, the expression of HIF-2α was increased in VE-cadherin$^+$ cells compared to the VE-cadherin$^-$ fraction *in vivo* or to *in vitro* cultured MM cells (Fig. 4F). The retention of pimonidazole and the expression level of HIF-1α were also elevated in the VE-cadherin$^+$ cell fraction (Fig. 4G, H). These results indicated that HIF-2αspecifically induced MM cells to express VE-cadherin in the BM. This HIF-2α-VE-cadherin pathway is activated in a subset of MM cells in response to hypoxia and might contribute to the maintenance and drug resistance of MM *in vivo*. A recent study has reported that lenalidomide, which is approved for the treatment of MM and myelodysplastic syndromes associated with deletion of the long arm of chromosome 5q, inhibited hypoxia-induced endothelial cell cord formation and HIF-1α accumulation [30]. lenalidomide

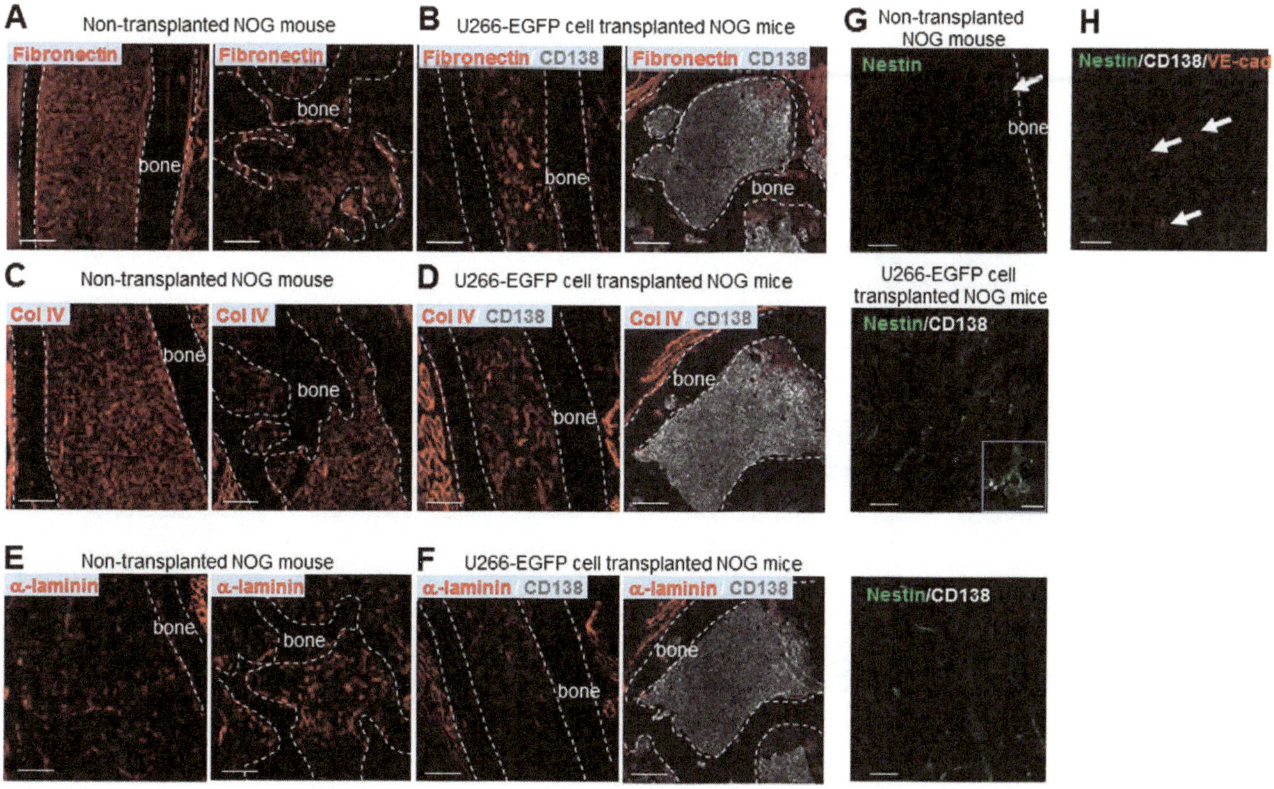

Figure 5. Disorganized ECM components and increased mesenchymal cells in the MM niche. A, B. IHC of fibronectin (red; **A**), or fibronectin (red) and human CD138 (gray; **B**), at the diaphyseal region (left) or metaphyseal region (right) of long bones of a non-transplanted NOG mouse (**A**) or U266-EGFP cell-transplanted NOG mice (**B**). Representative data from five fields from the BM of one non-transplanted NOG mouse and five U266-EGFP cell-transplanted mice in two independent experiments are shown. Bars = 200 μm. **C, D.** IHC of type IV collagen (red; **C**), or type IV collagen (red) plus human CD138 (gray; **D**), at the diaphyseal region (left) or metaphyseal region (right) of the long bones of a non-transplanted NOG mouse (**C**) or U266-EGFP cell-transplanted NOG mice (**D**). Representative data from five fields from the BM of one non-transplanted NOG mouse and five U266-EGFP cell-transplanted mice from two independent experiments are shown. Bars = 200 μm. **E, F.** IHC of α-laminin (red; **E**), or α-laminin (red) plus human CD138 (gray; **F**), at the diaphyseal region (left) or metaphyseal region (right) of the long bones of a non-transplanted NOG mouse (**E**) or U266-EGFP cell-transplanted NOG mice (**F**). Representative data from five fields from the BM of one non-transplanted NOG mouse and five U266-EGFP cell-transplanted mice from two independent experiments are shown. Bars = 200 μm. **G.** IHC of nestin (green; upper panel), or nestin (green) plus human CD138 (gray; middle and lower panels), of the long bones of a non-transplanted NOG mouse (upper panel) or U266-EGFP cell-transplanted NOG mice (middle and lower panels). Nestin^{+} mesenchymal cells were rare in normal NOG BM (upper panel; arrow) but increased in U266-EGFP cell-transplanted mice independent of vascular association (lower two panels). Representative images from five fields from the BM of one non-transplanted NOG mouse and five U266-EGFP cell-transplanted mice from two independent experiments are shown. Bars = 40 μm. (Magnified figure bar = 20 μm.) **H.** Triple IHC of nestin (green), CD138 (gray) and VE-cadherin (red) within the metaphyseal regions at 4 weeks after U266-EGFP cell transplantation. Arrows indicate vessels. Representative data from 10 to 20 fields from the BM of two mice from three independent experiments are shown. Bar = 40 μm.

also inhibited VE-cadherin and another adherens junction protein, β-catenin, in a dose-dependent manner [30]. Combination therapy including anti-angiogenic agents such as lenalidomide may overcome the drug resistance in MM. Recently, the stem cell-like fraction in glioblastoma has been shown to induce a subset of VE-cadherin-expressing endothelial progenitors [31], which form vascular-like structures [32] and maintain tumorigenesis. Thus, the tumor derived or associated vascular cells should be a target of cancer therapy.

During MM progression, in the metaphysical region of the BM, increased numbers of osteoclasts were localized near to, and made contact with, MM cells (Fig. 2B). Because inhibition of osteoclasts reduces angiogenesis and tumor burden in MM [33], both osteoclastogenesis and angiogenesis are considered to progress in parallel to the growth of MM cells. Therefore, these histological findings are in accordance with the current opinion that there is a close relationship between progression of MM, osteoclast formation, and angiogenesis.

ECM proteins play a crucial role in hematopoietic stem cell (HSC) regulation, especially as scaffold proteins [34]. Our observation that ECM structure, especially fibronectin, was increased and disorganized in the non-MM occupied diaphyseal area (Fig. 5B) may indicate migration of MM cells from the metaphysis to the diaphysis. Previous studies have reported that binding MM cells with fibronectin protected MM cells from drug-induced apoptosis [35,36]. Therefore, targeting not only tumor cells but also the BM niche that sustains tumor growth and survival is an effective treatment strategy for MM.

It is well known that osteoblasts are suppressed by MM cells [37]. We observed disruption of the osteoblast lining on the bone surface in MM mice (Fig. 6A), which suggested a functional decline in osteoblasts, which differentiate from MSCs. It has been reported that MM cells inhibit osteoblastogenesis by blocking the differentiation capacity of mesenchymal and osteoprogenitor cells [38]. According to these previous findings, the increased nestin^{+} mesenchymal cells in the MM BM (Fig. 4G) could be a result of

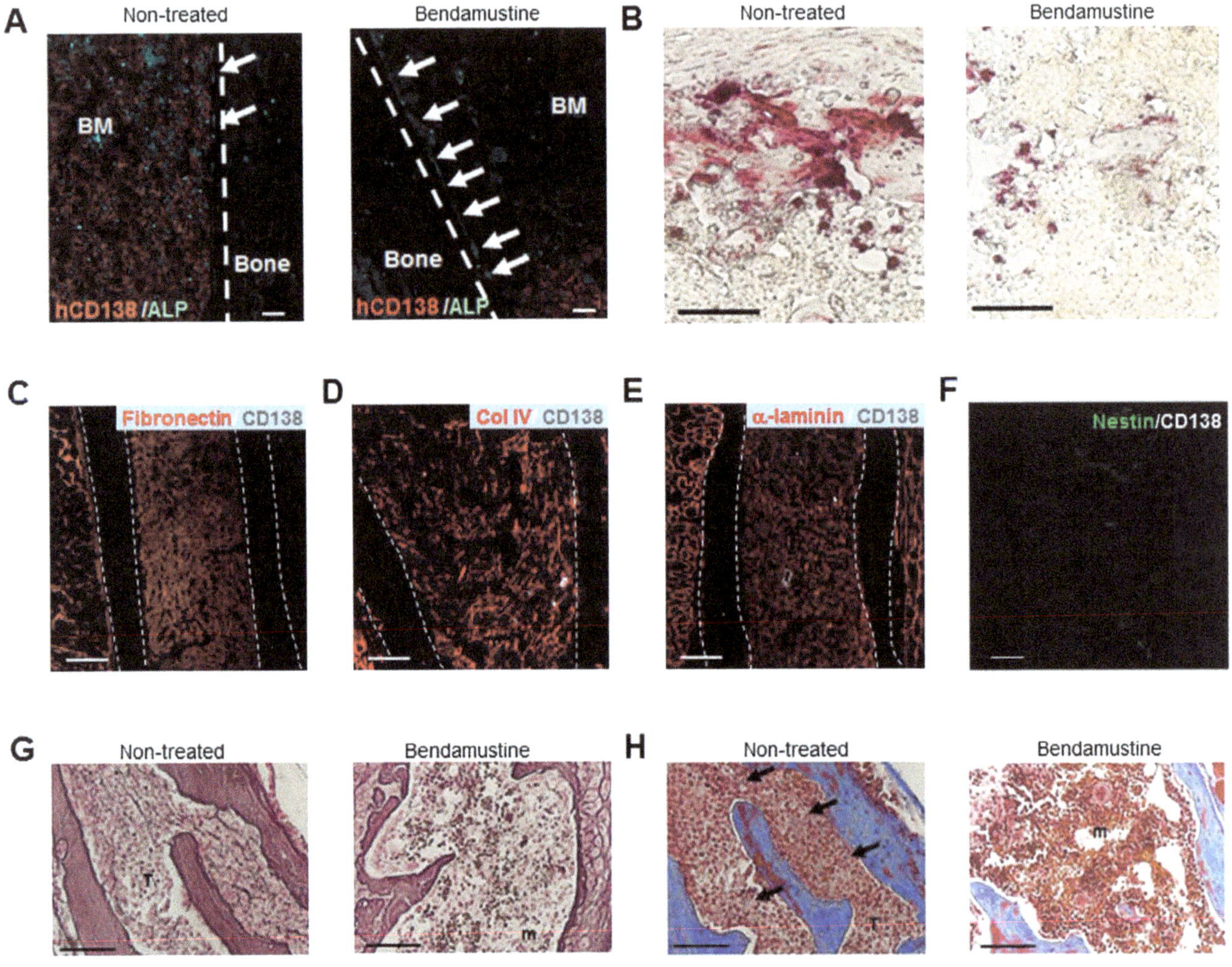

Figure 6. Bendamustine maintains the normal BM niche *in vivo*. A. Double IHC of human CD138 (red) and ALP (cyan) at 4 weeks after treatment in bendamustine-treated mice (right panel) or non-treated mice (left panel). The arrows indicate the osteoblast lining on the bone surface. Representative data from seven fields of the BM of two mice per group from two independent experiments are shown. Bars = 60 μm. **B.** Representative photomicrographs of TRAP staining of the metaphyseal region of the femur at 4 weeks after treatment in bendamustine-treated mice (right panel) or non-treated mice (left panel). Representative data from three fields from the BM of four non-treated mice or two bendamustine-treated mice from two independent experiments are shown. Bars = 100 μm. **C–E.** Double IHC of fibronectin (red; **C**), type IV collagen (**D**) or α-laminin (**E**) with human CD138 (gray) at 4 weeks after bendamustine treatment. Representative data from five fields of the BM of two bendamustine-treated mice from two independent experiments are shown. Bars = 200 μm. **F.** Double IHC of nestin (green) and human CD138 (gray) at 4 weeks after bendamustine treatment. Representative data from five fields of the BM of two bendamustine-treated mice from two independent experiments are shown. Bar = 40 μm. **G.** Histological studies of the thoracic vertebrae of NOG mice 4 weeks after treatment in bendamustine-treated mice (right panel) or non-treated mice (no treatment; left panel). Reticulin staining: T, tumor; m, marrow. Representative data from five fields of the BM of five mice per group from two independent experiments are shown.Bars = 100 μm. **H.** Histological studies of the thoracic vertebrae of NOG mice 4 weeks after treatment in bendamustine-treated mice (right panel) or non-treated mice (left panel). Masson trichrome staining: T, tumor; m, marrow. Representative data from five fields of the BM of five mice per group from two independent experiments are shown. Bars = 100 μm.

the inhibition of osteoblastogenesis and may have a role in the disease progression of MM. As nestin$^+$ mesenchymal cells produce various chemokines and cytokines, the disruption of normal hematopoiesis in MM pathophysiology might be caused by spatial occupancy of tumor growth, disorganized ECM, or reductions in HSC numbers, the latter of which may result from the reduction in osteoblast numbers or from MSC signaling in a paracrine manner.

The present study also clarified the specific molecular effects of bendamustine on MM cells and the MM niche using the NOG-hMM model. Bendamustine reduced VEGF and IL-6 levels in the NOG-hMM model (Fig. 4I). Any direct effects of bendamustine on MM niche cells are not detected at this time, but our results demonstrate that bendamustine could ameliorate MM-induced dysregulation of the BM niche. Future studies will address the direct and indirect effects of bendamustine on MM cells and MM niche cells in the patients and further evaluation of neovascular niches for MM in human samples.

In this study, the mice were not rescued from hind leg paralysis. Nor was the condition of the already diseased mice improved by bendamustine treatment. Bendamustine treatment only delayed the onset of hind leg paralysis (data not shown). The result is possibly due to the remaining MM cells being sufficient to induce clinical symptoms, including hind leg paralysis. In future studies, we will modify our hNOG-MM system by using fewer MM cells for transplantation and a treatment protocol designed to improve MM symptoms.

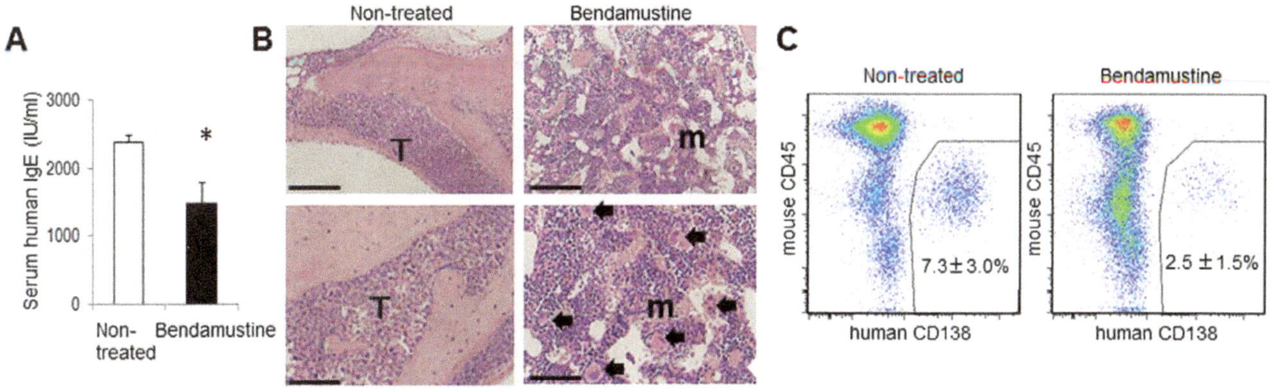

Figure 7. Bendamustine suppresses MM cells *in vivo*. A. Serum levels of human IgE. Human IgE levels in the serum of NOG mice 4 weeks after treatment with bendamustine were analyzed by ELISA. Non-treated mice were injected with PBS (n = 5, mean ± SD). The experiment was performed three times with similar results. **B.** Histological studies of the thoracic vertebrae of NOG mice 4 weeks after treatment with bendamustine (right panel) or non-treatment (left panel). Massive infiltration of U266-EGFP cells was observed in non-treated mice. However, an overall reduction of U266-EGFP cells and maintenance of normal hematopoiesis were observed in bendamustine-treated mice. HE staining: T, tumor; m, marrow; arrow, megakaryocyte. Representative data from five fields from the BM of five mice per group from two independent experiments are shown. Upper panel bars = 200 μm. Lower panel bars = 100 μm. **C.** FACS analysis of U266-EGFP cells at 4 weeks after treatment in bendamustine-treated or non-treated mice (n = 5, mean ± SD). Representative FACS plots of at least 10 mice from two independent experiments are shown.

In conclusion, this study characterized the myeloma niche in the NOG-hMM model and examined the effects of bendamustine on both myeloma cells and the surrounding microenvironment *in vivo*. The vascular component of the MM niche plays an important role in supporting MM cells, especially with regard to chemoresistance. Interestingly, these results demonstrated that VE-cadherin^{+} cells

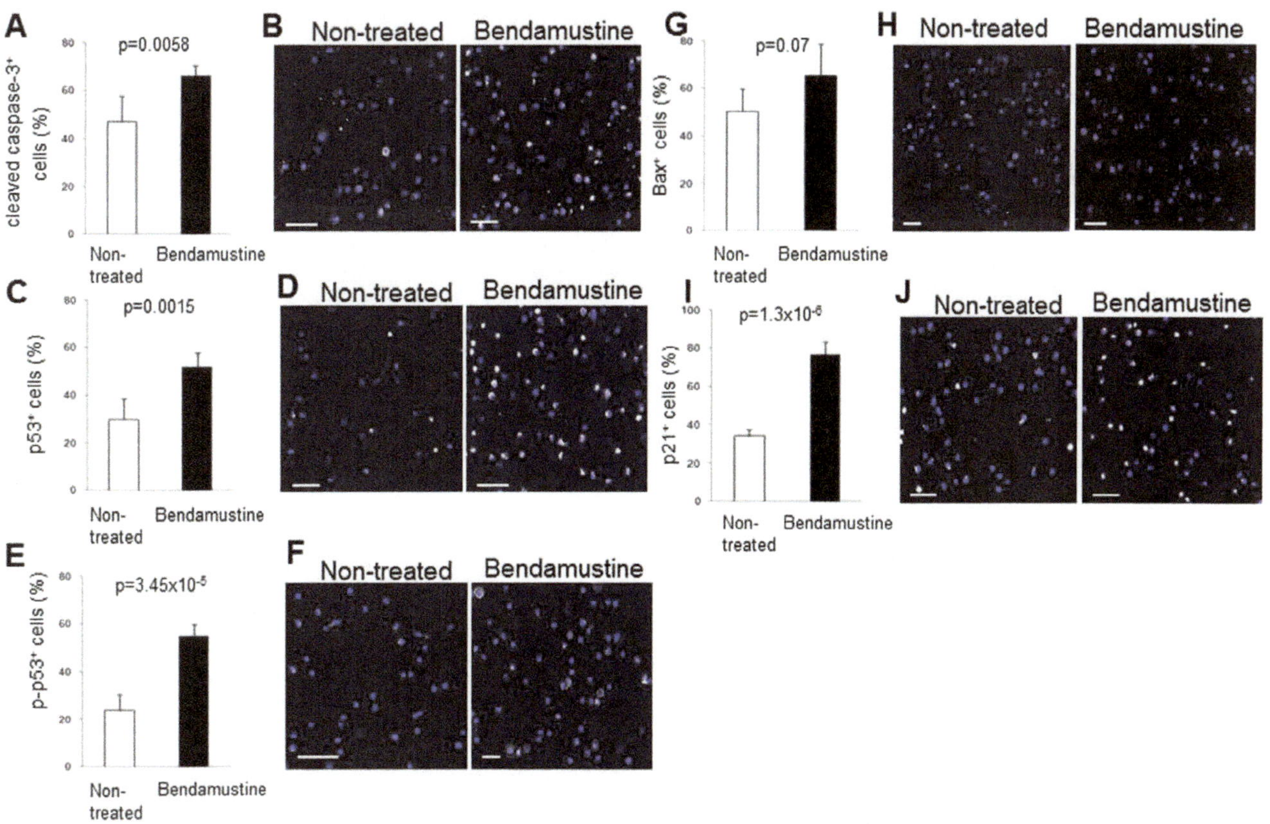

Figure 8. Bendamustine induces p53-dependent apoptosis. Human CD138^{+} mouse CD45^{-} MM cells from non-treated or bendamustine-treated mice were sorted and immunocytochemistry was performed to analyze cleaved caspase-3 (**A, B**), p53 (**C, D**), phosphorylated-p53 (**E, F**), Bax (**G, H**), and p21 (**I, J**). Each group of MM cells was stained with DAPI and anti-fibronectin antibody, anti-p53 antibody, anti-phosphorylated-p53 antibody, anti-Bax antibody, or anti-p21 antibody. At least 100 cells/sample were counted (mean ± SD, n = 10). Bars = 50 μm.

are derived from MM cells. Thalidomide [39]; lenalidomide [40]; and bortezomib [41] have all been shown to have anti-angiogenic effects. However, these agents have not been sufficient for the effective treatment of MM. The drug-resistant hypoxic VE-cadherin$^+$ HIF-2α$^+$ MM fraction identified in this model presents a candidate target for the adjustment of bendamustine dose, combination therapy, or selective targeting (Fig. 9). The NOG-hMM model described here is a useful system for the analysis of the *in vivo* dynamics and kinetics of myeloma cell pathophysiology and for observing the interactions of MM cells with other components of the microenvironment, as well as for the development of novel anti-MM therapies.

Materials and Methods

Mice

NOG (NOD/SCID/γ_c^{null}) mice [12] were purchased from the Central Institute for Experimental Animals. All animal experiments were approved by the Keio University School of Medicine's ethical review board (approval ID: 08104).

Reagents and antibodies

Bendamustine was kindly provided by SymBio Pharmaceuticals Ltd. The following antibodies (Abs) labeled with fluorophores were used for flow cytometric analysis and cell sorting: anti-mouse CD45 (30-F11; BD Biosciences), anti-human CD138 (BD Biosciences), and anti-human VE-cadherin (16B1; eBioscience). For immunohistochemical staining of BM sections or immunocytochemical staining of MM cells, the following Abs were used: mouse anti-CD138 (AbD seroTec), rabbit anti-ALP (R&D), anti-MMP9 (Chemicon), anti-GFP (MBL), rabbit anti-fibronectin (Dako), rabbit anti-type IV collagen (AbD seroTec), rabbit anti-α-laminin (Sigma), rat anti-nestin (BioAcademia), FITC-conjugated anti-pimonidazole (Chemicon), rabbit anti-HIF-1α (Santa Cruz), and rabbit anti-HIF-2α (Santa Cruz).

Quantitative RT-PCR

Quantitative PCR was performed as described previously [42]. Total RNA was prepared with the RNeasy Mini Kit (Qiagen) and was reverse-transcribed with Superscript VILO (Invitrogen) to prepare cDNA. Diluted cDNA samples were analyzed with SYBR Premix Ex Taq II (TaKaRa) using readymade primer sets for each gene (TaKaRa), according to the manufacturer's instructions. Primer sets were used for human IL-6 (HA032507), VEGFA (HA110047), FGF-2 (HA035991), or β-actin (HA031582), which served as an endogenous control. Data were analyzed using 7500 Fast System SDS software, version 1.3.1.

Human MM model

The human myeloma cell line, U266, was purchased from the American Tissue Culture Collection (Manassas, VA [13]; and was stably tagged with EGFP with a lentiviral vector. 2×10^6 U266-EGFP cells were intravenously inoculated into irradiated NOG mice (2.4 Gy). After transplantation, mice were given sterile water containing hydrochloric acid and G418 disulfate in aqueous solution (Nacalai Tesque).

Flow cytometry

Stained cells were analyzed and sorted on a SORP FACS Aria (BD Biosciences).

Immunohistochemistry

Femurs were fixed in 4% paraformaldehyde, decalcified in EDTA, and embedded in OCT. Frozen sections were cut using a cryostat (MICROME, model HM550). Slides were washed three

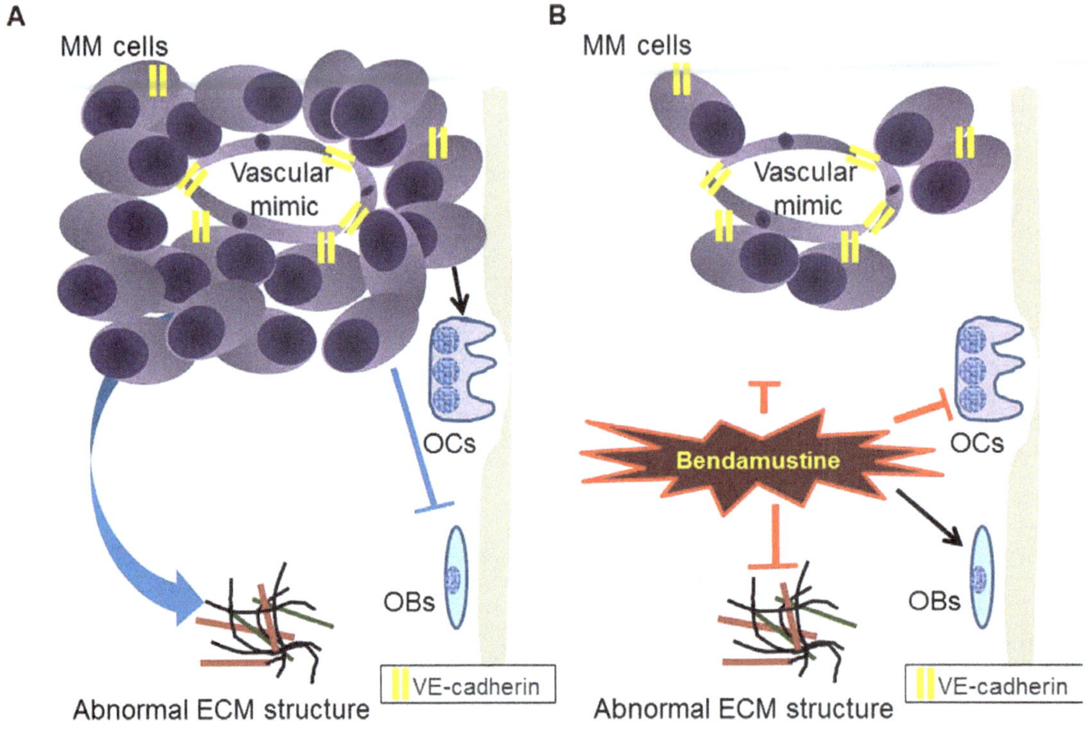

Figure 9. Anti-MM effects of bendamustine on MM cells and the BM niche. MM interacts with several BM microenvironments (**A**). Within the MM BM niche, bendamustine affects both MM cells and the surrounding niche *in vivo* (**B**). OBs, osteoblast cells; OCs, osteoclast cells.

times in PBS and stained for TRAP activity (Primary Cell Co., Ltd.). For immunohistochemistry, femoral frozen sections were washed three times in PBS, blocked with a protein blocker (DAKO), and then incubated with primary antibodies overnight in humidified chambers at 4°C. The sections were then washed three times in PBS and reacted with fluorophore-labeled secondary antibodies and a nuclear stain (TOTO3 or DAPI; Molecular Probes). Fluorescence images were obtained using a confocal laser-scanning microscope (FV1000; Olympus) in the linear range to avoid fluorescence saturation. Scanning was performed in the sequential laser emission mode to avoid cross-talk between the fluorescence channels. For detection of cellular hypoxia, six weeks after MM cell transplantation, NOG mice were injected with 60 mg/kg pimonidazole (Pimo; Chemicon) 90 min before sacrifice. Human CD138-gated VE-cadherin–positive or –negative fractions were sorted for immunocytochemistry.

Histological evaluation

Thoracic vertebra were fixed in 4% PFA and decalcified in EDTA, followed by paraffin embedding and sectioning. Morphological evaluation of the sections was performed following hematoxylin and eosin (HE) staining, reticulin staining, and Masson trichrome staining.

Human IgE measurement

Serum levels of human IgE in NOG recipients was measured using a human IgE ELISA kit (Phadia, SW) following the manufacturer's instructions.

Statistical analysis

P-values were calculated using two-tailed unpaired Student's t-tests (for experiments with normal distribution), Wilcoxon tests (for two-group experiments with non-normal distribution), or Tukey's multiple comparison tests (for multiple-group experiments).

Supporting Information

Table S1 U266-GFP cells rarely fused with mouse endothelial cells. Fluorescence in situ hybridization (FISH) analysis of VE-cadherin positive and VE-cadherin negative cell fractions, and cultured U266-GFP cells. Each fusion rate is represented.

Acknowledgments

We thank M. Suematsu for FACS resources and T. Muraki and T. Hirose for essential support.

Author Contributions

Conceived and designed the experiments: KT TS. Performed the experiments: HI KT Y. Miyakawa AN-I Y. Miyauchi NF KM TM. Analyzed the data: HI KT EI TS. Contributed reagents/materials/analysis tools: MK YN. Wrote the paper: HI KT TS.

References

1. Kyle RA, Rajkumar SV (2004) Multiple myeloma. N Engl J Med 351: 1860–73.
2. Basak GW, Srivastava AS, Malhotra R, Carrier E (2009) Multiple myeloma bone marrow niche. Curr Pharm Biotechnol 10: 345–346.
3. De Raeve HR, Vanderkerken K (2005) The role of the bone marrow microenvironment in multiple myeloma. Histol Histopathol 20: 1227–1250.
4. Nooka A, Gleason C, Lonial S (2010) Improving induction therapy in multiple myeloma. Curr Hematol Malig Rep 5: 119–128.
5. Cheson BD, Rummel MJ (2009) Bendamustine: rebirth of an old drug. J Clin Oncol 27: 1492–1501.
6. Leoni LM, Bailey B, Reifert J, Bendall HH, Zeller RW, et al. (2008) Bendamustine (Treanda) displays a distinct pattern of cytotoxicity and unique mechanistic features compared with other alkylating agents. Clin Cancer Res 14: 309–317.
7. Gandhi V (2002) Metabolism and mechanisms of action of bendamustine: rationales for combination therapies. Semin Oncol 29: 4–11.
8. Friedberg JW, Cohen P, Chen L, Robinson KS, Forero-Torres A, et al. (2008) Bendamustine in patients with rituximab-refractory indolent and transformed non-Hodgkin's lymphoma: results from a phase II multicenter, single-agent study. J Clin Oncol 26: 204–210.
9. Friedberg JW, Vose JM, Kelly JL, Young F, Bernstein SH, et al. (2011) The combination of bendamustine, bortezomib and rituximab for patients with relapsed/refractory indolent and mantle cell non-Hodgkin lymphoma. Blood 117: 2807–2812.
10. Ponisch W, Mitrow PS, Merkle K, Herold M, Assmann M, et al. (2006) Treatment of bendamustine and prednisone in patients with newly diagnosed multiple myeloma results in superior complete response rate, prolonged time to treatment failure and improved quality of life compared to treatment with melphalan and prednisone–a randomized phase III study of the East German Study Group of Hematology and Oncology (OSHO). J Cancer Res Clin Oncol 132: 205–212.
11. Knop S, Straka C, Haen M, Schwedes R, Hebart H, et al. (2005) The efficacy and toxicity of bendamustine in recurrent multiple myeloma after high-dose chemotherapy. Haematologica 90: 1287–1288.
12. Ito M, Hiramatsu H, Kobayashi K, Suzue K, Kamahata M, et al. (2002) NOD/SCID/gamma(c)(null) mouse: an excellent recipient mouse model for engraftment of human cells. Blood 100: 3175–3182.
13. Miyakawa Y, Ohnishi Y, Tomisawa M, Monnai M, Kohmura K, et al. (2004) Establishment of a new model of human multiple myeloma using NOD/SCID/gammac(null) (NOG) mice. Biochem Biophys Res Commun 313: 258–262.
14. Rajkumar SV, Mesa RA, Fonseca R, Schroeder G, Plevak MF, et al. (2002) Bone marrow angiogenesis in 400 patients with monoclonal gammopathy of undetermined significance, multiple myeloma, and primary amyloidosis. Clin Cancer Res 8: 2210–2216.
15. Rana C, Sharma S, Agrawal V, Singh U (2010) Bone marrow angiogenesis in multiple myeloma and its correlation with clinicopathological factors. Ann Hematol 89: 789–794.
16. Bisping G, Leo R, Wenning D, Dankbar B, Padró T, et al. (2003) Paracrine interactions of basic fibroblast growth factor and interleukin-6 in multiple myeloma. Blood 101: 2775–2783.
17. Bellamy WT, Richter L, Frutiger Y, Grogan TM (1999) Expression of vascular endothelial growth factor and its receptors in hematopoietic malignancies. Cancer Res 59: 728–733.
18. Mortensen K, Lichtenberg J, Thomsen PD, Larsson LI (2004) Spontaneous fusion between cancer cells and endothelial cells. Cell Mol Life Sci 61: 2125–2131.
19. Takubo K, Goda N, Yamada W, Iriuchishima H, Ikeda E, et al. (2010) Regulation of the HIF-1alpha level is essential for hematopoietic stem cells. Cell Stem Cell 7: 391–402.
20. Le Bras A, Lionneton F, Mattot V, Lelièvre E, Caetano B, et al. (2007) HIF-2alpha specifically activates the VE-cadherin promoter independently of hypoxia and in synergy with Ets-1 through two essential ETS-binding sites. Oncogene 26: 7480–7489.
21. Mendez-Ferrer S, Michurina TV, Ferraro F, Mazloom AR, Macarthur BD, et al. (2010) Mesenchymal and haematopoietic stem cells form a unique bone marrow niche. Nature 466: 829–834.
22. Abildgaard N, Bendix-Hansen K, Kristensen JE, Vejlgaard T, Risteli L, et al. (1997) Bone marrow fibrosis and disease activity in multiple myeloma monitored by the aminoterminal propeptide of procollagen III in serum. Br J Haematol 99: 641–648.
23. Nyangoga H, Mercier P, Libouban H, Baslé MF, Chappard D (2011) Three-dimensional characterization of the vascular bed in bone metastasis of the rat by microcomputed tomography (MicroCT). PLoS One 6: e17336.
24. Ellis SL, Grassinger J, Jones A, Camenisch T, Haylock D, et al. (2011) The relationship between bone, hemopoietic stem cells, and vasculature. Blood 118: 1516–1524.
25. Jiang Y, Bonig H, Ulyagova T, Chang K, Papayannopoulou T (2009) On the adaptation of endosteal stem cell niche function in response to stress. Blood 114: 3773–3782.
26. Roux S, Mariette X (2000) Hematological malignancies and the bone (myeloma excluded). Joint Bone Spine 67: 264–271.
27. Kataoka N, Iwaki K, Hashomoto K, Mochizuki S, Ogasawara Y, et al. (2002) Measurements of endothelial cell-to-cell and cell-to-substrate gaps and micromechanical properties of endothelial cells during monocyte adhesion. Proc Natl Acad Sci U S A 99: 15638–15643.
28. Jakob C, Sterz J, Zavrski I, Heider U, Kleeberg L, et al. (2006) Angiogenesis in multiple myeloma. Eur J Cancer 42: 1581–1590.

29. Vacca A, Ribatti D, Roccaro AM, Ria R, Palermo L, et al. (2001) Bone marrow angiogenesis and plasma cell angiogenic and invasive potential in patients with active multiple myeloma. Acta Haematol 106: 162–169.
30. Lu L, Payvandi F, Wu L, Zhang LH, Hariri RJ, et al. (2009) The anti-cancer drug lenalidomide inhibits angiogenesis and metastasis via multiple inhibitory effects on endothelial cell function in normoxic and hypoxic conditions. Microvasc Res 77: 78–86.
31. Wang R, Chadalavada K, Wilshire J, Kowalik U, Hovinga KE, et al. (2010) Glioblastoma stem-like cells give rise to tumour endothelium. Nature 468: 829–833.
32. Ricci-Vitiani L, Pallini R, Biffoni M, Todaro M, Invernici G, et al. (2010) Tumour vascularization via endothelial differentiation of glioblastoma stem-like cells. Nature 468: 824–828.
33. Croucher PI, De Hendrik R, Perry MJ, Hijzen A, Shipman CM, et al. (2003) Zoledronic acid treatment of 5T2MM-bearing mice inhibits the development of myeloma bone disease: evidence for decreased osteolysis, tumor burden and angiogenesis, and increased survival. J Bone Miner Res 18: 482–492.
34. Nilsson SK, Debatis ME, Dooner MS, Madri JA, Quesenberry PJ, et al. (1998) Immunofluorescence characterization of key extracellular matrix proteins in murine bone marrow in situ. J Histochem Cytochem 46: 371–377.
35. Vincent T, Mechti N (2005) Extracellular matrix in bone marrow can mediate drug resistance in myeloma. Leuk Lymphoma 46: 803–811.
36. Nefedova Y, Cheng P, Alsina M, Dalton WS, Gabrilovich DI (2004) Involvement of Notch-1 signaling in bone marrow stroma-mediated de novo drug resistance of myeloma and other malignant lymphoid cell lines. Blood 103: 3503–3510.
37. Roodman GD (2011) Osteoblast function in myeloma. Bone 48: 135–140.
38. Giuliani N, Colla S, Morandi F, Lazzaretti M, Sala R, et al. (2005) Myeloma cells block RUNX2/CBFA1 activity in human bone marrow osteoblast progenitors and inhibit osteoblast formation and differentiation. Blood 106: 2472–2483.
39. Kumar S, Witzig TE, Dispenzieri A, Lacy MQ, Wellik LE, et al. (2004) Effect of thalidomide therapy on bone marrow angiogenesis in multiple myeloma. Leukemia 18: 624–627.
40. Dredge K, Marriott JB, Macdonald CD, Man HW, Chen R, et al. (2002) Novel thalidomide analogues display anti-angiogenic activity independently of immunomodulatory effects. Br J Cancer 87: 1166–1172.
41. Roccaro AM, Hideshima T, Raje N, Kumar S, Ishitsuka K, et al. (2006) Bortezomib mediates antiangiogenesis in multiple myeloma via direct and indirect effects on endothelial cells. Cancer Res 66: 184–191.
42. Takubo K, Ohmura M, Azuma M, Nagamatsu G, Yamada W, et al. (2008) Stem cell defects in ATM-deficient undifferentiated spermatogonia through DNA damage-induced cell-cycle arrest. Cell Stem Cell 2: 170–182.

8

Erk1 Positively Regulates Osteoclast Differentiation and Bone Resorptive Activity

Yongzheng He[1,2], Karl Staser[1,2], Steven D. Rhodes[2,3], Yaling Liu[1,2], Xiaohua Wu[1,2], Su-Jung Park[1,2], Jin Yuan[1,2], Xianlin Yang[1,2], Xiaohong Li[1,2], Li Jiang[1,2], Shi Chen[1,2], Feng-Chun Yang[1,2,3]*

1 Departments of Pediatrics, Indiana University School of Medicine, Indianapolis, Indiana, United States of America, **2** Herman B Wells Center for Pediatric Research, Indiana University School of Medicine, Indianapolis, Indiana, United States of America, **3** Anatomy and Cell Biology, Indiana University School of Medicine, Indianapolis, Indiana, United States of America

Abstract

The extracellular signal-regulated kinases (ERK1 and 2) are widely-expressed and they modulate proliferation, survival, differentiation, and protein synthesis in multiple cell lineages. Altered ERK1/2 signaling is found in several genetic diseases with skeletal phenotypes, including Noonan syndrome, Neurofibromatosis type 1, and Cardio-facio-cutaneous syndrome, suggesting that MEK-ERK signals regulate human skeletal development. Here, we examine the consequence of *Erk1* and *Erk2* disruption in multiple functions of osteoclasts, specialized macrophage/monocyte lineage-derived cells that resorb bone. We demonstrate that Erk1 positively regulates osteoclast development and bone resorptive activity, as genetic disruption of *Erk1* reduced osteoclast progenitor cell numbers, compromised pit formation, and diminished M-CSF-mediated adhesion and migration. Moreover, WT mice reconstituted long-term with *Erk1*$^{-/-}$ bone marrow mononuclear cells (BMMNCs) demonstrated increased bone mineral density as compared to recipients transplanted with WT and *Erk2*$^{-/-}$ BMMNCs, implicating marrow autonomous, Erk1-dependent osteoclast function. These data demonstrate Erk1 plays an important role in osteoclast functions while providing rationale for the development of Erk1-specific inhibitors for experimental investigation and/or therapeutic modulation of aberrant osteoclast function.

Editor: Jose Alberola-Ila, Oklahoma Medical Research Foundation, United States of America

Funding: This work was supported in part by the Department of Defense (http://www.defense.gov/) NF043032 (FCY) and NF073112 (FCY). KS was additionally supported by a pre-doctoral training grant from the National Institutes of Health (http://www.nih.gov/) Grant T32 CA111198. SR is a Pre-Doctoral Trainee of Indiana CTSI (Career Development Award from NCCR 5TL1RR025759-03). The funders had no role in study design, data collection and analysis, decision to publish, or preparation of the manuscript.

Competing Interests: The authors have declared that no competing interests exist.

* E-mail: fyang@iupui.edu

Introduction

Normal bone physiology, as well as bone repair following injury, depends upon the productive and destructive interactions between osteoblasts and osteoclasts, whereby osteoblast-mediated bone production repairs localized defects created by osteoclasts. Many skeletal diseases result from an imbalance between osteoclast and osteoblast numbers and/or function [1]. Generally, increased osteoblast numbers and/or functions lead to abnormal bone mineralization while increased osteoclast numbers and/or functions underlie osteoporotic conditions. Multinucleated osteoclasts are continuously formed from the monocyte/macrophage lineage of hematopoietic cells [2,3], and osteoclastogenesis and normal osteoclast function depend upon multiple cytokines and growth factors, including macrophage colony stimulating factor (M-CSF), receptor activator for nuclear factor kappa-B ligand (RANKL), and transforming growth factor beta (TGFβ) [4,5,6]. These factors near-ubiquitously induce phosphorylation of Erk1 and Erk2 [4,5,6]. Intriguingly, alterations in the MAPK/ERK1/2 cascade contribute to cardio-facio-cutaneous syndrome (CFC), Noonan syndrome, LEOPARD syndrome, and Neurofibromatosis type 1. These pathophysiological observations suggest roles for ERK1 and ERK2 in human skeletal development [7,8,9].

ERK1 and ERK2 are serine/threonine-specific protein kinases sharing 84% homology [10,11]. Upon extracellular mitogen stimulation, the Ras-Raf-MEK cascade phosphorylates and activates ERK1 and ERK2, which then phosphorylate cytoplasmic and nuclear factors that execute normal and malignant cell functions, including gene expression, mitosis, movement, and the regulation of apoptosis [12,13,14,15,16]. *In vivo* genetic studies have shown differential and/or combined roles for Erk1 and Erk2 in multiple cell lineages, including T cells, B cells, and osteoblasts [17,18,19,20,21,22,23]. Specifically, dual *Erk1/2* disruption in osteoblast lineages results in reduced RANKL production, leading to a subsequent reduction in osteoclastogenesis. Likewise, studies using pharmacologic kinase inhibitors (e.g. U0126, Wortmannin, LY294002) have suggested the importance of these pathways to osteoclast formation and function [24,25]. However, no genetic study has examined Erk1 or Erk2's direct regulation of osteoclast physiology, although recent inquiries in other cell lineages have discovered isoform-specific roles for Erk1 and Erk2 [7,17,23].

In the present study, we evaluated the consequence of *Erk1* and *Erk2* disruption in osteoclast differentiation, migration, and bone resorptive activity *in vitro* and *in vivo*. To accomplish these aims, we performed functional assays on osteoclasts generated from bone marrow progenitor cells of *Erk1*$^{-/-}$ and hematopoietic *Erk2* conditional knockout ($Mx1Cre^{+}Erk2^{flox/flox}$) mice, and we assessed bone mineral density in WT mice transplanted long-term with bone marrow mononuclear cells (BMMNCs) of WT, $Erk1^{-/-}$, or $Erk2^{-/-}$ mice. We conclude that Erk1 plays a preponderant role in modulating osteoclast differentiation, migration, bone resorption, and bone mineral density.

Materials and Methods

Animals

Previously described $Erk1^{-/-}$ mice and $Erk2^{flox/flox}$ mice [18,22] were crossed with *Mx1Cre* transgenic mice ($Mx1Cre^{+}$ $Erk2^{fl/fl}$), allowing inducible disruption of *Erk2* in all hematopoietic cells. Cre expression was induced by intraperitoneal injections of poly I poly C (polyIC) (300 µg at 1 mg/mL in PBS; Sigma) every two days for a total of five injections. Genetic disruption of the *Erk2* gene in $Mx1Cre^{+}$ mice was verified by PCR of the recombinant *Erk2* gene and the absence of total Erk2 protein by western blot of mouse BMMNCs (Figure S1 and Figure S2, respectively). For simplicity, mice containing the disrupted $Erk2^{flox/flox}$ allele henceforth will be referred to as $Erk2^{-/-}$ mice. Animal care and experiments were conducted according to the guidelines established by the Indiana University Animal Care and Use Committee (IACUC). Age- and sex-matched WT, $Erk1^{-/-}$, and $Erk2^{-/-}$ mice were used for each experiment.

Bone marrow transplantation

2×10^{6} BMMNCs from WT, $Erk1^{-/-}$ and $Erk2^{-/-}$ mice were injected intravenously into lethally-irradiated (1100 cGy) 8-week old BoyJ mice [26]. Successful marrow reconstitution was confirmed by flow cytometry of CD45.2 expression in peripheral white blood cells, and stable *Erk2* allele deletion was confirmed by western blot. Bone mineral density (BMD) was measured six months after bone marrow transplantation.

BMD quantification

Bone mineral density (BMD) was measured by dual-energy X-ray absorptiometry (DEXA) with a Lunar Piximus densitometer (GE Medical Systems, software version 1.4 Lunar) [27]. The mice were anesthetized with avertin/tribromoethanol (0.25 mg/kg) and placed into the scanner in the prone position with arms and legs extended. The BMD of the left femoral metaphysis was measured by defining a region of interest of 11 pixels × 10 pixels proximal to the distal growth plate, a region containing high content of trabecular bone.

Micro computed tomography (µCT)

To evaluate trabecular microarchitecture in the distal femoral metaphysis, fixed femurs (stored in 70% EtOH) were scanned using a high-resolution desktop microcomputed tomography imaging system (µCT-20; Scanco Medical AG, Basserdorf, Switzerland). Scanning for the femur was started at 15% of the total femur length measured from the tip of femoral condyle and extended proximally for 200 slices with an increment of 9 µm, which were then reconstructed, filtered ($\sigma = 0.8$ and support = 1.0), and thresholded (at 22% of the possible gray scale value) for analysis, as described previously [28]. The trabecular region was outlined within the trabecular compartment, excluding the cortical shell. Parameters of microarchitecture for bone volume fraction (BV/TV, %), trabecular number (Tb.N, mm^{-1}), trabecular thickness (Tb.Th, mm), as well as and trabecular separation (Tb.Sp, mm) were measured.

Clonogenic progenitor assays

Colony-forming unit-macrophage/monocyte (CFU-M) of BMMNCs were assayed, as described previously [27]. Briefly, 2.5×10^{4} BMMNCs were seeded onto a 35-mm gridded dish containing methylcellulose supplemented with murine recombinant macrophage-colony stimulating factor (M-CSF, 30 ng/mL) and murine recombinant RANKL (20 ng/mL) for 7 days at 37°C in a 5% CO_2 incubator. Colonies were scored using an inverted light microscope. All cytokines were purchased from PeproTech (Rocky Hills, NC).

Generation of murine osteoclasts and tartrate resistant acid phosphatase (TRACP) staining

Mouse osteoclasts were obtained *in vitro* using BMMNCs, as described previously [27]. BMMNCs from 8-week old WT, $Erk1^{-/-}$, and $Erk2^{-/-}$ mice were isolated by long bone marrow flush and Ficoll density gradient isolation and cultured in α-MEM supplemented with 10% fetal bovine serum (FBS, Sigma), 30 ng/mL M-CSF and 20 ng/mL RANKL for 3 days. On day 4, cell culture media was switched to α-MEM supplemented with 10% FBS, M-CSF (30 ng/mL), and 60 ng/mL RANKL for another 3 days. To identify osteoclasts after this culture period, adherent cells were fixed with a solution containing 25 mL citrate solution, 65 mL acetone, and 8 mL of 3.7% formaldehyde, and stained for TRACP. Osteoclasts were visualized with a Nikon TE2000-S microscope (Nikon Inc., Melville, NY). Images were taken by a QImaging camera and QCapture-Pro software (Fryer Company Inc., Cincinnati, OH). Multinucleated $TRACP^{+}$ cells containing more than three nuclei were scored as mature osteoclasts. The area of multinucleated, $TRACP^{+}$ osteoclasts and the number of nuclei per osteoclast were calculated using MetaMorph Offline software (Molecular Devices, Inc. Sunnyvale, CA).

Bone resorption assay

Osteoclasts were dissociated from tissue culture plates using 0.5% Trypsin-EDTA. Single-cell suspensions of purified osteoclasts were seeded at a density of 1×10^{4}/well on dentine slices (ALPCO Diagnostic, Windham, NH) pre-wetted with α-MEM for 2 hours and then incubated at 37°C/5% CO_2 in the presence of 30 ng/mL M-CSF and 60 ng/mL RANKL, as previously described [27]. Following 7 days of culture, the slices were rinsed with PBS, immersed overnight in 1 M ammonium hydroxide, and stained with a 1% toluidine blue/0.5% sodium tetraborate solution. At the same time, cells on dentine slices in the independent cultures were fixed and stained with TRACP for osteoclast counting. Microphotographs were taken under a reflective light microscopy at a 100× magnification, and the resorptive areas or "pits" in low-power field were analyzed by the MetaMorph Offline software. Six fields per condition were scored.

Migration assay

Migration of preosteoclasts was evaluated with a transwell assay, as described previously [27]. Equivalent numbers of cells were loaded onto the upper chamber of an 8 µm polycarbonate transwell (Corning Inc., Lowell, MA) coated with vitronectin (Takara, Japan) for 15 hours in a humidified incubator at 37°C/5% CO_2. The lower chamber contained α-MEM supplemented with 0.1% bovine serum albumin and M-CSF (30 ng/mL). Cells that migrated to the bottom chamber were stained with crystal violet and the number of migrated cells per field was counted. Six fields per condition were counted.

Preosteoclast adhesion assay

A single-cell suspension of osteoclast precursors (1×10^{4} cells/well) were placed into 96-well plates pre-coated with vitronectin as previously described [29]. After 30 minutes of incubation, nonattached cells were gently washed away with PBS and adherent cells were fixed and counted.

Western blotting analysis

Western blot using phospho-specific antibodies was conducted to determine the phosphorylation levels of Erk1/2 and p90^{rsk}, (Cell Signaling, Danvers, MA) in preosteoclasts [29]. Phosphorylation levels were compared to total-ß-actin levels (Cell Signaling). Briefly, cells were deprived of growth factors for 12 hours in α-MEM supplemented with 0.5% BSA, stimulated with or without 30 ng/mL M-CSF for 5 minutes and lysed in ProteoJET lysis buffer (Fermentas, Glen Burnie, MD) supplemented with Complete Mini protease inhibitor cocktail (Roche, Indianapolis, IN). The intensity of the bands was measured with Fluorchem Software (Cell Biosciences, Inc., Santa Clara, CA) and standardized with beta-actin for arbitrary intensity comparison.

Detection of C-terminal telopeptide of type I collagen (CTX) in plasma

Blood was collected from the retrobulbar venous plexus and kept in EDTA coated tubes, which were immediately cooled on ice and centrifuged within 30 min. Plasma samples were stored at −80°C before being tested. All samples were analyzed in the same experiment. CTX concentrations were determined using a commercial enzyme immunoassay kit (Ratlaps^{TM} EIA, Immunodiagnostic systems Inc., Fountain Hills, AZ).

Histomorphometric measurements

Upon sacrifice, femurs were harvested for histomorphometric analyses. The isolated bones were fixed in 10% neutral buffered formalin for 48 hours, dehydrated in graded ethanols, and embedded undecalcified in methyl methacrylate. Sagittal sections (5 µm thick) were cut from the middle of the femur. TRACP staining was performed using a leukocyte acid phosphatase kit (Sigma Diagnostics, St. Louis, Missouri) and McNeal Staining was performed using McNeal's Tetrachrome kit (Polysciences, Warrington, Pennsylvania), both according to manufacturers' protocols. One section per femur was viewed at 100× magnification on a Leitz DMRXE microscope (Leica Mikroskopie und System GmbH, Wetzlar, Germany) and the image captured using a QImaging camera and QCapture-Pro software (Fryer Company Inc., Cincinnati, OH). The measurement area for the metaphysis was determined by a region beginning 0.5 mm proximal to the midpoint of the growth plate, non-inclusive of cortical bone, and extending proximally for a total area of approximately 2.8 mm^2.

Alpha V (αv) integrin detection by flow cytometry

Expression of αv integrin was assessed by flow cytometry. Preosteoclasts were blocked using CD16/32 (BD Biosciences), washed and incubated with PE-linked anti-CD51 (αv integrin) antibody (BD Biosciences) for 60 min at 4°C. After three further washing steps, CD51 expression was measured using a FACS-Calibur^{TM} flow cytometer (Becton-Dickinson, San Jose, USA). Data were analyzed with FlowJo Software (version 7.6, TreeStar Inc.).

Statistical analyses

Unpaired or paired student's *t*-tests or ANOVA with appropriate post hoc corrections were used, as indicated, to evaluate differences among genotypic groups. *P* values less than 0.05 were considered significant. Statistical analyses were performed with Prism 5.0 software (GraphPad, La Jolla, CA).

Results

Deletion of *Erk1* or *Erk2* in BMMNCs and cultured osteoclasts

PCR was conducted to assay the presence of the *Erk1* null allele (*Erk1*$^{-/-}$), *Mx1Cre* transgene, and flanking loxP (*Erk2*$^{flox/flox}$) alleles. Figure S1 depicts the genomic PCR analysis for homozygous null *Erk1* (600 bp) and homozygous floxed *Erk2* (432 bp).To induce Cre expression and genetic disruption of *Erk2*, mice were treated with polyIC, as described in the Materials and Methods. Western blot analysis demonstrated undetectable Erk1 or Erk2 in protein isolates from BMMNCs extracted from genomic-verified *Erk1*$^{-/-}$ or *Mx1Cre*$^{+}$ *Erk2*$^{flox/flox}$ mutant mice (Figure S2, top panels). Likewise, western blot of protein from cultured osteoclasts demonstrated no detectable Erk1 or Erk2 protein (Figure S2 lower panels). For simplicity throughout, we refer to the genotypes of BMMNCs and osteoclasts derived from polyIC-treated *Mx1Cre*$^{+}$ *Erk2*$^{flox/flox}$ mice as *Erk2*$^{-/-}$.

Decreased multinucleated osteoclast formation from *Erk1*$^{-/-}$ BMMNCs

To evaluate the consequence of *Erk1* or *Erk2* disruption in osteoclast differentiation, we cultured osteoclasts from BMMNCs in M-CSF- and RANKL-supplemented α-MEM, followed by TRACP staining to evaluate cellular morphology. Compared with wildtype (WT) cultures, *Erk1*$^{-/-}$ BMMNCs demonstrated significantly decreased osteoclast-forming areas, as shown qualitatively and quantitatively in Figure 1A and 1B, respectively. In addition, the average number of nuclei per osteoclast was significantly less in *Erk1*$^{-/-}$ cultures than that in WT or *Erk2*$^{-/-}$ cultures (Figure 1C). Although we found no difference in the size of osteoclasts between *Erk2*$^{-/-}$ and WT cultures, the number of nuclei of *Erk2*$^{-/-}$ osteoclasts were slightly decreased as compared to WT osteoclasts. *Erk1*$^{-/-}$ cells display impaired osteoclast differentiation while Erk2 level should remain at least as WT cell level. It is possible that ERK2 expression in osteoclasts is not high enough to compensate for the loss of ERK1.

Genetic deletion of *Erk1* impairs osteoclast migration and bone resorption

Osteoclast bone resorptive capacity requires that osteoclast progenitor cells (preosteoclasts) migrate across the bone surface. To evaluate whether genetic disruption of *Erk1* or *Erk2* affects preosteoclast migration *in vitro*, we assessed transwell migration of preosteoclasts in response to recombinant M-CSF, a chemotactic signal for monocytic cells [27,29]. *Erk1*$^{-/-}$ preosteoclasts migrated at a lower number than both WT and *Erk2*$^{-/-}$ preosteoclasts in response to M-CSF, as shown by representative microphotograph of migrated cells and by quantification (Figure 2A). By contrast, *Erk2*$^{-/-}$ preosteoclasts did not demonstrate alterations in M-CSF-induced migratory capacity.

The initiation of osteoclastic bone resorption depends on osteoclasts' ability to bind to the bone surface through the interaction of cell surface receptors, such as the αvβ3 integrin, with extracellular bone proteins [27,30,31,32]. We examined whether deficiency of *Erk1* or *Erk2* affects αvβ3- and M-CSF-mediated preosteoclast adhesion. We found that fewer *Erk1*$^{-/-}$ preosteoclasts adhered to vitronectin during stimulation with M-CSF (Figure 2B), while the expression of integrin αv (CD51) was similar between the different genotypes (data not shown). We found no difference between WT and *Erk2*$^{-/-}$ osteoclasts in their capacity to adhere to vitronectin in cell culture.

To functionally assess the consequence of *Erk1* or *Erk2* disruption on osteoclast bone lytic activity, we cultured osteoclasts

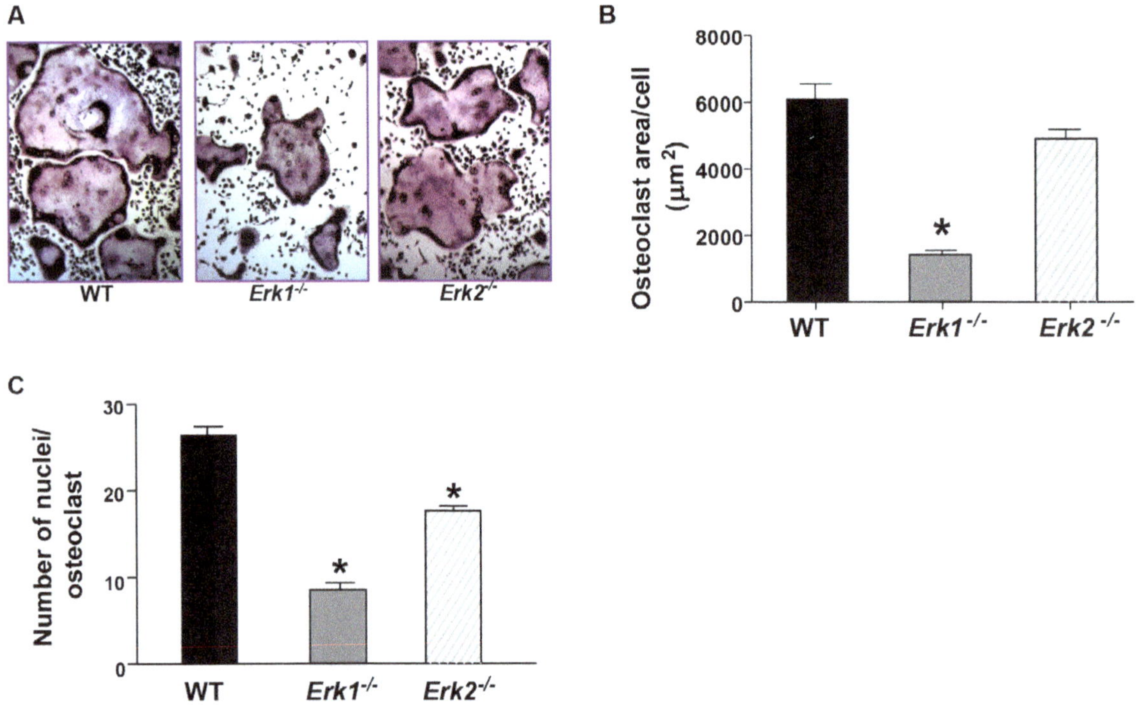

Figure 1. Genetic deletion of *Erk1* hinders osteoclast development. (**A**) Representative microphotograph of osteoclast formation of the indicated genotypes generated *in vitro* following culture in a-MEM, 10% FBS, M-CSF 30 ng/mL and RANKL 60 ng/mL for 6 days. Osteoclasts were identified by TRACP staining. (**B**) Quantitative analysis of the area of osteoclasts is shown. $^*P<0.01$ for *Erk1*$^{-/-}$ vs. WT and *Erk2*$^{-/-}$ by ANOVA followed by post-hoc *t*-tests. (**C**) Quantitative analysis of the number of nuclei per osteoclast is shown. Data represents Mean ± SEM of six fields per condition in triplicates. Experiments were conducted on three independent occasions with similar results. $^*P<0.01$ for *Erk1*$^{-/-}$ vs. WT and *Erk2*$^{-/-}$ vs. WT as assessed by ANOVA followed by post-hoc *t*-tests.

on dentine slices and examined the number and area of "pits" formed by osteoclast resorptive activity, as previously described [27,29]. Representative microphotographs of bone resorption are shown (Figure 2C). The quantitative data represents the total resorptive area (Figure 2C, upper panel). The resorptive area per osteoclast is shown quantitatively (Figure 2D). *Erk1*$^{-/-}$ osteoclast culture demonstrated a three-fold reduction in resorbed area and the *Erk2*$^{-/-}$ osteoclast culture demonstrated an approximate two-fold reduction, as compared to the WT osteoclast culture.

Collectively, these data indicate that *Erk1* positively regulates osteoclast differentiation and M-CSF-mediated migration and pit formation. Deletion of *Erk2* also reduces osteoclast nucleation and bone resorptive activity (albeit less substantially than Erk1). *Erk1*$^{-/-}$ cultures show stronger phenotypic changes although Erk2 exists. This may be explained by ERK2 expression in osteoclasts is not high enough to compensate for the loss of ERK1. Nevertheless, our cell culture data suggests important and preponderant contributions of Erk1 toward osteoclast differentiation and function.

Genetic deletion of *Erk1* in osteoclasts reduces total kinase activity

To examine biochemical alterations in the MAPK pathway in the context of *Erk1* or *Erk2* disruption, we stimulated cultured preosteoclasts with M-CSF (30 ng/mL), lysed the cells, and extracted protein for western blot. We assessed total and phosphorylated levels of Erk1, Erk2, and p90^{rsk}, a downstream Erk1/2 effector. Following M-CSF stimulation, Erk1 phosphorylation increased dramatically in WT and Erk2$^{-/-}$ cells, while no pErk1 was detected in *Erk1*$^{-/-}$ cells (Figure 3A). Interestingly, a slight, perhaps compensatory, increase in pErk1 was observed in *Erk2*$^{-/-}$ cells, as compared to WT. Similarly, we observed a moderate increase in pErk2 levels in M-CSF-stimulated *Erk1*$^{-/-}$ preosteoclasts, as compared to WT cells. As expected, no pErk2 was observed in Erk2$^{-/-}$ cells.

We also found a substantial reduction in phospho-p90^{rsk} in M-CSF-stimulated *Erk1*$^{-/-}$ preosteoclasts, as compared to stimulated WT and *Erk2*$^{-/-}$ cells (Figure 3B). Since PI3-K has been shown to regulate osteoclast development [33], we also examined phosphorylation of Akt in the cultured preosteoclasts. Similar levels of Akt phosphorylation were observed among WT, *Erk1*$^{-/-}$, and *Erk2*$^{-/-}$ preosteoclasts (data not shown), suggesting that the functional aberrancies observed in *Erk1*-deficient osteoclasts are Akt independent. Quantitative analysis of the western blot result is shown in Figure S4.

Genetic deletion of *Erk1* reduces osteoclast progenitors

Since osteoclasts are tissue-specific progeny of the monocyte/macrophage lineage, we quantitatively evaluated the number of macrophage and osteoclast progenitors per femur in *Erk1*$^{-/-}$, *Erk2*$^{-/-}$, and WT mice using established clonogenic assays [27]. Following culture in semisolid media supplemented with osteoclast-promoting cytokines (i.e. M-CSF, RANKL), the number of osteoclast and macrophage progenitor colonies were scored. *Erk1*$^{-/-}$ BMMNCs developed approximately one-fourth to one-third fewer macrophage colonies as compared to the number of colonies formed from *Erk2*$^{-/-}$ and WT BMMNCs (Figure 4A). Although the osteoclast progenitors are decreased in *Erk2*$^{-/-}$ also, the result showed that Erk1 plays a more vital role than Erk2 in osteoclastogenesis. Of note, there was no significant difference in

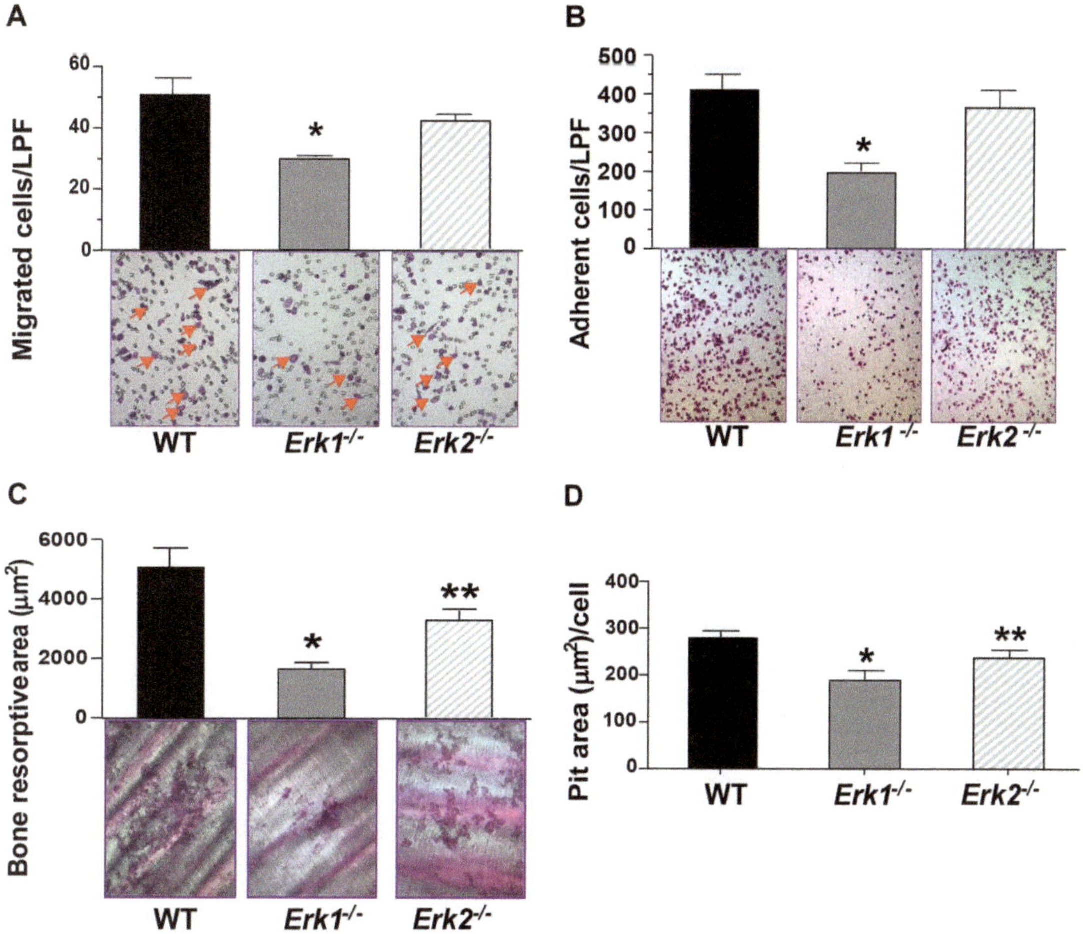

Figure 2. Effect of *Erk1* deletion on osteoclast haptotaxis, adhesion, and bone resorption in response to M-CSF. (**A**) Haptotaxis of preosteoclasts from WT, *Erk1*$^{-/-}$, *Erk2*$^{-/-}$ cultures in response to M-CSF. Representative microphotographs of low power field (100× magnifications) from 1 of 3 experiments are shown. Quantitative evaluation of migration in response to M-CSF was performed. Result represents the mean ± SEM of six fields per condition in triplicates. Three independent experiments were conducted with similar results. **P*<0.01 by ANOVA. (**B**) Quantitative evaluation of M-CSF mediated preosteoclast adhesion (30 minutes) to αVβ3 is shown. Data represents mean ± SEM of six fields per condition of triplicates. Representative microphotographs (100× magnification) are shown. **P*<0.01 by ANOVA followed by post-hoc *t*-tests. Experiment conducted on three independent occasions with similar results. (**C**) Representative microphotographs of the bone resorption on dentine slices, referred to as 'pits', are shown. Bar graph indicates the average of "pit" area per dentine slice. Data represents mean+standard error of the mean (SEM). **P*<0.01 for *Erk1*$^{-/-}$ vs. WT, ***P*<0.05 for *Erk2*$^{-/-}$ vs. WT and *Erk1*$^{-/-}$ as assessed by ANOVA followed by post-hoc *t*-tests. (**D**) Quantitative analysis of bone resorption following culture of osteoclasts on dentine slices. The area of the resorbed regions per osteoclasts was quantified. Data represents one of three independent experiments with similar results. **P*<0.01 for *Erk1*$^{-/-}$ vs. WT, ***P*<0.05 for *Erk2*$^{-/-}$ vs. WT and *Erk1*$^{-/-}$ as assessed by ANOVA followed by post-hoc *t*-tests.

total bone marrow cellularity between *Erk1*$^{-/-}$, *Erk2*$^{-/-}$, and WT mice (data not shown), indicating a primary reduction in the frequency of monocyte/osteoclast progenitor cells in *Erk1*$^{-/-}$ bone marrow.

Reduced TRACP^{+} osteoclast development in *Erk1*$^{-/-}$ mice

Given the impaired osteoclast differentiation *in vitro* and reduced number of osteoclast progenitors in *Erk1*$^{-/-}$ bone marrow, we next assayed the number of mature osteoclasts in *Erk1*$^{-/-}$ mice *in vivo*. The femurs of 8-week old syngeneic WT, *Erk1*$^{-/-}$ and *Erk2*$^{-/-}$ mice were fixed and embedded in methyl methacrylate, and histological sections from the distal metaphysis were stained with the osteoclast enzyme TRACP. Compared to WT mice, the TRACP^{+} area per low power field (100× magnification) of trabecular surface in *Erk1*$^{-/-}$ mice was decreased as qualitatively and quantitatively shown in Figure 4B and Figure 4C, respectively. To determine if deletion of *Erk1* additionally alters osteoblast formation, McNeal staining was performed on the methyl methacrylate processed histological sections, revealing no significant change in osteoblast numbers between WT, *Erk1*$^{-/-}$, and *Erk2*$^{-/-}$ bone sections (Figure S3).

Reduced C-terminal telopeptide of type I collagen (CTX) in *Erk1*$^{-/-}$ mice

Type I Collagen, which constitutes more than 90% of the organic matrix of bone, can be degraded and released during osteoclastic bone resorption. Thus, the level of CTX production in plasma is a sensitive marker of bone loss [34]. The level of CTX production in plasma was substantially reduced in *Erk1*$^{-/-}$ mice as compared with that in WT and *Erk2*$^{-/-}$ mice (Figure 4D), suggesting a reduced osteoclast bone resorptive activity in *Erk1*$^{-/-}$ mice *in vivo*.

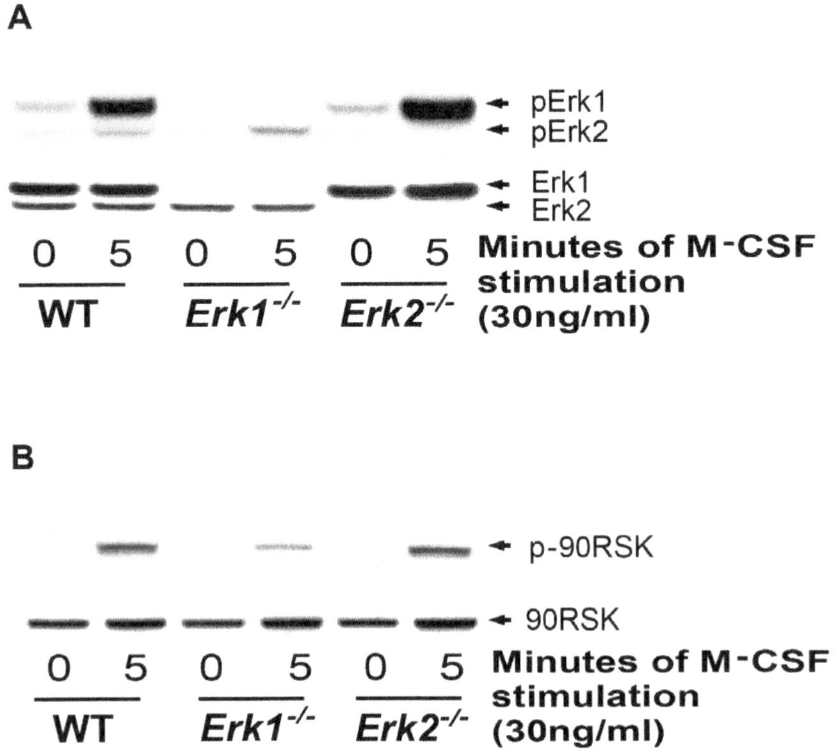

Figure 3. Effect of *Erk1* genetic deletion on MAPK activation in preosteoclasts. Phosphorylation of Erk1/2 (Figure 3A) and p90RSK (Figure 3B) in preosteoclasts of WT, *Erk1*$^{-/-}$ and *Erk2*$^{-/-}$ mice was measured at the indicated times following stimulation with M-SCF. Representative blots are shown.

Increased bone mineral density in *Erk1*$^{-/-}$ mice and *Erk1*$^{-/-}$ bone marrow mononuclear cell transplanted recipients

Given that alteration in osteoclast bone resorptive activity affects bone structure, we hypothesized that *Erk1*$^{-/-}$ mice would demonstrate increased bone mineral density (BMD). To test this hypothesis, we acquired BMD data using dual-energy X-ray absorptiometry (DEXA) with a Lunar Piximus densitometer. We specifically analyzed a region of interest with a high content of trabecular bone, located proximal to the distal growth plate of the left femur of each mouse. *Erk1*$^{-/-}$ male mice demonstrated increased BMD, as measured monthly after birth (Figure 5A). *Erk1*$^{-/-}$ female mice also displayed increased BMD as compared to WT littermates (Figure 5B), though the difference was milder than in the male mice. However, the cause of the different BMD between male and female mice remains unclear.

To compare the long bone mass between the WT and *Erk1*$^{-/-}$ mice, micro-computed tomography (μCT) was utilized to examine the bone volume and architecture. *Erk1*$^{-/-}$ mice exhibited an ~80% increase (**$P<0.05$) in trabecular bone volume fraction (BV/TV), (Figure 5C and 5D); an ~15% increase (**$P<0.05$) in trabecular thickness, an ~50% increase (**$P<0.05$) in trabecular number, and an ~30% decrease (**$P<0.05$) in trabecular separation, as compared to the WT controls (Figure S6A–C). This increased bone volume in *Erk1*$^{-/-}$ mice is consistent with the increase of BMD in *Erk1*$^{-/-}$ mice.

Based on our tissue culture and *in vivo* findings, we hypothesized that aberrant formation and function of *Erk1*$^{-/-}$ osteoclasts directly results in increased BMD. To test this hypothesis, we performed long-term transplantation [26] of BMMNCs from WT, *Erk1*$^{-/-}$ and *Erk2*$^{-/-}$ mice into lethally-irradiated WT BoyJ recipient mice, thus isolating our analysis to cells derived from the donor hematopoietic cells. For complete reconstitution of hematopoietic cells, we waited six months after the transplantation to confirm successful reconstitution of hematopoietic stem cells and *Erk2* allele deletion by flow cytometry-based detection of CD45.2 expression (data not shown) and by western blot of peripheral blood (Figure S5), respectively. We then measured BMD in the recipient mice, finding that *Erk1*$^{-/-}$ bone marrow reconstitution produced increased BMD as compared to WT recipients (Figure 6), while transplantation of *Erk2*$^{-/-}$ BMMNCs did not alter BMD as compared to WT recipients. These data imply a marrow-autonomous role for *Erk1* in regulating osteoclast development and bone resorptive activity *in vivo*.

Discussion

Alterations of the Ras/MAPK pathway have been observed in disease models of Paget's bone disease, bone metastasis, and Neurofibromatosis type 1 (NF1) [35,36,37,38]. Moreover, congenital disorders including Noonan syndrome, Noonan-like/multiple giant cell lesion syndrome, NF1, LEOPARD syndrome, Costello syndrome, and Cardio-facio-cutaneous syndrome carry germline mutations that variously affect genes within the MAPK signaling cascades [39]. These studies broadly implicate deregulation of Ras signals in skeletal pathologies. However, the interaction between and contribution of individual cell lineages (e.g. osteoblasts, osteoclasts, mesenchymal stromal cells) to specific pathologies, as well as their potential dependence on a specific Erk isoform, require further delineation.

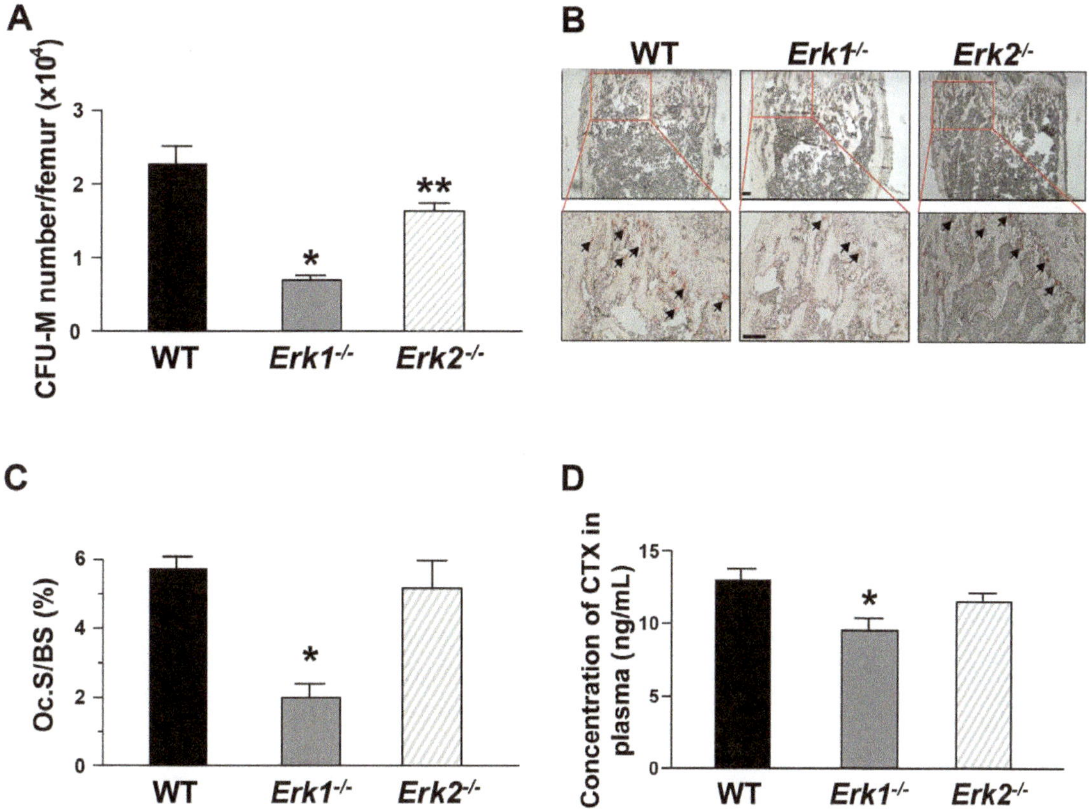

Figure 4. Genetic deletion of Erk1 affects osteoclast progenitor frequency and osteoclast formation *in vivo*. (**A**) BMMNCs of the indicated genotypes were cultured in agar-based media containing M-CSF (30 ng/mL) and RANKL (20 ng/mL) for 7 days and CFU-macrophage (M) were counted based on morphology. Y-axis indicated CFU-M number per femur. Data represents mean ± SEM of triplicate cultures. *$P<0.01$ for *Erk1*$^{-/-}$ vs. WT, **$P<0.05$ for *Erk2*$^{-/-}$ vs. WT and *Erk1*$^{-/-}$, as evaluated by ANOVA followed by post-hoc *t*-tests. Experiments were conducted on three independent occasions with similar results. (**B**) Representative microphotographs (40×, 100× magnification) of WT, *Erk1*$^{-/-}$ and *Erk2*$^{-/-}$ distal femoral metaphyses following TRACP staining. Arrows indicate selected osteoclasts. Scale bar = 100 µm. (**C**) Data represent the mean ± SEM of 5 independent experiments. Ten high-power fields per experimental mouse were scored. *$P<0.01$ for *Erk1*$^{-/-}$ vs. WT and *Erk2*$^{-/-}$, as analyzed by ANOVA followed by post-hoc *t*-tests. (D) Detection of CTX in plasma of WT, *Erk1*$^{-/-}$ and *Erk2*$^{-/-}$ mice (N = 4–6 mice in each group).*$P<0.05$ for *Erk1*$^{-/-}$ vs. WT, as analyzed by ANOVA followed by post-hoc *t*-tests.

Previously, we found that the Mek-Erk inhibitor PD98059 reduces osteoclast development and belt formation [29]. Since PD98059 inhibits phosphorylation of both Erk1 and Erk2, and perhaps exhibits a high degree of non-selectivity at its applied concentration, we were unable to delineate if Erk1, Erk2, both, or, potentially, neither isoform modulates osteoclast differentiation. Here, we show that genetic disruption of *Erk1* versus *Erk2* preferentially impairs osteoclast formation and function *in vitro* and *in vivo*. Important to note, this phenotype arises in a marrow-autonomous manner, implicating *Erk1's* importance to the marrow-derived osteoclast and its regulation of normal bone physiology. Although we show that Erk2 cannot compensate, either functionally or biochemically, for loss of *Erk1* in the osteoclast, we still suspect that Erk2 can positively contribute to osteoclastogenesis and osteoclast function. Supporting this notion, we have found that *Erk1/2* dual disruption ablates early myelopoiesis and precludes the study of osteoclastogenesis, a phenotype which will be reported in detail elsewhere. By contrast, Erk1 appears largely capable of compensating for *Erk2* disruption in the observed biochemical and functional phenotypes. Thus, we have concluded that Erk1 plays the preponderant role in regulating osteoclastogenesis and osteoclast function. However, it remains unknown whether this phenotype results from isoform functional specificity or solely from osteoclast-intrinsic dependence on increased Erk1 expression and/or activation.

Biochemical, pharmacological, and genetic models have broadly implicated ERK1/2 activity in proliferation, survival, migration, and protein synthesis in diverse cell types (reviewed in [40]). However, lineage- and isoform-specific functions are less known, and genetic murine studies have been limited, thus far demonstrating *Erk1*-specific requirements for thymocyte development [18], erythropoiesis [41], adipogenesis [19], and skin tumor development [17]. Other studies have suggested a negative regulatory role for Erk1, whereby *Erk1* disruption enhances fibroblast and neuron function by dis-inhibiting Mek-Erk2 signals [42,43]. These data suggest the preponderance of Erk2 over Erk1 function in these cell types. Accordingly, *Erk2* disruption is embryonically lethal [44] while, grossly, *Erk1*$^{-/-}$ mice demonstrate no profound phenotypes [18]. However, as reported elsewhere and as we show here for the osteoclast, homeostatic processes in particular organ systems may depend upon Erk1, and generalizations as to Erk1 versus Erk2's functional importance should not be derived from observations in one cell type. Our results showed that Ekr1 had higher expression level than Erk2 in preosteoclasts; it is most likely that Erk1 has higher affinity than Erk2 does for the antibody.

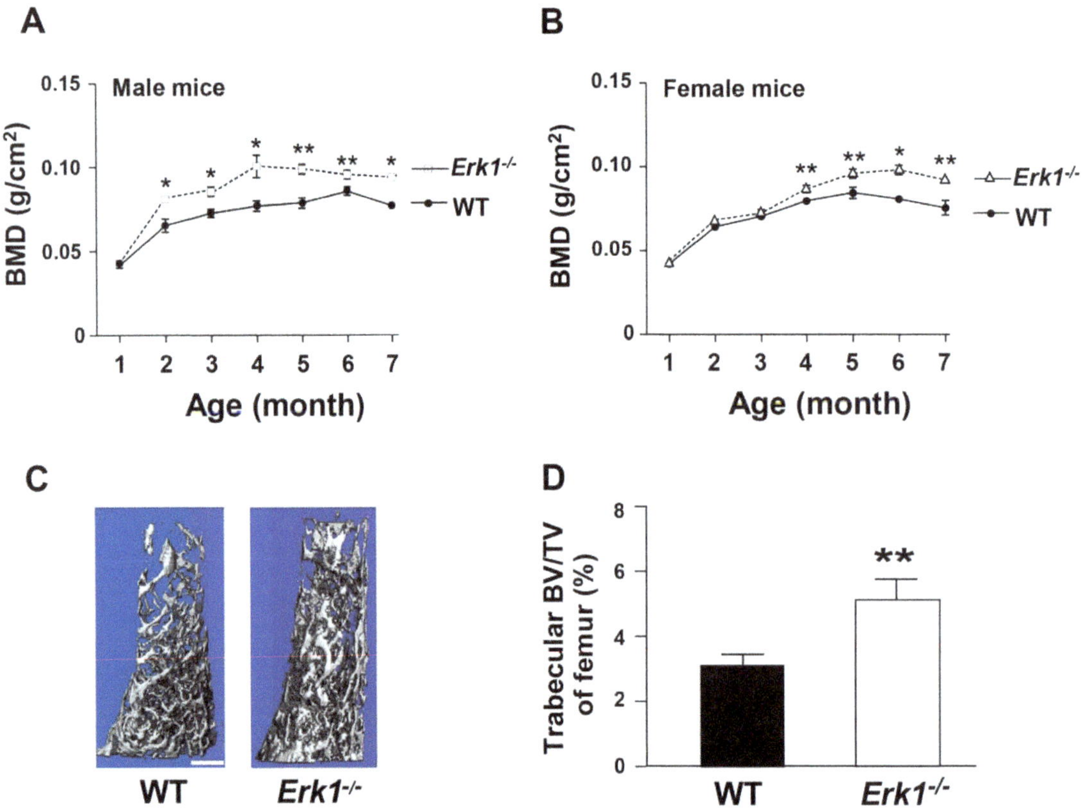

Figure 5. *Erk1*$^{-/-}$ mice have increased BMD and BV/TV. BMD of age and sex matched *Erk1*$^{-/-}$ and WT mice was measured from birth to 7 months of age. The BMD of male (**A**) and female (**B**) WT and *Erk1*$^{-/-}$ mice is shown (N = 5 mice in each group). (**C**) Representative μCT reconstructions of WT and *Erk1*$^{-/-}$ femurs are shown. Scale bar = 1 mm. (**D**) Quantitative data comparing the left femur BV/TV between WT and *Erk1*$^{-/-}$ mice.

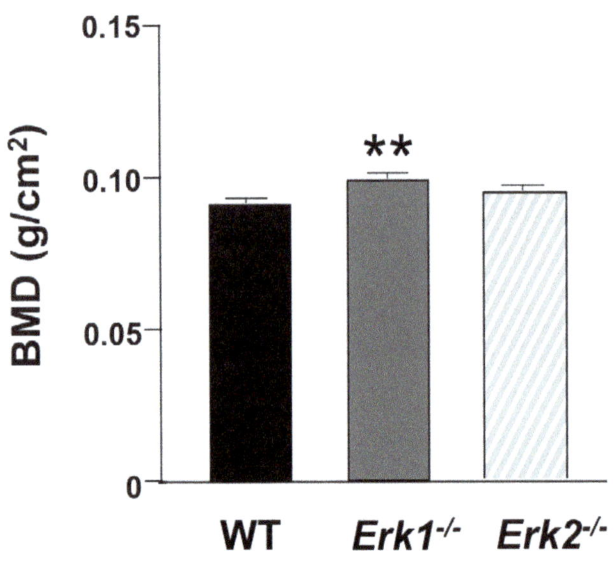

Figure 6. Transplantation of *Erk1*$^{-/-}$ bone marrow increases BMD in WT recipients. Six months after transplantation with WT, *Erk1*$^{-/-}$ or *Erk2*$^{-/-}$BMMNCs into WT recipient mice, BMD was measured (N = 5 mice in each group). **$P<0.05$ for *Erk1*$^{-/-}$ vs. WT recipients, as analyzed by ANOVA followed with post-hoc *t*-tests.

Different cell lineage- and isoform-specific studies *in vitro* and *in vivo* will produce crucial insights into the subtleties of MAPK signaling, thus informing therapeutic strategies. Accordingly, ERK isoform-specific chemical inhibition may prove pivotal to targeted therapy. Though bisphosphonates have been the cornerstone of osteoporosis therapy since the 1960's, recent work has focused on more selective compounds [45]. Molecular targets to Ras itself, such as farnesyl transferase inhibitors, have been disappointing, as K-ras and N-ras, the isoforms prevalent in myeloid lineages, do not depend on farnesylation. Because disruption of *Erk1* dampens osteoclast function to a degree sufficient to increase bone mineral density *in vivo*, an Erk1-targeted chemical kinase inhibitor may be an effective therapeutic agent for the diminished bone mineral density found in multiple skeletal pathologies, including hormonal loss-dependent osteoporosis. This strategy may selectively modulate osteoclast function while producing fewer off-target and detrimental effects potentially associated with dual Erk1/2 inhibition. Of note, a recent crystal structure of human ERK1 revealed substantial differences in D-motif and backside binding sites, as compared to ERK2, indicating the feasibility of a selective ERK1 inhibitory agent [46].

In conclusion, osteoclastogenesis and osteoclast functions depend upon Erk1 to a greater degree than Erk2, and singular genetic inhibition of *Erk1* mitigates osteoclast function *in vitro* and *in vivo*. This loss-of-function phenotype appears to proceed in a marrow autonomous manner, thus implicating a primary defect within the *Erk1*-disrupted osteoclast. These results uniquely demonstrate a positive regulator role for Erk1 while suggesting the potential for Erk isoform-targeted therapy of osteoporotic conditions.

Supporting Information

Figure S1 Genotypic analysis. PCR was performed to confirm the genotype of WT (lane 1), *Erk1*$^{-/-}$ (lane 2) and *Mx1Cre*$^{+}$ *Erk2*$^{fl/fl}$ (lane 3) mice.

Figure S2 Western Blot. Representative western blot of three independent experiments shows the total protein level of Erk1 or Erk2 in bone marrow mononuclear cells (BMMNCs) and osteoclast. β-actin was utilized as a loading control.

Figure S3 (**A**) Representative microphotographs (100× magnification) of WT, *Erk1*$^{-/-}$ and *Erk2*$^{-/-}$ distal femoral metaphyses following McNeal Staining. Arrows indicate selected osteoblasts. (**B**) Data represent the mean ± SEM of 5 independent experiments. Six high-power fields per experimental mouse were scored. Scale bar = 50 μm.

Figure S4 Quantitative evaluation of Erk1 phosphorylation over ß-actin level of Figure 3. (**A**), Erk2 phosphorylation (**B**), and phosphorylation of p90RSK (**C**) in WT, *Erk1*$^{-/-}$ and *Erk2*$^{-/-}$ preosteoclasts is shown.

Figure S5 Western blot shows the protein levels of Erk1 and Erk2 in peripheral blood of the WT and *Erk1*$^{-/-}$ transplanted WT recipients. Scale bar = 1 mm.

Figure S6 Quantitative data comparing the left femur Tb.Th, Tb.N and Tb.Sep between WT and *Erk1*$^{-/-}$ mice (N = 5 in each group). **$P<0.05$ for *Erk1*$^{-/-}$ vs. WT mice.

Acknowledgments

We thank Lisa Tully for administrative support.

Author Contributions

Conceived and designed the experiments: F-CY YH KS. Performed the experiments: YH KS SDR YL XW S-JP JY XY XL LJ SC. Analyzed the data: YH KS SDR YL S-JP SC XW F-CY JY XY XL LJ. Wrote the paper: YH F-CY.

References

1. Raisz LG (2005) Pathogenesis of osteoporosis: concepts, conflicts, and prospects. J Clin Invest 115: 3318–3325.
2. Datta HK, Ng WF, Walker JA, Tuck SP, Varanasi SS (2008) The cell biology of bone metabolism. J Clin Pathol 61: 577–587.
3. Chambers TJ (2000) Regulation of the differentiation and function of osteoclasts. J Pathol 192: 4–13.
4. Lacey DL, Timms E, Tan HL, Kelley MJ, Dunstan CR, et al. (1998) Osteoprotegerin ligand is a cytokine that regulates osteoclast differentiation and activation. Cell 93: 165–176.
5. Yasuda H, Shima N, Nakagawa N, Yamaguchi K, Kinosaki M, et al. (1998) Osteoclast differentiation factor is a ligand for osteoprotegerin/osteoclastogenesis-inhibitory factor and is identical to TRANCE/RANKL. Proc Natl Acad Sci U S A 95: 3597–3602.
6. Cohen MM, Jr. (2006) The new bone biology: pathologic, molecular, and clinical correlates. Am J Med Genet A 140: 2646–2706.
7. Aoki Y, Niihori T, Narumi Y, Kure S, Matsubara Y (2008) The RAS/MAPK syndromes: novel roles of the RAS pathway in human genetic disorders. Hum Mutat 29: 992–1006.
8. Newbern J, Zhong J, Wickramasinghe RS, Li X, Wu Y, et al. (2008) Mouse and human phenotypes indicate a critical conserved role for ERK2 signaling in neural crest development. Proc Natl Acad Sci U S A 105: 17115–17120.
9. Stevenson D, Schwarz E, Carey J, Viskochil D, Hanson H, et al. Bone resorption in syndromes of the Ras/MAPK pathway. Clin Genet.
10. Leevers SJ, Paterson HF, Marshall CJ (1994) Requirement for Ras in Raf activation is overcome by targeting Raf to the plasma membrane. Nature 369: 411–414.
11. Leevers SJ, Marshall CJ (1992) Activation of extracellular signal-regulated kinase, ERK2, by p21ras oncoprotein. EMBO J 11: 569–574.
12. Shaul YD, Gibor G, Plotnikov A, Seger R (2009) Specific phosphorylation and activation of ERK1c by MEK1b: a unique route in the ERK cascade. Genes Dev 23: 1779–1790.
13. Paroo Z, Ye X, Chen S, Liu Q (2009) Phosphorylation of the human microRNA-generating complex mediates MAPK/Erk signaling. Cell 139: 112–122.
14. Fiil BK, Petersen K, Petersen M, Mundy J (2009) Gene regulation by MAP kinase cascades. Curr Opin Plant Biol 12: 615–621.
15. Subramaniam S, Unsicker K (2009) ERK and cell death: ERK1/2 in neuronal death. FEBS J 277: 22–29.
16. Bates ME, Sedgwick JB, Zhu Y, Liu LY, Heuser RG, et al. (2010) Human airway eosinophils respond to chemoattractants with greater eosinophil-derived neurotoxin release, adherence to fibronectin, and activation of the Ras-ERK pathway when compared with blood eosinophils. J Immunol 184: 7125–7133.
17. Bourcier C, Jacquel A, Hess J, Peyrottes I, Angel P, et al. (2006) p44 mitogen-activated protein kinase (extracellular signal-regulated kinase 1)-dependent signaling contributes to epithelial skin carcinogenesis. Cancer Res 66: 2700–2707.
18. Pages G, Guerin S, Grall D, Bonino F, Smith A, et al. (1999) Defective thymocyte maturation in p44 MAP kinase (Erk 1) knockout mice. Science 286: 1374–1377.
19. Bost F, Aouadi M, Caron L, Even P, Belmonte N, et al. (2005) The extracellular signal-regulated kinase isoform ERK1 is specifically required for in vitro and in vivo adipogenesis. Diabetes 54: 402–411.
20. Matsushita T, Chan YY, Kawanami A, Balmes G, Landreth GE, et al. (2009) Extracellular signal-regulated kinase 1 (ERK1) and ERK2 play essential roles in osteoblast differentiation and in supporting osteoclastogenesis. Mol Cell Biol 29: 5843–5857.
21. Yasuda T, Sanjo H, Pages G, Kawano Y, Karasuyama H, et al. (2008) Erk kinases link pre-B cell receptor signaling to transcriptional events required for early B cell expansion. Immunity 28: 499–508.
22. Fischer AM, Katayama CD, Pages G, Pouyssegur J, Hedrick SM (2005) The role of erk1 and erk2 in multiple stages of T cell development. Immunity 23: 431–443.
23. D'Souza WN, Chang CF, Fischer AM, Li M, Hedrick SM (2008) The Erk2 MAPK regulates CD8 T cell proliferation and survival. J Immunol 181: 7617–7629.
24. Bradley EW, Oursler MJ (2008) Osteoclast culture and resorption assays. Methods Mol Biol 455: 19–35.
25. Kim HH, Chung WJ, Lee SW, Chung PJ, You JW, et al. (2003) Association of sustained ERK activity with integrin beta3 induction during receptor activator of nuclear factor kappaB ligand (RANKL)-directed osteoclast differentiation. Exp Cell Res 289: 368–377.
26. Yang FC, Ingram DA, Chen S, Zhu Y, Yuan J, et al. (2008) Nf1-dependent tumors require a microenvironment containing Nf1+/− and c-kit-dependent bone marrow. Cell 135: 437–448.
27. Yang FC, Chen S, Robling AG, Yu X, Nebesio TD, et al. (2006) Hyperactivation of p21 and PI3K cooperate to alter murine and human neurofibromatosis type 1-haploinsufficient osteoclast functions. J Clin Invest 116: 2880–2891.
28. Munugalavadla V, Vemula S, Sims EC, Krishnan S, Chen S, et al. (2008) The p85alpha subunit of class IA phosphatidylinositol 3-kinase regulates the expression of multiple genes involved in osteoclast maturation and migration. Mol Cell Biol 28: 7182–7198.
29. Yan J, Chen S, Zhang Y, Li X, Li Y, et al. (2008) Rac1 mediates the osteoclast gains-in-function induced by haploinsufficiency of Nf1. Hum Mol Genet 17: 936–948.
30. Aubin JE (1992) Osteoclast adhesion and resorption: the role of podosomes. J Bone Miner Res 7: 365–368.
31. McHugh KP, Hodivala-Dilke K, Zheng MH, Namba N, Lam J, et al. (2000) Mice lacking beta3 integrins are osteosclerotic because of dysfunctional osteoclasts. J Clin Invest 105: 433–440.
32. Chellaiah MA, Hruska KA (2003) The integrin alpha(v)beta(3) and CD44 regulate the actions of osteopontin on osteoclast motility. Calcif Tissue Int 72: 197–205.
33. Munugalavadla V, Borneo J, Ingram DA, Kapur R (2005) p85alpha subunit of class IA PI-3 kinase is crucial for macrophage growth and migration. Blood 106: 103–109.
34. Seibel MJ (2005) Biochemical markers of bone turnover: part I: biochemistry and variability. Clin Biochem Rev 26: 97–122.
35. Yip KH, Feng H, Pavlos NJ, Zheng MH, Xu J (2006) p62 ubiquitin binding-associated domain mediated the receptor activator of nuclear factor-kappaB ligand-induced osteoclast formation: a new insight into the pathogenesis of Paget's disease of bone. Am J Pathol 169: 503–514.
36. Abbas S, Clohisy JC, Abu-Amer Y (2003) Mitogen-activated protein (MAP) kinases mediate PMMA-induction of osteoclasts. J Orthop Res 21: 1041–1048.

37. Yamanaka Y, Abu-Amer Y, Faccio R, Clohisy JC (2006) Map kinase c-JUN N-terminal kinase mediates PMMA induction of osteoclasts. J Orthop Res 24: 1349–1357.
38. Wu X, Estwick SA, Chen S, Yu M, Ming W, et al. (2006) Neurofibromin plays a critical role in modulating osteoblast differentiation of mesenchymal stem/progenitor cells. Hum Mol Genet 15: 2837–2845.
39. Tumurkhuu M, Saitoh M, Sato A, Takahashi K, Mimaki M, et al. Comprehensive genetic analysis of overlapping syndromes of RAS/RAF/MEK/ERK pathway. Pediatr Int 52: 557–562.
40. Meloche S, Pouyssegur J (2007) The ERK1/2 mitogen-activated protein kinase pathway as a master regulator of the G1- to S-phase transition. Oncogene 26: 3227–3239.
41. Guihard S, Clay D, Cocault L, Saulnier N, Opolon P, et al. The MAPK ERK1 is a negative regulator of the adult steady-state splenic erythropoiesis. Blood 115: 3686–3694.
42. Vantaggiato C, Formentini I, Bondanza A, Bonini C, Naldini L, et al. (2006) ERK1 and ERK2 mitogen-activated protein kinases affect Ras-dependent cell signaling differentially. J Biol 5: 14.
43. Mazzucchelli C, Vantaggiato C, Ciamei A, Fasano S, Pakhotin P, et al. (2002) Knockout of ERK1 MAP kinase enhances synaptic plasticity in the striatum and facilitates striatal-mediated learning and memory. Neuron 34: 807–820.
44. Saba-El-Leil MK, Vella FD, Vernay B, Voisin L, Chen L, et al. (2003) An essential function of the mitogen-activated protein kinase Erk2 in mouse trophoblast development. EMBO Rep 4: 964–968.
45. Boyle WJ, Simonet WS, Lacey DL (2003) Osteoclast differentiation and activation. Nature 423: 337–342.
46. Kinoshita T, Yoshida I, Nakae S, Okita K, Gouda M, et al. (2008) Crystal structure of human mono-phosphorylated ERK1 at Tyr204. Biochem Biophys Res Commun 377: 1123–1127.

9

Targeting Bone Alleviates Osteoarthritis in Osteopenic Mice and Modulates Cartilage Catabolism

Thomas Funck-Brentano[1], Hilène Lin[1], Eric Hay[1], Marie-Dominique Ah Kioon[1], Corinne Schiltz[1], Didier Hannouche[2], Rémy Nizard[2], Frédéric Lioté[1], Philippe Orcel[3], Marie-Christine de Vernejoul[1], Martine Esther Cohen-Solal[1]*

1 INSERM U606, Centre Viggo Petersen and Université Paris-Diderot Paris 7, Hôpital Lariboisière, Paris, France, **2** Department of Orthopedics, Centre Viggo Petersen and Université Paris-Diderot Paris 7, Hôpital Lariboisière, Paris, France, **3** Department of Rheumatology, Centre Viggo Petersen and Université Paris-Diderot Paris 7, Hôpital Lariboisière, Paris, France

Abstract

Objective: Subchondral bone modifications occur early in the development of osteoarthritis (OA). The level of bone resorption might impact cartilage remodeling. We therefore assessed the in vivo and in vitro effects of targeting bone resorption in OA and cartilage metabolism.

Methods: OA was induced by meniscectomy (MNX) in ovariectomized osteopenic mice (OP) treated with estradiol (E2), pamidronate (PAM), or phosphate buffered saline (PBS) for 6 weeks. We assessed the subchondral bone and cartilage structure and the expression of cartilage matrix proteases. To assess the involvement of bone soluble factors in cartilage metabolism, supernatant of human bone explants pre-treated with E2 or PAM were transferred to cartilage explants to assess proteoglycan release and aggrecan cleavage. OPG/RANKL mRNA expression was assessed in bone explants by real-time quantitative PCR. The role of osteoprotegerin (OPG) in the bone-cartilage crosstalk was tested using an OPG neutralizing antibody.

Results: Bone mineral density of OP mice and osteoclast number were restored by E2 and PAM ($p<0.05$). In OP mice, E2 and PAM decreased ADAMTS-4 and -5 expression, while only PAM markedly reduced OA compared to PBS (2.0 ± 0.63 vs 5.2 ± 0.95; $p<0.05$). OPG/RANKL mRNA was increased in human bone explants treated with both drugs (2.2–3.7-fold). Moreover, supernatants from bone explants cultured with E2 or PAM reduced aggrecan cleavage and cartilage proteoglycan release ($73\pm8.0\%$ and $80\pm22\%$ of control, respectively, $p<0.05$). This effect was reversed with osteoprotegerin blockade.

Conclusion: The inhibition of bone resorption by pamidronate in osteopenic mice alleviates the histological OA score with a reduction in the expression of aggrecanases. Bone soluble factors, such as osteoprotegerin, impact the cartilage response to catabolic factors. This study further highlights the importance of subchondral bone in the regulation of joint cartilage damage in OA.

Editor: Jean-Marc Vanacker, Institut de Génomique Fonctionnelle de Lyon, France

Funding: TFB was supported by INSERM, "Société Française de Rhumatologie" and "Fondation pour la Recherche Médicale". The funders had no role in study design, data collection and analysis, decision to publish, or preparation of the manuscript.

Competing Interests: The authors have declared that no competing interests exist.

* E-mail: martine.cohen-solal@inserm.fr

Introduction

Osteoarthritis (OA) is a common disease responsible for high morbidity related to functional disability and pain. Although cartilage lesions are the main feature of OA, other joint structures also contribute to progression of the disease via several mechanisms. Radin *et al.* [1,2] was the first to suggest that subchondral bone could trigger degradation of the overlying cartilage. Subsequently, studies on humans and animal models have revealed concomitant changes in bone and cartilage structures, particularly during the late stages of OA. In patients with established OA, trabecular bone volume is high, and bone accretion is correlated with the severity of cartilage damage [3]. Subchondral bone lesions appear during the early stages of OA, as demonstrated by the presence of bone marrow lesions that are factors predictive of OA progression [4,5]. The natures of such bone lesions are still poorly established, although trabecular fractures or enhanced trabecular bone remodeling are suspected. Early stages of OA are accompanied by a decrease in bone volume, which suggests that initial bone resorption might trigger OA [6–9]. Indeed, OA can be prevented in rats by inhibiting bone resorption with alendronate [6]. Several molecules may mediate osteoclastic bone resorption, and thus have an impact on cartilage remodeling [10]. We and others have demonstrated that osteoprotegerin (OPG), a decoy receptor of Receptor Activator for Nuclear Factor κB Ligand (RANKL) produced by osteoblasts, could decrease joint cartilage degradation in a murine model of joint instability [10,11]. Reducing bone remodeling in Runx2 transgenic mice prevents from cartilage breakdown [12].

The role of bone resorption related to estrogen failure in the development of OA is still a matter of debate. In humans, estrogen deficiency is reported to be a risk factor for OA, and estrogen deficiency/polymorphism appears to increase the incidence of OA in postmenopausal women [13–16], although this remains controversial [17]. In mice, the deletion of estrogen receptors does not affect the cartilage structure [18], whereas protective effects of estradiol in the development of OA have been shown in other animal models [19,20]. Estrogens are powerful osteoclast inhibitors [21], and might contribute to OA protection via their effects in bone.

The aim of this study was to assess whether cartilage protection could be achieved by inhibiting bone remodeling in mice with high bone resorption induced by estrogen deficiency. We therefore investigated the impact of reducing bone resorption in osteopenic mice (OP) with joint instability, and the effects of bone-secreted cytokines on cartilage catabolism.

Results

Inhibitors of bone resorption restore subchondral bone architecture in OP mice

The bodyweight of mice remained stable in each group throughout the study (Table 1). Uterus weight declined after ovariectomy in the Phosphate Buffered Saline (PBS)-treated and Pamidronate (PAM)-treated mice, but was maintained in the mice treated with estradiol. Total body BMD decreased significantly in OP mice ($p<0.05$), and this was reversed by both pamidronate and estradiol. These results indicate an appropriate systemic response to both anti-resorptive therapies. BMD changes in the knee were in line with those of total body BMD.

Bone indices were measured at the tibia 6 weeks after MNX. Bone volume (BV/TV) was lower in OP mice than in controls, which was consistent with the increase in Tb.Sp and osteoclast number, and the lower Tb.Th (Table 2). Estradiol prevented the local bone loss observed in the OP-PBS mice (48.8±4.8% vs 27.6±3%, $p=0.005$), and also prevented the increase in trabecular spacing and osteoclast number. The effects of estrogens on the local microarchitecture were in line with their effects on systemic bone. In contrast, pamidronate-treated mice had significantly lower osteoclast numbers, but no significant changes were observed in BV/TV (30.7±4.6% vs 27.6±3%, $p=0.48$), although BMD data indicated that this treatment did prevent systemic bone loss.

Anti-resorptive agents protected mice against OA

The histological OA score was significantly greater after MNX than in the sham-operated knees (5.1±0.47 vs 0.5±0.18, respectively; $p=0.018$) (Figure 1). However, OP did not produce any further increase in the OA score compared to controls (5.2±0.95; $p=0.86$). In MNX knees, pamidronate provided significant reduction of cartilage degradation compared to PBS treatment (OARSI 2010 score: 2.0±0.63 vs 5.2±0.95; $p=0.042$). In contrast, the effect of estradiol was not significant, although a similar trend was observed (3.7±1.30; $p=0.18$) (Figure 1). These results show that pamidronate reduced OA in a context of high systemic bone resorption whereas estradiol deficiency or supplementation had no significant structural effects on cartilage degradation induced by MNX.

To further investigate the biochemical changes in cartilage in each group, we analyzed the expression of ADAMTS by immunohistochemistry (Figure 2). MNX increased the expression of ADAMTS-4 and ADAMTS-5 in chondrocytes compared to controls (positive cells for ADAMTS-4 and -5: 58.1±3.5% vs 38.8±5.8%; $p=0.017$; 22.9±4.7% vs 7.5±4.3%; $p=0.027$, respectively). The number of ADAMTS-4 expressing cells was lower after estradiol and pamidronate than in PBS-treated mice (45.2±5.9%, and 37.0±5.6%, vs 60.2±3.0%, $p=0.025$ and $p=0.01$ respectively). Similar results were observed with ADAMTS-5 (14.2±2.9% and 7.10±4.7% vs 34.5±6.1%, $p=0.025$ and $p=0.039$, respectively, Figure 2).

Thus, estradiol and pamidronate both reduced aggrecanase expression, whereas only pamidronate significantly decreased the OA score induced by MNX.

Bone supernatants reduced human cartilage explants breakdown

To further understand the crosstalk between bone and cartilage, we investigated whether the conditioned media of bone explants contributed to the cartilage breakdown. IL-1β alone or in addition to the supernatants of control bone explants induced a significant increase in proteoglycan release from cartilage explants (123.9±2.4% and 132±16% of controls, respectively, $p<0.05$) (Figure 3). Moreover, culture supernatant from bone pre-treated with estradiol at 0.01 μM or 1 μM, or with pamidronate at 1 μM, was able to reverse cartilage breakdown (102±8.0%, 73±8.0% and 80±22% of control, respectively, $p<0.05$) (Figure 3A). The expression of aggrecan neoepitopes ($ARGS^{374}$ sequences) was high in baseline conditions, the cartilage explants being harvested from patients with severe OA. However, this level was reduced by adding the supernatant of bone cultured with pamidronate, but not with the 2 doses of estradiol (Figure 3B).

Table 1. Effect of bone resorption inhibitors on bone indices in osteopenic mice with joint instability.

	Controls	Osteopenic mice		
		PBS	E2	PAM
Body weight (g)	22.1±0.52	22.4±0.64	23.9±0.50	21.4±0.42
Uterus weight (mg)	47±3	25±4§	68±6*	35±15
ΔBMD Total body (g/cm²)	0.039±0.006	−0.027±0.023§	0.124±0.014§*	0.119±0.0 18§*
ΔBMD Left knee (g/cm²)	0.053±0.024	−0.065±0.035§	0.178±0.048§*	0.189±0.010§*
ΔBMD Right knee (g/cm²)	0.141±0.023	−0.063±0.048§	0.216±0.043§*	0.231±0.028§*

§: compared to controls, $p<0.05$.
*: compared to PBS, $p<0.05$.

Table 2. Histomorphometric parameters in the meniscectomized knees.

	Controls	Osteopenic mice		
		PBS	E2	PAM
BV/TV (%)	42±2.8	27.6±3§	48.8±4.8*	30.7±4.6
Tb.Th (μm)	12.5±0.98	9.8±0.53§	11.4±1.03	10.03±0.88
Tb.Sp (μm)	17.5±13.6	28.6±3.4§	12.6±1.7*	24.5±4.8
Tb.N (/μm)	0.034±0.002	0.028±0.003	0.043±0.004*	0.030±0.004
Oc.N/BV (/mm^2)	17.4±6.3	45.7±10.5§	21.4±10.6*	19.9±7.9*

§: compared to controls, p<0.05.
*: compared to PBS, p<0.05.

OPG contributes to the bone-cartilage crosstalk

To find out whether cytokines were involved in this effect, the expressions of RANKL and OPG transcripts were measured. Adding IL-1β did not increase the OPG/RANKL mRNA ratio in bone explants (1.2±0.55 times control, p = 0.43, Figure 4A). Bone cultured with E2 showed a significant, dose-dependent increase in the OPG/RANKL ratio (2.9±0.16 and 3.7±1.3 times control, at 0.01 and 1 μM, respectively, p = 0.019), as did those cultured with PAM (2.2±0.9 times control, p = 0.028). To find out whether the effect of conditioned bone cultures was mediated by OPG, OPG neutralizing antibody was added to the bone culture medium before it was transferred onto cartilage explants. We observed that OPG neutralization reversed the protective effects of E2 and PAM on aggrecanase neoepitopes expression (Figure 4B).

Discussion

In this study, we show that regulating the level of bone remodeling in OP mice modulates the response of cartilage to meniscetomy. The inhibition of high bone resorption, here induced by ovariectomy, reduced cartilage lesions and the increase in both ADAMTS-4 and ADAMTS-5, the main aggrecanases involved in OA [22,23]. These results are consistent with our previous observations showing that pamidronate reduced cartilage damage in Runx-2 transgenic mice with high bone resorption, but had no effect in control littermates with normal bone remodeling

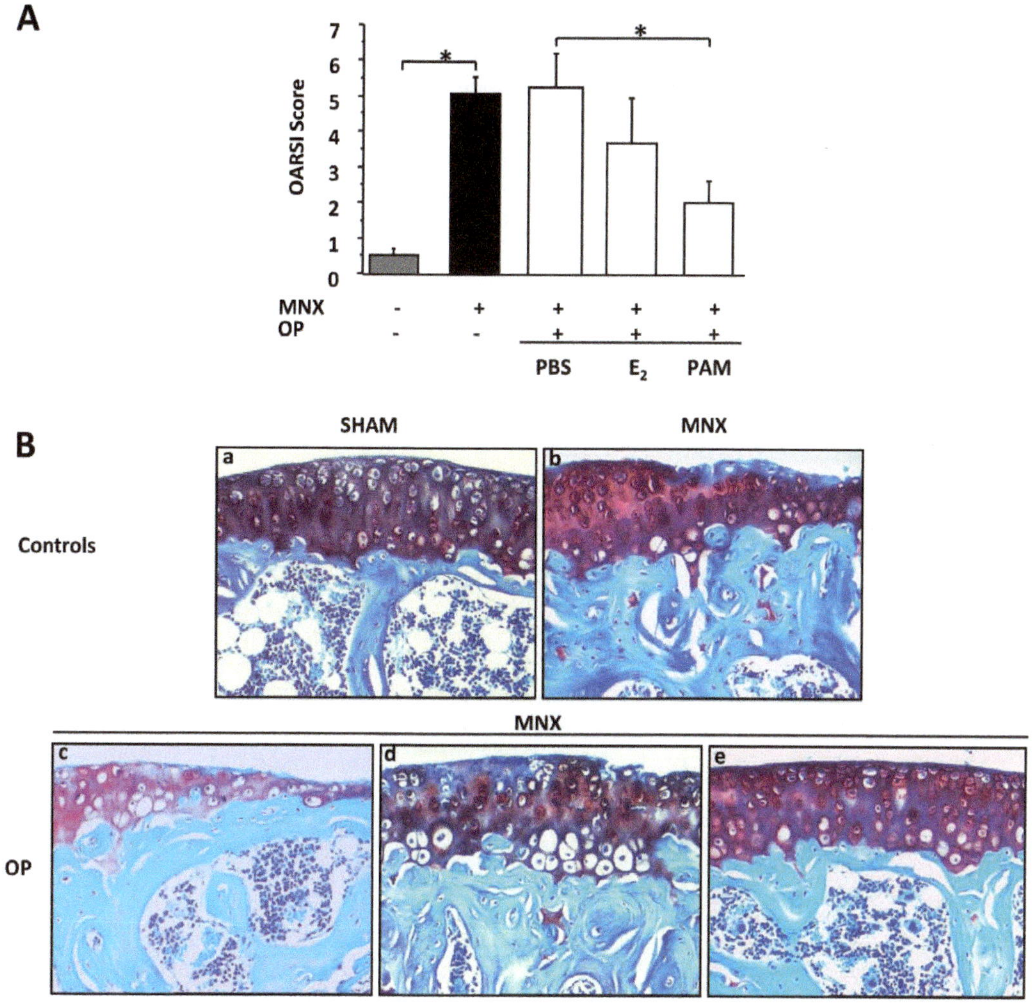

Figure 1. Histological assessment of cartilage lesions. A. OA scored according to the 2010 OARSI recommendations. The score represents the sum of the grades at the tibia and femur in sagittal sections. B. Magnifications of slides stained with safranin-O (40×) in control mice (a: Sham operated knees; b: MNX knees; n = 8) and osteopenic (OP) mice treated with phosphate buffered saline (PBS) (c; n = 10), estradiol (E_2) (d; n = 6), or pamidronate (PAM) (e; n = 5). *: p<0.05.

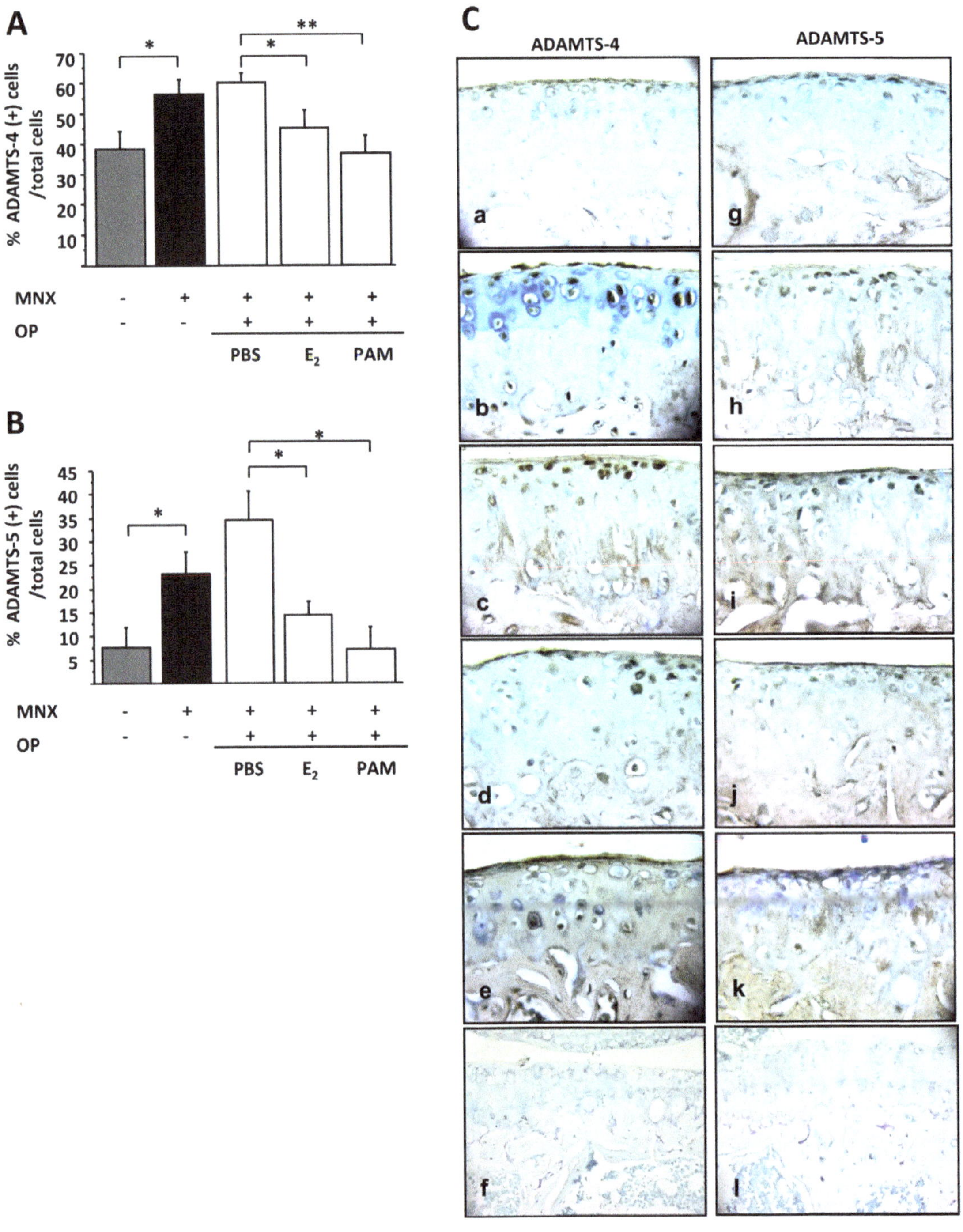

Figure 2. Expression of ADAMTS-4 and ADAMTS-5 in joint cartilage. A. Immunostaining for ADAMTS-4 in cartilage. Bars represent the percentage of positive cells. B. Immunostaining for ADAMTS-5 in cartilage. C. 40× magnification of ADAMTS-4 & ADAMTS-5 expression in the tibial joint cartilage in Sham operated knees (a–g), and MNX knees (b–h) of control mice, and in MNX knees from OP mice treated with phosphate buffered saline (PBS) (c–i), estradiol (E_2) (d–j) or pamidronate (PAM) (e–k), with corresponding negative controls (f–l). *: $p<0.05$. **: $p<0.01$.

[12]. Altogether, these results show that pamidronate was effective only in mice with high resorption, suggesting that its action is driven by bone. Thus, in the murin model of OA by joint instability, the inhibition of high osteoclast activity has some protective effects on the overlying cartilage.

At 6 weeks after MNX, ovariectomy induced no additional damage, in contrast with previous observations in rats or rabbits [24,25]. In our study, the effect of ovariectomy could have been minimized by the local effect of MNX. Mice were treated with estrogens or with pamidronate to target osteoclast formation. Along with the reduction of osteoclast number, pamidronate reduces cartilage structural lesions both at the tissue and cellular level. Estrogens, that inhibit osteoclasts, failed to provide significant protection against cartilage structural lesions, despite reducing ADAMTS expression. However, subchondral bone was restored with estrogens along with the prevention of systemic bone

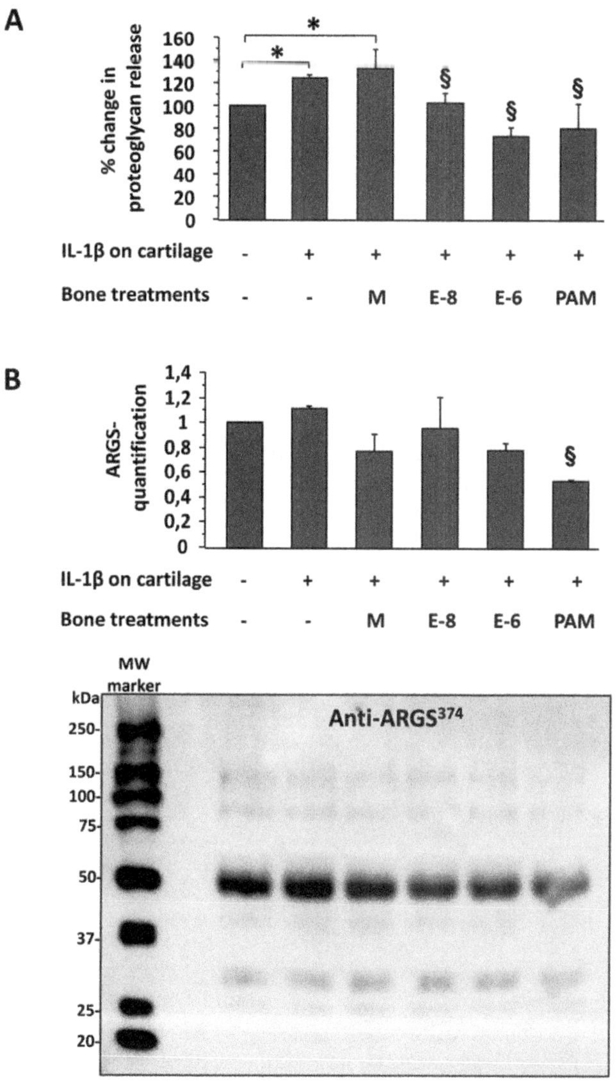

Figure 3. Bone mediated effects of estradiol and pamidronate on proteoglycan and aggrecan neoepitopes release by human cartilage explants. A. Proteoglycan release in cartilage supernatants. IL1-β stimulated cartilage explants were cultured with media from bone explants previously cultured with estradiol at 0.01 μM (E-8) or 1 μM (E-6) or pamidronate at 1 μM (PAM) or with control medium (M). Results are the mean ± SEM of 3 different experiments performed in triplicate. B. Aggrecan neoepitopes expression (ARGS^{374} sequences) in cartilage supernatants. Image of a representative Western blot. The overlying graph represents the mean quantification ± SEM of 3 different experiments. Quantification was done on the 50 kDa bands. *: compared to control, $p<0.05$. §: compared to IL-1β stimulation of cartilage, $p<0.05$.

loss. These differences suggest that these drugs may have differential impacts on subchondral and trabecular bone in OP mice. These results demonstrate the role of subchondral bone, and in particular of osteoclast activity, in the initiation of OA lesions.

Despite clinical evidence showing that OA is more frequent in women, the contribution of estrogen in the pathogenesis of OA remains unclear and might be mediated by the effects of bone resorption. Estradiol modulates the chondrocyte phenotype *in vitro* via both the ERα and ERβ receptors [26–29]. *In vivo*, studies have shown that ovariectomy has harmful effects on joint cartilage [8], but conflicting findings have also been reported [19,30]. Osteoporosis induced in rabbits using both ovariectomy and corticosteroids experienced cartilage damage [8] further indicating that cartilage lesions might be induced by bone signals in addition to a direct effect on chondrocytes.

To investigate the mechanisms by which bone cell activity could modulate cartilage metabolism, we transferred supernatant of human subchondral bone cultures on cartilage explants. Indeed, we found that the release of proteoglycan and aggrecan neoepitopes in cartilage cultures was reduced by bone supernatants cultured with estradiol and pamidronate, indicating that bone-secreted soluble factors are involved in regulating cartilage catabolism. Since chondrocytes express RANK and RANKL [31–34] and treatment with OPG showed protective effects in the joint instability model [10,11], we speculated that OPG could mediate the effect of estradiol or pamidronate. Hence, we found that the OPG/RANKL ratio was significantly higher in bone explants cultured in the presence of estradiol and pamidronate. The inhibition of OPG in the bone culture medium transferred into cartilage cultures resulted in a marked increase in aggrecanase activity, demonstrating the role of OPG in the regulation of cartilage catabolism. Indeed, OPG/RANKL ratio is reduced in subchondral bone of OA rabbits with osteoporosis [8] as well as in rat mandibular condyles [33]. The effect of OPG can be mediated by its interaction with TRAIL, and thus via regulation of chondrocyte apoptosis, as suggested by Shimizu et al. [11]. Taken together, these data indicate that OPG and RANKL are involved in a two-way crosstalk between bone and joint cartilage, regulating both cartilage catabolism and subchondral bone resorption. How these tissues can communicate has long been a subject of debate given the absence of vascularization in cartilage, and the high mineralization of calcified cartilage. In addition to the neo-vascularization of subchondral bone, the diffusion of local factors through bone clefts or through canaliculae in calcified cartilage seems likely to occur [35].

In conclusion, our study shows that bone is implicated in the mechanisms leading to OA, and that the level of bone remodeling modulates how cartilage responds to joint instability. Moreover, OPG is an essential factor that regulates cartilage catabolism. This study further highlights bone as a target for the treatment of OA.

Methods

Animals

Ten week-old female C57/Bl6 mice underwent medial meniscectomy (MNX) of the right knee to induce joint instability, as previously described [10]. A sham operation was performed on the left knee. To increase bone resorption, we induced osteopenia (OP) by ovariectomy and treated mice by two different bone resorption inhibitors: estradiol and a bisphosphonate (pamidronate) to inhibit osteoclast activity. All ovariectomies were performed in a random order regardless of the groups. After meniscectomy, mice were divided into 4 groups:

- 3 groups of 5–10 animals underwent bilateral ovariectomy to induce OP. These mice received either subcutaneous daily injections of 17β estradiol (15 μg/kg/d, OP-E2), or intraperitoneal injections of pamidronate (30 mg/kg/w, OP-PAM), or Phosphate buffered saline (100 μl, OP-PBS).
- 1 group was sham operated without ovariectomy, and was used as the control group.

Mice were pair-fed in order to control for bodyweight, and were sacrificed 6 weeks after surgery. The uterus was removed and weighed.

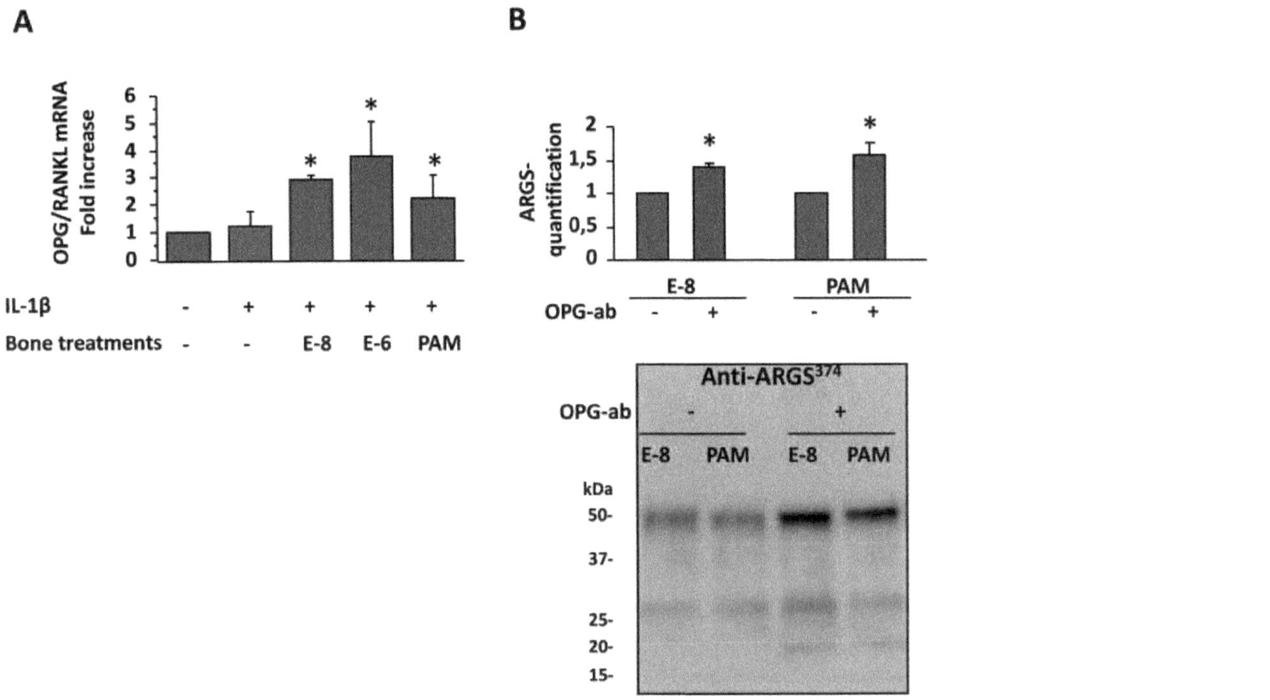

Figure 4. OPG exerts protective effects on cartilage catabolism. A. OPG/RANKL mRNA ratio in IL1-β stimulated bone explants cultured with estradiol at 0.01 μM (E-8) and 1 μM (E-6), and with pamidronate (PAM). The graph represents the mRNA ratio to controls in 3 different experiments. **B.** Effect of OPG blockade by a neutralizing antibody (OPG-ab) on $ARGS^{374}$ sequences expression in supernatants of cartilage explants cultured with conditioned bone media. Image of a representative Western blot, and the graph shows the mean quantifications ± SEM of 4 different experiments. Quantification was done on the 50 kDa bands. *: $p<0.05$.

Whole-body bone mineral density was measured using a GE Lunar Piximus (GE Healthcare, WI, USA) at baseline and at sacrifice (BMD, g/cm^2) in order to assess whether the doses of estradiol and bisphosphonate were appropriate. The relative change in BMD from baseline to sacrifice (ΔBMD) was calculated as (BMD at sacrifice - BMD at baseline)/BMD at baseline.

The experiments complied with the Guidelines for Animal Experimentation issued by the local Ethics Committee on Animal Care and Experimentation (Ethical committee Lariboisière-Villemin, Paris, France). This committee specifically approved this study.

Preparation of mouse joint samples

Whole knee joints were dissected free of soft tissues. Specimens were fixed with 4% PFA (pH 7.4) for 24 h at 4°C, and then decalcified with 1% PFA-0.2 M EDTA (pH 7.4, 4°C) for 2 weeks, changing the solution twice a week. The specimens were then dehydrated using increasing concentrations of ethanol, before being embedded in paraffin. Five-µm thick serial sagittal sections were cut in the medial femoro-tibial compartment for histology and immunohistochemistry procedures.

Histology and immunohistochemistry

We assessed the histological OA score on slides stained with safranin-O. Sections were deparaffinized by two successive 20-minute immersions in xylene baths. They were then rehydrated by immersion for 1 min in each of 3 successive baths containing 100%, 70%, and 40% alcohol, respectively, before being washed twice by 5-min immersions in baths of distilled water. Sections were stained using Mayer-Hemalum staining for 5 min to stain the nuclei, and then counterstained with 0.125% Fast Green for 2 minutes to visualize bone tissue. After being rinsed in two successive 1% acetic acid baths, they were stained in 0.5% Safranin-O in the same bath, and then rinsed in 95% ethanol. All stained sections were then rinsed with distilled water. Osteoarthritic lesions were determined using the OARSI 2010 score with a scale ranging from stage 0 (normal) to 6 (vertical clefts/erosion to the calcified cartilage extending over >75% of the joint surface) on both the tibial and femoral articular cartilage, resulting in a global score of 0 to 12 [36].

Immunohistochemistry was performed on serial sections, as previously described [10]. Vector kit (PK-6101, from Abcys, France) was used according to the Manufacturer's instructions, and sections were counterstained with toluidine blue. Primary polyclonal antibodies directed against murine ADAMTS-4 and ADAMTS-5 (ab28285 and ab41037, respectively, Abcam, United-Kingdom) were used to assess aggrecanase expression and activity. Positive cells were counted on the tibial joint cartilage surface (25× magnification), and expressed as a percentage of the total cell count.

Histomorphometry of subchondral bone

Bone parameters were measured on slides stained with Fast-Green. Microarchitectural indices of the underlying bone were assessed in total epiphyses by an image analyzer using specially designed software (Bonolab, Microvision®, France). For each section, the bone between the cartilage and the growth plate was analyzed, and measured as follows:

- Bone Volume/Tissue Volume (BV/TV, %)
- Trabecular Thickness (Tb.Th, µm), which reflects bone formation

- Trabecular Separation (Tb.Sp, μm), which reflects bone resorption.
- Osteoclast number (N. Oc/BV, /mm^2)

Human explant cultures

Human cartilage samples were harvested from patients who were undergoing total knee replacement surgery for medial OA, in accordance with the French National Authority Legislation for the collection of human tissues. This study was specifically approved by the Institutional Review Board: IRB N° 0000383). As required by the French bioethics law and the local IRB, the need for informed consent was waived since these tissues were surgical waste of routine joint replacement surgery, and since there was no patient private information being collected. All participants received an information note explaining the purpose of the study and were asked for their non opposition to participate.

Samples were collected from the posterior surface of the unaffected femoral condyle, using a bone-marrow trephine that ensured that the explants removed were equal in size (3.5-mm diameter). Bone and cartilage explants were separated mechanically, and cultured separately. All cultures were conducted in a humidified atmosphere of 95% air-5% CO2. After culturing for 72 h in BGJb medium (US Biological, MA, USA), bone explants were serum starved for 24 h hours, and the pre-stimulated with IL-1β at 10 ng/ml for 24 hours (R&D systems, France). They were then cultured for 48 h with 0.01 or 1 μM (E^{-8} or E^{-6}) 17β-estradiol (Sigma-Aldrich, MO, USA), or 1 μM pamidronate (PAM). The explants were then washed and cultured in fresh medium for 24 hours. Cartilage explants were cultured in phenol-red free DMEM with 10% FCS and a cocktail of antibiotics until being subjected to stimulation with IL-1β at 10 ng/ml for 24 hours. Bone culture supernatants were then transferred onto cartilage explants for 72 h.

The proteoglycan content in the media was measured as sulfated glycosaminoglycan by a colorimetric assay using dimethylmethylene blue [37]. Aggrecan neoepitopes were analyzed by Western blotting using a monoclonal antibody that recognizes the human aggrecan neoepitopes $ARGS^{374}$ sequences (ab3773, Abcam). The culture media (15 μl) used for each condition were deglycosylated with hyaluronidase at 0.3 mg/ml for 30 min, and then with chondroitinase ABC (Sigma-Aldrich) at 0.1 U/ml in a buffer containing 50 nM sodium acetate, 0.1 M Tris-HCl, pH 6.5, at 37°C for 90 min [38]. Samples were then analyzed by SDS-PAGE on 8% polyacrylamide gels following standard procedures.

Finally, to investigate the role of OPG released from bone in cartilage breakdown, OPG neutralizing antibody, OPG-ab (MAB805, R&D systems, France) or isotype control was added to the supernatant of bone cultures, and then transferred to cartilage explants for 72 hours. Supernatants were then tested for aggrecan neoepitopes by Western blotting.

Bone mRNA extraction and gene expression

Human bone explants were then collected and processed for RNA extraction. Bone samples were ground in liquid nitrogen, and placed in 1 ml Trizol (Invitrogen, UK) for RNA extraction by centrifuging in chloroform and isopropanol, according to the manufacturing protocol. Total RNA were transcripted into cDNA by the cDNA verso Kit (Thermo Fisher Scientific, UK). Relative mRNA levels were evaluated by quantitative PCR analysis using LightCycler (Roche Applied Science, France) in Absolute Blue qPCR SYBR Green (Thermo Fisher Scientific), at a fusion temperature of 60°C, with 40 cycles and normalized to GAPDH mRNA using the following primers:

OPG-F: CTTTGGTCTCCTGCTAACTC
OPG-R: GAAGAATGCCTCCTCACACA
RANKL-F: GGCCTTTCAAGGAGCTGTGCAAAA
RANKL-R: AGCTTGCTCCTCTTGGCCAGATCTAA
GAPDH-F: ACAACAGCCTCAAGATCATCAG
GAPDH-R: CTGTGGTCATGAGTCCTTCCA

Statistical analysis

All statistical analyzes were performed using STATVIEW® software (SAS Institute, NC, USA). Results are expressed as the mean ± SEM of at least 3 different experiments. The effects of meniscectomy and bone resorption inhibitors were analyzed using the Wilcoxon rank and Mann-Whitney tests. The latter test was also used to analyze the different conditions of culture of the human explants.

Author Contributions

Conceived and designed the experiments: TFB EH MECS. Performed the experiments: TFB HL CS DH MDAK. Analyzed the data: TFB EH MCDV FL PO MECS. Contributed reagents/materials/analysis tools: RN. Wrote the paper: TFB EH MECS.

References

1. Radin EL, Rose RM (1986) Role of subchondral bone in the initiation and progression of cartilage damage. Clin Orthop Relat Res. pp 34–40.
2. Radin EL, Parker HG, Pugh JW, Steinberg RS, Paul IL, et al. (1973) Response of joints to impact loading. 3. Relationship between trabecular microfractures and cartilage degeneration. J Biomech 6: 51–57.
3. Bobinac D, Spanjol J, Zoricic S, Maric I (2003) Changes in articular cartilage and subchondral bone histomorphometry in osteoarthritic knee joints in humans. Bone 32: 284–290.
4. Crema MD, Roemer FW, Zhu Y, Marra MD, Niu J, et al. (2010) Subchondral cystlike lesions develop longitudinally in areas of bone marrow edema-like lesions in patients with or at risk for knee osteoarthritis: detection with MR imaging–the MOST study. Radiology 256: 855–862.
5. Roemer FW, Guermazi A, Javaid MK, Lynch JA, Niu J, et al. (2009) Change in MRI-detected subchondral bone marrow lesions is associated with cartilage loss: the MOST Study. A longitudinal multicentre study of knee osteoarthritis. Ann Rheum Dis 68: 1461–1465.
6. Hayami T, Pickarski M, Wesolowski GA, McLane J, Bone A, et al. (2004) The role of subchondral bone remodeling in osteoarthritis: reduction of cartilage degeneration and prevention of osteophyte formation by alendronate in the rat anterior cruciate ligament transection model. Arthritis Rheum 50: 1193–1206.
7. Pelletier JP, Boileau C, Brunet J, Boily M, Lajeunesse D, et al. (2004) The inhibition of subchondral bone resorption in the early phase of experimental dog osteoarthritis by licofelone is associated with a reduction in the synthesis of MMP-13 and cathepsin K. Bone 34: 527–538.
8. Bellido M, Lugo L, Roman-Blas JA, Castaneda S, Caeiro JR, et al. (2010) Subchondral bone microstructural damage by increased remodelling aggravates experimental osteoarthritis preceded by osteoporosis. Arthritis Res Ther 12: R152.
9. Botter SM, van Osch GJ, Clockaerts S, Waarsing JH, Weinans H, et al. (2011) Osteoarthritis induction leads to early and temporal subchondral plate porosity in the tibial plateau of mice: an in vivo microfocal computed tomography study. Arthritis Rheum 63: 2690–2699.
10. Kadri A, Ea HK, Bazille C, Hannouche D, Liote F, et al. (2008) Osteoprotegerin inhibits cartilage degradation through an effect on trabecular bone in murine experimental osteoarthritis. Arthritis Rheum 58: 2379–2386.
11. Shimizu S, Asou Y, Itoh S, Chung UI, Kawaguchi H, et al. (2007) Prevention of cartilage destruction with intraarticular osteoclastogenesis inhibitory factor/osteoprotegerin in a murine model of osteoarthritis. Arthritis Rheum 56: 3358–3365.
12. Kadri A, Funck-Brentano T, Lin H, Ea HK, Hannouche D, et al. (2010) Inhibition of bone resorption blunts osteoarthritis in mice with high bone remodelling. Ann Rheum Dis 69: 1533–1538.
13. Bergink AP, van Meurs JB, Loughlin J, Arp PP, Fang Y, et al. (2003) Estrogen receptor alpha gene haplotype is associated with radiographic osteoarthritis of the knee in elderly men and women. Arthritis Rheum 48: 1913–1922.

14. Fytili P, Giannatou E, Papanikolaou V, Stripeli F, Karachalios T, et al. (2005) Association of repeat polymorphisms in the estrogen receptors alpha, beta, and androgen receptor genes with knee osteoarthritis. Clin Genet 68: 268–277.
15. Jin SY, Hong SJ, Yang HI, Park SD, Yoo MC, et al. (2004) Estrogen receptor-alpha gene haplotype is associated with primary knee osteoarthritis in Korean population. Arthritis Res Ther 6: R415–421.
16. Lian K, Lui L, Zmuda JM, Nevitt MC, Hochberg MC, et al. (2007) Estrogen receptor alpha genotype is associated with a reduced prevalence of radiographic hip osteoarthritis in elderly Caucasian women. Osteoarthritis Cartilage 15: 972–978.
17. Cirillo DJ, Wallace RB, Wu L, Yood RA (2006) Effect of hormone therapy on risk of hip and knee joint replacement in the Women's Health Initiative. Arthritis Rheum 54: 3194–3204.
18. Sniekers YH, van Osch GJVM, Ederveen AGH, Inzunza J, Gustafsson JA, et al. (2009) Development of osteoarthritic features in estrogen receptor knockout mice. Osteoarthritis Cartilage 17: 1356–1361.
19. Sniekers YH, Weinans H, Bierma-Zeinstra SM, van Leeuwen JP, van Osch GJ (2008) Animal models for osteoarthritis: the effect of ovariectomy and estrogen treatment - a systematic approach. Osteoarthritis Cartilage 16: 533–541.
20. Ma HL, Blanchet TJ, Peluso D, Hopkins B, Morris EA, et al. (2007) Osteoarthritis severity is sex dependent in a surgical mouse model. Osteoarthritis Cartilage 15: 695–700.
21. Riggs BL (2000) The mechanisms of estrogen regulation of bone resorption. J Clin Invest 106: 1203–1204.
22. Glasson SS, Askew R, Sheppard B, Carito B, Blanchet T, et al. (2005) Deletion of active ADAMTS5 prevents cartilage degradation in a murine model of osteoarthritis. Nature 434: 644–648.
23. Stanton H, Rogerson FM, East CJ, Golub SB, Lawlor KE, et al. (2005) ADAMTS5 is the major aggrecanase in mouse cartilage in vivo and in vitro. Nature 434: 648–652.
24. Oestergaard S, Sondergaard BC, Hoegh-Andersen P, Henriksen K, Qvist P, et al. (2006) Effects of ovariectomy and estrogen therapy on type II collagen degradation and structural integrity of articular cartilage in rats: implications of the time of initiation. Arthritis Rheum 54: 2441–2451.
25. Calvo E, Castaneda S, Largo R, Fernandez-Valle ME, Rodriguez-Salvanes F, et al. (2007) Osteoporosis increases the severity of cartilage damage in an experimental model of osteoarthritis in rabbits. Osteoarthritis Cartilage 15: 69–77.
26. Richette P, Dumontier MF, Tahiri K, Widerak M, Torre A, et al. (2007) Oestrogens inhibit interleukin 1beta-mediated nitric oxide synthase expression in articular chondrocytes through nuclear factor-kappa B impairment. Ann Rheum Dis 66: 345–350.
27. Richmond RS, Carlson CS, Register TC, Shanker G, Loeser RF (2000) Functional estrogen receptors in adult articular cartilage: estrogen replacement therapy increases chondrocyte synthesis of proteoglycans and insulin-like growth factor binding protein 2. Arthritis Rheum 43: 2081–2090.
28. Claassen H, Schluter M, Schunke M, Kurz B (2006) Influence of 17beta-estradiol and insulin on type II collagen and protein synthesis of articular chondrocytes. Bone 39: 310–317.
29. Ushiyama T, Ueyama H, Inoue K, Ohkubo I, Hukuda S (1999) Expression of genes for estrogen receptors alpha and beta in human articular chondrocytes. Osteoarthritis Cartilage 7: 560–566.
30. Roman-Blas JA, Castaneda S, Largo R, Herrero-Beaumont G (2009) Osteoarthritis associated with estrogen deficiency. Arthritis Res Ther 11: 241.
31. Kwan Tat S, Amiable N, Pelletier JP, Boileau C, Lajeunesse D, et al. (2009) Modulation of OPG, RANK and RANKL by human chondrocytes and their implication during osteoarthritis. Rheumatology (Oxford) 48: 1482–1490.
32. Moreno-Rubio J, Herrero-Beaumont G, Tardio L, Alvarez-Soria MA, Largo R (2010) Nonsteroidal antiinflammatory drugs and prostaglandin E(2) modulate the synthesis of osteoprotegerin and RANKL in the cartilage of patients with severe knee osteoarthritis. Arthritis Rheum 62: 478–488.
33. Jiao K, Niu LN, Wang MQ, Dai J, Yu SB, et al. (2011) Subchondral bone loss following orthodontically induced cartilage degradation in the mandibular condyles of rats. Bone 48: 362–371.
34. Byron CR, Barger AM, Stewart AA, Pondenis HC, Fan TM (2010) In vitro expression of receptor activator of nuclear factor-kappaB ligand and osteoprotegerin in cultured equine articular cells. Am J Vet Res 71: 615–622.
35. Funck-Brentano T, Cohen-Solal M (2011) Crosstalk between cartilage and bone: when bone cytokines matter. Cytokine Growth Factor Rev 22: 91–97.
36. Glasson S, Chambers M, Van Den Berg W, Little C (2010) The OARSI histopathology initiative - recommendations for histological assessments of osteoarthritis in the mouse. Osteoarthritis Cartilage 18 Suppl 3: S17–23.
37. Farndale RW, Buttle DJ, Barrett AJ (1986) Improved quantitation and discrimination of sulphated glycosaminoglycans by use of dimethylmethylene blue. Biochim Biophys Acta 883: 173–177.
38. Tortorella MD, Malfait AM, Deccico C, Arner E (2001) The role of ADAM-TS4 (aggrecanase-1) and ADAM-TS5 (aggrecanase-2) in a model of cartilage degradation. Osteoarthritis Cartilage 9: 539–552.

Cthrc1 Is a Positive Regulator of Osteoblastic Bone Formation

Hiroaki Kimura[1], Kin Ming Kwan[2,4], Zhaoping Zhang[2], Jian Min Deng[2], Bryant G. Darnay[3], Richard R. Behringer[2], Takashi Nakamura[1], Benoit de Crombrugghe[2], Haruhiko Akiyama[1]*

1 Department of Orthopaedics, Kyoto University, Kyoto, Japan, **2** Department of Molecular Genetics, The University of Texas M. D. Anderson Cancer Center, Houston, Texas, United States of America, **3** Department of Experimental Therapeutics, The University of Texas M. D. Anderson Cancer Center, Houston, Texas, United States of America, **4** Department of Biology, The Chinese University of Hong Kong, Shatin, Hong Kong SAR, China

Abstract

Background: Bone mass is maintained by continuous remodeling through repeated cycles of bone resorption by osteoclasts and bone formation by osteoblasts. This remodeling process is regulated by many systemic and local factors.

Methodology/Principal Findings: We identified collagen triple helix repeat containing-1 (Cthrc1) as a downstream target of bone morphogenetic protein-2 (BMP2) in osteochondroprogenitor-like cells by PCR-based suppression subtractive hybridization followed by differential hybridization, and found that *Cthrc1* was expressed in bone tissues *in vivo*. To investigate the role of Cthrc1 in bone, we generated *Cthrc1*-null mice and transgenic mice which overexpress *Cthrc1* in osteoblasts (*Cthrc1* transgenic mice). Microcomputed tomography (micro-CT) and bone histomorphometry analyses showed that *Cthrc1*-null mice displayed low bone mass as a result of decreased osteoblastic bone formation, whereas *Cthrc1* transgenic mice displayed high bone mass by increase in osteoblastic bone formation. Osteoblast number was decreased in *Cthrc1*-null mice, and increased in *Cthrc1* transgenic mice, respectively, while osteoclast number had no change in both mutant mice. *In vitro*, colony-forming unit (CFU) assays in bone marrow cells harvested from *Cthrc1*-null mice or *Cthrc1* transgenic mice revealed that Cthrc1 stimulated differentiation and mineralization of osteoprogenitor cells. Expression levels of osteoblast specific genes, *ALP*, *Col1a1*, and *Osteocalcin*, in primary osteoblasts were decreased in *Cthrc1*-null mice and increased in *Cthrc1* transgenic mice, respectively. Furthermore, BrdU incorporation assays showed that Cthrc1 accelerated osteoblast proliferation *in vitro* and *in vivo*. In addition, overexpression of Cthrc1 in the transgenic mice attenuated ovariectomy-induced bone loss.

Conclusions/Significance: Our results indicate that Cthrc1 increases bone mass as a positive regulator of osteoblastic bone formation and offers an anabolic approach for the treatment of osteoporosis.

Editor: Suzannah Rutherford, Fred Hutchinson Cancer Research Center, United States of America

Funding: This work was supported by a Grant-in-aid for Scientific Research from the Japanese Ministry of Education, Culture, Sports, Science, and Technology (#18390413).

Competing Interests: The authors have declared that no competing interests exist.

* E-mail: hakiyama@kuhp.kyoto-u.ac.jp

Introduction

Bone modeling is initiated by osteoblastic differentiation of mesenchymal cells into preosteoblasts. Preosteoblasts then differentiate into functional osteoblasts producing bone matrix proteins, including type I collagen, osteopontin, and osteocalcin to form bone tissues. Bone is constantly remodeled through bone formation by functional osteoblasts and bone resorption by osteoclasts which arise from monocytic cells, and bone mass is maintained by their precise balance [1–3]. Recently, significant advances have been made in our understandings of the factors that regulate the balance between osteoblastic bone formation and osteoclastic bone resorption, but the mechanisms have not been fully elucidated.

Bone morphogenetic proteins (BMPs) are potent osteogenic agents that induce differentiation of mesenchymal cells toward an osteoblastic lineage and stimulate the differentiation and functions of osteoblasts during a process of bone modeling [4–6]. Postnatally, BMP signaling regulates osteoblastic bone formation and osteoclastic bone resorption in bone remodeling [7]. Recent studies show that osteoblast-specific inhibition of BMP signals in mice affects postnatal bone mass [8–12]. Osteoblast-specific *Bmpr1a* deficient mice show reduced bone volume and bone formation rates with normal osteoblast number due to impaired osteoblast function at 3 months old and increased bone volume probably due to reduced osteoclastic bone resorption at 10 months old [11]. Transgenic mice that osteoblast-specifically overexpress *noggin*, the BMP inhibitor, display reduced bone mineral densities and bone formation rates due to impaired osteoblast function [8,9]. Mice carrying a targeted deletion of *Tob*, which is a member of a new antiproliferative protein family and represses BMP-induced Smad-dependent transcription in osteoblasts, have increased bone mass due to increased osteoblast numbers and acceleration of the bone formation rates [12]. Thus, BMPs are key molecules that control bone modeling and bone remodeling.

To identify the molecules that regulate bone modeling and/or bone remodeling as a downstream target of BMP signaling, we compared the mRNAs expressed in BMP2-untreated and BMP2-treated ATDC5 osteochondroprogenitor-like cells by PCR-based suppression subtractive hybridization followed by differential hybridization, and identified a cDNA upregulated by BMP2, that encoded Collagen triple helix repeat containing protein 1 (Cthrc1). Cthrc1 is a 30-kD glycosylated secreted protein containing a short collagen-like motif with 12 Gly-X-Y repeats similar to the collagen domains present in the C1q/tumor necrosis factor α related proteins [13]. *Cthrc1* is transiently expressed in the arterial wall in response to injury, suggesting that Cthrc1 is involved in vascular remodeling by limiting collagen matrix deposition and promoting cell migration [13]. A recent study shows that neointimal lesion formation and adventitial collagen deposition in response to carotid artery ligation are reduced in transgenic mice overexpressing *Cthrc1* under the control of cytomegalovirus promoter [14]. According to expression analysis of *Cthrc1*, abundant expression of *Cthrc1* is observed in developing skeleton during embryogenesis and in the bone matrix and periosteum in adult mice [15].

In this study, we generated *Cthrc1*-null mice and transgenic mice that overexpress *Cthrc1* under the control of *Col1a1* osteoblast-specific promoter. *Cthrc1*-null mice developed a low-bone-mass-phenotype as a result of reduced bone formation, while the transgenic mice exhibited a high-bone-mass-phenotype caused by enhanced bone formation. *In vitro* analyses showed that Cthrc1 stimulated osteoblast proliferation and differentiation. Thus, our results indicate that Cthrc1 is a positive regulator of osteoblastic bone formation.

Results

Cthrc1 is expressed in bone

To identify potential osteoblast-specific proteins as downstreams of BMPs, we performed two-step screening consisting of PCR-based suppression subtractive hybridization followed by differential hybridization using the poly(A)$^+$ RNA extracted from BMP2-untreated and BMP2-treated ATDC5 cells, and identified a cDNA encoding Cthrc1(Figure S1A). *In vitro*, *Cthrc1* was expressed in MC3T3-E1 osteoblastic cells and differentiated ATDC5 cells, but not in C3H10T1/2 fibroblastic cells and C2C12 myoblastic cells (Figure S1B). We next assessed the expression of *Cthrc1* in various adult mouse tissues by northern blot analysis, and *Cthrc1* was expressed in bone but not in the other adult mouse tissues examined (Figure S1C). During the skeletogenesis in the limb buds of mouse embryos, *Cthrc1* was expressed in the mesenchymal condensation in E13.5 and in the bone tissues in E16.5 (Figure S1D). In addition, the expression levels of *Cthrc1* increased during mouse embryogenesis (Figure S1E). These results suggest that Cthrc1 plays an important role in bone modeling or remodeling.

Low bone mass and decreased bone formation in *Cthrc1*-null mice

To investigate the physiological role of Cthrc1 in bone, we inactivated the *Cthrc1* gene in mouse embryonic stem cells by homologous recombination. In the target strategy, an *IRES-lacZ-pA-loxP*-flanked neomycin resistance expression cassette was introduced into exon 2 which codes a short Gly-X-Y collagen triple helix repeat domain (Figure 1 A and B). As shown in Figure 1C, Cthrc1 RNA was absent in E16.5 *Cthrc1*-null embryo, indicating that the mutation was a null mutation. Homozygous *Cthrc1* mutant mice were born at the expected Mendelian ratio and grew normally in comparison with their wild-type littermates (data not shown). X-gal staining of heterozygous *Cthrc1* mutant embryos revealed the expression of *Cthrc1* in bone-forming tissues in E12.5 embryos and in bones and periarticular cartilages in E16.5 embryos, which corresponded to the results of *in situ* hybridization (Figure 1D and Figure S2A). Skeletal preparations showed no obvious skeletal phenotypes in *Cthrc1*-null newborn mice (Figure S2B). *In situ* hybridization analyses showed comparable expression of osteoblast marker genes, *Runx2* and *Col1a1*, and chondrocyte marker genes, *Col2a1* and *Col10a1* between E16.5 *Cthrc1*-null embryos and their wild-type littermates (Figure S3A), suggesting that Cthrc1 has no apparent effect on skeletal development. However, histological analyses of decalcified adult bone tissues revealed that the number and thickness of trabecular bones were reduced in *Cthrc1*-null mice, compared with their wild-type littermates (data not shown). This result suggested that Cthrc1 may regulate bone remodeling postnatally. To test this hypothesis, we performed bone histomorphometric analyses and microcomputed tomography (micro-CT) analyses of 2-month-old *Cthrc1*-null and wild-type mice. Micro-CT analyses of tibiae showed that the trabecular bone mass in *Cthrc1*-null mice was approximately 70% of that in wild-type mice (Figure 2 A and B). Bone histomorphometric and micro-CT analyses showed a significant decrease in trabecular number (Tb.N) and osteoblast number (Ob.N/BS) in *Cthrc1*-null mice, while trabecular thickness (Tb.Th) and tartrate-resistant acid phosphatase (TRAP)-positive osteoclast number (Oc.N/BS) had no change in *Cthrc1*-null mice (Figure 2C–E and Figure S4A). In addition, the osteoblast surface (Ob.S/BS) in *Cthrc1*-null mice, which represents the proportion of the bone surface covered with osteoblasts, was approximately 40% less than that in wild-type mice, and the osteoclast surface (Oc.S/BS), which represents the proportion of the bone surface covered with osteoclasts, showed no significant difference between *Cthrc1*-null and wild-type mice (Figure 2F and Figure S4A). To analyze osteoblast proliferation *in vivo*, we performed BrdU incorporation assays in the calvaria of *Cthrc1*-null and wild-type littermates, and found that the percentage of proliferating cells was decreased by approximately 30% in *Cthrc1*-null mice (Figure 2G). Moreover, double-labeling analyses with calcein, a marker of newly formed bone, showed that the bone formation rate was significantly decreased in *Cthrc1*-null mice (Figure 2H). Thus, these results indicate that the decreased bone mass in *Cthrc1*-null mice is due to the suppression of osteoblastic bone formation, not due to an acceleration of osteoclastic bone resorption.

High bone mass and increased bone formation in transgenic mice overexpressing *Cthrc1* in osteoblasts

To determine if Cthrc1 is sufficient to increase bone mass, we next generated transgenic mice that specifically overexpressed 3×HA tagged *Cthrc1* in osteoblasts under the control of the *Col1a1* 2.3 kb osteoblast-specific promoter (Figure 3A). Immunohistochemistry with antibody against the HA-epitope tag showed specific expression of 3×HA tagged protein in bone collars, periosteum, and trabecular bones (Figure 3B). Hemizygous *Cthrc1* transgenic mice were born at the expected Mendelian ratio and grew normally in comparison with their wild-type littermates (data not shown). Skeletal preparations showed no apparent skeletal phenotypes in newborn hemizygous transgenic mice (Figure S2C). In addition, *in situ* hybridization analyses revealed that overexpression of Cthrc1 in osteoblasts did not affect the expression of the osteoblast markers, *Runx2* and *Col1a1*, and chondrocyte markers, *Col2a1* and *Col10a1*, in E16.5 mouse embryos (Figure S3B). As we found an osteopenic phenotype in adult *Cthrc1*-null mice, we analyzed bone in adult *Cthrc1* transgenic mice. Micro-CT analyses of tibiae showed that the trabecular bone mass in

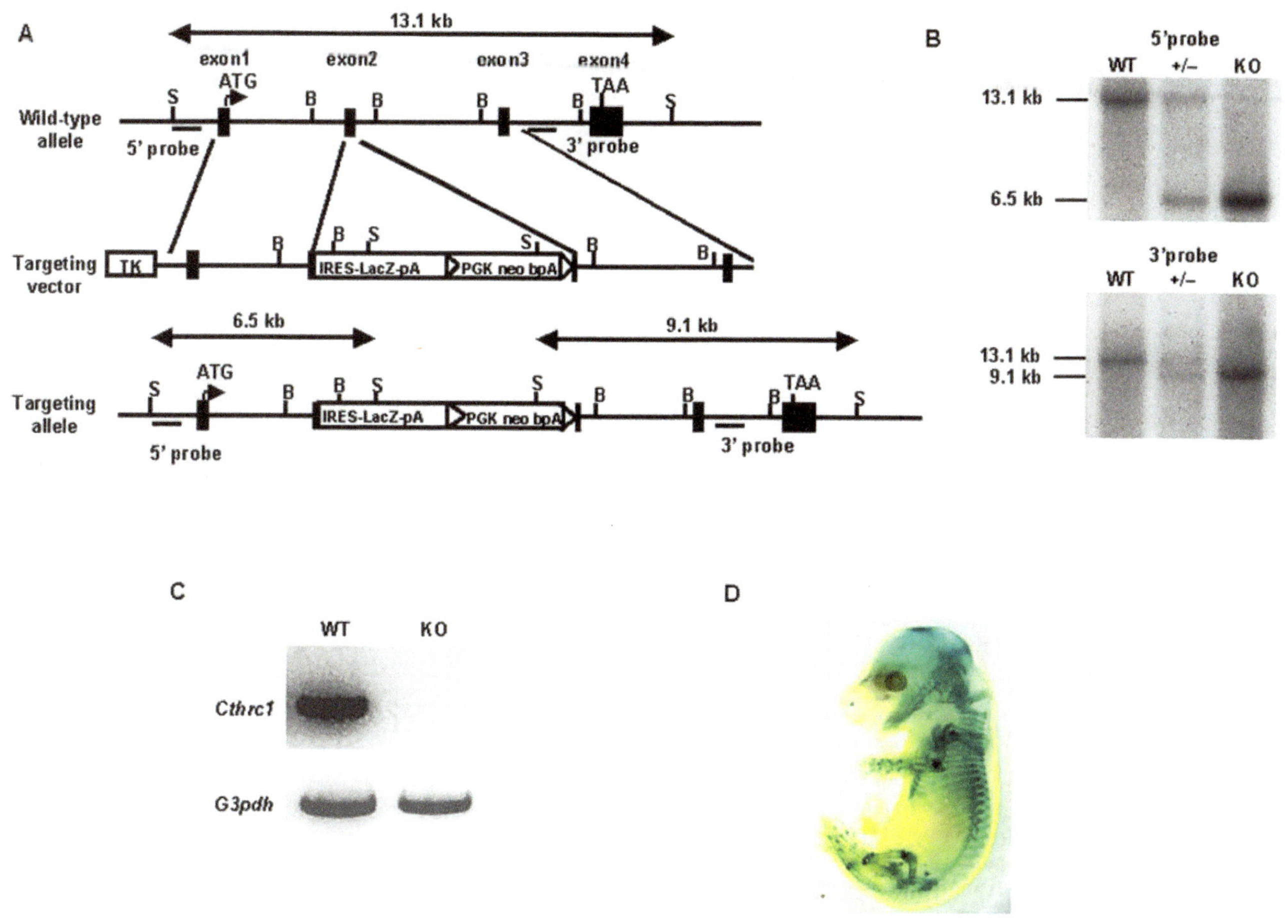

Figure 1. Generation of *Cthrc1*-null mice. (A) Structure of the genomic *Cthrc1* locus, targeting vector, and targeting allele. Exons are depicted as closed boxes, and intronic sequences are shown as solid lines. IRES-LacZ-pA-loxP-flanked PGK-neo-bpA cassettes are depicted as open boxes. S, SacI; B, BamHI. (B) Southern blot analysis of fetal genomic DNA. Genomic DNA isolated from the skin was digested with SacI and then hybridized with the 5′ or 3′ probe. The wild-type and the mutant allele were detected with the 5′ probe as 13.1-kb and 6.5-kb fragments and with the 3′ probe as 13.1-kb and 9.1-kb fragments, respectively. (C) RT-PCR analysis of *Cthrc1* transcript in E16.5 wild-type and *Cthrc1*-null littermates. (D) Whole-mount X-gal staining of E16.5 heterozygous *Cthrc1* embryo. WT: wild-type mice; KO: *Cthrc1*-null mice; +/−: *Cthrc1* heterozygous mice.

hemizygous *Cthrc1* transgenic mice was approximately 25% greater than that in wild-type mice (Figure 3C and D). Likewise, bone histomorphometric and micro-CT analyses showed significant increase in trabecular number (Tb.N) and osteoblast number (Ob.N/BS) in transgenic mice, while trabecular thickness (Tb.Th) and TRAP-positive osteoclast number (Oc.N/BS) had no change between transgenic mice and wild-type mice (Figure 3E–G and Figure S4C). The osteoblast surface (Ob.S/BS) in transgenic mice was approximately 40% greater than that in wild-type mice, while there was no difference in the osteoclast surface (Oc.S/BS) between transgenic mice and wild-type mice (Figure 3H and Figure S4C). BrdU incorporation assays showed that the percentage of proliferating osteoblasts was increased by approximately 35% in transgenic mice (Figure 3I). Furthermore, double-labeling analyses with calcein showed a marked increase in the bone formation rate in transgenic mice (Figure 3J). Thus, these data indicate that the increase in bone mass in *Cthrc1* transgenic mice is due to the stimulation of osteoblastic bone formation.

Cthrc1 stimulates osteoblast proliferation and differentiation

Both the loss-of-function and gain-of-function analyses using mouse genetics approaches indicate that Cthrc1 positively regulates osteoblastic bone formation *in vivo*. To clarify the functions of Cthrc1 in osteoblasts, we isolated osteoblasts from the calvaria of wild-type (*Cthrc1*$^{+/+}$ osteoblasts) and *Cthrc1*-null (*Cthrc1*$^{-/-}$ osteoblasts) newborn mice and analyzed the effects of Cthrc1 on osteoblast proliferation and differentiation *in vitro*. BrdU incorporation in *Cthrc1*$^{-/-}$ osteoblasts was 40% less than that in *Cthrc1*$^{+/+}$ osteoblasts (Figure 4A). Real-time PCR analyses confirmed that the mRNA levels of the osteoblast marker genes, *ALP*, *Col1a1*, and *Osteocalcin* were all decreased in *Cthrc1*$^{-/-}$ osteoblasts, whereas the expression level of receptor activator of nuclear factor κB ligand (*RANKL*), a major determinant of osteoclastogenesis, did not differ (Figure 4B and Figure S4B). We further performed *in vitro* analyses of osteoprogenitor frequency and differentiation capacity by colony-forming unit (CFU) assays. CFU-ALP assays demonstrated that *Cthrc1*$^{-/-}$ bone marrow cells had dramatically reduced osteoprogenitors, and mineralized area of CFU-osteoblast (CFU-O) was also reduced by more than half in *Cthrc1*$^{-/-}$ bone marrow cells, consistent with decreased functional progenitors (Figure 4C and D). Likewise, we examined osteoblast proliferation and differentiation in osteoblasts derived from *Cthrc1* transgenic mice (Tg-osteoblasts) *in vitro*. As shown in Figure 4A, BrdU incorporation in Tg-osteoblasts was 25% greater than that in wild-type osteoblasts. The mRNA levels

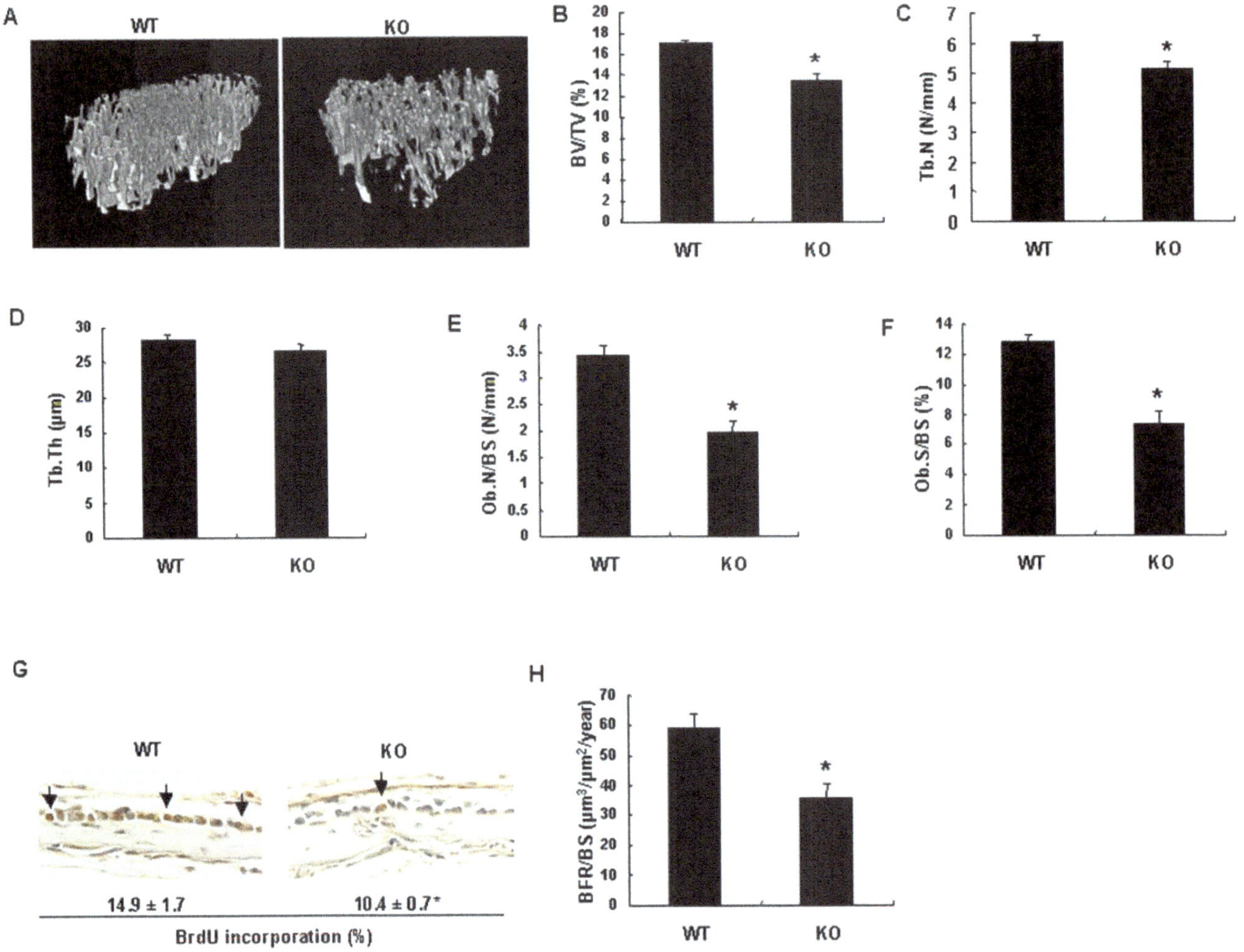

Figure 2. Bone phenotypes of *Cthrc1*-null mice. (A–D) Micro CT analyses of tibiae in 2-month-old *Cthrc1*-null and wild-type mice (n = 6). Bone volume/total volume (BV/TV), trabecular number (Tb.N), trabecular thickness (Tb.Th) are shown. (E and F) Bone histomorphometric analyses of vertebrae in 2-month-old *Cthrc1*-null and wild-type mice (n = 6). Osteoblast number/bone surface (Ob.N/BS) and osteoblast surface/bone surface (Ob.S/BS) are shown. (G) Analyses of osteoblast proliferation in calvaria of 1-week-old *Cthrc1*-null and wild-type mice by BrdU incorporation assays. Arrows indicate BrdU positive osteoblasts. (H) Calcein double-labeling of vertebrae in 2-month-old *Cthrc1*-null and wild-type mice. BFR : Bone formation rate. WT: wild-type mice; KO: *Cthrc1*-null mice. Data are shown as the mean±SEM ($^*p<0.05$).

of *ALP*, *Col1a1*, and *Osteocalcin* were all increased in Tg-osteoblasts, whereas the expression level of *RANKL* did not differ (Figure 4B and Figure S4D). CFU assays showed that the frequency of osteoprogenitors and mineralized area of CFU-O were significantly increased in *Cthrc1* transgenic mice (Figure 4C and D). Thus, these results indicate that Cthrc1 accelerates bone formation by stimulating osteoblast proliferation and differentiation, resulting in increased postnatal bone volume.

Cthrc1 attenuates ovariectomy (OVX)-induced bone loss

In view of an anabolic effect of Cthrc1 on bone formation, we tested whether Cthrc1 may impact bone mass in the OVX mice, an established preclinical disease model of postmenopausal osteoporosis [16]. Eight-week-old *Cthrc1* transgenic and wild-type mice were ovariectomized or sham-operated, and four weeks after operation, metaphyseal regions of tibiae were analyzed by micro-CT. OVX induced 47% trabecular bone loss in wild-type mice, and 38%, in transgenic mice (Figure 5A and B), and trabecular bone mass in OVX transgenic mice was only 17% less than that in sham-operated wild-type mice. Trabecular number, which was reduced by ovariectomy in both wild-type and transgenic mice, did not significantly differ between sham-operated wild-type mice and OVX transgenic mice (Figure 5C). Trabecular thickness, which was reduced in OVX wild-type mice, had no significant difference between sham-operated and OVX transgenic mice (Figure 5D). These results indicated that stimulatory effect of Cthrc1 on bone formation partly prevents reduction in bone volume by ovariectomy. Indeed, increase in bone formation rates was maintained after ovariectomy in transgenic mice. (Figure 5E). Thus, Cthrc1 attenuates estrogen deficiency-induced bone loss by enhanced osteoclastic bone resorption through stimulating osteoblastic bone formation.

Discussion

Bone mass is regulated by continuous remodeling which is based on the balanced action between osteoblastic bone formation and osteoclastic bone resorption [2]. This process is precisely coordinated to maintain the bone mass homeostasis mediated by multiple signaling pathways such as parathyroid hormone, transforming growth factor-β (TGF-β) and BMP [3,7]. In this

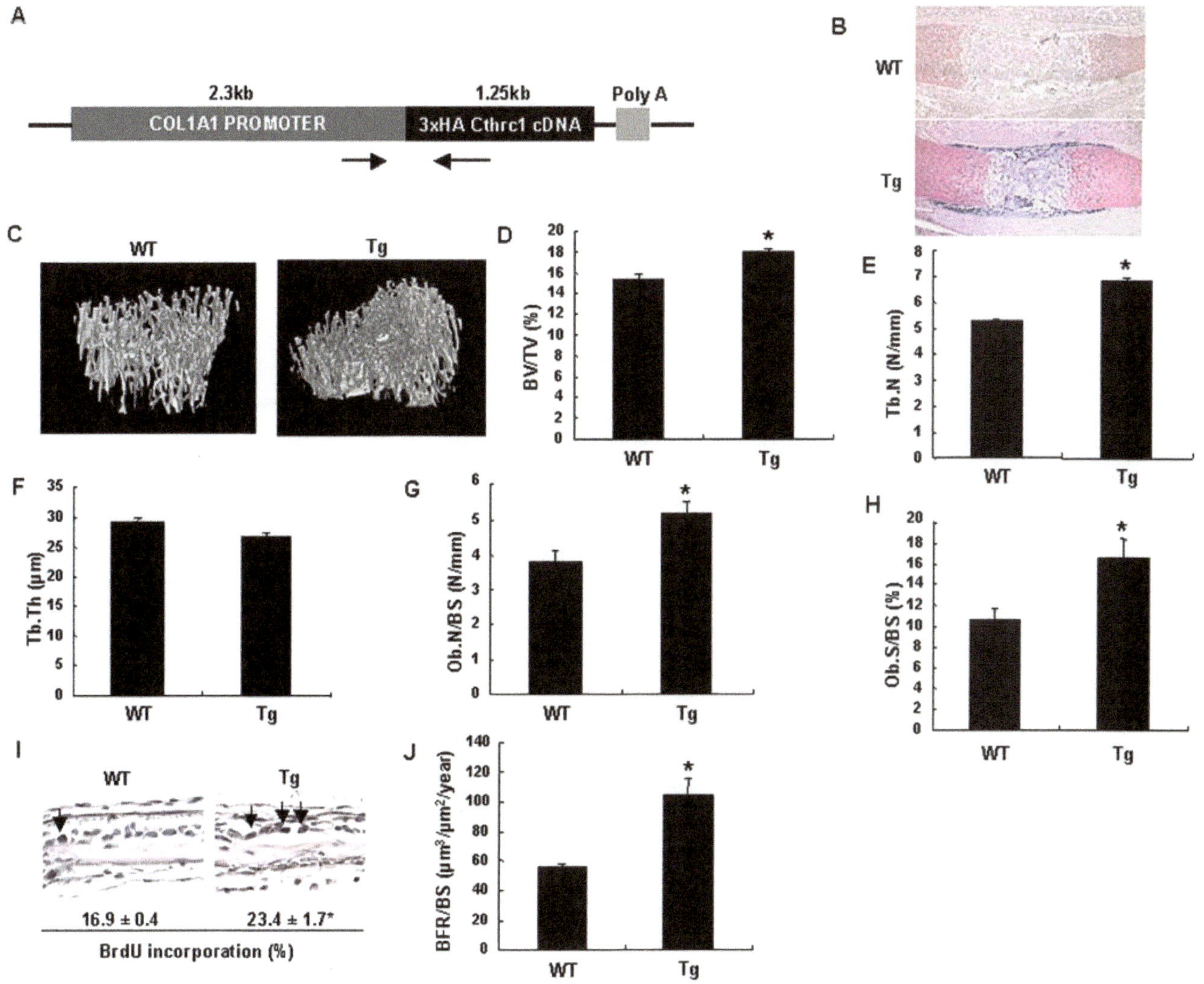

Figure 3. Generation of *Cthrc1* transgenic mice and analyses of bone phenotypes. (A) Schematic representation of the *Col1a1-Cthrc1* transgene. Poly A: SV40 polyadenylation signal. Arrows indicate the primers for genotyping. (B) Expression of 3×HA-tagged Cthrc1 protein in humeri of E16.5 *Cthrc1* transgenic mice. (C–F) Micro-CT analyses of tibiae in 2-month-old *Cthrc1* transgenic and wild-type mice (n = 6). Bone volume/total volume (BV/TV), trabecular number (Tb.N) and trabecular thickness (Tb.Th) are shown. (G and H) Bone histomorphometric analyses of vertebrae in 2-month-old *Cthrc1* transgenic and wild-type mice (n = 6). Osteoblast number/bone surface (Ob.N/BS) and osteoblast surface/bone surface (Ob.S/BS) are shown. (I) Analyses of osteoblast proliferation in calvaria of 1-week-old *Cthrc1* transgenic and wild-type mice by BrdU incorporation assays. Arrows indicate BrdU positive osteoblasts. (J) Calcein double-labeling of vertebrae in 2-month-old *Cthrc1* transgenic and wild-type mice. BFR: Bone formation rate. WT: wild-type mice; Tg: *Cthrc1* transgenic mice. Data are shown as the mean±SEM ($^*p<0.05$).

study, we show that Cthrc1 is involved in postnatal bone formation. In *Cthrc1*-null mice, bone volume, trabecular number, osteoblast number, and bone formation rates were significantly decreased. In *Cthrc1* transgenic mice, bone volume, trabecular number, osteoblast number and bone formation rates were increased. *In vitro*, CFU assays in bone marrow cells and analyses of expression of osteoblast specific genes, *ALP*, *Col1a1*, and *Osteocalcin*, in osteoblasts revealed that Cthrc1 stimulates differentiation of osteoprogenitor cells and osteoblasts. Furthermore, BrdU incorporation assays showed that Cthrc1 stimulates osteoblast proliferation *in vitro* and *in vivo*. In contrast, Cthrc1 did not affect either TRAP-positive osteoclast number and osteoclast surface *in vivo*, or *RANKL* expression levels in primary osteoblasts. These findings indicate that Cthrc1 acts as a stimulator of osteoblastic bone formation, but has no effect on osteoclastic bone resorption.

BMPs have potent osteogenic effects and control osteoblast proliferation and differentiation during osteogenesis [6,12,17]. Several studies of cell-specific inactivation or activation of BMP signals in mice have shown that BMPs regulate postnatal bone remodeling [8–12]. As shown in previous studies, Cthrc1 is regulated by TGF-β and BMP4, and a putative Smad binding site is identified in the promoter region of *Cthrc1* [13,18]. We show that Cthrc1, which is induced by BMP2, is not required for skeletal development, but is for the maintainance of bone homeostasis, suggesting that Cthrc1 may act as one of the downstream targets of BMP-Smad signaling, followed by enhanced expression of osteoblast specific genes including *ALP*, *Col1a1 and Osteocalcin.*

The detail mechanism of Cthrc1 during bone formation is unclear. Cthrc1 inhibited TGF-β signaling in smooth muscle cells but not in endotherial cells [14]. Contrary to the effect of Cthrc1 on osteoblasts in *Col1a1* expression in our study, overexpression of

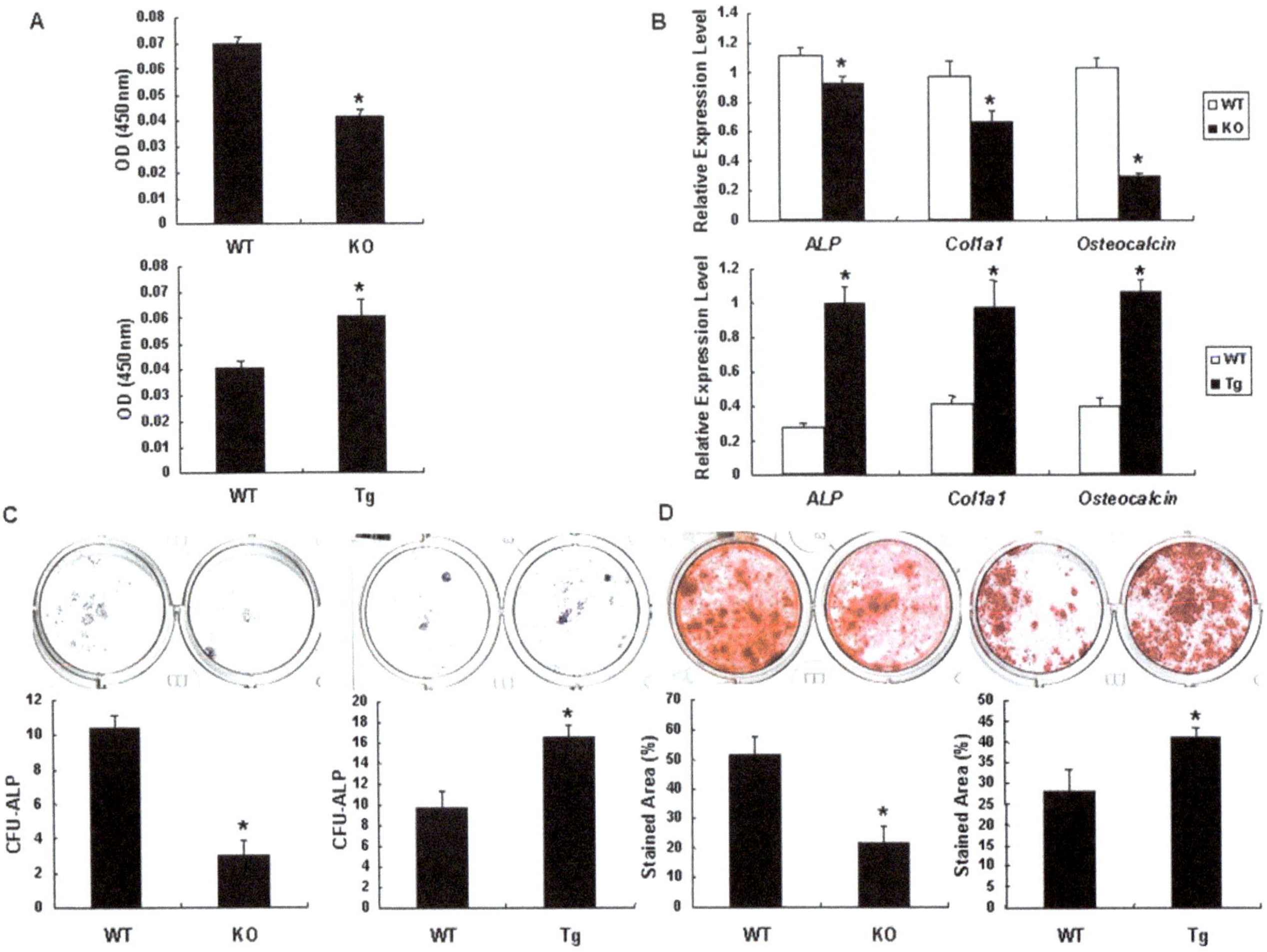

Figure 4. Effects of Cthrc1 on osteogenesis. (A) Cell proliferation in primary osteoblasts harvested from *Cthrc1*-null mice (upper panel) and from *Cthrc1* transgenic mice (lower panel) as shown by BrdU incorporation assays. (B) Expression of early and late osteoblast marker genes in primary osteoblasts harvested from *Cthrc1*-null mice (upper panel) and *Cthrc1* transgenic mice (lower panel). (C) The total numbers of CFU-ALP in bone marrow cell cultures derived from *Cthrc1*-null mice (left) and *Cthrc1* transgenic mice (right). (D) The mineralized area of CFU-O in bone marrow cell cultures derived from *Cthrc1*-null mice (left) and *Cthrc1* transgenic mice (right). WT: wild-type mice; KO: *Cthrc1*-null mice; Tg: *Cthrc1* transgenic mice. Data are shown as the mean±SEM ($^{*}p<0.05$).

Cthrc1 in PAC1 cells, smooth muscle cell line, reduced mRNA levels of *Col1a1*, and collagen deposition [13,14]. These results suggest that the function of Cthrc1 differs among cell types, or that Cthrc1 signals through its own signaling pathway which is functional in a cell-type specific manner. In addition, there are discrepancies of phenotypes between *Cthrc1* transgenic mice which we generated in this study and the transgenic mice overexpressing *Cthrc1* previously reported [14]. First, transgenic mice we generated display a high-bone-mass phenotype, whereas transgenic mice previously reported show an osteopenic phenotype. Second, transgenic mice previously reported are smaller in size and have a higher rate of postnatal mortality, whereas transgenic mice we generated are fertile and normal in appearance and body weight. A possible explanation for these discrepancies is that transgenic mice we generated overexpress *Cthrc1* specifically in osteoblasts under the control of the *Col1a1* 2.3kb osteoblast-specific promoter to focus on the function of Cthrc1 in bones, while transgenic mice previously reported ubiquitously overexpress *Cthrc1* under the control of cytomegalovirus promoter.

Ovariectomy leads to a deficit in bone mineral densities due to cortical bone modeling and resorption of cancellous bone [19,20]. This change largely results in severe cancellous osteopenia. Dempster et al. demonstrated that the primary mechanism of ovariectomy-induced bone loss is osteoclast perforation and removal of the trabecular plates [21]. Furthermore, a recent study showed that selective ablation of estrogen receptor α in differentiated osteoclasts induced trabecular bone loss, similar to the osteoporotic bone phenotype, caused by inhibition of osteoclast apoptosis [22]. Thus, ovariectomy-induced bone loss, a model of postmenopausal osteoporosis, results from an acceleration of osteoclastic bone resorption, followed by high bone turnover in which bone resorption exceeds bone formation. *Cthrc1*-null mice exhibit cancellous bone loss, and *Cthrc1* transgenic mice increase cancellous bone with no change in osteoclastic bone resorption. In addition, Cthrc1 stimulates osteoblast proliferation and differentiation and increases bone formation rates, suggesting that Cthrc1 prevents cancellous bone loss in ovariectomized mice by stimulating osteoblastic bone formation. Indeed, bone volume and trabecular number in OVX transgenic mice were higher than those in OVX wild-type mice, and the loss of trabecular thickness by ovariectomy was protected in transgenic mice. Moreover, increased bone formation rates in transgenic mice were maintained after OVX. Considering that Cthrc1 does not affect

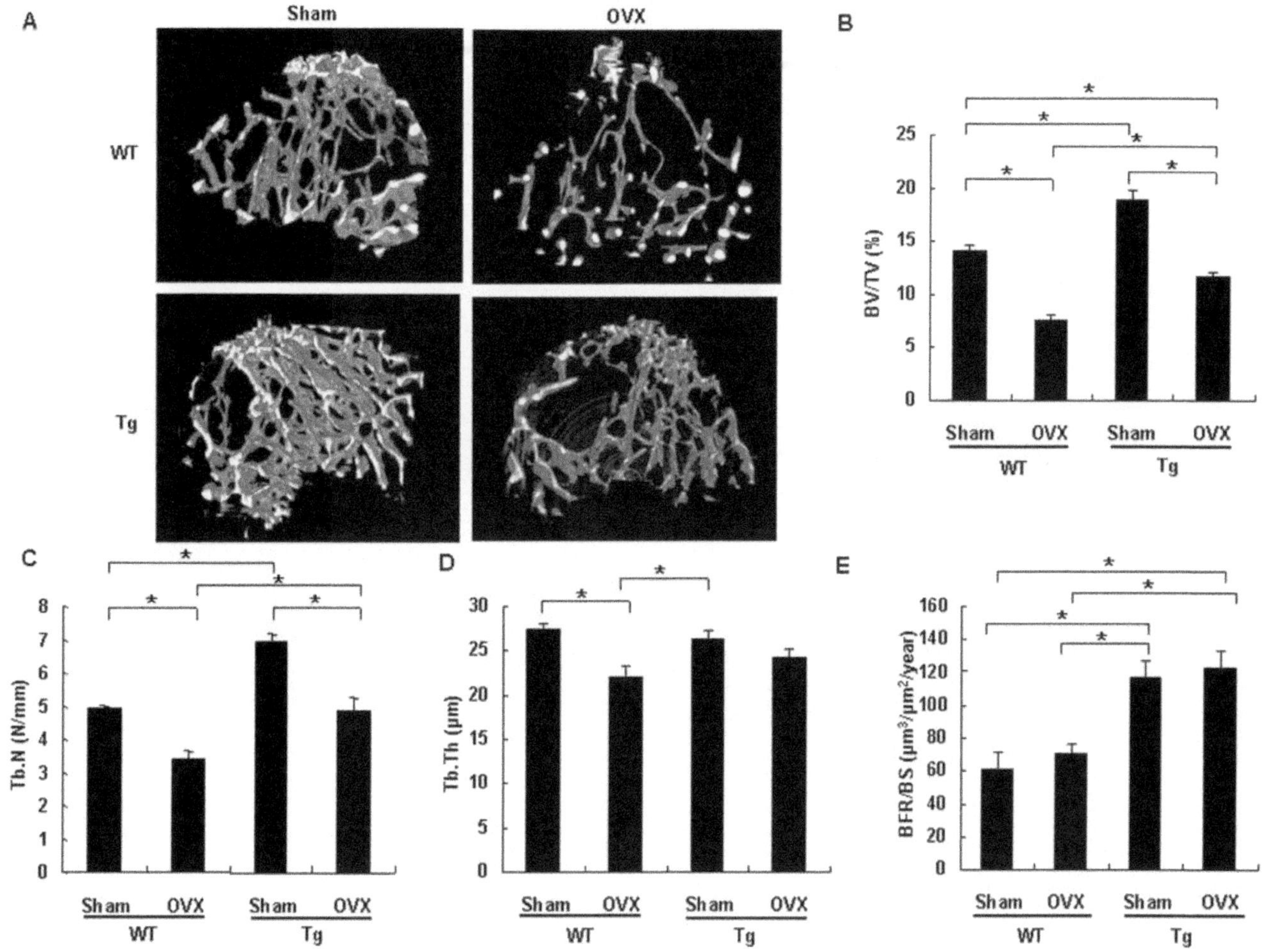

Figure 5. OVX-induced bone loss is attenuated in *Cthrc1* transgenic mice. (A) micro-CT of tibiae from 3-month-old *Cthrc1* transgenic and wild-type mice which were sham-operated or ovariectomized at 2 months of age (n = 5). (B–E) Bone volume/total volume (BV/TV) (B), trabecular number (Tb.N) (C), trabecular thickness (Tb.Th) (D) and bone formation rate (BFR) (E) were assessed by micro-CT or bone histomorphometry. WT: wild-type mice; Tg: *Cthrc1* transgenic mice. Data are shown as the mean±SEM ($^*p<0.05$).

osteoclastogenesis, enhanced bone formation by overexpression of Cthrc1 may attenuate bone loss caused by enhanced osteoclastic bone resorption induced by OVX.

It is noteworthy in this article that Cthrc1 may have a potential role in treating osteoporosis, because we observed that osteoblast-specific overexpression of *Cthrc1* in mice attenuates bone loss which is induced by OVX, an accepted preclinical disease model of postmenopausal osteoporosis. The function of Cthrc1 as a stimulator of bone formation without affecting bone resorption is very promising, because most types of drugs which are currently used for the treatment of osteoporosis are antiresorptive in nature and insufficient for restoring bone volume in osteoporotic patients [23]. Although anabolic agents improve bone mass by stimulating osteoblast-mediated bone formation, only a single anabolic agent, parathyroid hormone 1–34 is available to treat osteoporosis at present [24,25]. Herein, we indicate that Cthrc1 attenuates estrogen deficiency-induced bone loss by stimulating osteoblastic bone formation. Hence, Cthrc1 constitutes a potential target of an anabolic therapy for osteoporosis and the therapeutic effects are expected to be enhanced with antiresorptive drugs.

Materials and Methods

Suppression subtractive hybridization

ATDC5 cells were cultured for a total of 5 days in DMEM/Ham's F12 medium supplemented with 5% FBS and 10 μg/ml insulin with medium change every other day. Cells were exposed to 1 μg/ml BMP2 or vehicle for 10 hr. Poly $(A)^+$ RNA was isolated from BMP2 -untreated and BMP2 -treated ATDC5 cells by a single-step method as previously described [26] and analyzed by suppression subtractive hybridization according to the manufacturer's instruction (PCR-Select cDNA Subtractions Kit, Clontech). After subtraction, the cDNAs were ligated into pCR2.1 (Invitrogen), and these subtracted cDNA libraries were further screened by differential hybridization (differential screening kit, Clontech). The cDNA fragment of approximately 500-bp expressed at a high level in BMP2 -treated ATDC5 cells was identified. Oligo (dT) primed cDNA library from poly$(A)^+$ RNA of BMP2 -treated ATDC5 cells was constructed in λZAP Express vector (Stratagene), and 1×10^6 plaques were screened with the 500-bp fragment as a probe as previously described [26].

Generation of mutant mice

A Cthrc1 genomic clone was isolated from a mouse 129SvEv genomic DNA library. The targeting vector was constructed by inserting an IRES-LacZ-pA-loxP-flanked neomycin resistance expression cassette into exon 2 of the *Cthrc1* gene. Homologous recombination in 129SvEv ES clones harboring *Protamine 1-Cre* transgenes was identified by Southern blot analysis of SacI-digested genomic DNA using 5′ and 3′ probes located outside the homology regions used for gene recombination [27]. Mouse chimeras were generated by C57BL/6 host blastocyst injection of mutant embryonic stem cell clones, and the chimeras obtained were bred with C57BL/6 mice to generate heterozygous *Cthrc1* mice. Heterozygous mutants were then backcrossed eight times with C57BL/6 mice to generate mutant mice with a C57BL/6 genetic background. We then performed RT-PCR to determine the presence of *Cthrc1* transcripts. We used the following primers of *Cthrc1* for RT-PCR, based on exon3 and exon4: 5′-CTGCG-AGTTCTGTTCAGTGG-3′ and 5′-GGGACTGAAATCGTC-AGAGG-3′. *Cthrc1* transgenic mice were generated using an osteoblast-specific 2.3-kb *Col1a1* promoter, the 1.25-kb 3×HA-tagged full-length mouse *Cthrc1* cDNA, and the 240-bp SV40 polyadenylation signal [28]. DNAs were injected into pronuclei of fertilized C57BL/6×DBA/2 hybrid eggs, and the injected eggs were then transferred into CD1 foster mothers. Hemizygous mutants were backcrossed eight times with C57BL/6 mice to generate transgenic mice with a C57BL/6 genetic background. The tissue specificity of transgene expression was examined in immunohistochemistry studies. Routine mouse genotyping was performed by PCR. The following primer pairs were used: 5′-CATCAAGATGGTATAAAAGG-3′ and 5′-GCAGCAGCAG-CACAAGGAAG-3′. The experimental protocols were approved by the Animal Care and Use Committee of Kyoto University.

Histological analyses

Whole mount X-gal staining of embryos was performed as previously described [29]. For the histological analyses, we fixed embryos with 4% paraformaldehyde, embedded them in paraffin, and sectioned them into 7-μm-thick slices. Immunohistochemical staining was performed using peroxidase chromogens (Zymed)/ TrueBlue substrate (KPL) with rabbit polyclonal anti-HA antibody (1:500, Covance). For *in vivo* BrdU labeling, 1-week-old mice were injected intraperitoneally with 100 μg/kg BrdU (Amersham) and sacrificed 3 hr later. Sections were stained with anti-BrdU antibody (Amersham) and were counterstained with hematoxylin according to the manufacturer's instruction.

Micro-CT Analyses

High-resolution micro-CT scanning (SMX-100CT; Shimazu) was performed to measure morphological indices of metaphyseal regions of tibia as previously described [30]. Metaphyseal regions were scanned 100 times with a slice increment of 8 μm. The most proximal slice was defined as the plane where the growth plate had just disappeared. Material properties were calculated using a commercial software package (VG Studio Max1.2: Visual Science) [30].

Bone Histomorphometry

The mice were injected subcutaneously with calcein (20 mg/kg body weight; Sigma) 10 and 3 days before sacrifice. Fifth lumber vertebrae were fixed with 4% paraformaldehyde for 18 hr at 4°C. Undecalcified bones were embedded in methylmethacrylate, and 4-μm-thick sections were prepared for bone histomorphometric analyses of adult mice as previously described [31]. Sections were stained with 1% toluidine blue. Static and dynamic histomorphometric analyses were performed according to standard protocols using Histometry RT (SYSTEM-SUPPLY) [32,33].

Osteoblast Isolation and Culture

Primary osteoblasts were harvested from calvaria of newborn mice by sequential collagenase digestion (Roche) and were maintained in α-MEM containing 10% FBS. BrdU incorporation was measured using the cell proliferation ELISA Biotrack kit (Amersham).

Real-Time PCR

Primary osteoblasts were cultured in α-MEM containing 10% FBS, 50 μg/ml ascorbic acid, and 10 nM β-glycerophosphate for 10 days, and total RNA was isolated from the cultured cells by RNeasy Mini Kit (Qiagen) according to the manufacturer's instruction. Two μg of total RNA was reverse transcribed to cDNA with the use of Transcriptor First Strand cDNA Synthesis Kit (Roche). Real-time PCR was performed using the LightCycler system with the FastStart DNA Master SYBR Green (Roche). The following primers were used: *G3pdh*, 5′-TGTCCGTCGTGGAT-CTGAC-3′ and 5′-CCTGCTTCACCACCTTCTTG-3′; *ALP*, 5′-ACTCAGGGCAATGAGGTCAC-3′ and 5′-CACCCGAGT-GGTAGTCACAA -3′; *Col1a1*, 5′-CTCCTGGCAAGAATGGA-GAT-3′ and 5′-AATCCACGAGCACCCTGA-3′; *Osteocalcin*, 5′-AGACTCCGGCGCTACCTT-3′ and 5′-CTCGTCACAAG-CAGGGTTAAG-3′.

Measurement of CFU-ALP and CFU-O

Bone marrow cells were isolated as previously described [26]. Bone marrow cells from 5-week-old mice were plated into 12-well plates at 2.5×10^6 cells per well for CFU-ALP assays and at 5×10^6 cells per well for CFU-O assays, and were cultured in α-MEM containing 10% FBS, 50 μg/ml ascorbic acid, and 10 nM β-glycerophosphate. For CFU-ALP assays, cultures were stained at day 10 with Sigma alkaline phosphatase kit (Sigma), and colonies with >20 cells were counted. Cultures were stained with 1% alizarin red S (Wako) at day 20 for the CFU-O assay of *Cthrc1*-null mice, and at day 16 for that of *Cthrc1* transgenic mice, respectively. The stained area was calculated using the freeware Image-J (NIH).

Ovariectomy

Mice were ovariectomized or sham-operated at 2 months of age, and all of the mice were killed 4 weeks later and the tibiae and vertebrae were removed for analyses.

Statistical analyses

Statistical analysis was performed by Student's t test to determine the significance between groups. Wild-type and transgenic OVX and sham-operated mice were analyzed by ANOVA followed by Fisher's protected least significant difference. Values were considered statistically significant at $p<0.05$.

More methods were shown in Supporting Information Text S1.

Supporting Information

Figure S1 Analyses of Cthrc1 expression in vitro and in vivo by northern blot and in situ hybridization. (A) Effect of BMP2 (1 μg/ ml) on Cthrc1 expression in ATDC5 cells. Cthrc1 expression is upregulated by BMP2. (B) Expression of Cthrc1 in various cell lines. (C) Expression of Cthrc1 in adult mouse tissues. (D) In situ hybridization analysis of Cthrc1 expression in limb buds of E13.5

and E16.5 mouse embryos. (E) Expression of Cthrc1 during embryogenesis.

Figure S2 Skeletal preparation of Cthrc1-null and Cthrc1 transgenic mice. (A) Whole-mount X-gal staining of heterozygous Cthrc1 embryos during embryogenesis. (B and C) Skeletons of newborn Cthrc1-null mice (B) and Cthrc1 transgenic mice (C) stained by alcian blue followed by alizarin red. WT: wild-type mice; KO: Cthrc1-null mice; Tg: Cthrc1 transgenic mice.

Figure S3 In situ hybridization analyses of osteoblast and chondrocyte marker genes in Cthrc1-null and Cthrc1 transgenic mouse embryos. Runx2, Col1a1, Col2a1 and Col10a1 expression in humeri of E16.5 embryos. (A) Cthrc1-null mouse embryos. (B) Cthrc1 transgenic mouse embryos. WT: wild-type mice; KO: Cthrc1-null mice; Tg: Cthrc1 transgenic mice.

Figure S4 Effect of Cthrc1 on osteoclastogenesis. (A) TRAP staining of vertebrae of 2-month-old Cthrc1-null and wild-type mice. TRAP-positive osteoclast number/bone surface (Oc.N/BS) and osteoclast surface/bone surface (Oc.S/BS) are shown (n = 6). (B) Expression of RANKL in primary osteoblasts harvested from Cthrc1-null mice, assessed by real-time PCR. (C) TRAP staining of vertebrae of 2-month-old Cthrc1 transgenic and wild-type mice. TRAP-positive osteoclast number/bone surface (Oc.N/BS) and osteoclast surface/bone surface (Oc.S/BS) are shown (n = 6). (D) Expression of RANKL in primary osteoblasts harvested from Cthrc1 transgenic mice, assessed by real-time PCR. WT: wild-type mice; KO: Cthrc1-null mice; Tg: Cthrc1 transgenic mice. Data are shown as the mean±SEM (*$p<0.05$).

Text S1 Supplementary Methods.

Acknowledgments

We thank Janie Finch for editorial assistance, Neung-Seon Seo and Magnus Hook for technical support, and Steve O'Gorman for PC3 mouse ES cells.

Author Contributions

Conceived and designed the experiments: BdC HA. Performed the experiments: HK KMK BGD HA. Analyzed the data: HK BGD RRB TN HA. Contributed reagents/materials/analysis tools: ZZ JMD RRB BdC. Wrote the paper: HK BdC HA.

References

1. Olsen BR, Reginato AM, Wang W (2000) Bone development. Annu Rev Cell Dev Biol 16: 191–220.
2. Karsenty G, Wagner EF (2002) Reaching a genetic and molecular understanding of skeletal development. Dev Cell 2: 389–406.
3. Harada S, Rodan GA (2003) Control of osteoblast function and regulation of bone mass. Nature 423: 349–355.
4. Hughes FJ, Collyer J, Stanfield M, Goodman SA (1995) The effects of bone morphogenetic protein-2, -4, and -6 on differentiation of rat osteoblast cells in vitro. Endocrinology 136: 2671–2677.
5. Abe E, Yamamoto M, Taguchi Y, Lecka-Czernik B, O'Brien CA, et al. (2000) Essential requirement of BMPs-2/4 for both osteoblast and osteoclast formation in murine bone marrow cultures from adult mice: antagonism by noggin. J Bone Miner Res 15: 663–673.
6. Kronenberg HM (2003) Developmental regulation of the growth plate. Nature 423: 332–336.
7. Abe E (2006) Function of BMPs and BMP antagonists in adult bone. Ann N Y Acad Sci 1068: 41–53.
8. Devlin RD, Du Z, Pereira RC, Kimble RB, Economides AN, et al. (2003) Skeletal overexpression of noggin results in osteopenia and reduced bone formation. Endocrinology 144: 1972–1978.
9. Wu XB, Li Y, Schneider A, Yu W, Rajendren G, et al. (2003) Impaired osteoblastic differentiation, reduced bone formation, and severe osteoporosis in noggin-overexpressing mice. J Clin Invest 112: 924–934.
10. Zhao M, Harris SE, Horn D, Geng Z, Nishimura R, et al. (2002) Bone morphogenetic protein receptor signaling is necessary for normal murine postnatal bone formation. pp 1049–1060.
11. Mishina Y, Starbuck MW, Gentile MA, Fukuda T, Kasparcova V, et al. (2004) Bone morphogenetic protein type IA receptor signaling regulates postnatal osteoblast function and bone remodeling. J Biol Chem 279: 27560–27566.
12. Yoshida Y, Tanaka S, Umemori H, Minowa O, Usui M, et al. (2000) Negative regulation of BMP/Smad signaling by Tob in osteoblasts. Cell 103: 1085–1097.
13. Pyagay P, Heroult M, Wang Q, Lehnert W, Belden J, et al. (2005) Collagen triple helix repeat containing 1, a novel secreted protein in injured and diseased arteries, inhibits collagen expression and promotes cell migration. Circ Res 96: 261–268.
14. LeClair RJ, Durmus T, Wang Q, Pyagay P, Terzic A, et al. (2007) Cthrc1 is a novel inhibitor of transforming growth factor-beta signaling and neointimal lesion formation. Circ Res 100: 826–833.
15. Durmus T, LeClair RJ, Park KS, Terzic A, Yoon JK, et al. (2006) Expression analysis of the novel gene collagen triple helix repeat containing-1 (Cthrc1). Gene Expr Patterns 6: 935–940.
16. Kalu DN (1991) The ovariectomized rat model of postmenopausal bone loss. Bone Miner 15: 175–191.
17. Wozney JM, Rosen V, Celeste AJ, Mitsock LM, Whitters MJ, et al. (1988) Novel regulators of bone formation: molecular clones and activities. Science 242: 1528–1534.
18. Tang L, Dai DL, Su M, Martinka M, Li G, et al. (2006) Aberrant expression of collagen triple helix repeat containing 1 in human solid cancers. Clin Cancer Res 12: 3716–3722.
19. Wronski TJ, Cintron M, Dann LM (1988) Temporal relationship between bone loss and increased bone turnover in ovariectomized rats. Calcif Tissue Int 43: 179–183.
20. Turner RT, Vandersteenhoven JJ, Bell NH (1987) The effects of ovariectomy and 17 beta-estradiol on cortical bone histomorphometry in growing rats. J Bone Miner Res 2: 115–122.
21. Dempster DW, Birchman R, Xu R, Lindsay R, Shen V (1995) Temporal changes in cancellous bone structure of rats immediately after ovariectomy. Bone 16: 157–161.
22. Nakamura T, Imai Y, Matsumoto T, Sato S, Takeuchi K, et al. (2007) Estrogen prevents bone loss via estrogen receptor alpha and induction of Fas ligand in osteoclasts. Cell 130: 811–823.
23. Rodan GA, Martin TJ (2000) Therapeutic approaches to bone diseases. Science 289: 1508–1514.
24. Canalis E, Giustina A, Bilezikian JP (2007) Mechanisms of anabolic therapies for osteoporosis. N Engl J Med 357: 905–916.
25. Garrett IR (2007) Anabolic agents and the bone morphogenetic protein pathway. Curr Top Dev Biol 78: 127–171.
26. Kimura H, Akiyama H, Nakamura T, de Crombrugghe B (2007) Tenascin-W inhibits proliferation and differentiation of preosteoblasts during endochondral bone formation. Biochem Biophys Res Commun 356: 935–941.
27. O'Gorman S, Dagenais NA, Qian M, Marchuk Y (1997) Protamine-Cre recombinase transgenes efficiently recombine target sequences in the male germ line of mice, but not in embryonic stem cells. Proc Natl Acad Sci U S A 94: 14602–14607.
28. Rossert J, Eberspaecher H, de Crombrugghe B (1995) Separate cis-acting DNA elements of the mouse pro-alpha 1(I) collagen promoter direct expression of reporter genes to different type I collagen-producing cells in transgenic mice. J Cell Biol 129: 1421–1432.
29. Nakashima K, Zhou X, Kunkel G, Zhang Z, Deng JM, et al. (2002) The novel zinc finger-containing transcription factor osterix is required for osteoblast differentiation and bone formation. Cell 108: 17–29.
30. Nakanishi R, Shimizu M, Mori M, Akiyama H, Okudaira S, et al. (2006) Secreted frizzled-related protein 4 is a negative regulator of peak BMD in SAMP6 mice. J Bone Miner Res 21: 1713–1721.
31. Hahn M, Vogel M, Delling G (1991) Undecalcified preparation of bone tissue: report of technical experience and development of new methods. Virchows Arch A Pathol Anat Histopathol 418: 1–7.
32. Parfitt AM (2002) Physiologic and pathogenetic significance of bone histomorphometric data. In: Coe FL, Favus MJ, eds. Disorders of Bone Miner Metabolism, 2nd ed. Philadelphia, PA, USA: Lippincott Williams & Wilkins. pp 469–485.
33. Parfitt AM, Drezner MK, Glorieux FH, Kanis JA, Malluche H, et al. (1987) Bone histomorphometry: standardization of nomenclature, symbols, and units. Report of the ASBMR Histomorphometry Nomenclature Committee. J Bone Miner Res 2: 595–610.

Accelerated Postero-Lateral Spinal Fusion by Collagen Scaffolds Modified with Engineered Collagen-Binding Human Bone Morphogenetic Protein-2 in Rats

Xinglong Han[1]☯, Wen Zhang[2]☯, Jun Gu[3]☯, Huan Zhao[1], Li Ni[1], Jiajun Han[1], Yun Zhou[1], Yannan Gu[1], Xuesong Zhu[1], Jie Sun[4], Xianglin Hou[5], Huilin Yang[1], Jianwu Dai[5]*, Qin Shi[1]*

1 Orthopedic Department, the First Affiliated Hospital of Soochow University, Suzhou, P.R. China, **2** Orthopedic Institute of Soochow University, Suzhou, P.R. China, **3** Orthopedic Department, the Second Affiliated Hospital of Soochow University, Suzhou, P.R. China, **4** Division of Nanobiomedicine, Suzhou Institute of Nano-Tech and Nano-Bionics, Chinese Academy of Sciences, Suzhou, P.R. China, **5** State Key Laboratory of Molecular Developmental Biology, Institute of Genetics and Developmental Biology, Chinese Academy of Sciences, Beijing, P.R. China

Abstract

Bone morphogenetic protein-2 (BMP-2) is a potent osteoinductive cytokine that plays a critical role in bone regeneration and repair. However, its distribution and side effects are major barriers to its success as therapeutic treatment. The improvement of therapy using collagen delivery matrices has been reported. To investigate a delivery system on postero-lateral spinal fusion, both engineered human BMP-2 with a collagen binding domain (CBD-BMP-2) and collagen scaffolds were developed and their combination was implanted into Sprague-Dawley (SD) rats to study Lumbar 4–5 (L4–L5) posterolateral spine fusion. We divided SD rats into three groups, the sham group (G1, n = 20), the collagen scaffold-treated group (G2, n = 20) and the BMP-2-loaded collagen scaffolds group (G3, n = 20). 16 weeks after surgery, the spines of the rats were evaluated by X-radiographs, high-resolution micro-computed tomography (micro-CT), manual palpation and hematoxylin and eosin (H&E) staining. The results showed that spine L4–L5 fusions occurred in G2(40%) and G3(100%) group, while results from the sham group were inconsistent. Moreover, G3 had better results than G2, including higher fusion efficiency (X score, G2 = 2.4±0.163, G3 = 3.0±0, $p<0.05$), higher bone mineral density (BMD, G2: 0.3337±0.0025g/cm3, G3: 0.4353±0.0234g/cm3. $p<0.05$) and more bone trabecular formation. The results demonstrated that with site-specific collagen binding domain, a dose of BMP-2 as low as 0.02mg CBD-BMP-2/cm^3 collagen scaffold could enhance the posterolateral intertransverse process fusion in rats. It suggested that combination delivery could be an alternative in spine fusion with dramatically decreased side effects caused by high dose of BMP-2.

Editor: Xiaohua Liu, Texas A&M University Baylor College of Dentistry, United States of America

Funding: This work was supported by National Nature Science Foundation of China (81101369), the "Strategic Priority Research Program of the Chinese Academy of Sciences" (Grant No. XDA01030000), SRF for ROCS of SEM (QS), PH.D. Program Foundation of SEM (20113201110013), Jiangsu Provincial Special Program of Medical Science (BL2012004, BK2011264), and the State Key Laboratory Cultivation Base of Stem Cell and Bio-medical Materials. The funders had no role in study design, data collection and analysis, decision to publish, or preparation of the manuscript.

Competing Interests: The authors have declared that no competing interests exist.

* E-mail: shiqin@suda.edu.cn (QS); jwdai@genetics.ac.cn (JD)

☯ These authors contributed equally to this work.

Introduction

Low back pain caused by instability of spine is a common disease as the population ages and life styles change. Various factors, such as trauma, tumor, deformity, and degenerative disease, may play prominent roles in spine instability [1,2]. Spinal fusion is one of the most popular procedures to correct unstable parts of the spine. In the US alone, there are approximately 500,000 spinal fusion surgeries performed annually to recover biomechanical stability, and the numbers are increasing [3,4]. Spine fusion has become one of the most common surgical interventions for spine reconstruction.

Since their introduction by Albee and Hibbs in 1911 for the treatment of disseminated tuberculosis of the spine, the materials for spine fusion have evolved tremendously [1]. Autogenous iliac crest bone graft has long been considered the "gold standard" used in spinal fusion procedures because its characteristics, such as osteogenesis, osteoinduction, and osteoconduction, are ideal for promoting fusion from a biological perspective [3]. But a series of complications accompanied by autogeneous bone grafting are inevitable. In addition, the limited source of autogenous iliac crest bone graft largely restricts its application to patients, especially the elderly and children [5]. Allogeneic bone is another possible source of the materials. Although allograft bone may be obtained in greater quantities, the problems of complex processing, low biocompatibility and the risk of disease transfer also hinder its applications [6]. Consequently, tissue engineering products have been considerated as the favorable alternative strategy.

Much of attention has been focused on composite materials for spine fusion because of their advantages of biocompatibility, safety, operability. Collagen is the most abundant protein in the body and is also one of the most important components of extracellular matrix. Scaffold manufactured with collagen has shown its excellent biocompatibility and biodegradability [7]. Furthermore, as a carrier, collagen scaffold can provide physical support for cells and also appropriate incorporation sites for mineral substances and cytokines [7]. A number of applications with collagen scaffolds have been extensively accepted in clinic [4,6,7].

Bone morphogenetic protein-2 (BMP-2) is a potent osteoinductive cytokine that plays a critical role in bone regeneration and repair. Both basic researches and clinic trials have demonstrated its repair efficacy in bone fractures, nonunion and defects [7]. Its safety in clinical application has also been well studied. In 2002, BMP-2 was approved by American Food and Drug Administration (FDA) to apply to spine fusion for patients [8]. However, some recent clinical reports mention that 30% of BMP-2 was released in burst upon initial implantation because conventional collagen materials have no specific binding affinity to BMP-2. Quick degradation and unsustainability have also been reported as a consequence of burst release [6]. The others found cancer risk showing an upward trend after the doctors used a high dose of BMP-2. These findings raise concerns that this growth factor may act as a cancer promoter [9]. To avoid of the side effects of high dose of BMP-2 in vivo, a collagen binding domain (CBD) has been added to the N-terminal of BMP-2 (CBD-BMP-2), which consequently can enhance the binding of BMP-2 to collagen scaffolds and results in a remarkably sustained release action [10,11,12].

To achieve better therapeutic effect and to avoid the local or systemic adverse effects in vivo, here we developed collagen scaffolds from bovine aponeurosis and implanted the collagen scaffolds incorporated with CBD-BMP-2 in a rat spine fusion model and explored the feasibility of this delivery matrices for clinical application.

Materials and Methods

Preparation of Collagen scaffolds

Collagen scaffolds were prepared followed a well-established method as previously described [13,14]. In brief, fresh bovine aponeurosis was separated and its muscles, connective tissues and fats were removed. Next, the cellular components and soluble proteins from aponeurosis were extracted, freeze-dried and made into granular shape. The materials were sterilized by 15 kGy Co^{60} irradiation and weighted. The morphology of the scaffolds was taken photographs by the scanning electron microscope (FEG-SEM, XL-30, Philips, Holland).

Preparation of CBD-BMP-2

The fusion protein CBD-rhBMP-2 consists of a 6×his purification tag, a collagen binding domain (WREPSFCALS) and mature human BMP2 fragment. It was prepared following the steps in the references [10,11]. A reconstructed BMP-2 DNA sequence cloned by PCR procedure was linked to a bacterial expression plasmid pET-28a (Novagen, Germany), and then was transfected into the BL21 (DE3) strain of E.Coli. The bacteria were cultured and proliferated in the container at 200 rpm and then induced with 1mM isopropyl β-D-thiogalactopyranoside (IPTG) to express recombinant protein at 37°C for 4 h. The target protein was separated as inclusion body from the lysate of the E.Coli, collected by centrifugation, and purified using chromatography. After being renatured, the fusion protein was concentrated by ultrafiltration. After the activity of CBD-BMP-2 was assessed, the protein was freeze-dried and weighted. 2hrs before the implantation, CBD-BMP-2 was dissolved in normal saline and then loaded into the Collagen scaffolds at 4°C (0.02mg CBD-BMP-2/cm^3 scaffold).

The biological activity of the CBD-BMP-2 in vitro. The MC-3T3-E1 (the Cell Bank of the Chinese Academy of Sciences, Shanghai, China) were used to evaluate the osteoinduction activity of CBD-BMP-2 and commercial BMP2 (East China Pharmaceutical Group Co. LTD, Hangzhou, China). Cells were seed at a density of 2×10^4 cells/well in 24-well plates and maintained in α-MEM containing 10% FBS for 24h. Then, cells were treated with the osteoblast inducing medium supplemented with 0.5%FBS and CBD-BMP-2 or commercial BMP-2 for additional 3 days. After washed with PBS, the treated cells were lysed with 0.1% TritonX-100/PBS and repeatedly frozen/thawed for three times to disrupt the cell membranes. Alkaline phosphatase (ALP) activities were determined using an alkaline phosphatase reagent kit (ANASPEC, Fremont, CA, USA) and Protein concentrations was measured by the Bicinchoninic Acid (BCA) protein assay reagent (Santa Cruz Biotechnology, USA) [9,11].

The binding and release assay of CBD-BMP-2 in vitro. The collagen scaffolds were sterilized by 15 kGy Co^{60} irradiation, and divided into 10 with an equal volume ($8mm^3$). CBD-BMP-2 and commercial BMP-2 (East China Pharmaceutical Group, Hangzhou, China) solutions with an amount of 5 μg (10 μl/scaffold) were added to sterility eppendorf tube and incubated at 37°C for 2 h. Then all the tubes were extensively washed with PBS, and the unconjugated proteins were measured by the Bicinchoninic Acid protein assay reagent [9,15].

The pre-treated scaffolds were divided 2 groups: the commercial BMP-2 group (n = 5), and the CBD-BMP-2 group (n = 5), were placed respectively in tubes containing 100 μl PBS at 37°C. At various time points (6h, 12h, 24h, 4d, 7d), the scaffolds was removed and the released protein amount was determined by using the Bicinchoninic Acid protein assay reagent (Santa Cruz Biotechnology, USA) [16,17].

Construction of rat Lumbar 4-Lumbar 5 (L4-L5) posterolateral spine fusion model

All experimental procedures were performed following the Guide for the Care and Use of Laboratory Animals of the US National Institutes of Health (NIH), and were approved by the Animal Research Committee of Soochow University (No. 20120406–022).

60 male Sprague-Dawley rats (150±27g, Shanghai Slac laboratory animal Co. Ltd, Shanghai, China.) were divided into 3 groups randomly: the sham group (G1, n = 20), the collagen scaffold group (G2, n = 20) and collagen scaffold with CBD-BMP-2 group (G3, n = 20). The posterior-lateral lumbar spine fusion technique was performed as previously described [3,6,7,18]. The animals were anesthetized with intraperitoneal injection of 3% pentobarbital (50mg/kg of body weight), and placed on the operating table in the prone position. A vertical incision was made in the skin and muscle tissue was dissected. Two separate paramedian incisions were made 3 mm from the midline in the lumbar fascia, and then the transverse processes of L4 and L5 were exposed. After decorticated with a high-speed burr, the transverse processes of G2 and G3 were implanted with collagen scaffolds (5mm×3mm×10mm/side) on both left and right sides or with CBD-BMP-2 (3 μg/side) separately, while the control group was untreated. The fascial and skin incisions were closed with a 4–0 absorbable suture after implantation. The surgery was completed by the same person. All animals survived without nerve injury during the surgical procedure. All rats were housed in separate cages and fed rat chow, water and antibiotics to avoid infection ad libitum, and were monitored for general health on a daily basis.

There were also no abnormal behavior appearing after the surgical procedure and no death due to infection or other reasons. After 16 weeks, all rats were sacrificed and samples were collected for further research.

Manual palpation

Manual palpation is an easy and specific way for assessing rat postero-lateral spinal fusion [1,19,20,21]. 16 weeks after surgery, all rats were killed and the spines were collected and the segments from T12 (Thoracic) to sacrum were preserved. After removing soft tissues around the bone masses and facet joints, the explanted lumbar spines for intersegmental motion were blindly tested by three independent orthopedists manually. Only the bilateral fusion without any left or right motion was considered a successful fusion. Any motion detected between either the transverse processes or the facets, or unilateral fusion was regarded as a fusion failure. The spines of all rats were recorded as motion, partial motion or no motion. Motion and partial motion were considered as not fused and no motion as fused.

X-Ray analysis

At 8 and 16 weeks after surgery, posteroanterior radiographs were taken for each spine (full digital molybdenum targeted photographic scanner, Giotto image MD, Italy). Three independent orthopedists assessed the fusion between the L4 and L5 transverse processes in each rat. If the transverse processes were fused completely, there were a quantity of bone bridges appear and no gap could be found [22,23]. Unilateral or incomplete fusion was considered as a partial fusion and the lack of bone bridges indicated a failed case, which is scored via the following system: 0 = no osteogenesis(bone filling less than 25% of the area); 1 = slight osteogenesis without fusion(bone filling 25% to 50% of the area); 2 = osteogenesis with partial fusion(bone filling 50% to 90% of the area); 3 = osteogenesis with complete fusion (bone filling more than 90% of the area)[7,13].

Micro-CT analysis

The L4 and L5 of the rats were scanned using micro-CT (Skyscan 1176, Belgium) in the spine position at 8 and 16 weeks, and high resolution scanograms (9–20 μm) were obtained (resolution:18 μm, Source Voltage:65KV, Source Current:385μA, Rotation Step:0.7°). The selected images of L4 and L5 were used for 3D reconstruction, meanwhile we chose a cylinder with 1mm diameter, 1.8mm thick (100 continuous slices) in the image to analyze the bone mineral density (BMD) in the fusion area. Well-known standard substances offered by the factory (Skyscan, Belgium) were used to quantify the BMD.[7,18,24].

Hematoxylin-eosin (H&E) staining

After the explanted spines were collected, they were fixed in 10% formaldehyde solution with a volume that was nine times that of the spine tissues. Bone tissues were decalcified in 5% EDTA solution for 4 weeks, and then embedded in paraffin. The specimens near the transverse processes were sliced sagittally at the level of the transverse process. The sections were stained with hematoxylin and eosin (H&E). Images were recorded by fluorescence microscopy (Axio imager. M1, zeiss, Germany). Histologically, the spine fusion could be observed in the presence of the bony trabeculae from one transverse process to another [7,25].

Statistical analysis

The software Statiscal Package for the Social Sciences (SPSS) 13.0 (Chicago, IL, USA) was used to analyze the experimental data. Quantitative data were presented as means ± standard deviation. For the results of radiographic and manual palpation, three groups were compared by rank-sum test or nonparametric *chi*-square test. For the continuous data of BMD and release assay, we used ANOVA in one group at different time points and *t* test or parametric *chi*-square test for different groups at same time point, and any *p*-value less than 0.05 was considered to be statistically significant.

Results

Collagen scaffolds were prepared in porosity

As we expected, the collagen scaffolds were prepared from fresh bovine aponeurosis and characterized by a proper porosity (65%). The pore size ranged from 100 μm to 300 μm (Fig.1)[11,12].

The biological activity of the CBD-BMP-2 in vitro. The biological activities of the CBD-BMP-2 and commercial BMP-2 were tested by the ALP activity assay using the MC-3T3-E1 cells. After incubating for 3 days with CBD-BMP-2 or commercial BMP-2 over a range of 0.5–5 μg, we found that ALP activities were increased significantly in a dose-dependent manner. And there is a statistical differences in 1, 2, 5 μg/well between the two groups, while no difference in 0.5 μg/well. It shows that the CBD-BMP-2 has a slight higher inductive osteogenesis potential than the commercial BMP-2 (Fig.2A).

The binding and release assay of CBD-BMP-2 in vitro. Collagen scaffolds in the CBD-BMP-2 solution resulted in a binding rate of 98.89±0.26% 2hrs after immersion. It showed statistically significant difference with the collagen scaffolds in the commercial BMP-2 solution, whose binding rate was 94.37±0.53% (Fig.2B). The release profiles of CDB-BMP-2 and the commercial BMP-2 are displayed in Fig.2C. At the initial stage (less than 6h), both of them showed slightly burst release. But the cumulative drug release in CBD-BMP-2 was significantly lower than that of commercial BMP-2. There still is a lower released protein content in CBD-BMP-2 group within 24 hours. After 24 hours, the releasing amount and rate in the commercial BMP-2 group was higher than the CBD-BMP-2 group. It indicated that this sustained system could significantly slow down the release of the BMP-2 in vitro.

Spine fusion occurred in G2 and G3 group by manual palpation

Manual palpation for fusion evaluation was performed by three orthopedists blindly. The results are shown in Table 1. G1 group showed no or partial spine fusion and still reserved the ability of scoliosis. It indicated that no fusion happened without any external factors in the process of rats' recovery. In G2 group, only a few fused spines could be found. But all spines in G3 group were assessed as fused by manual palpation. There were significant differences among three groups. The biological advantages of collagen promoted spine fusion and the incorporation of CBD-BMP-2 at a level of 3 μg/side increased this promotion.

New bone formation was observed by X-Ray and Micro-CT

X-ray was used to study the fusion between the L4 and L5 transverse processes, as shown in Fig. 3. According to the orthopedists' judgment, no bony bridge was detected in G1 (Fig. 3, G1). In contrast, a significant amount of bone bridges were

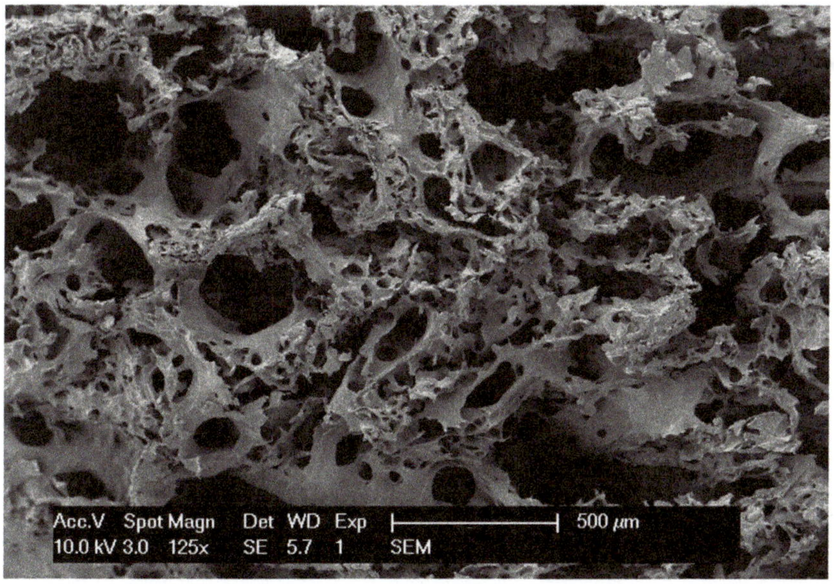

Figure 1. The morphology of the processed collagen scaffolds. This granular scaffolds were taken photographs under the scanning electron microscope (125×). The micropores size range from 100 μm to 300 μm.

found both in G2 and G3 groups, and the bone bridges in G3 group were much denser (Fig.3, G2, G3). After the rats were sacrificed, radiographs of all the SD rat spines were obtained in vitro (Fig. 4) and the same results were observed as from the images obtained in vivo. Differences were significant among three groups (Table 2, score: $G1 = 0.8 \pm 0.133$, $G2 = 2.4 \pm 0.163$, $G3 = 3.0 \pm 0$, $p < 0.05$).

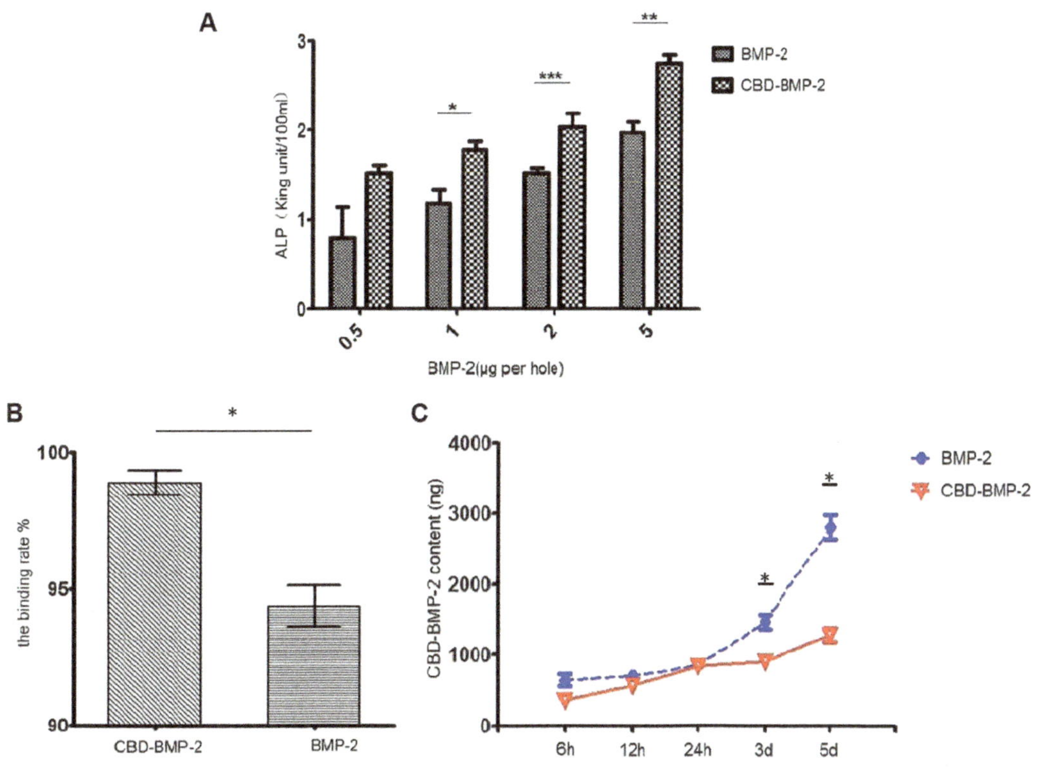

Figure 2. The release profile and bioactivity assay of BMP-2 in vitro. A: The CBD-BMP-2 shows a higher biological activity than the commercial BMP-2 (*:$p<0.05$; **:$p<0.01$; ***:$p<0.001$;). B: The binding rate of CBD-BMP-2 to the collagen scaffolds is higher than that of commercial BMP-2($p<0.05$). C: The releasing amount and rate in the commercial BMP-2 group was higher than those of the CBD-BMP-2 group.(*, Compare to the control group, $p<0.05$).

Table 1. Assessment of postero-lateral fusion via manual palpation (n = 10 per each group).

	manual palpation (Number)		
	G1	**G2**	**G3**
Motion	10	0	0
Partial motion	0	4	0
No motion	0	6	10

There were significant differences among three groups (G2 *vs* G1,$p<0.05$; G3 *vs* G1, $p<0.05$; G3 *vs* G2, $p<0.05$). It indicated that both collagen scaffolds and the CBD-BMP-2-loaded collagen scaffolds can promote a postero-lateral fusion in rats and the latter presented a higher fusion efficiency.

Micro-CT was also used for bone formation assessment. BMD in Fig.5 showed that the gaps between the L4 and L5 transverse processes were filled with new bone tissues in G2 and G3 groups, but the similar phenomenon did not appear in G1 group. The volume of new bone formation was much larger in G3 compared to G2. Moreover, the new bone formed in the area where the scaffolds were implanted, but did not migrated or had ectopic osteogenesis, suggesting that collagen scaffolds retained the migration of CBD-BMP-2. The BMD analysis of the spines demonstrated substantial bones emerged between the transverse processes in G3 group. A statistical analysis of BMD showd a significant difference among three groups (Fig. 6A, G1: 0g/cm^3, G2: 0.3337±0.0025g/cm^3, G3: 0.4353±0.0234g/cm^3. $p<0.05$). Furthermore, we found that the increased BMD between 4 and 8 weeks was less than that between 8 and 16 weeks (Fig. 6B), which may be a result of collagen degradation. We randomly selected a cylindrical area of 1mm in diameter and 100 layers in thickness from the scanograms of Micro-CT to quantify the ratio of bone volume to tissue volume, representing the quantity of new bone formation. The results showed that the collagen/CBD-BMP-2 composites led to much more new bone formation than collagen alone (Fig. 6C, G3: 77.68±14.76%, G2: 53.28±6.499%, $p<0.05$). Meanwhile, the degradation of collagen scaffolds was clearly observed at 16 weeks after the surgery compared to the one at 8 weeks.

New bone formation was assessed by histologic analysis

H&E staining provided an objective assessment on collagen degradation and bone formation. As shown in Fig.7, trabeculae were barely observed in G1 group, while a great quantity of trabeculae were found in G2 and G3 groups. Chondrocytes and osteoblasts around the new bone area were also detected, indicating an active process of new bone formation. The amount of trabeculae and osteoblasts in G3 group was much greater compared to G2 group. Same as previous study [12,13], the partially degraded collagen scaffolds were also observed (Fig. 7).

Discussion

In recent years, an increasing number of patients have been receiving spine fusion operations to prevent further instability and insult to the cord. Autogenous iliac crest was used as a substitute to provide the osteoinductive and osteoconductive effect for the new bone formation in the traditional spinal fusion procedures. But the volume of bone harvested from the donor site is limited and the harvest of autograft may be associated with various complications [26,27]. Allografting does not have these complications. However, it increases the risk of disease transfer. An attractive strategy is to combine osteoinductive cytokine with osteoconductive vehicle as an alternative to stimulate new bone formation [9].

BMP-2 has been shown to be successful in achieving spinal fusion in animals and humans. Subsequent pre-clinical studies have shown that the interbody spinal fusion rate in BMP-2 group

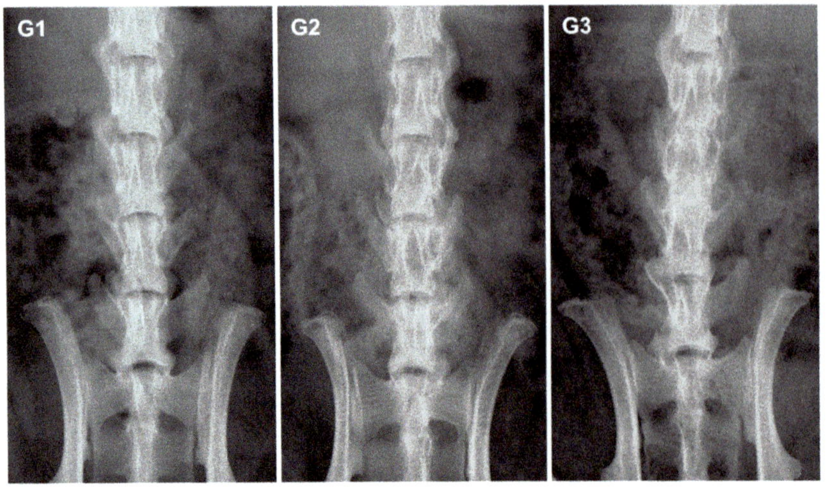

Figure 3. X-Radiographs of SD rat spines in vivo. Representative images of rats in each group are shown (coronal view). 8 weeks after the implantation, the spines appeared fused in G3, partially fused in G2 and no fused in G1.

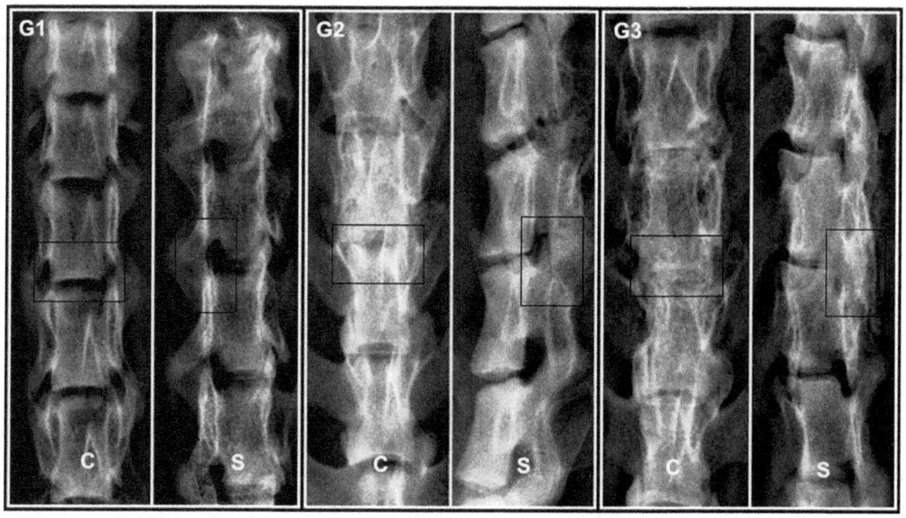

Figure 4. X-radiographs of SD rat spines in vitro. The Representative images showed that visible fusion occurred in both G2 and G3 groups at 16 weeks after the implantation (coronal view (C) and sagittal view (S)). The intervertebral space in G3 was hid under the new bone. A great quantity of new bone could be found and the processus transversus were joined to form a whole from a posterior lateral aspect between L4 and L5. There was a similar, but slightly imperfect result in G2.

was almost 100% while only 30%–50% fusion rates in the autograft controls and a similar outcome were obtained in clinical studies [28,29]. Favorable results of BMP-2 in improving the rates of interbody spinal fusion stimulated the increased use of BMP-2 in analogous spine procedures. According to a report, by 2007, more than 50% of primary anterior interbody lumbar fusion (ALIF), 43% of posterior lumbar interbody fusion (PLIF)/ transforaminal lumbar interbody fusion (TLIF), and 30% of posterolateral lumbar fusion (PLF) were reported to use BMP-2 [29]. These reports suggest that BMP-2 has been accepted as an effective inducing factor of osteogenesis.

However, controversies are still associated with the clinical applications of BMP-2. A number of reported complications include osteolysis, seroma with radiculopathy, soft-tissue swelling, increased infections, cage subsidence or migration and so on [30]. Bae HW et al. provided strong support that excessive BMP-2 could cause trachea edema, and even death. Some of patient developed retroperitoneal hematoma (7.2%) [31]. Devine JG et al. reviewed the cancer risk of rhBMP-2 used in spine fusion as published and came to a conclusion that cancer risk with BMP-2 may be dose dependent and a higher dose cause a higher risk of cancer, even when collage scaffold are used to slow the release of BMP-2, while the risk of cancer reduced to the level of control groups in a dose of BMP-2 (4.2–4.8mg) [32]. Furthermore, the excessive dosage of BMP-2 could create other potential risks, such as excessive bone formation and adverse immune responses [33]. Thus, it is critical to maintain the therapeutic function with the dosage of BMP-2 as low as possible in clinical application.

It has been well established that BMP-2 requires a suitable delivery vehicle to be effective. In 2002, the Federal Drug Administration (FDA) approved a device called INFUSE, which contained a porous resorbable collagen sponge to retain the BMP-2 [34,35]. However, the open porous structure of the collagen carrier failed to reduce the dosage and some side effects of BMP-2. Spilled cytokines cause not only significant waste but also many kinds of sequelae [32]. Further investigations focus on improving the BMP-2 efficacy in INFUSE. A great number of new biomaterials have emerged in recent years such as bacterial cellulose, PEGylated fibrinogen, hydroxyapatite (HA), supramolecular nanofibers [6,8,10]. In addition to the ability of sustaining release of the BMP-2 for sufficient time, these biomaterials also can partially avoid the complications caused by BMP-2. Thus, to

Table 2. Score evaluation of postero-lateral fusion via radiographs (n = 10 per each group).

	X-ray (Number)		
score	G1	G2	G3
0	2	0	0
1	8	0	0
2	0	6	0
3	0	4	10
Mean±SD:	0.8±0.133	2.4±0.163	3.0±0

There were significant differences among three groups (G2 *vs* G1, $p<0.05$; G3 *vs* G1, $p<0.05$; G3 *vs* G2, $p<0.05$). It indicated the collagen scaffolds had a positive effect on spine fusion and CBD-BMP-2 accelerated the fusion.

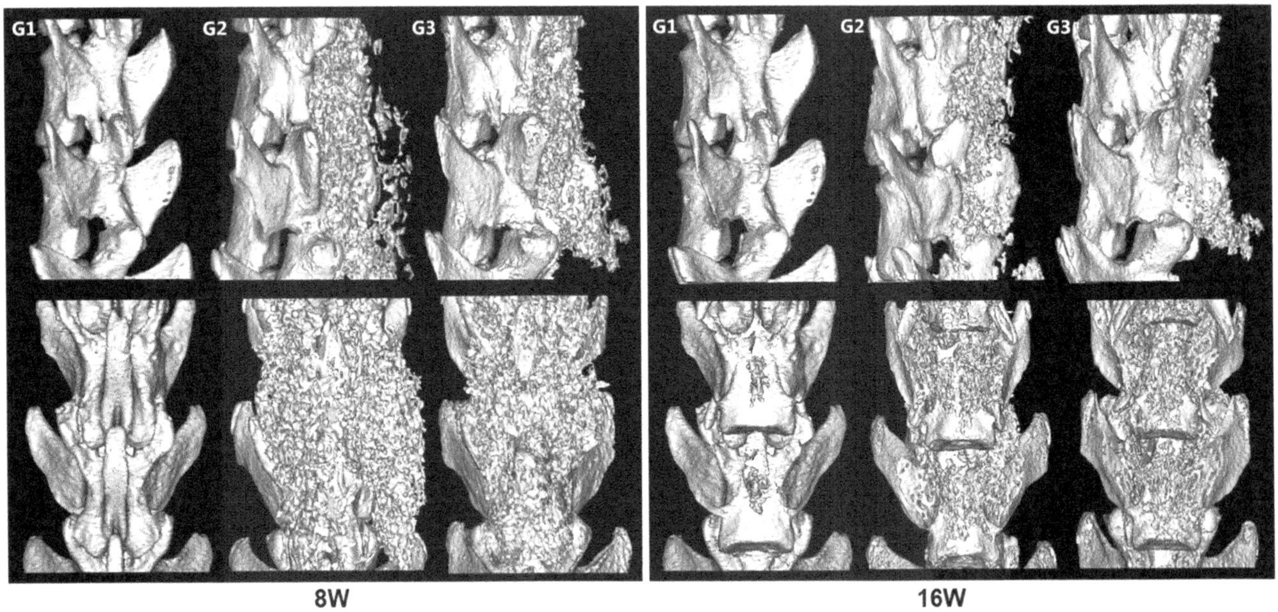

Figure 5. Representative 3D reconstruction images of Micro-CT images. 8W: The images of 8 weeks after the implantation showed that obvious new bone formed in G2 and G3 while a similar phenomenon did not appear in G1. 16W: The images of 16weeks after the implantation showed that the spines of all the rats exhibited considerable new bone formation in G3 and fusion masses were significantly larger and denser than G2. There was still no new bone found in G1.

reduce the negative effect, we introduced collagen scaffolds incorporated with CBD-BMP-2 to enhance posterolateral inter-transverse process fusion in rats.

In this study, we prepared the collagen scaffolds from bovine aponeurosis. As previously described, the processed material showed good cell compatibility and low immunogenisity[14]. Meanwhile, the collagen scaffolds were characterized by a proper porosity (65%) and micropores size (100–300 μm), which showed excellent osteoconduction [31]. The data of histology and imageology showed that new bone formation was appeared in collagen-treated group, indicating that collagen scaffolds has clear osteoconduction and play a positive role in spine fusion.

Although the collagen scaffolds can retain the BMP-2, partially avoiding problems of the complications caused by the high focal concentration of BMP-2, some studies have reported the phenomena of burst release upon initial implantation. Here we modified the BMP-2 by adding a collagen binding domain (CBD). By the site-specific combination, the modified BMP-2 could be incorporated to the collagen scaffolds and achieve a sustained release. In our previous and present study, the CBD-BMP-2 showed a higher affinity to collagen scaffolds than that of the commercial BMP-2. Without burst release and quick degradation, it suggested that engineered CBD-BMP-2 be administrated at a lower dose compared to traditional BMP-2. The INFUSE contains 1.5 mg BMP-2 per milliliter, which exceed the physiological levels of BMP-2 (1 μg/kg). In clinic, it is also generally recognized that the average BMP-2 dosage per implant site was 12–40 mg, and the BMP-2 concentration showed a gradual decrease over time [24,36,37]. To enhance posterolateral intertransverse process fusion in rats, we administrated CBD-BMP-2 at a dose of 20 μg per milliliter collagen scaffold, which was much less than the commercial INFUSE. As we respected, the group with collagen scaffolds incorporated CBD-BMP-2 had better results than with collagen scaffolds alone, including higher fusion efficiency, higher bone mineral density (BMD) and more bone trabecular formation. We speculated that the sustained-release system developed here reduced the BMP-2 burst release because of site-specific collagen binding domain. It was benefited to avoid of heterotopic bone

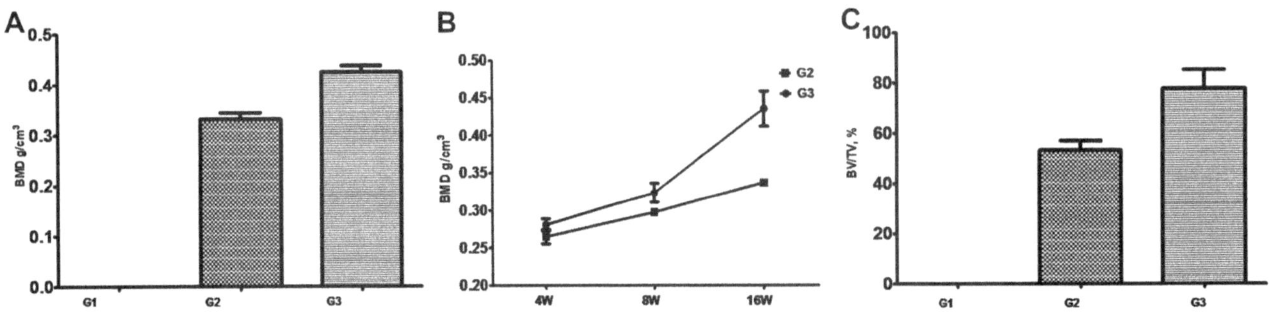

Figure 6. Bone mineral density (BMD) analysis by Micro-CT. A: BMD analysis at 16 weeks after surgery. B: The BMD at different time points. C: The ratio of new bone volume (BV) to tissue volume (TV) at 16weeks. Data are expressed as the mean±SD (n = 10 per each group).

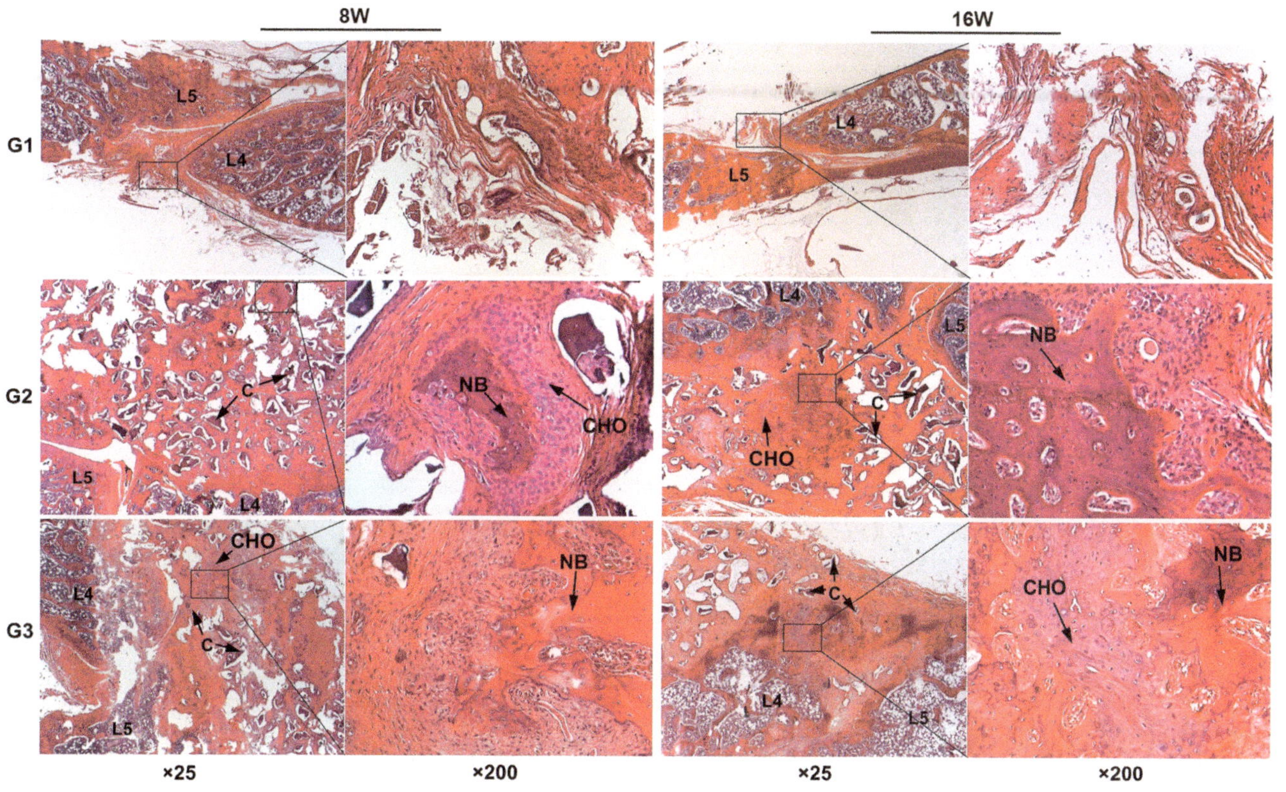

Figure 7. The H&E staining for L4–L5 posterolateral space in rats. There were plenty of trabeculae between spongy bone which mean a fusion in G2 and G3 and no new bone were found in G1 (C: incompletely degraded collagen scaffolds, CHO: chondrocyte, NB: new bone).

formation in the clinical application. Meanwhile, CBD-BMP-2 was released into surrounding environment during the collagen scaffold degraded. It was helpful for BMP-2 being an osteoinduction factor as long as possible. However, further investigations on controlling the BMP2 release via the collagen scaffolds are necessary.

We did not observe overgrowth and heterotopic bone formation in the experiments. All rats survived without infection and did not suffer inflammation at the site of implantation. Our results indicated that CBD-BMP-2 can stimulate the new bone formation and promote spine fusion without any detectable side effects of BMP-2. It suggested that combination delivery could be an alternative candidate in spine fusion with decreased dramatically side effects caused by high dose of BMP-2. This advantage needs investigation and verification in future application.

However, there still have many variables which were not taken into consideration. The fusions in SD rats have been limited to posterolateral fusion and can not provide enough iliac crest bone for posterolateral fusion as controls. Larger animals can offer advantages for experiments that study internal fixation devices and biomechanics[38]. So we need larger animal model to further confirm our results. Meanwhile tetrapods like rats can not reflect the condition of the spine in bipedality because lumbars are not the highest load bearing region[39]. Methods used in our experiments need to be further improved, such as the BMD date should be optimized to reflect the bone density. In addition, we need further to compare the effects of different dose of CBD-BMP-2 on spine fusion in vivo. All the problems would be solved in future.

Conclusion

Collagen scaffolds loaded with CBD-BMP-2 enhanced a posterolateral intertransverse process fusion. With site-specific collagen binding domain, BMP-2 could be adhensive to carries for a longer time than commercial BMP-2, which suggested a potential delivery system to promote bone regeneration and to increase the probability of spine fusion.

Acknowledgments

The authors thank Dr. Zongping Luo for invaluable comments.

Author Contributions

Conceived and designed the experiments: JD QS. Performed the experiments: X. Han WZ JG HZ LN. Analyzed the data: HY. Contributed reagents/materials/analysis tools: JS JH YZ YG XZ X. Hou. Wrote the paper: X. Han.

References

1. Reid JJ, Johnson JS, Wang JC (2011) Challenges to bone formation in spinal fusion. J Biomech. 44: 213–220.
2. Kettler A, Rohlmann F, Ring C, Mack C, Wilke HJ (2011) Do early stages of lumbar intervertebral disc degeneration really cause instability? Evaluation of an in vitro database. Eur Spine J. 20: 578–584.
3. Alsaleh KA, Tougas CA, Roffey DM, Wai EK (2012) Osteoconductive bone graft extenders in posterolateral thoracolumbar spinal fusion. Spine(Phila Pa 1976) 37: 993–1000.
4. Geiger M, Li RH, Friess W (2003) Collagen sponges for bone regeneration with rhBMP-2. Adv Drug Deliv Rev 55: 1613–1629.

5. Dewan AK, Dewan RA, Calderon N, Fuentes A, Lazard Z, et al. (2010) Assessing mechanical integrity of spinal fusion by in situ endochondral osteoinduction in the murine model. J Orthop Surg Res 5: 58–67.
6. Lee SS, Huang BJ, Kaltz SR, Sur S, Newcomb CJ, et al. (2013) Bone regeneration with low dose BMP-2 amplified by biomimetic supramolecular nanofibers within collagen scaffolds. Biomaterials 34: 452–459.
7. Miyazaki M, Morishita Y, He W, Hu M, Sintuu C, et al. (2009) A porcine collagen-derived matrix as a carrier for recombinant human bone morphogenetic protein-2 enhances spinal fusion in rats. Spine J 9: 22–30.
8. Ben-David D, Srouji S, Shapira-Schweitzer K, Kossover O, Ivanir E, et al. (2013) Low dose BMP-2 treatment for bone repair using a PEGylated fibrinogen hydrogel matrix. Biomaterials 34: 2902–2910.
9. Carragee EJ, Chu G, Rohatgi R, Hurwitz EL, Weiner BK, et al. (2013) Cancer risk after use of recombinant bone morphogenetic protein-2 for spinal arthrodesis. J Bone Joint Surg Am 95: 1537–1545.
10. Shi Q, Li Y, Sun J, Zhang H, Chen L, et al. (2012) The osteogenesis of bacterial cellulose scaffold loaded with bone morphogenetic protein-2. Biomaterials 33: 6644–6649.
11. Chen B, Lin H, Zhao Y, Wang B, Zhao Y, et al. (2007) Activation of demineralized bone matrix by genetically engineered human bone morphogenetic protein-2 with a collagen binding domain derived from von Willebrand factor propolypeptide. J Biomed Mater Res A 80: 428–434.
12. Chen B, Lin H, Wang J, Zhao Y, Wang B, et al. (2007) Homogeneous osteogenesis and bone regeneration by demineralized bone matrix loading with collagen-targeting bone morphogenetic protein-2. Biomaterials 28: 1027–1035.
13. Zhao H, Guan HG, Gu J, Luo ZP, Zhang W, et al. (2013) Collagen membrane alleviates peritendinous adhesion in the rat Achilles tendon injury model. Chin Med J (Engl) 126: 729–733.
14. Lin H, Chen B, Wang B, Zhao Y, Sun W, et al. (2006) Novel nerve guidance material prepared from bovine aponeurosis. J Biomed Mater Res A 79: 591–598.
15. Hsieh CY, Hsieh HJ, Liu HC, Wang DM, Hou LT (2006) Fabrication and release behavior of a novel freeze-gelled chitosan/gamma-PGA scaffold as a carrier for rhBMP-2. Dent Mater 22: 622–629.
16. Kempen DH, Lu L, Hefferan TE, Creemers LB, Maran A, et al. (2008) Retention of in vitro and in vivo BMP-2 bioactivities in sustained delivery vehicles for bone tissue engineering. Biomaterials 29:3245–3252.
17. Hannink G, Geutjes PJ, Daamen WF, Buma P (2013) Evaluation of collagen/heparin coated TCP/HA granules for long-term delivery of BMP-2. J Mater Sci Mater Med 24: 325–332.
18. Lopez MJ, McIntosh KR, Spencer ND, Borneman JN, Horswell R, et al. (2009) Acceleration of Spinal Fusion Using Syngeneic and Allogeneic Adult Adipose Derived Stem Cells in a Rat Model. J Orthop Res 27: 366–373.
19. Crandall DG, Revella J, Patterson J, Huish E, Chang M, et al. (2013) Transforaminal lumbar interbody fusion with rhBMP-2 in spinal deformity, spondylolisthesis and degenerative disease – Part 2: BMP dosage related complications and long-term outcomes in 509 patients. Spine (Phila Pa 1976) 38: 1137–1145.
20. Dmitriev AE, Farhang S, Lehman RA Jr, Ling GS, Symes AJ (2010) Bone morphogenetic protein-2 used in spinal fusion with spinal cord injury penetrates intrathecally and elicits a functional signaling cascade. Spine J 10: 16–25.
21. Hsu HP, Zanella JM, Peckham SM, Spector M (2006) Comparing Ectopic Bone Growth Induced by rhBMP-2 on an Absorbable Collagen Sponge in Rat and Rabbit Models. J Orthop Res 24: 1660–1669.
22. Lee JW, Lee S, Lee SH, Yang HS, Im GI, et al. (2011) Improved spinal fusion efficacy by long-term delivery of bone morphogenetic protein-2 in a rabbit model. Acta Orthop 82: 756–760.
23. Park BH, Song KJ, Yoon SJ, Park HS, Jang KY, et al. (2011) Acceleration of spinal fusion using COMP-angiopoietin 1 with allografting in a rat model. Bone 49: 447–454.
24. Zhu W, Rawlins BA, Boachie-Adjei O, Myers ER, Arimizu J, et al. (2004) Combined Bone Morphogenetic Protein-2 and -7 Gene Transfer Enhances Osteoblastic Differentiation and Spine Fusion in a Rodent Model. J Bone Miner Res 19: 2021–2032.
25. Lu J, Bhargav D, Wei AQ, Diwan A (2008) Posterolateral Intertransverse Spinal Fusion Possible in Osteoporotic Rats With BMP-7 in a Higher Dose Delivered on a Composite Carrier. Spine (Phila Pa 1976) 33: 242–249.
26. Liao SS, Guan K, Cui FZ, Shi SS, Sun TS (2003) Lumbar Spinal Fusion With a Mineralized Collagen Matrix and rhBMP-2 in a Rabbit Model. Spine (Phila Pa 1976) 28: 1954–1960.
27. Rao RD, Bagaria V, Gourab K, Haworth ST, Shidham VB, et al. (2008) Autograft containment in posterolateral spine fusion. Spine J 8: 563–569.
28. Gupta MC, Khan SN (2005) Application of bone morphogenetic proteins in spinal fusion. Cytokine Growth Factor Rev 16: 347–355.
29. Carragee EJ, Hurwitz EL, Weiner BK (2011) A critical review of recombinant human bone morphogenetic protein-2 trials in spinal surgery: emerging safety concerns and lessons learned. Spine J 11: 471–491.
30. Poynton AR, Lane JM (2002) Safety profile for the clinical use of bone morphogenetic proteins in the spine. Spine (Phila Pa 1976) 27: S40–S48.
31. Bae HW, Strenge KB, Ashraf N, Badura JM, Peckham SM, et al. (2012) Transient soft-tissue edema associated with implantation of increasing doses of rhBMP-2 on an absorbable collagen sponge in an ectopic rat model. J Bone Joint Surg Am 94: 1845–1852.
32. Devine JG, Dettori JR, France JC, Brodt E, McGuire RA (2012) The use of rhBMP in spine surgery: is there a cancer risk? Evid Based Spine Care J 3: 35–41.
33. Glassman SD, Carreon LY, Campbell MJ, Johnson JR, Puno RM, et al. (2008) The perioperative cost of Infuse bone graft in posterolateral lumbar spine fusion. Spine J 8: 443–448.
34. Koo KH, Lee JM, Ahn JM, Kim BS, La WG, et al. (2013) Controlled Delivery of Low-Dose Bone Morphogenetic Protein-2 Using Heparin-Conjugated Fibrin in the Posterolateral Lumbar Fusion of Rabbits. Artif Organs 37: 487–494.
35. Glassman SD, Carreon L, Djurasovic M, Campbell MJ, Puno RM, et al. (2007) Posterolateral lumbar spine fusion with INFUSE bone graft. Spine J 7: 44–49.
36. Park DK, Kim SS, Thakur N, Boden SD (2013) Use of Recombinant Human Bone Morphogenetic Protein-2 with Local Bone Graft Instead of Iliac Crest Bone Graft in Posterolateral Lumbar Spine Arthrodesis. Spine (Phila Pa 1976) 38:E738–E747
37. Boerckel JD, Kolambkar YM, Dupont KM, Uhrig BA, Phelps EA, et al. (2011) Effects of protein dose and delivery system on BMP-mediated bone regeneration. Biomaterials 32: 5241–5251.
38. Drespe IH, Polzhofer GK, Turner AS, Grauer JN (2005) Animal models for spinal fusion. Spine J 5: 209S–216S.
39. Schimandle JH, Boden SD (1994) Spine update. The use of animal models to study spinal fusion. Spine (Phila Pa 1976) 19: 1998–2006.

12

Growth Hormone Improves Growth Retardation Induced by Rapamycin without Blocking Its Antiproliferative and Antiangiogenic Effects on Rat Growth Plate

Óscar Álvarez-García[1,2], Enrique García-López[3], Vanessa Loredo[3], Helena Gil-Peña[3], Natalia Mejía-Gaviria[1], Julián Rodríguez-Suárez[1,3], Flor Á. Ordóñez[3], Fernando Santos[1,2,3]*

1 Department of Pediatrics, University of Oviedo, Oviedo, Spain, **2** Laboratory of Growth and Cancer, Instituto Universitario de Oncología del Principado de Asturias, Oviedo, Asturias, Spain, **3** Department of Pediatrics, Hospital Universitario Central de Asturias, Oviedo, Spain

Abstract

Rapamycin, an immunosuppressant agent used in renal transplantation with antitumoral properties, has been reported to impair longitudinal growth in young individuals. As growth hormone (GH) can be used to treat growth retardation in transplanted children, we aimed this study to find out the effect of GH therapy in a model of young rat with growth retardation induced by rapamycin administration. Three groups of 4-week-old rats treated with vehicle (C), daily injections of rapamycin alone (RAPA) or in combination with GH (RGH) at pharmacological doses for 1 week were compared. GH treatment caused a 20% increase in both growth velocity and body length in RGH animals when compared with RAPA group. GH treatment did not increase circulating levels of insulin-like growth factor I, a systemic mediator of GH actions. Instead, GH promoted the maturation and hypertrophy of growth plate chondrocytes, an effect likely related to AKT and ERK1/2 mediated inactivation of GSK3β, increase of glycogen deposits and stabilization of β-catenin. Interestingly, GH did not interfere with the antiproliferative and antiangiogenic activities of rapamycin in the growth plate and did not cause changes in chondrocyte autophagy markers. In summary, these findings indicate that GH administration improves longitudinal growth in rapamycin-treated rats by specifically acting on the process of growth plate chondrocyte hypertrophy but not by counteracting the effects of rapamycin on proliferation and angiogenesis.

Editor: Frank Beier, University of Western Ontario, Canada

Funding: This study was supported by Fondo de Investigacion Sanitaria (FIS, PI08-1723), Fondo Europeo de Desarrollo Regional (FEDER), Fundacion para el Fomento en Asturias de la Investigacion Cientifica Aplicada y Tecnología (FICYT, PC07-004), Instituto Universitario de Oncología del Principado de Asturias (IUOPA) and Fundación Nutrición y Crecimiento. The funders had no role in study design, data collection and analysis, decision to publish, or preparation of the manuscript.

Competing Interests: The authors have declared that no competing interests exist.

* E-mail: fsantos@uniovi.es

Introduction

Rapamycin or sirolimus (Rapamune, Wyeth Pharmaceuticals, Philadelphia, PA, USA) is used as immunosuppressant in transplanted patients. Rapamycin directly inhibits mammalian target of rapamycin (mTOR), a ubiquitous kinase that controls different pathways related with cell proliferation, growth and metabolism [1]. On the basis of its potent immunosuppressive, antiproliferative and antitumor effects, rapamycin is able to treat multiple conditions simultaneously [2]. Experimental and clinical studies have showed that rapamycin is able not only to provide a low rate of acute rejection and a significant improvement in kidney allograft function, but also to significantly decrease the incidence of posttransplant malignancies [3,4]. In addition, rapamycin has the potential to interfere with fibrotic processes that often accompany transplant rejection and to influence the preferential development of immunological tolerance [2]. However, the use of rapamycin is associated with many side effects, including increases in serum cholesterol and triglycerides, anemia, proteinuria, skin rashes, retard of wound healing and diarrhea, which can eventually lead to rapamycin withdrawal [5].

In pediatric renal transplantation, rapamycin is mainly used as a substitute for calcineurin inhibitors when nephrotoxicity or proliferative diseases occur [6]. In this group of patients, preservation and improvement of height potential, which can be severely reduced due to multiple factors, is a major challenge [7]. Longitudinal growth is the result of new bone formation during endochondral ossification, in which proliferation and differentiation of epiphyseal growth plate chondrocytes directly correlate with bone elongation. Recent studies from our group found that rapamycin impairs longitudinal growth in young rats, causing marked alterations in the growth plate [8], and that rapamycin disrupts angiogenesis and decreases proliferation and hypertrophy of growth cartilage chondrocytes [9]. In humans, Gonzalez et al [10] reported lower growth rate in a small series of kidney transplanted children treated with rapamycin in comparison with a control group not treated with rapamycin. Therefore, there is growing evidence that rapamycin can adversely affect longitudinal growth this undesirable effect being of special relevance in pediatric renal transplantation.

Over the past two decades, introduction of recombinant human growth hormone (hereafter referred as GH) treatment has been used to improve growth retardation in children with chronic renal disease, including transplanted patients [7]. It is unknown whether the growth promoting effect of GH remains in the presence of rapamycin and, on the contrary, the growth inhibiting effect of rapamycin may be counterbalanced by GH treatment.

The study presented here was designed to find out the effect of GH therapy on longitudinal growth in a model of young rat with growth retardation induced by rapamycin administration.

Results

GH Effects on Growth and Nutrition

As shown in Table 1, animals treated with rapamycin and GH (RGH) had a significantly greater increase in both nose to tail-tip length gain and longitudinal bone growth rate when compared with those treated with rapamycin (RAPA). Representative images of tibial growth plate sections illustrating the differences in longitudinal bone growth rate are shown in Figure 1A. GH treatment was not associated to higher levels of circulating IGF-I in RGH group when compared with RAPA (C: 288±27 ng/ml; RAPA: 524±32 ng/ml; RGH: 516±93 ng/ml). Trough rapamycin levels were similar in both groups (RAPA: 19.4±4.0 ng/ml *vs* RGH: 18.1±3.8 ng/ml).

GH Effects on Growth Plate Morphology

As shown in Figure 1B, RAPA animals exhibited marked morphological alterations in the proliferative and hypertrophic zones of the epiphyseal cartilage, including disorganization of the proliferative layer with loss of the columnar pattern, hardly noticeable transition zone from proliferative to hypertrophic strata, and highly irregular chondro-osseus junction. These alterations were also found in RGH growth plates. In addition, Von Kossa staining revealed an abnormal pattern of mineralization in both groups of rats evidenced by a wide area of extracellular mineralized matrix as well as presence of both transverse bands of mineralized matrix (red arrows) and numerous chondrocytes totally surrounded by mineralized tissue (Figure 1C).

As resumed in Table 2, histomorphometrical analysis revealed that the height of tibial growth cartilage was greater in RGH than in RAPA animals. These differences were also found in the height of the hypertrophic zone. However, the ration of hypertrophic zone to cartilage height was not significantly different between the three groups. Interestingly, the height of the terminal chondrocyte was significantly higher in RGH animals when compared with RAPA.

Finally, chondrocyte proliferation was assessed in growth cartilage by immunodetection of bromodeoxyuridine (BrdU). BrdU-labelled chondrocytes were localized in the proliferative zone in all groups (Figure 2A). Although there were a significant decrease in the percentage of positive cells between rapamycin treated groups and control animals, no statistical differences between RAPA and RGH groups were found [C: 35±1 positive cells/100 cells; RAPA: 28±3 positive cells/100 cells ($p \leq 0.05$ *vs* C); RGH: 31±2 positive cells/100 cells ($p \leq 0.05$ *vs* C)].

Table 1. Growth of rats treated with vehicle (C), rapamycin (RAPA) or with rapamycin and growth hormone (RGH).

	C (n = 10)	RAPA (n = 10)	RGH (n = 10)
Length gain (cm)	2.4±0.2	2.0±0.2[a]	2.5±0.1[b]
Longitudinal growth rate (μm/day)	164±7	82±6[a]	102±5[a,b]

Values are expressed as mean±SEM.
[a]Means statistically different from C group ($P \leq 0.05$).
[b]Means statistically different from RAPA group ($P \leq 0.05$).

GH Effects on Growth Plate Angiogenesis

Picrosirius red/alcian blue staining showed morphological anomalies in the primary spongiosa of both groups treated with rapamycin (Figure 2B). In contrast with the typical arrangement of longitudinal trabeculae seen in the primary spongiosa of C rats, numerous transverse unresorbed septa were found in both groups (yellow arrows), strongly depicting the pattern of the invading capillary sprouts (red arrows).

Tartrate-resistant acid phosphatase (TRAP) positive cells were found in the primary spongiosa and along the vascular invasion front in all groups (Figure 2C). In the area between the chondro-osseous junction and 50 mm deep in the primary spongiosa, there was a significant decrease in the number of TRAP-reactive cells per mm^2 between both groups treated with rapamycin and C animals [C: 262±6; RAPA: 139±21 ($p \leq 0.05$ *vs* C); RGH: 103±6 ($p \leq 0.05$ *vs* C)].

VEGF immunohistochemical signal was localized within the cytoplasm of hypertrophic chondrocytes from the early hypertrophic zone to the distal end of the cartilage in all groups (Figure 2D). This pattern of VEGF protein distribution was also observed at mRNA level as disclosed by in situ hybridization experiments (Figure 2E). In rapamycin treated animals, it is of note that several chondrocytes adjacent to distal end of the growth cartilage did not express VEGF, despite being metabolically active, as evidenced by normal collagen X expression and alkaline phosphatase activity (see Figure S1). Accordingly, the percentage of terminal VEGF immunopositive cells showed a significant decrease in both rapamycin treated groups when compared with controls [C: 92±1 positive cells/100 terminal chondrocytes; RAPA: 62±4 positive cells/100 terminal chondrocytes ($p \leq 0.05$ *vs* C); RGH: 68±3 positive cells/100 terminal chondrocytes ($p \leq 0.05$ *vs* C)].

GH Effects on Chondrocyte Autophagy and Metabolism

Autophagy was studied in growth cartilage of rapamycin treated rats using two different approaches. First, fluorescent immunodetection of total microtubule-associated protein light chain 3 (LC3) revealed a strong signal mostly in the cytoplasm of early hypertrophic chondrocytes in both groups (Figure 3A). This signal, often detected as punctual staining (arrows in Figure 3B), indicated induction of autophagy in these cells. Second, conversion of LC3-I isoform to LC3-II, as indicative of autophagosome formation, was assessed by western blotting. No differences in LC3-II/LC3-I ratio were found between groups (Figure 3C), suggesting that GH administration did not modify autophagy in the epiphyseal chondrocytes.

Periodic acid-Schiff (PAS) stain was used to identify glycogen deposits, as an index of the energetic reserves of growth plate chondrocytes. As shown in Figure 4A, PAS positive cytoplasmatic granules were mostly seen in chondrocytes of the upper hypertrophic zone, and positively marked cells were gradually disappearing toward the distal end of the cartilage in all groups. In C and RGH samples, PAS-positive granules were more abundant and more intense stained than in RAPA animals suggesting increased glycogen content.

Expression and phosphorylation of several proteins related to glycogen biosynthesis and chondrocyte hypertrophy were studied. IGF-I expression, assessed by immunohistochemistry and in situ hybridization, was confined to the hypertrophic zone of growth cartilage without differences between groups (data not shown). As

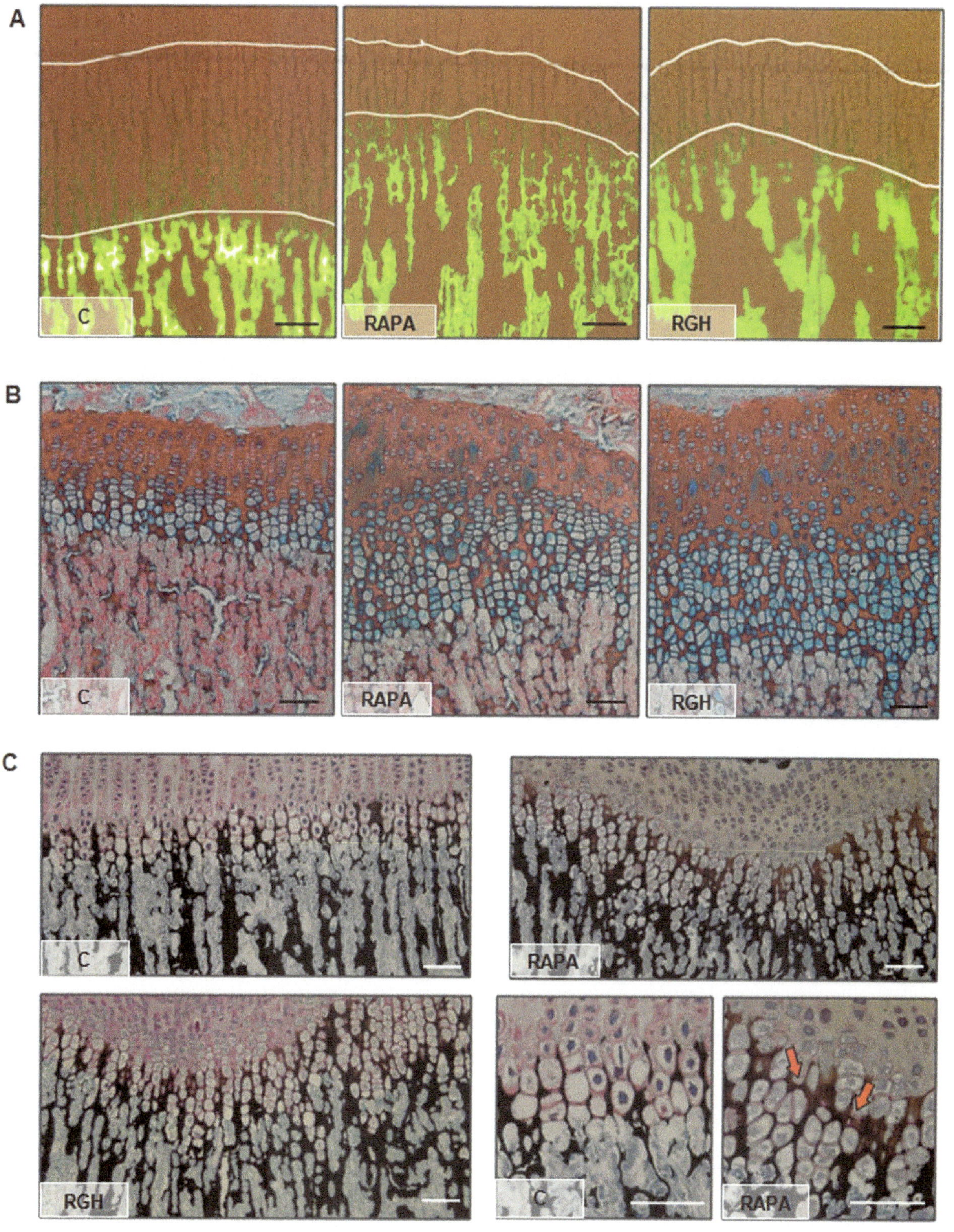

Figure 1. GH effects on longitudinal growth rate and growth plate morphology. (A) Representative images showing the distance between the metaphyseal end of the growth cartilage and the fluorescent calcein front, which indicates longitudinal bone growth rate during the last 3 days of the study, in control rats (C), rats treated with rapamycin (RAPA) or rapamycin and GH (RGH). (B) Representative alcian blue/safranine stained sections showing tibial growth cartilage morphology of C, RAPA and RGH animals. (C) Representative Von Kossa stained sections showing the pattern of extracellular matrix mineralization in proximal tibial growth plate of C, RAPA and RGH animals. Mineralized transverse septa (Red arrows) were often found in RAPA and RGH animals and not in C group. Magnification bars = 100 μm.

Table 2. Growth plate characteristics of rats treated with vehicle (C), rapamycin (RAPA) or with rapamycin and growth hormone (RGH).

	C (n = 10)	RAPA (n = 10)	RGH (n = 10)
Epiphyseal cartilage height (μm)	396±27	471±10[a]	579±40[a,b]
Hypertrophic zone height (μm)	232±21	271±11[a]	345±28[a,b]
Terminal chondrocyte height (μm)	26±1	25±0	27±1[b]

Values are expressed as mean±SEM.
[a]Means statistically different from C group (P≤0.05).
[b]Means statistically different from RAPA group (P≤0.05).

shown in Figure 4B, GH treatment strongly increased phosphorylation of GSK3β (Ser9), a kinase that inhibits glycogen synthesis and that is inactive upon phosphorylation. In addition, in RGH animals GSK3β inactivation was associated with increased levels of β-catenin (Figure 4C), one of the main GSK3β substrates that is known to be degraded upon phosphorylation. Finally, marked increases of p-AKT (Thr308) and p-ERK1/2 (Thr202/Tyr204) were also found in RGH animals with regard to RAPA group (Figure 4D).

Discussion

This study shows for the first time that GH administration increases longitudinal growth in young individuals treated with rapamycin at therapeutic doses. We [8,9] and others [11,12] have previously reported that rapamycin impairs longitudinal growth in young rats. In the present study, RAPA animals were markedly growth retarded in comparison with control rats. GH treatment caused a 20% increase in both growth velocity and nose to tail tip length in RGH animals when compared with RAPA group. In a recent case report, Rangel et al showed that GH therapy induced catch up growth in a kidney transplanted child with growth failure associated with sirolimus treatment [13]. Taken together, these data suggest that GH administration has the potential to improve longitudinal growth in transplanted children receiving rapamycin. Prospective clinical trials are needed to confirm this assumption.

The present work also shows that GH acts locally in the growth plate to promote linear growth in rapamycin treated animals. GH is known to bind to specific receptors located in the epiphyseal chondrocytes to increase longitudinal growth [14]. In our study, GH treatment did not increase IGF-I circulating levels in RGH animals when compared with RAPA, indicating that GH effects on growth are exerted at local level in the growth plate rather than mediated by an increase of systemic IGF-I. On the other hand, it is unlikely that GH action was mediated by stimulus of the local expression of IGF-I because *in situ* hybridization and immunostaining for IGF-I showed no differences between groups. As we have previously shown [9], IGF-I levels were increased in rapamycin treated animals when compared with control group suggesting a resistance to systemic IGF-I. Since IGF-I levels have been reported to control GH secretion through a negative feedback loop [14], it could be argued that some of rapamycin effects on growth may be the result of lower levels of circulating GH. As GH is secreted in pulsatile form, further studies including repeated serum samples and assessment of the GH profile and the secretory bursts are required to confirm o reject this hypothesis.

An important finding of this study was that GH enhanced chondrocyte hypertrophy in rapamycin treated animals, as disclosed by a significant increase in the height of the terminal chondrocyte. Similar effects on chondrocyte hypertrophy have also been found in uremic young rats receiving GH [15]. Given that chondrocyte enlargement supports nearly 60% of longitudinal bone growth in young rats [16], and height of terminal chondrocytes and longitudinal growth rate have been shown to be positively correlated [17], it is likely that the increase in longitudinal growth seen in RGH animals was mainly produced by terminal chondrocyte enlargement. Although chondrocyte hypertrophy is the major contributor to longitudinal growth [16], numerous aspects of chondrocyte physiology contribute to bone growth, and we cannot rule out that GH could target others than those adversely affected by rapamycin. In fact, GH administration rescued only partially longitudinal growth velocity of rapamycin treated animals, indicating that some rapamycin adverse effects on growth plate biology were still persistent. Indeed, GH administration did not increase chondrocyte proliferation in the growth cartilage and did not normalize the alterations in vascular invasion described in RAPA animals, further supporting this notion.

Chondrocyte hypertrophy is a complex process regulated by largely unknown molecular mechanisms. We have previously shown that mTOR inhibition by rapamycin decreased chondrocyte hypertrophy in the growth plate [8,9]. Indeed, Akt/mTOR pathway has been found to regulate chondrocyte autophagy [18], a process thought to increase chondrocyte survival and maturation within the epiphyseal cartilage [19]. As shown by immunofluorescent detection of LC3, a major component of autophagosomes and a marker of autophagy [20], we found that chondrocytes in the early hypertrophic cartilage zones exhibited a distinctive autophagic phenotype. This immunofluorescent labeling and the western blot analysis of LC3-II/LC3-I ratio were not different between both groups of animals, indicating that modulation of autophagy is not involved in the effects of GH on growth plate.

A recent report has showed that hypertrophic differentiation of growth plate chondrocytes during skeletal growth is promoted by phosphorylation and inactivation of GSK-3β [21]. PIP3/Akt and MAPK signalling pathways are both downstream of GH and IGF-I receptors [22], and have been found to directly phosphorylate and inactivate GSK3β [23]. In addition, inactivation of GSK3β upon phosphorylation in Ser9 has been shown to increase glycogen synthesis and to stabilize β-catenin in chondrocytes [21]. β-catenin is a well known mediator of the canonical Wnt signalling pathway, a major promoter of both chondrocyte hypertrophy and final maturation [24]. In our study, we demonstrated that GH administration increases GSK3β phosphorylation, cytoplasmatic glycogen deposits and β-catenin protein levels in growth plate chondrocytes of rapamycin treated rats. Moreover, we also reported a marked increase in Akt and ERK 1/2 phosphorylation in GH treated animals when compared with RAPA group. In the light of these findings, we propose that GH would signal through PIP3/Akt and MAPK pathways to phosphorylate and inactivate GSK3β in epiphyseal chondrocytes (Figure 5). This would lead to an increase of glycogen synthesis and stabilization of β-catenin, which eventually would enhance chondrocyte hypertrophy. However, the role of GSK3 in cartilage physiology is not completely understood. GSK3 protein family consist of two different isoforms, GSK3α and GSK3 β with both overlapping and distinct roles. A recent report by Gillespie *et al.* showed that cartilage-specific inactivation of GSK3β in mice does not affect bone growth [25]. Conversely, the authors report that GSK3α expression levels were increased in these mice suggesting the existence of a compensatory mechanism to counteract the loss

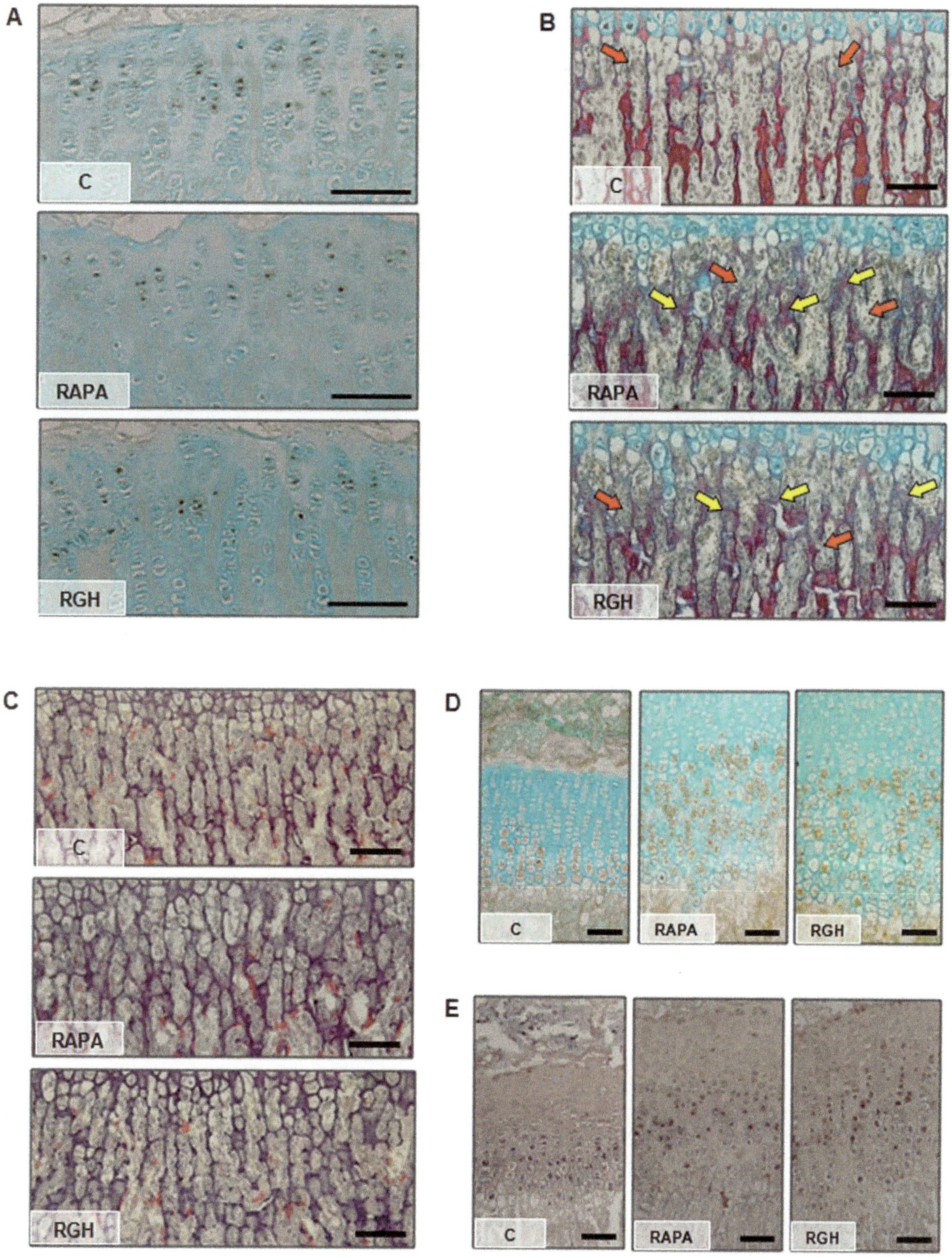

Figure 2. GH effects on growth plate cell proliferation and angiogenesis. (A) Representative images of BrdU immunodetection in the proliferative zone of the epiphyseal cartilage of control rats (C), rats treated with rapamycin (RAPA) or rapamycin and GH (RGH). (B) Representative sections of proximal tibial growth plates stained with picrosirius red/alcian blue showing trabeculae and vascular sprouts arrangement in the primary spongiosa of C, RAPA and RGH animals. Transverse unresorbed septa are indicated with yellow arrows. Vascular sprouts are indicated with red arrows. (C) Representative sections of proximal tibial growth plates stained with tartrate-resistant acid phosphatase (TRAP) showing positive chondroclasts/osteoclasts in the chondro-osseous junction of C, RAPA and RGH animals. Representative images of immunohistochemistry (D) and *in situ* hybridization (E) experiments showing VEGF expression in growth plates of C, RAPA and RGH animals. Magnification bars = 100 μm.

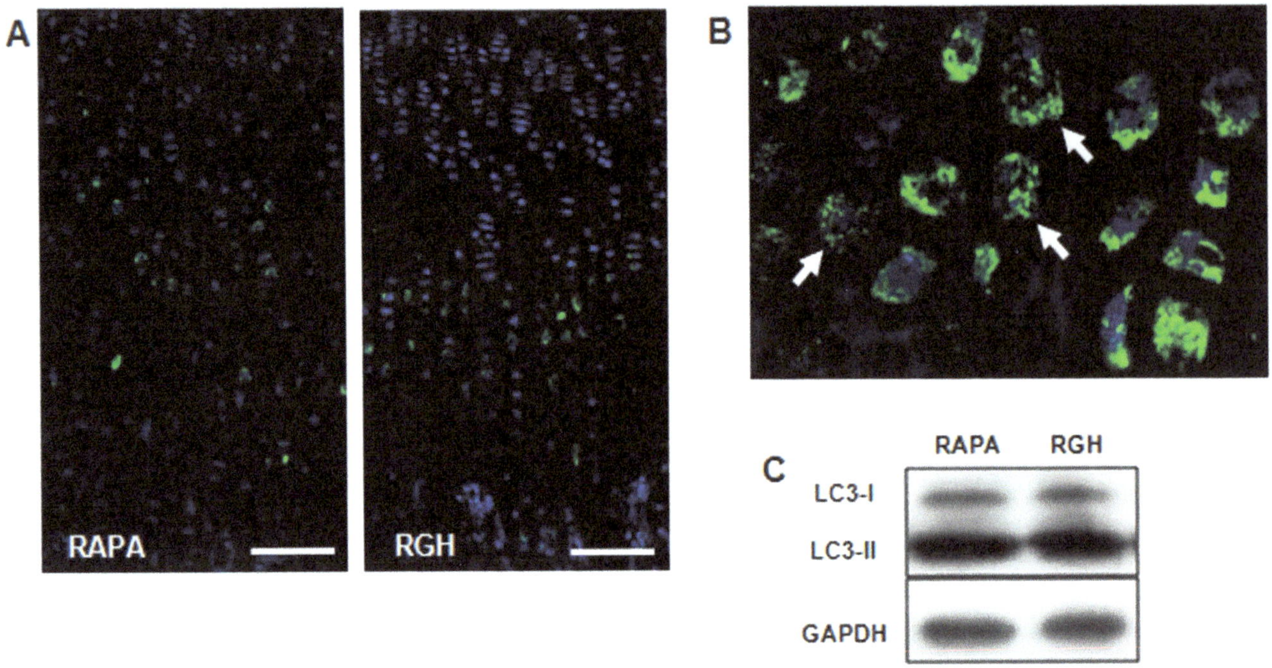

Figure 3. GH effects on chondrocyte autophagy. (A) Immunofluorescent detection of LC3, a marker of autophagy, in the growth plates of rats treated with rapamycin (RAPA) or rapamycin and GH (RGH). Fluorescent signal was observed in prehypertrophic chondrocytes often displaying a punctuate distribution (white arrows in B). (C) Western blot of LC3-I (18 kDa) and LC3-II (16 kDa) in the growth cartilage of rats treated with rapamycin (RAPA) or rapamycin and GH (RGH). GAPDH was used as loading control. Image is representative of three blots giving similar results.

of GSK3β in cartilage. We cannot rule out the possibility that GH administration is also inhibiting GSK3α activity in our study, thus resulting in an overall inhibition of GSK3 signalling pathway. In addition, it is of note that activation of the ERK1/2 pathway has been shown to repress endochondral bone growth [26] which is not consistent with the above hypothesis. Further experiments are needed to clarify the role of the various intracellular pathways and its functional interrelationship into the processes of cell growth and maturation.

It is worth to mention that rapamycin antiproliferative and antiangiogenic activities remained in the growth plate of RGH animals. Despite being a well known mitotic agent, GH did not increase cell proliferation in the growth cartilage of RGH animals. In addition, alterations in vascular invasion seen in rapamycin treated animals, such as abnormal arrangement of septa and blood vessels in primary spongiosa, decreased VEGF expression in terminal chondrocytes, and reduction of TRAP positive cells near chondro-osseous junction, were also found in RGH group. Antitumoral effects of rapamycin are thought to be related to inhibition of cell proliferation and angiogenesis. Our study importantly indicates that GH treatment can promote growth without interfering with these effects, at least at the growth plate level. Further studies are needed to clarify whether the potential of GH to increase the risk of malignancy in kidney transplanted children [27] persists in the presence of rapamycin treatment.

In summary, our study reports that GH administration improves longitudinal growth in young rats treated with rapamycin. This GH promoting effect is not related to antagonism of the antiproliferative and antiangiogenic actions of rapamycin, but to an increase in the growth cartilage chondrocyte hypertrophy which involves GSK3β inactivation and β-catenin stabilization.

Materials and Methods

Animals

Female Sprague–Dawley rats aged 4 weeks and weighing 70±5 g were housed in individual cages under controlled conditions of light (12 h light/dark cycle) and temperature (21–23°C). All animals received standard rat chow (A03, Panlab, Barcelona, Spain) and tap water. Control animals were fed *ad libitum* and RAPA and RGH were *pair fed* with C group. The study complied with the Directive 86/609/EEC on the protection of Animals used for Experimental and other scientific purposes in the European Union. The protocol was approved by the Ethics Committee on Animal Research of the University of Oviedo, Spain.

Experimental Protocol and Sample Collection

After 3 days of adaptation to the experimental area, 1 mg/kg/day of rapamycin diluted in 5% dimethyl sulfoxide (DMSO, Sigma, St Louis, MO, USA) was administered intraperitoneally at 10.00 am for seven days to 20 animals whereas control (C, n = 10) rats were injected with 5% DMSO. On day 0 of the protocol, rapamycin treated animals were classified into two groups of 10 individuals each: RAPA and RGH. From day 0 to 6 of the protocol, in addition to rapamycin injection, RGH animals received also 10 IU/kg/day of intraperitoneal recombinant human GH (Norditropin, Novo Nordisk Pharma, Madrid, Spain) at 09.00 and 17.00 h, whereas C and RAPA received vehicle. Animals were killed under anesthesia on day 7 of the protocol. Three days before sacrifice, each animal received 20 mg/kg of calcein (Sigma) by intraperitoneal route for calculation of osseous front advance as an index of longitudinal bone growth rate [9]. BrdU (100 mg/kg; Sigma) was also injected intraperitoneally at 1, 9, and 17 h before animals' death. Blood samples were collected

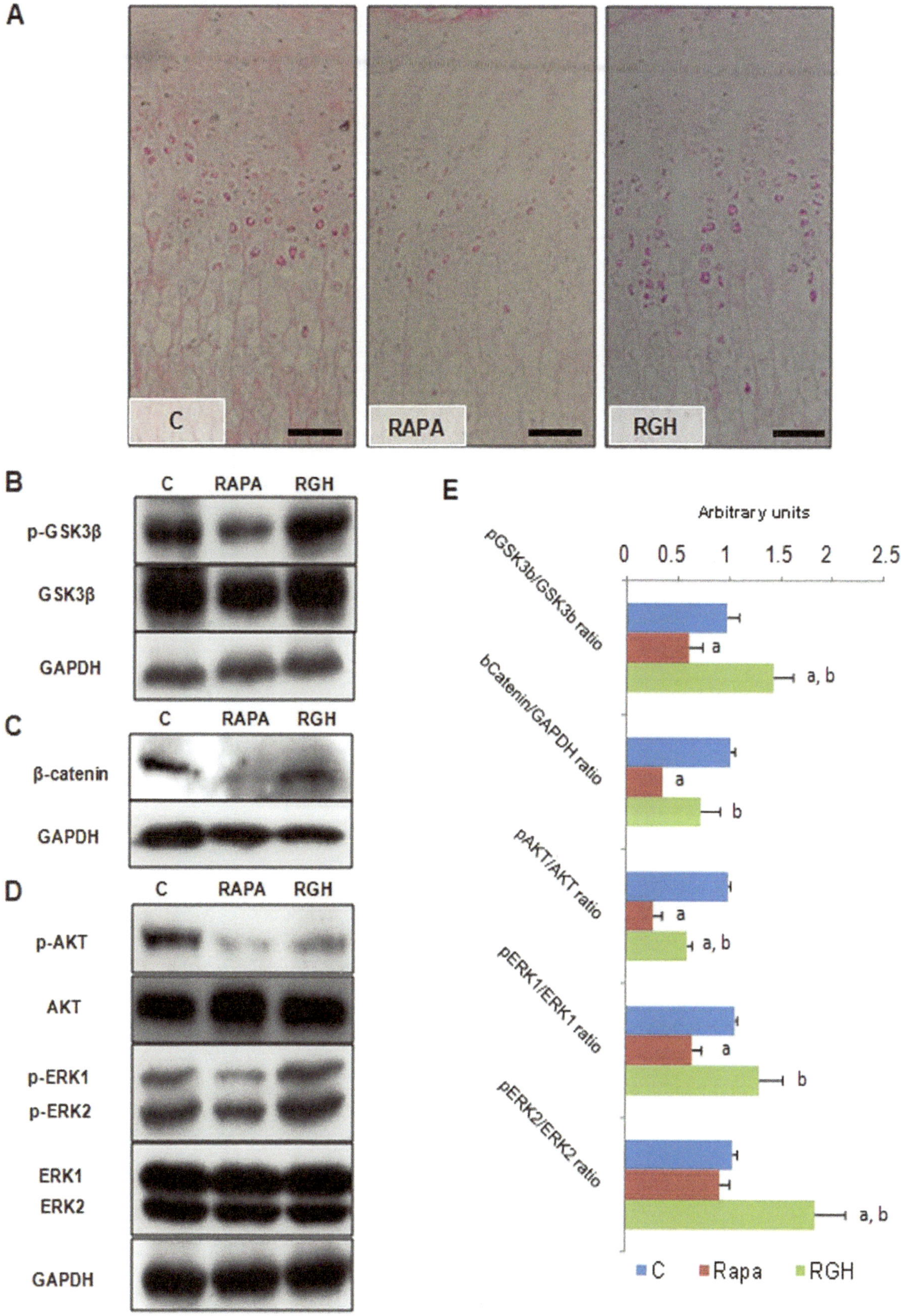

Figure 4. GH effects on chondrocyte metabolism. (A) Periodic acid-Schiff (PAS) reaction in the proximal tibial growth plate of control rats (C), rats treated with rapamycin (RAPA) or rapamycin and GH (RGH). Magnification bars = 100 μm. (B) Western blot of p-GSK3β (Ser9) and GSK3β in the

growth cartilage of C, RAPA and RGH animals. (C) Western blot of β-catenin in the growth cartilage of C, RAPA and RGH animals. (D) Western blot of p-AKT (Thr308), AKT, p-ERK1/2 (Thr202/Tyr204) and ERK1/2 in the growth cartilage of C, RAPA and RGH animals. GAPDH was used as loading control. Images are representative of three blots giving similar results. (E) Densitometry analysis of the western blot experiments shown in B,C and D. At least four animals per group were used per experiment and each assay was repeated at least three times. [a]Means statistically different from C group ($P \leq 0.05$). [b]Means statistically different from RAPA group ($P \leq 0.05$).

and stored at −20°C until the measurement of rapamycin and circulating IGF-I concentrations. Proximal ends of right tibiae were immediately frozen in liquid nitrogen for protein expression studies. Proximal ends of left tibiae were embedded in methyl metacrilate as previously described [15]. Samples from half the animals were fixed in 40% ethanol and used for analysis of calcein and BrdU staining. The remaining samples were fixed in 4% paraformaldehyde and used for histomorphometry, immunohistochemistry, immunofluorescence and *in situ* hybridization studies.

Blood Measurements

Concentrations of rapamycin were measured in whole-blood samples using an Abbott Imx analyzer (Abbott Cientifica, Madrid, Spain) as previously described [8,9]. IGF-I serum concentrations were measured by enzyme-linked immunosorbent assay using a commercial kit and following manufacturer's instructions (Immunodiagnostic Systems, Boldon, UK). Inter- and intra-assay variation coefficients were below 7%.

Growth

Nose to tail-tip length was measured under anesthesia on days 0 and 7. Longitudinal growth rate was measured in 10 µm-thick frontal sections of the proximal end of tibiae as described elsewhere [8].

Growth Plate Histology and Histomorphometry

Frontal sections (5 mm thick) of proximal tibiae fixed in formalin were stained by the following methods: alcian blue/safranine (Merck, Darmstadt, Germany) for morphometric analysis, alkaline phosphatase stain (Roche, Basel, Switzerland) for chondrocyte maturation, TRAP stain (Sigma) for osteoclast identification, periodic acid-Schiff (PAS) reaction to stain glycogen deposits (Merck), and picrosirius red/alcian blue/hematoxylin (Merck) for analysis of bone and cartilage extracellular matrix. Heights of the growth cartilage and its hypertrophic zone were identified following morphological criteria and measured at regular intervals using an image analysis system previously described [8]. Height of the hypertrophic chondrocytes placed in three most distal rows, those adjacent to the metaphyseal bone, was measured in alternate columns using the same system. Approximately, twenty five measurements were made per section for a total of fifty measurements per animal. The number of TRAP positive cells at the vascular invasion front was measured in an area extending 50 mm from the distal end of the growth cartilage into the primary spongiosa. Two slides per animal were used and results were expressed as the number of positive cells per mm^2.

Growth Plate Immunohistochemistry and *in situ* Hybridization

Immunodetection of BrdU, VEGF, IGF-I and collagen X were carried out as described elsewhere [9]. For the immunohistochemical detection of LC3, after overnight incubation with primary antibody (dilution 1:10, MBL International, Woburn, MA, USA), sections were treated with Alexa Fluor 488–labeled secondary antibody (dilution 1:500, Fisher-Invitrogen, Barcelona, Spain), counterstained with 4,6-diamidino-2-phenylindole (Vectashield, Vector Laboratories Inc., Peterborough, UK), and examined by confocal microscopy. Two sections per animal were

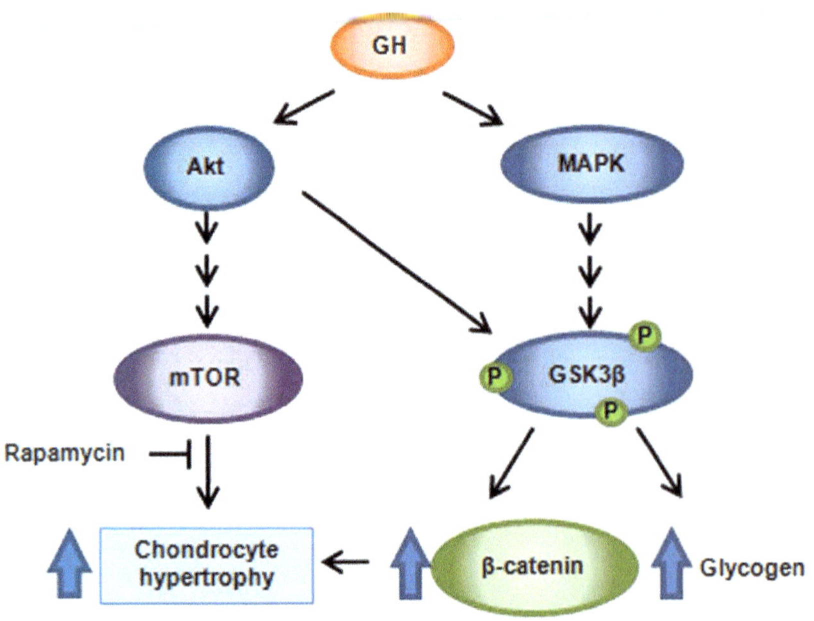

Figure 5. Proposed mechanism of the stimulating effect of GH on the hypertrophy of growth cartilage chondrocytes. GH would signal through PIP3/Akt and MAPK pathways to phosphorylate and inactivate GSK3β in growth plate chondrocytes. This would lead to an increase of glycogen synthesis and stabilization of β-catenin that, eventually, would enhance chondrocyte hypertrophy.

analyzed. The proliferating activity was expressed as the number of positive cells per 100 cells in the proliferative zone, previously defined as the band of tissue between the resting zone and a line traced by the most distal BrdU-labeled cells. VEGF immunohistochemical signal was measured in the three most distal rows of chondrocytes and expressed as number of positive cells per 100 terminal chondrocytes.

In situ hybridization was used to define the mRNA distribution pattern of VEGF and IGF-I in the growth cartilage following a methodology previously described [9].

Western Blot

A total of 30 μg of protein, extracted from tibial frozen samples as previously described [9], were resolved in SDS-PAGE and transferred to polyvinylidene difluoride membrane (Immobilon-P; Millipore Iberica, Madrid, Spain). After blocking the membranes in 5% (w/v) non-fat dry milk in TBST (Tris-buffered saline, pH 7.4, containing 0.05% Tween 20) at room temperature for 1 h, blots were incubated with primary antibody specific to LC3 (MBL), p-AKT (ser473), AKT, p-ERK 1/2 (Thr202/Tyr204), ERK 1/2, p-GSK3β (ser9), GSK3β, and β-catenin (Cell Signaling, Danvers, MA, USA) diluted 1:1000 in TBST at 4°C overnight. Immunoblots were then incubated at room temperature for 1 h with the corresponding secondary antibody (Sigma). Peroxidase activity was visualized using a chemiluminescent HRP substrate commercial kit (Immobilon Western; Millipore Iberica) following manufacturer's instructions.

Statistical Analysis

Data are given as mean ± SEM. Differences between groups were assessed by ANOVA. Comparisons between two groups were performed by Student t test. A P value ≤0.05 was considered significant. All data sets were analyzed using SPSS 15.0 software package (SPSS, Chicago, IL, USA).

Supporting Information

Figure S1 GH effects on chondrocyte expression of collagen type X and alkaline phosphatase activity. (A) Representative images of immunohistochemistry experiments showing collagen type X expression in growth plates of control rats (C), rats treated with rapamycin (RAPA) or rapamycin and GH (RGH). (B) Representative sections of proximal tibial growth plates showing alkaline phosphatase activity in hypertrophic chondrocytes of C, RAPA and RGH animals.

Acknowledgments

We gratefully thank the technical assistance of Teresa Usín. We also thank Lourdes Tricas for her help in measuring rapamycin levels, Verdad Curto-Reyes for western blot technical support and Ana Gutierrez for her invaluable assistance in immunofluorescence techniques.

Author Contributions

Conceived and designed the experiments: OAG FS. Performed the experiments: OAG EGL VL HGP NMG JRS FO. Analyzed the data: OAG. Wrote the paper: OAG FS.

References

1. Wullschleger S, Loewith R, Hall MN (2006) TOR signaling in growth and metabolism. Cell 124: 471–484.
2. Geissler EK, Schlitt HJ (2010) The potential benefits of rapamycin on renal function, tolerance, fibrosis, and malignancy following transplantation. Kidney Int 78: 1075–1079.
3. Koehl GE, Andrassy J, Guba M, Richter S, Kroemer A, et al. (2004) Rapamycin protects allografts from rejection while simultaneously attacking tumors in immunosuppressed mice. Transplantation 77: 1319–1326.
4. Hudes G, Carducci M, Tomczak P, Dutcher J, Figlin R, et al. (2007) Temsirolimus, interferon alfa, or both for advanced renal-cell carcinoma. N Engl J Med 356: 2271–2281.
5. Cravedi P, Ruggenenti P, Remuzzi G (2009) Sirolimus to replace calcineurin inhibitors? Too early yet. Lancet 373: 1235–1236.
6. Ibáñez JP, Monteverde ML, Goldberg J, Diaz MA, Turconi A (2005) Sirolimus in pediatric renal transplantation. Transplant Proc 37: 682–684.
7. Fine RN (2007) Management of growth retardation in pediatric recipients of renal allografts. Nat Clin Pract Nephrol 3: 318–324.
8. Alvarez-Garcia O, Carbajo-Pérez E, Garcia E, Gil H, Molinos I, et al. (2007) Rapamycin retards growth and causes marked alterations in the growth plate of young rats. Pediatr Nephrol 22: 954–961.
9. Alvarez-García O, García-López E, Loredo V, Gil-Peña H, Rodríguez-Suárez J, et al. (2010) Rapamycin induces growth retardation by disrupting angiogenesis in the growth plate. Kidney Int 78: 561–518.
10. González D, García CD, Azócar M, Waller S, Alonso A, et al. (2011) Growth of kidney-transplanted pediatric patients treated with sirolimus. Pediatr Nephrol 26: 961–966.
11. Sanchez CP, He YZ (2009) Bone growth during rapamycin therapy in young rats. BMC Pediatr 9: 3.
12. Phornphutkul C, Lee M, Voigt C, Wu KY, Ehrlich MG, et al. (2009) The effect of rapamycin on bone growth in rabbits. J Orthop Res 27: 1157–1161.
13. Rangel GA, Ariceta G (2009) Growth failure associated with sirolimus: case report. Pediatr Nephrol 24: 2047–2050.
14. van der Eerden BC, Karperien M, Wit JM (2003) Systemic and local regulation of the growth plate. Endocr Rev 24: 782–801.
15. Molinos I, Santos F, Carbajo-Perez E, Garcia E, Rodriguez J, et al. (2006) Catch-up growth follows an abnormal pattern in experimental renal insufficiency and growth hormone treatment normalizes it. Kidney Int 70: 1955–1961.
16. Wilsman NJ, Farnum CE, Leiferman EM, Fry M, Barreto C (1996) Differential growth by growth plates as a function of multiple parameters of chondrocytic kinetics. J Orthop Res 14: 927–936.
17. Cobo A, López JM, Carbajo E, Santos F, Alvarez J, et al. (1999) Growth plate cartilage formation and resorption are differentially depressed in growth retarded uremic rats. J Am Soc Nephrol 10: 971–979.
18. Bohensky J, Leshinsky S, Srinivas V, Shapiro IM (2010) Chondrocyte autophagy is stimulated by HIF-1 dependent AMPK activation and mTOR suppression. Pediatr Nephrol 25: 633–642.
19. Srinivas V, Bohensky J, Shapiro IM (2009) Autophagy: a new phase in the maturation of growth plate chondrocytes is regulated by HIF, mTOR and AMP kinase. Cells Tissues Organs 189: 88–92.
20. Mizushima N, Yoshimori T, Levine B (2010) Methods in mammalian autophagy research. Cell 140: 313–326.
21. Kawasaki Y, Kugimiya F, Chikuda H, Kamekura S, Ikeda T, et al. (2008) Phosphorylation of GSK-3beta by cGMP-dependent protein kinase II promotes hypertrophic differentiation of murine chondrocytes. J Clin Invest 118: 2506–2515.
22. Le Roith D, Bondy C, Yakar S, Liu JL, Butler A (2001) The somatomedin hypothesis: 2001. Endocr Rev 22: 53–74.
23. Cohen P, Frame S (2001) The renaissance of GSK3. Nat Rev Mol Cell Biol 2: 769–776.
24. Guo X, Mak KK, Taketo MM, Yang Y (2009) The Wnt/beta-catenin pathway interacts differentially with PTHrP signaling to control chondrocyte hypertrophy and final maturation. PLoS One 4: e6067.
25. Gillespie JR, Ulici V, Dupuis H, Higgs A, Dimattia A, et al. (2011) Deletion of glycogen synthase kinase-3β in cartilage results in up-regulation of glycogen synthase kinase-3α protein expression. Endocrinology 152: 1755–1766.
26. Murakami S, Balmes G, McKinney S, Zhang Z, Givol D, et al. (2004) Constitutive activation of MEK1 in chondrocytes causes Stat1-independent achondroplasia-like dwarfism and rescues the Fgfr3-deficient mouse phenotype. Genes Dev 18: 290–305.
27. Dharnidharka VR, Talley LI, Martz KL, Stablein DM, Fine RN (2008) Recombinant growth hormone use pretransplant and risk for post-transplant lymphoproliferative disease–a report of the NAPRTCS. Pediatr Transplant 12: 689–695.

13

Phase II Open Label Study of Valproic Acid in Spinal Muscular Atrophy

Kathryn J. Swoboda[1]*, Charles B. Scott[2], Sandra P. Reyna[1], Thomas W. Prior[3], Bernard LaSalle[1], Susan L. Sorenson[1], Janine Wood[1], Gyula Acsadi[4], Thomas O. Crawford[5], John T. Kissel[3], Kristin J. Krosschell[6], Guy D'Anjou[7], Mark B. Bromberg[1], Mary K. Schroth[8], Gary M. Chan[1], Bakri Elsheikh[3], Louise R. Simard[9]

1 Departments of Neurology, Pediatrics, Neonatology and General Clinical Research Center, University of Utah School of Medicine, Salt Lake City, Utah, United States of America, **2** CBS Squared, Inc, Fort Washington, Pennsylvania, United States of America, **3** Departments of Molecular Pathology and Neurology, Ohio State University Medical Center, Columbus, Ohio, United States of America, **4** Departments of Neurology and Pediatrics, Wayne State University School of Medicine, Detroit, Michigan, United States of America, **5** Departments of Neurology and Pediatrics, Johns Hopkins University School of Medicine, Baltimore, Maryland, United States of America, **6** Department of Physical Therapy and Human Movement Sciences, Feinberg School of Medicine, Northwestern University, Chicago, Illinois, United States of America, **7** Division of Pediatric Neurology, Hôpital Sainte-Justine Montréal, Montréal, Québec, Canada, **8** Department of Pediatrics, University of Wisconsin School of Medicine, Madison, Wisconsin, United States of America, **9** Department of Biochemistry and Medical Genetics, University of Manitoba, Winnipeg, Manitoba, Canada

Abstract

Preliminary in vitro and in vivo studies with valproic acid (VPA) in cell lines and patients with spinal muscular atrophy (SMA) demonstrate increased expression of *SMN*, supporting the possibility of therapeutic benefit. We performed an open label trial of VPA in 42 subjects with SMA to assess safety and explore potential outcome measures to help guide design of future controlled clinical trials. Subjects included 2 SMA type I ages 2–3 years, 29 SMA type II ages 2–14 years and 11 type III ages 2–31 years, recruited from a natural history study. VPA was well-tolerated and without evident hepatotoxicity. Carnitine depletion was frequent and temporally associated with increased weakness in two subjects. Exploratory outcome measures included assessment of gross motor function via the modified Hammersmith Functional Motor Scale (MHFMS), electrophysiologic measures of innervation including maximum ulnar compound muscle action potential (CMAP) amplitudes and motor unit number estimation (MUNE), body composition and bone density via dual-energy X-ray absorptiometry (DEXA), and quantitative blood SMN mRNA levels. Clear decline in motor function occurred in several subjects in association with weight gain; mean fat mass increased without a corresponding increase in lean mass. We observed an increased mean score on the MHFMS scale in 27 subjects with SMA type II ($p \leq 0.001$); however, significant improvement was almost entirely restricted to participants <5 years of age. Full length SMN levels were unchanged and Δ7SMN levels were significantly reduced for 2 of 3 treatment visits. In contrast, bone mineral density ($p \leq 0.0036$) and maximum ulnar CMAP scores ($p \leq 0.0001$) increased significantly.

Conclusions: While VPA appears safe and well-tolerated in this initial pilot trial, these data suggest that weight gain and carnitine depletion are likely to be significant confounding factors in clinical trials. This study highlights potential strengths and limitations of various candidate outcome measures and underscores the need for additional controlled clinical trials with VPA targeting more restricted cohorts of subjects.

Trial Registration: ClinicalTrials.gov NCT00374075

Editor: Brian D. McCabe, Columbia University, United States of America

Funding: This work was funded by Families of Spinal Muscular Atrophy. This investigation was also supported by the Public Health Services research grant numbers UL1-RR025764 and C06-RR11234 from the National Center for Research Resources. The funders had no role in study design, data collection and analysis, decision to publish, or preparation of the manuscript.

Competing Interests: The authors have declared that no competing interests exist.

* E-mail: Swoboda@genetics.utah.edu

Introduction

Spinal muscular atrophy (SMA) is the most common inherited motor neuron disease, and a leading cause of infant and childhood mortality [1,2]. With an incidence of 1 in 10,000 births, it is an autosomal recessive disorder associated with severe neuromuscular weakness and premature death in the majority of patients [3–6]. More than 96% of affected individuals demonstrate a homozygous deletion/mutation involving exon 7 in *SMN1* (survival motor neuron 1), resulting in the biochemical deficiency of the SMN protein, part of a complex that functions in the assembly of small nuclear ribonucleoprotein particles (snRNP) [7,8]. A genomic duplication at this locus has resulted in a nearly identical gene, *SMN2* (survival motor neuron 2). *SMN2* differs from *SMN1* by a nucleotide substitution that promotes exon 7 exclusion. Consequently, SMN2 produces a fraction of the identical full length protein. Phenotypic variation in SMA correlates with the number of *SMN2* gene copies and the level of SMN protein in cells [9–15].

The broad range of phenotypes has led to classification into clinical types including the most common severe infantile form (SMA type I), non-ambulatory variants of intermediate severity (SMA type II), and ambulatory variants (SMA types III, IV). The majority of subjects develop symptoms in infancy or early childhood.

An opportunity for therapeutic intervention has arisen from the discovery of small molecule compounds which target *SMN2* gene copies present in all SMA patients to produce increased amounts of full-length SMN protein. Several compounds demonstrated to up-regulate SMN expression in SMA patient-derived cell lines, including valproic acid (VPA), sodium phenylbutyrate (NaPB) and hydroxyurea (HU), have been in clinical use for decades. These histone deacetylase (HDAC) inhibitors variably increase expression of many genes, including the SMN gene [16–20]. Preliminary in vivo data in human subjects supports up-regulation of SMN by both VPA and NaPB [21,22]. VPA up-regulates *SMN2* expression at the promoter via inhibition of HDAC2, and both VPA and HU appear to alter splicing to increase full-length SMN protein [20,23]. VPA has demonstrated neuroprotective properties on glutamate-induced excitotoxicity via up-regulation of alpha-synuclein and increases neurite outgrowth in vitro[24,25]. Both VPA and NaPB have been reported to increase survival in ALS animal models [26,27]. More recently, VPA administration in an SMA mouse model resulted in apparent improved motor function, larger evoked motor potentials, less degeneration of spinal motor neurons and improved neuromuscular junction innervation in treated animals compared to age-matched controls [28,29]. Finally, two small open label trials of VPA in human subjects have reported modest strength or functional benefit in a subset of those patients [30,31]. Such observations support the potential benefit of small molecule therapeutics not only for SMA, but for other forms of motor neuron disease, such as ALS. This preliminary in vivo and in vitro evidence encouraged us to proceed with an open label study of VPA in SMA patients as a first step towards more formal efficacy studies. Our primary objectives were to determine the safety of VPA in SMA patients and to assess the utility of a number of exploratory outcome measures for future clinical trials.

Methods

The protocol for this trial and supporting CONSORT checklist are available as supporting information; see Checklist S1 and Protocol S1.

Study population

Subjects participating in a natural history study at the University of Utah were recruited for an open label study of VPA (Clinicaltrials.gov ID NCT00374075). All subjects at least 2 years of age receiving <16 hours/day ventilator support were invited to participate. Fifty-eight subjects were enrolled in the natural history study. At the start of VPA study enrollment, thirteen type I subjects were deceased, required full-time mechanical ventilation, or were less than 2 years of age. Two subjects were excluded for prior noncompliance with natural history study visits. Two subjects declined due to the burden of study visits. Three additional subjects declined due to perceived risks. Enrollment was then opened in the order of calls received to recruit 4 additional subjects. Type I subjects were not specifically excluded but enrollment was discontinued following recruitment of 40 type II and type III subjects. Two subjects had a severe phenotype (SMA type I ages 2–3 years), 29 subjects had an intermediate phenotype (SMA type II ages 2–14 years) and 11 had a mild phenotype (SMA type III ages 2–31 years). Additional details of baseline study population characteristics are shown in Tables S1 and S2. The progress of all participants through the trial is diagrammed in Figure S1.

Consent and adverse event grading

Written informed consent (subjects ≥18 years), parental consent (subjects <18 years) and assent (subjects ≥7 years) were obtained for all subjects. The study was approved by the University of Utah Institutional Review Board and General Clinical Research Center Advisory Committees. Adverse events were graded using Common Terminology Criteria for Adverse Events v3.0 (CTCAE v3.0). An independent Data and Safety Monitoring Committee provided oversight for the study.

Study design

Inclusion criteria were age ≥2 years and confirmed genetic diagnosis of SMA. Exclusion criteria were ventilator support for ≥16 hours or concomitant medications with known hepatotoxicity or potential benefit in SMA. Each subject had to complete ≥2 natural history assessments within a 3–6 month period to qualify for enrollment in the VPA trial. Treatment assessments were performed at 3 (V1), 6 (V2) and 12 (V3) months. Divalproex sodium coated particles (Depakote® sprinkle capsules, 125 mg per capsule) were administered in divided doses two to three times daily sufficient to maintain overnight trough levels of 50–100 mg/dL. Dosing was typical of that used in epilepsy patients (15–50 mg/kg/day). Laboratory testing, which included a basic chemistry profile, CBC with platelets, transaminases, carnitine profile, amylase, lipase, and trough VPA levels, was performed at baseline, 2–3 weeks following initiation, and at each treatment visit.

Primary outcome measures were laboratory safety and adverse event data. Exploratory outcome measures included change from baseline assessments of motor function, pulmonary function (subjects ≥5 years), degree of denervation via maximum ulnar compound motor action potential (CMAP) and motor unit number estimation (MUNE) values, dual-energy X-ray absorptiometry (DEXA) of body composition and bone density and quantitative assessment of SMN mRNA.

Gross motor function was assessed with the Modified Hammersmith Functional Motor Scale for SMA (MHFMS). This scale contains the same 20 gross motor items as the original clinical scale, but was modified for use in the research setting [32,33]. A version of this scale has been successfully used in a multicenter trial with SMA subjects [34]. Each item is scored from 0–2, with a hierarchy of skills ranging from rolling to sitting to standing. Unfortunately, this scale as it stands in its present form is inadequate for testing subjects across the full range of SMA phenotypes, due to significant floor and ceiling effects for subjects with SMA types I and III, respectively (additional details available at http://www.smaoutcomes.org). The degree of denervation in the hand was estimated using maximum ulnar CMAP amplitude and MUNE negative peak area values [12,35]. In children ≥5 years, pulmonary function testing (PFT) was performed in an accredited pediatric laboratory, and included forced vital capacity (FVC), forced expiratory volume in 1 second (FEV1), and maximum expiratory and inspiratory pressures (MEP and MIP, respectively). We analyzed absolute values rather than corrected values due to concerns regarding accurate measurements of length due to contractures in many subjects. Norland DEXA XR-36 software version 3.3.1 for small subjects was used to assess whole body composition and bone mineral density and content.

SMN2 copy numbers were determined as previously described [11]. Whole blood was drawn into PAXgene tubes at baseline and each visit. Quantitative SMN mRNA levels were performed with slight modifications to the prior protocol [36]. Assays were carried out on a 7500 Real Time PCR system (Applied Biosystems). To increase efficiency on this apparatus, full-length SMN was amplified by primers 5′-GCTTTGGGAAGTATGTTAATTT-CATGGT-3′ (exon 6) and 5′-TGTGAGCACCTTCCTTC-TTTTTGAT-3′ (exon 7), and detected by the 5′FAM-TC-TGAAACCCATATAATAGCC-MGBNFQ-3′ exon 6–7 junction probe. Delta-7 (Δ7) SMN was detected as published [36]. Human RPLPO (large ribosomal protein) and PGK1 (phosphoglycerate kinase 1) were run as endogenous controls. Patients missing baseline data or who had only one treatment visit were excluded from this analysis. Results are reported as relative amounts of full-length (fl) or Δ7SMN transcripts normalized against the relative amount of RPLPO.

Statistical Analysis

The analysis of variance (ANOVA) test was used to evaluate the differences between means for function tests. When a factor level is empty and only two levels exists, ANOVA defaults to t-test. Linear regression analysis was used to examine the relationship between function parameters and genetic variables at baseline. The dependent variables in the linear regressions were evaluated for normality using the Shapiro-Wilk test and the paired t-test was used to test change from baseline in follow-up. If the dependent variable was not normally distributed then an appropriate transformation was used. A two-sided p-value less than 0.05 was considered statistically significant.

Results

All 42 subjects completed *at least* 6 months of treatment. Five subjects discontinued treatment after the V2 visit at 6 months due to drug-related side effects, as detailed below. The remaining 37 subjects continued on treatment for a full year.

Evaluation of safety and tolerability

For the most part, VPA was well tolerated and drug-related side effects mild. Grade I mood alteration was reported in three subjects. Grade II weight gain associated with functional decline led to discontinuation of VPA after V2 (6 months) in 2 subjects (both 9 year old girls, one with type II, the other with type IIIa but non-ambulatory). Poor compliance or lack of perceived benefit led to discontinuation in 3 additional subjects after V2 (2 siblings with type II, a 5 year old girl and 7 year old boy, and a poorly compliant 3 year old boy with type II who repeatedly refused oral dosing). One subject developed grade IV acidosis and carnitine depletion with respiratory failure requiring intubation and mechanical ventilation (3 year old type I subject). No deaths occurred during the study. Mean overnight (minimum 12 hour) trough VPA levels were 52 mg/dL (V1), 64 mg/dL (V2), and 59 mg/dL (V3). Abnormal laboratory values at baseline and during treatment are depicted in table 1; grade I elevations in transaminases without clinical correlate were present at baseline in 3 subjects and in 20 subjects (48%) for at least one visit. Transient grade I thrombocytopenia occurred in 2 subjects in association with illness. Grade I anemia was observed in 8 subjects at baseline and 19 subjects (45%) on treatment. Grade I leukopenia was frequent (36%) but absolute neutrophil counts remained $>1.0\times10^3$/uL in all subjects. Two subjects had low carnitine levels at baseline and a substantial proportion of the first thirteen subjects enrolled demonstrated reductions in total or free plasma carnitine within the first 3 months of treatment (Figure S2). In two subjects, this was associated with transient worsening of gross motor function which reversed with carnitine supplementation. Our Data Safety and Monitoring Board recommended supplementation of carnitine 50 mg/kg/day in all subjects subsequent to the first interim safety analysis.

Evaluation of gross motor function

Gross motor function was assessed using the MHFMS in a subgroup of 27 of 29 non-ambulatory SMA II subjects; one 14.9 year old subject with severe contractures who was no longer able to sit unsupported, and one uncooperative 2.8 year-old toddler were not evaluated with the MHFMS. Mean age of the remaining 27 subjects was 4.58 years. All subjects completed V1 and V2 visits and 25 (86%) completed all three visits. V1 was performed at 3.2 (2.3–4.3) months; V2 at 6.8 (5.5–9.9) months and V3 at 13 (8.7–15.6) months following treatment initiation. Mean MHFMS scores improved by 2.15; 2.92; and 4.65 at V1, V2 and V3 visits respectively, compared to baseline (table 2, $p\leq0.001$). Motor function in type II subjects was then defined as stable, deteriorated or improved using a three or six point change in the MHFMS score. Each time point was examined for frequency of that change from baseline for the entire cohort (table 3, part I). We further explored the effect of age on change in motor function (table 3, part II). Of note, 8/16 (50%) children <5 years of age achieved at least a 6 point improvement after 1 year, while no children ≥5 years of age demonstrated a six point improvement. The most significant change in scores was observed in 5 SMA type II children ages 25–34 months at enrollment who gained from 8–15 points. Table 4 further documents the effect of age on change in motor function for those children who achieved at least a 3 point improvement on the MHFMS.

Gross motor function was assessed using the MHFMS in a subgroup 10 of 11 ambulatory SMA III subjects. Increase in MHFMS scores in this cohort was limited by ceiling effects since several scored maximally at baseline (table 2).

Evaluation of pulmonary function measures

Pulmonary function testing was performed in 14 subjects ≥5 years of age, comprised of 10 type II subjects and 4 type III subjects. We observed a significant improvement in MIP values at the V1 and V2 visits, and in FVC, FEV1 and MIP values at the V3 visit in type II subjects (table 5).

Table 1. Percent of Subjects With Abnormal Lab Values Before and During Treatment All Patients (n = 42).

Laboratory Parameter	Baseline Incidence	Treatment Incidence
ALT	7%	19%
AST	10%	38%
WBC	12%	36%
HGB	17%	45%
HCT	17%	48%
Platelets	0%	5%
Neutrophils	36%	57%

ALT = alanine aminotransferase; AST = aspartate aminotransferase; WBC = total white blood count; HGB = hemoglobin; HCT = hematocrit.

Table 2. Change in MHFMS Score by Time Point.

Time	Type II Subjects				Type III Subjects			
	Avg Change	Range	SD	p-value[1]	Avg Change	Range	SD	p-value[1]
V1	2.15 N = 27	−5/7	3.02	0.0010	1.0 n = 10	−2/9	3.20	NS
V2	2.92 N = 26	−4/13	3.78	0.0006	1.4 n = 10	−4/11	3.92	NS
V3	4.65 N = 23	−6/15	4.76	0.0001	1.44 n = 9	−2/9	3.24	NS
Baseline	13.7 N = 27	0/35	8.22		34.4 n = 10	10/40	9.40	

[1]P-Values based upon paired t-test.
V1 = 3 months; V2 = 6 months; V3 = 12 months; SD = standard deviation, NS = not significant.

Table 3. Deterioration vs. Improvement in MHFMS score, SMA type II.

Part I. Three vs. Six point change, All type II Subjects				
Criteria	**Change**	**V1**	**V2**	**V3**
Three-Point		N = 27	N = 26	N = 23
	Deterioration	2 (7%)	1 (4%)	1 (4%)
	Stable	14 (52%)	12 (46%)	6 (26%)
	Improvement	11 (41%)	13 (50%)	16 (70%)
Six-Point				
	Deterioration	0	0	1 (4%)
	Stable	23 (85%)	21 (81%)	14 (61%)
	Improvement	4 (15%)	5 (19%)	8 (35%)
Part II. Deterioration vs. Improvement by Age, Six-Point Change				
Criteria	**Change**	**V1**	**V2**	**V3**
Under 5 years		N = 18	N = 17	N = 16
	Deterioration	0	0	0
	Stable	14 (78%)	12 (71%)	8 (50%)
	Improvement	4 (22%)	5 (29%)	8 (50%)
5+ years		N = 9	N = 9	N = 7
	Deterioration	0	0	1 (14%)
	Stable	9 (100%)	9 (100%)	6 (86%)
	Improvement	0	0	0

Table 4. Deterioration vs. Improvement by Age: Three-Point Change, SMA type II.

Criteria	Change	V1	V2	V3
Under 5 years		N = 18	N = 17	N = 16
	Deterioration	1 (6%)	0	0
	Stable	9 (50%)	6 (35%)	2 (13%)
	Improvement	8 (44%)	11 (65%)	14 (87%)
5+ years		N = 9	N = 9	N = 7
	Deterioration	1 (11%)	1 (11%)	1 (14%)
	Stable	5 (56%)	6 (67%)	4 (57%)
	Improvement	3 (33%)	2 (22%)	2 (29%)

Evaluation of body composition and bone density

Total lean body mass was stable but fat mass increased 38% between the baseline and the one year visit in type II subjects; this is in contrast to a 14% increase in type III subjects (table 6). We observed progressive increases in total body bone mineral density and content (BMD, BMC) across all treatment visits in type II subjects ($p \leq 0.0034$) and at V2 and V3 in type III subjects ($p \leq 0.0066$). When change in MHFMS score was analyzed by change in fat mass, those with three or six point gains demonstrated a lower gain in fat mass than those who were stable or deteriorated (p = NS; table 7).

Evaluation of electrophysiologic measures of denervation

CMAP amplitude increased over baseline at each visit. The increase in mean values was significant for V2 and V3 in type II subjects and for all visits for type III subjects (table 8, $p \leq 0.0127$). There was also a significant difference in CMAP values by change in MHMFS. At V1, subjects showing at least a three point

Table 5. Change in Pulmonary Function Tests from Baseline by Time Point.

Time	Type II Subjects N = 10			Type III Subjects N = 4	
	Avg Change Range	**SD**	**p-value[1]**	**Avg Change Range**	**SD**
V1 (3 months)					
FVC (L)	0.04	0.10	NS	0.10	0.27
	−0.06/0.22			−0.10/0.41	
FEV1 (L)	0.00	0.12	NS	−0.03	0.09
	−0.13/0.22			−0.12/0.05	
MIP (cm H_2O)	−11.0	8.9	p = 0.0059	−5.7	20.0
	−24.0/1.0		−26/14.0		
MEP (cm H_2O)	18.0	27.9	NS	−9.3	23.2
	−7.0/81.0			−35.0/10.0	
V2 (6 months)					
FVC (L)	0.07	0.12	NS	0.09	0.23
	−0.12/0.21			−0.11/0.40	
FEV1 (L)	0.04	0.15	NS	−0.03	0.14
	−0.27/0.22			−0.10/0.22	
MIP (cm H_2O)	−16.6	17.4	p = 0.0212	−13.0	17.0
	−39.0/20.0			−38.0/0.0	
MEP (cm H_2O)	16.9	24.5	NS	7.25	17.9
	−4.0/74.0			−7.0/30.0	
FVC (L)	0.12	0.14	p = 0.0472	0.28	0.20
	−0.12/0.26			−0.14/0.42	
FEV1 (L)	0.12	0.14	p = 0.0467	0.26	0.21
	−0.12/0.26			−0.12/0.41	
MIP (cm H_2O)	−16.6	17.7	p = 0.0481	−16.6	30.2
	−35.0/18.0			−38.0/4.7	
MEP (cm H_2O)	14.3	16.9	NS	1.3	23.6
	−3.0/47.0			−15.0/18.0	

FVC = forced vital capacity; FEV1 = forced expiratory volume in 1 second; MIP = maximal inspiratory pressure; MEP = maximum expiratory pressure.

improvement demonstrated higher CMAP values, indicating the best response in those with less severe denervation (table 9; $p = 0.03$). Changes in MUNE negative peak area or amplitude values were not significant.

Evaluation of SMN2 copy number and quantitative measures of SMN mRNA in whole blood samples

A linear regression analysis was performed on the transformed MHFMS scores (square root transformation) to evaluate the influence of genetic variables, including SMN2 copy number and SMN mRNA levels on MHFMS (Table 10). The results indicate no statistically significant relationship between MHFMS score and SMN mRNA levels, but do indicate a positive relationship between SMN2 copy number and SMA type with MHFMS score. Subjects with 3 SMN2 copies had an average of 0.67 flSMN compared to 0.79 flSMN in subjects with 4 SMN2 copies (Table S3). Δ7SMN levels were on average 1.04 and 1.15 for SMN2 copies 3 and 4, respectively. These results indicate no relationship between SMN mRNA levels and SMN2 copy number. There was a trend toward an increased relative amount of Δ7SMN transcripts per SMA type (0.91 ± 0.47 for type 2 vs. 1.42 ± 1.11 for type 3; $p = 0.053$). The mean relative amount of flSMN and Δ7SMN transcripts was 0.67 ± 0.29 and 0.91 ± 0.47 for type II and 0.77 ± 13 and 1.42 ± 1.11 for type III, respectively. Baseline measures point to the high degree of inter-patient variability in the relative amount of SMN transcripts, as previously reported [36,37].

There were no significant changes in the relative amount of flSMN transcripts in response to drug treatment. There was a significant decrease in Δ7SMN transcripts between baseline and V2 ($p = 0.0053$) and V3 ($p = 0.0429$) for type II subjects (table 11). Similar results were observed when using PGK1 as endogenous control to normalize for amount of input cDNA template and RT-PCR efficiency (baseline data in Table S3, treatment data not shown). Finally, there was no relationship between decreased Δ7SMN transcripts and any physiological or functional measure.

Discussion

In this open label study, we enrolled a relatively heterogeneous group of SMA subjects, although we focused recruitment predominantly on children with SMA types II and III. Our experience emphasizes the need to stratify subjects by SMA type, age and current gross motor abilities in future trials since the majority of outcome measures examined in this study were optimal for only a subset of subjects which was highly dependent on the

Table 6. Change in Lean and Fat Mass and Bone Density by Time Point.

Time	Type II Subjects N = 29			Type III Subjects N = 10		
	Avg Change[1]	SD	p-value[2]	Avg Change[1]	SD	p-value[2]
V1 (3 months)						
Lean mass, grams	123	973	NS	−267	1865	NS
Fat mass, grams	1094	1034	0.0003	1269	1844	0.078
Total BMD, g/cm^2	0.05	0.06	0.0003	0.02	0.05	NS
Total BMC, grams	33.6	54.4	0.0036	71.0	80.0	0.0287
V2 (6 months)						
Lean mass, grams	−366	1174	NS	184	1582	NS
Fat mass, grams	2579	2013	<0.0001	2101	2213	0.0149
Total BMD, g/cm^2	0.05	0.06	<0.0001	0.03	0.03	0.0066
Total BMC, grams	99.5	68.1	<0.0001	90.5	76.2	0.0045
V3 (12 months)						
Lean mass, grams	−212	1029	NS	322	960	NS
Fat mass, grams	3680	2470	<0.0001	2596	3193	0.0406
Total BMD g/cm^2	0.07	0.06	<0.0001	0.07	0.04	0.0011
Total BMC, grams	145	66.4	<0.0001	124.2	98.1	0.0052

[1]Range at baseline in Table S1.
[2]P-values based upon paired t-test.
BMD = bone mineral density; BMC = bone mineral content; g/cm^2 = grams/centimeter squared; SD = standard deviation, NS = not significant.

subject's age, motor disability and the overall degree of medical fragility.

This study provides evidence that VPA can be used safely in SMA subjects >2 years of age, as long as carnitine status is closely monitored. VPA is known to alter enteral absorption, inhibit biosynthesis and secondarily deplete carnitine from muscle by direct binding and excretion in the urine [38]. Given the diminished lean body mass in SMA subjects, an increased susceptibility to carnitine depletion is not surprising. Decreased nutritional intake and depleted whole body carnitine stores related to an associated abnormality in fatty acid metabolism may be contributing factors [39,40]. Thus, treatment with VPA in the absence of close monitoring and supplemental carnitine therapy could increase risks for further muscle weakness or fatal hepatotoxicity [41]. In this study, we did not observe any serious clinical or laboratory evidence of hepatotoxicity with careful monitoring and supplementation but grade I elevations of transaminases were common. Infants and children less than two years of age, a group not included in the current study, theoretically have a greater risk of such complications.

Table 7. Change in MHFMS Score by Change in Fat Mass.

Criteria	Change	V1	V2	V3
Three-Point				
	Deterioration	2320	7541	9502
		N = 2	N = 1	N = 1
	Stable	1173	1995	4459
		N = 14	N = 12	N = 6
	Improvement	825	2318	2918
		N = 11	N = 13	N = 16
P-value[1]		0.73	0.22	0.09
Six-Point				
	Deterioration			9502.0
		N = 0	N = 0	N = 1
	Stable	1287	2584	3624
		N = 23	N = 21	N = 1
	Improvement	189	1460	2839
		N = 4	N = 5	N = 8
P-value[1]		0.10	0.27	0.18

[1]P-value based upon ANOVA.

The apparent positive effect of treatment on bone density is surprising since prolonged VPA treatment has been associated with decreased bone density in other populations [42–45]. Whether the observed increased bone density is spurious or relates to increased weight gain, weight bearing or other factors is unclear. The significant increase in fat mass in the absence of an increase in lean mass is concerning given the detrimental impact weight gain could have on gross motor function and potential long-term consequences for general health. Weight gain was not uniform across the population; rather, non-ambulatory subjects ≥5 years, or those already with such a tendency appear to be at greatest risk. Notably, children demonstrating the most significant improvement in gross motor function gained less fat mass compared to those who displayed stable or deteriorated motor function.

Maximum CMAP amplitudes showed a statistically significant increase from baseline, while MUNE values did not change. This would imply that axonal reinnervation did not account for the change, but that the observed changes may be due to reinnervation of muscle via "sprouting" from remaining motor units or a direct trophic effect on muscle. If future controlled trials confirm that increased CMAP amplitude is a consistent marker of

Table 8. Change in Maximum Ulnar CMAP Amplitude and MUNE Negative Peak Area from Baseline by Time Point.

Time	Type II Subjects (n = 29)				Type III Subjects (n = 10)			
	Avg Change	Range	SD	p-value[1]	Avg Change	Range	SD	p-value[1]
V1 (3 months)								
CMAP (mV)	0.12	−0.98/1.26	0.38	0.0909	1.03	−0.10/2.50	0.95	0.0074
MUNE (μVms)	−3.03	−95.0/10.0	18.6	NS	−0.50	−38.0/53.0	28.2	NS
V2 (6 months)								
CMAP (mV)	0.23	−0.96/1.12	0.39	0.0041	1.20	0.23/3.56	1.13	0.0085
MUNE (μVms)	−5.59	−117.0/7.0	22.2	NS	−16.4	−93.0/17.0	33.8	NS
V3 (12 months)								
CMAP (mV)	0.35	−0.52/1.58	0.54	0.0031	1.44	−0.24/3.75	1.35	0.0127
MUNE (μVms)	−8.58	−126.0/10.0	26.3	NS	−17.7	−93.0/17.0	51.0	NS

[1]P-values based upon paired t-test.
SD = standard deviation, NS = not significant.

biologic response that correlates with improvement in motor function, then this outcome measure could prove a powerful surrogate biomarker for future clinical trials.

Changes in pulmonary function were observed; however, the significance is limited by the small number of subjects ≥5 years in each cohort. Nonetheless, PFT measures are important with regard to clinical outcomes in patients with SMA, so other means of reliably determining pulmonary function in younger children is an important goal.

We had hypothesized that VPA might increase flSMN and Δ7SMN mRNA levels in blood samples in light of prior data demonstrating increased mRNA and protein levels in patient-derived cells [16–20]. When analyzed as a group, we observed a significant decrease in the relative amount of Δ7SMN mRNA in SMA type II subjects while flSMN transcripts were unchanged. However, flSMN and Δ7SMN mRNA levels fluctuated throughout drug treatment, with patients showing increased, decreased or unaltered relative amounts of both transcripts. This variability contrasts with the fairly stable SMN mRNA levels observed in untreated patients [21,36,37]. Consistent with previously published data, these results are suggestive of a VPA response and SMN mRNA could help discriminate between non-responders and responders [21]. Furthermore, the implication of decreased relative Δ7SMN mRNA levels in the absence of changes in flSMN would be to increase the ratio of flSMN to SMNΔ7, the major discriminator between SMA subjects and unaffected controls/carriers when using relative measures of SMN mRNA, suggesting that these changes could be important. Finally, in order for SMN mRNA levels in blood to inform us about VPA effects in spinal cord, there must be a significant relationship between SMN mRNA and a clinical outcome measure. We did not observe any relationship between changes in Δ7SMN and any of the outcome measures in this pilot open label study. One reason for this may be that blood may not be the appropriate tissue to screen for biomarkers of SMA. Alternatively, extensive variability in SMN mRNA levels during treatment trials may mask significant relationships in a sub-set of SMA patients. Fluctuations in SMN mRNA levels may be amplified by fluctuations in transcript levels produced by endogenous controls used normalize for the amount of input template and efficacy of RT-PCR. VPA is a non-specific drug target and may itself affect expression of genes used as endogenous controls. We observed similar

Table 9. Average Maximum Ulnar CMAP vs. Three-point and Six-point Change in MHFMS Score.

Criteria	Change	CMAP (mV)	CMAP (mV)	CMAP (mV)
		V1	V2	V3
3-Point				
	Deterioration	0.46	0.47	0.55
		N = 2	N = 1	N = 1
	Stable	1.59	1.70	1.22
		N = 14	N = 12	N = 6
	Improvement	2.05	2.11	2.00
		N = 11	N = 13	N = 16
P-value[1]		0.03	0.07	0.29
6-Point				
	Deterioration			0.55
		N = 0	N = 0	N = 1
	Stable	1.52	1.68	1.33
		N = 23	N = 21	N = 14
	Improvement	2.67	2.58	2.61
		N = 4	N = 5	N = 8
P-value[1]		0.29	0.24	0.24

[1]P-value based upon ANOVA.
Maximum ulnar CMAP (compound muscle action potential amplitude).

Table 10. Linear Regression of Square Root of MHFMS Total Score Versus Genetic Variables.

Term	Estimate	Std Error	t Ratio	Prob>|t|
Intercept	−0.77	1.07	−0.71	0.4818
flSMN	−0.19	0.82	−0.23	0.8177
Δ7SMN	−0.68	0.45	−1.50	0.1455
SMN2	0.52	0.25	2.05	0.0497
Type	2.35	0.48	4.93	<.0001

Table 11. Change in Quantitative SMN mRNA levels by Time Point.

Time	Type II Subjects (n = 25)				Type III Subjects (n = 11)			
	Avg Change	Range	SD	p-value[1]	Avg Change	Range	SD	p-value[1]
V1	N = 25				N = 11			
flSMN	0.10	−0.19/2.00	0.42	NS	−0.02	−0.17/0.04	0.06	NS
Δ7SMN	0.42	−1.17/10.91	2.26	NS	−0.47	−2.68/0.65	0.98	NS
V2	N = 25				N = 11			
flSMN	−0.01	−0.38/0.52	0.17	NS	−0.04	−0.25/0.12	0.11	NS
Δ7SMN	−0.35	−1.82/0.60	0.57	0.0053	−0.46	−3.17/1.25	1.26	NS
V3	N = 19				N = 9			
flSMN	−0.01	−0.34/0.33	0.16	NS	−0.30	−0.14/0.10	0.06	NS
Δ7SMN	−0.32	−1.61/1.01	0.64	0.0429	−0.30	−3.25/1.63	1.34	NS
Baseline values								
flSMN	0.67	0.05/1.27	0.29		0.77	0.63/1.05	0.13	
Δ7SMN	0.91	0.05/2.14	0.47		1.42	0.41/4.29	1.11	

[1]P-value based upon ANOVA.

results with two endogenous controls (RPLPO and PGK1) and do not have any evidence to suggest that these genes are affected by VPA treatment. Nonetheless, there is a need for an absolute quantification method to measure SMN mRNA in order to remove variability introduced by the use of endogenous controls to normalize data.

In conclusion, this study provides good evidence that VPA can be used safely in SMA subjects over 2 years of age in the setting of close monitoring of carnitine status. This being said, further studies of VPA in infants and young children are needed to better assess safety in this more vulnerable cohort. This study provides evidence in support of improvement in gross motor function in younger non-ambulatory type II children. This finding was unexpected and it is unclear whether this improvement reflects a therapeutic drug effect, maturation or increased cooperation on improved scores in the youngest subjects. These data suggest that further studies with VPA are warranted, although clearly such findings must be replicated in randomized, controlled efficacy studies. The data presented here emphasizes the benefit of a trial design with a less heterogenous population of younger SMA subjects, particularly in light of significantly increased fat mass and lack of apparent benefit of VPA treatment in older non-ambulatory subjects. Furthermore, our experience indicates that the MHFMS scale alone is not adequate to measure motor function in ambulatory SMA subjects, prompting us to explore other measures to assess functional change in this population. Future clinical trials targeted to this cohort should generate additional informative data as to the usefulness of PFTs, timed test modules, and biomarker data including electrophysiologic measures of denervation, which appear to have promise in this cohort.

Supporting Information

Protocol S1 Clinical trial protocol summary

Figure S1 CONSORT Flowchart

Figure S2 Free carnitine levels at enrollment and subsequent follow-up for the first thirteen subjects

Checklist S1 CONSORT Checklist

Table S1

Table S2

Table S3

Acknowledgments

The authors gratefully acknowledge the SMA patients and families who participated in this study, and members of the DSMB including Colin Van Orman, Nicola Longo, and Natalie Mellem.

Author Contributions

Conceived and designed the experiments: KJS CBS SPR SLS GA TC JTK KJK GD MBB MKS LRS. Performed the experiments: KJS TWP JW BE LRS. Analyzed the data: KJS CBS BL GMC. Contributed reagents/materials/analysis tools: KJS TWP LRS. Wrote the paper: KJS SPR BL SLS JW GA TC JTK KJK GD MBB MKS GMC.

References

1. Brahe C, Bertini E (1996) Spinal muscular atrophies: recent insights and impact on molecular diagnosis. J Mol Med 74: 555–562.
2. Roberts DF, Chavez J, Court SD (1970) The genetic component in child mortality. Arch Dis Child 45: 33–38.
3. Pearn J (1978) Incidence, prevalence, and gene frequency studies of chronic childhood spinal muscular atrophy. J Med Genet 15: 409–413.
4. Czeizel A, Hamula J (1989) A hungarian study on Werdnig-Hoffmann disease. J Med Genet 26: 761–763.

5. Emery AE (1991) Population frequencies of inherited neuromuscular diseases–a world survey. Neuromuscul Disord 1: 19–29.
6. Merlini L, Stagni SB, Marri E, Granata C (1992) Epidemiology of neuromuscular disorders in the under-20 population in Bologna Province, Italy. Neuromuscul Disord 2: 197–200.
7. Lefebvre S, Burgien L, Reboullet S, Clermont O, Burlet P, et al. (1995) Identification and Characterization of a Spinal Muscular Atrophy-determining Gene. Cell 80: 155–165.
8. Wan L, Battle DJ, Yong J, Gubitz AK, Kolb SJ, et al. (1995) The Survival of Motor Neurons Protein Determines the Capacity for snRNP Assembly: Biochemical Deficiency in Spinal Muscular Atrophy. Mol Cell Biol 25(13): 5543–51.
9. Lorson CL, Hahnen E, Androphy EJ, Wirth B (1998) A single nucleotide in the SMN gene regulates splicing and is responsible for spinal muscular atrophy. Proc Natl Acad Sci USA 96: 6307–6311.
10. Feldkotter M, Schwarzer V, Wirth R, Wienker TF, Wirth B. Quantitative Analyses of SMN1 and SMN2 Based on Real-Time LightCycler PCR: Fast and Highly Reliable Carrier Testing and Prediction of Severity of Spinal Muscular Atrophy (2002) Am J Hum Genet. 70(2): 358–368.
11. Mailman MD, Heinz JW, Papp AC, Snyder PJ, Sedra MS, et al. (2002) Molecular Analysis of Spinal Muscular Atrophy and Modification of the Phenotype by SMN2. Genet Med 4: 20–26.
12. Swoboda KJ, Prior TW, Scott CB, McNaught TP, Wride MC, et al. (2005) Natural history of denervation in SMA: relation to age, SMN2 copy number, and function. Ann Neurol 57: 704–712.
13. Wirth B, Brichta L, Schrank B, Lochmüller H, Blick S, et al. (2006) Mildly affected patients with spinal muscular atrophy are partially protected by an increased SMN2 copy number. Hum Genet 119: 422–428.
14. Prior TW, Swoboda KJ, Scott HD, Hejmanowski AQ (2004) Homozygous SMN1 deletions in unaffected family members and modification of the phenotype by SMN2. Am J Med Genet A 130: 307–310.
15. Lefebvre S, Burlet P, Liu Q, Bertrandy S, Clermont O, et al. (1997) Correlation between severity and SMN protein level in spinal muscular atrophy. Nat Genet 16: 265–269.
16. Chang JG, Hsieh-Li HM, Jong YJ, Wang NM, Tsai CH, et al. (2001) Treatment of spinal muscular atrophy by sodium butyrate. Proc Natl Acad Sci U S A 98: 9808–9813.
17. Brichta L, Hofmann Y, Hahnen E, Siebzehnrubl FA, Raschke H, et al. (2003) Valproic acid increases the SMN2 protein level: a well-known drug as a potential therapy for spinal muscular atrophy. Hum Mol Genet 12: 2481–2489.
18. Sumner CJ, Huynh TN, Markowitz JA, Perhac JS, Hill B, et al. (2003) Valproic acid increases SMN levels in spinal muscular atrophy patient cells. Ann Neurol 54: 647–654.
19. Andreassi C, Angelozzi C, Tiziano FD, Vitali T, De Vincenzi E, et al. (2004) Phenylbutyrate increases SMN expression in vitro: relevance for treatment of spinal muscular atrophy. Eur J Hum Genet 12: 59–65.
20. Grzeschik SM, Ganta M, Prior TW, Heavlin WD, Wang CH (2005) Hydroxyurea enhances SMN2 gene expression in spinal muscular atrophy cells. Ann Neurol 58: 194–202.
21. Brichta L, Holker I, Haug K, Klockgether T, Wirth B (2006) In Vivo Activation of SMN in Spinal Muscular Atrophy Carriers and Patients Treated with Valproate. Ann Neurol 59: 970–975.
22. Brahe C, Vitali T, Tiziano FD, Angelozzi C, Pinto AM, et al. (2005) Phenylbutyrate increases SMN gene expression in spinal muscular atrophy patients. Eur J Hum Genet 13: 256–259.
23. Kernochan LE, Russo ML, Woodling NS, Huynh TN, Avila AM, et al. (2005) The role of histone acetylation in SMN gene expression. Hum Mol Genet 14: 1171–1182.
24. Leng Y, Chuang DM (2006) Endogenous α-Synuclein is Induced by Valproic Acid through Histone Deacetylase Inhibition and Participates in Neuroprotection against Glutamate-Induced Excitotoxicity. J Neurosci 26(28): 7502–7512.
25. van Bergeijk J, Haastert K, Grothe C, Claus P (2006) Valproic acid promotes neurite outgrowth in PC12 cells independent from regulation of the survival of motoneuron protein. Chem Biol Drug Des 67: 244–247.
26. Sugai F, Yamamoto Y, Miyaguchi K, Zhou Z, Sumi H, et al. (2004) Benefit of valproic acid in suppressing disease progression of ALS model mice. Eur J Neurosci 20: 3179–3183.
27. Petri S, Kiaei M, Kipiani K, Chen J, Chalingasan NY, et al. (2006) Additive neuroprotective effects of a histone deacetylase inhibitor and a catalytic antioxidant in a transgenic mouse model of amyotrophic lateral sclerosis. Neurobiol Dis 22: 40–49.
28. Tsai LK, Tsai MS, Lin TB, Hwu WL, Li H (2006) Establishing a standardized therapeutic testing protocol for spinal muscular atrophy. Neurobiol Dis 24: 286–295.
29. Tsai LK, Tsai MS, Ting CH, Li H (2008) Multiple therapeutic effects of valproic acid in spinal muscular atrophy model mice. J Mol Med 86: 1243–1254.
30. Weihl CC, Connolly AM, Pestronk A (2006) Valproate may improve strength and function in patients with type III/IV spinal muscular atrophy. Neurology 67: 500–501.
31. Tsai LK, Yang CC, Hwu WL, Li H (2007) Valproic acid treatment in six patients with spinal muscular atrophy. Eur J Neurol 14: e8–e9.
32. Main M, Kairon K, Mercuri E, Muntoni F (2003) The Hammersmith functional motor scale for children with spinal muscular atrophy: a scale to test ability and monitor progress in children with limited ambulation. Eur J Paediatr Neurol 7: 155–159.
33. Krosschell KJ, Maczulski JA, Crawford TO, Scott C, Swoboda KJ (2006) A modified Hammersmith functional motor scale for use in multi-center research on spinal muscular atrophy. Neuromuscul Disord 16: 417–426.
34. Mercuri E, Messina S, Battini R, Berrardinelli A, Boffi P, et al. (2006) Reliability of the Hammersmith functional motor scale for spinal muscular atrophy in a Multicentric Study. Neuromuscul Disord 16: 93–98.
35. Bromberg MB, Swoboda KJ (2002) Motor unit number estimation in infants and children with spinal muscular atrophy. Muscle Nerve 25: 445–447.
36. Simard LR, Belanger M-C, Morrissette S, Wride M, Prior TW, et al. (2007) Preclinical validation of a multiplex real-time RT-PCR assay to quantify SMN transcripts in whole blood from SMA patients. Neurology 68: 451–456.
37. Sumner CJ, Kolb SJ, Harmison GG, Jeffries NO, Schadt K, et al. (2006) SMN mRNA and protein levels in peripheral blood. Neurology 66: 1067–1073.
38. Melegh B, Pap M, Morava E, Molnar D, Dani M, et al. (1994) Carnitine-dependent changes of metabolic fuel consumption during long-term treatment with valproic acid. J Pediatr 125: 317–321.
39. Tein I, Sloane AE, Donner EJ, Lehotay DC, Millington DS, et al. (1995) Fatty acid oxidation abnormalities in childhood-onset spinal muscular atrophy: primary or secondary defect(s)? Pediatr Neurol 12: 21–30.
40. Crawford TO, Sladky JT, Hurko O, Besner-Johnston A, Kelley RI (1999) Abnormal fatty acid metabolism in childhood spinal muscular atrophy. Ann Neurol 45: 337–343.
41. Coulter DL (1984) Carnitine deficiency: a possible mechanism for valproate hepatotoxicity. Lancet 1(8378): 689.
42. Kumandas S, Koklu E, Gümüs H, Koklu S, Kurtoglu S, et al. (2006) Effect of carbamezapine and valproic acid on bone mineral density, IGF-I and IGFBP-3. J Pediatr Endocrinol Metab 19: 529–534.
43. Boluk A, Guzelipek M, Savlı H, Temel I, Iın Ozık H, et al. (2004) The effect of valproate on bone mineral density in adult epileptic patients. Pharmacol Res 50: 93–97.
44. Ecevit C, Aydoğan A, Kavakli T, Altinöz S (2004) Effect of carbamazepine and valproate on bone mineral density. Pediatr Neurol 31: 279–282.
45. Leet AI, Mesfin A, Pichard C, Launay F, Brintzenhofeszoc K, et al. (2006) Fractures in children with cerebral palsy. J Pediatr Orthop 26: 624–627.

14

Mechanical Behaviour of Umbrella-Shaped, Ni-Ti Memory Alloy Femoral Head Support Device during Implant Operation: A Finite Element Analysis Study

Wei Yi[1], Qing Tian[2], Zhipeng Dai[3], Xiaohu Liu[4]*

1 Department of Mechanics, Huazhong University of Science and Technology, Wuhan, Hubei, China, **2** Tongji Medical College, Huazhong University of Science and Technology, Wuhan, Hubei, China, **3** Tongji Medical College, Huazhong University of Science and Technology, Wuhan, Hubei, China, **4** Department of Mechanics, Huazhong University of Science and Technology, Wuhan, Hubei, China

Abstract

A new instrument used for treating femoral head osteonecrosis was recently proposed: the umbrella-shaped, Ni-Ti memory femoral head support device. The device has an efficacy rate of 82.35%. Traditional radiographic study provides limited information about the mechanical behaviour of the support device during an implant operation. Thus, this study proposes a finite element analysis method, which includes a 3-step formal head model construction scheme and a unique material assignment strategy for evaluating mechanical behaviour during an implant operation. Four different scenarios with different constraints, initial positions and bone qualities are analyzed using the simulation method. The max radium of the implanted device was consistent with observation data, which confirms the accuracy of the proposed method. To ensure that the device does not unexpectedly open and puncture the femoral head, the constraint on the impact device should be strong. The initial position of sleeve should be in the middle to reduce the damage to the decompression channel. The operation may fail because of poor bone quality caused by severe osteoporosis. The proposed finite element analysis method has proven to be an accurate tool for studying the mechanical behaviour of umbrella-shaped, Ni-Ti memory alloy femoral head support device during an implant operation. The 3-step construct scheme can be implemented with any kind of bone structure meshed with multiple element types.

Editor: Mikko Lammi, University of Eastern Finland, Finland

Funding: This work was supported by the National Natural Science Foundation of China through the project No. 11172110. The funders had no role in study design, data collection and analysis, decision to publish, or preparation of the manuscript.

Competing Interests: The authors have declared that no competing interests exist.

* Email: xhliu@mail.hust.edu.cn

Introduction

Osteonecrosis of the femoral head is a devastating disease that typically presents in young patients between the ages of thirty and forty [1]. If osteonecrosis is not effectively treated, many patients will experience femoral head collapse [2]. Hip replacement is not an optimal choice for the younger patients because of the validity of the artificial joint. Therefore, several minimally invasive surgery modalities [3] have been used to prevent the collapse of the femoral head. The following treatments, in the order they've been introduced, have been used in therapy: transtrochanteric osteotomy [4], core compression [5], Nonvascularized bone graft [6], vascularized bone graft [7], porous tantalum implant [8], Ni-Ti superelastic cage implant [3]. Of these treatments, those that used implant techniques were much more effective than the others [3]. This is because the structural stiffness of the implanted device provides a high level of support. However, all of these devices come with certain limitations, including a support area that is too small. Recently, an umbrella-shaped, Ni-Ti alloy femoral head support device [9] was proposed to treat the early stage osteonecrosis of the femoral head. Based on 17 devices implanted in 10 patients, the device showed an 82.35% efficacy rate. As reported, the support area was much larger than the traditional implant treatment. Note, however, that there are also risks associated with this operation. The biomechanical mechanism was not entirely clear, and the operation process has not yet been perfected.

Ni-Ti shape memory alloy, as a functional metal material, has many advantages including a remarkable resistance to wear and corrosion, good biocompatibility, and other special mechanical characters: SME (shape memory effect) [10], PE (pseudo elastic) and pseudo plastic [11]. These distinct characteristics make the shape memory alloy very useful in bone surgery instrument design [12]. The many studies on the biomechanical characteristics of the Ni-Ti SMA (shape memory alloy) have increased its used in orthopedics. From the work of Auricchio [13], Lsdyna provides a linearized macroscopic phenomenological model for SMA spans, which is widely used for SMA simulation. Although this model did not include permanent strain, PE was still in effect.

The major focus on Ni-Ti surgery instruments has been in clinical practice, with few computational studies conducted on the instruments. This is particularly true for the umbrella-shaped formal head support device, which has yet to be computationally researched. The FEA (finite element analysis) can serve as the deformation field, strain field and stress field of the femoral head and support device, which is almost impossible to determine in a radiological imaging study. More importantly, the computational simulation study can predict the whole process without actually performing the surgery. Because the bone is damaged inside the femoral head, and a traditional static analysis is unable to address issues related to element failure, the explicit integration method is used.

The aim of present study is to propose a finite element analysis method based on Lsdyna to simulate the mechanical behaviour of the Ni-Ti umbrella-shaped femoral head support device during the implant process. This method includes 1) a 3-step model construction and particular material assignment strategy for the femoral head in FEA pre-processing and 2) a dynamic relaxation analysis (the normal step) in which the stress initialization file is derived from a pre-analysis (the pre-step) of the support device.

We attempted to illustrate the expanding process within the femoral head during surgery, and review the accuracy of the simulation method by comparing the literature data with the simulation. Two different cases of sleeve initial positions were simulated. The results suggested that the open shape might be similar, but different kinds of damage were found inside the femoral neck. Finally, we conducted a simulation of the same patient with moderate osteoporosis. The results show that moderate osteoporosis might lead to surgery failure because the femoral head was not strong enough to resist the expending of the implant device. Since the finite element simulation method was effective and accurate, it might also be used as a rehearsal for selecting both the best implant location and implant device size for patients with varying bone qualities. Equation Chapter 1 Section 1.

Materials and Methods

The FEA study is based on a 3-step model construction scheme, outlined below. Initially, the model is digitized based on a CT (Computed Tomography) scan experiment. Then, the geometric model is created with Mimics and Geomagic Studio. The finite element is then discretized and a special material assignment strategy is carried out. Finally, an analyses is conducted during which the pre-step simulates the reshape phase under 0°C in vitro and the normal step simulates the opening phase under 50°C in vivo. The Boundary conditions and loading are explained in a following subsection.

CT Scan Experiment

The first step of the 3-step construction scheme was to digitize the geometric and bone quality information of the femoral head. An anonymous 45-year-old male patient with Stage I femoral head osteonecrosis was CT scanned every two millimeters from the femoral head to the lesser trochanter and then at five millimeter intervals along the femur bone. A Brilliance 128 iCT scanner (Philips) was used to scan the patient. The CT slice image data were saved and exported in DICOM (Digital Imaging and Communications in Medicine) format.

The second step was to reconstruct a high quality 3D geometric model based on the digitized slice image data. The slice images were imported into Mimics software (Materialise, Leuven, Belgium) for the model reconstruction. Then, using Geomagic Studio V13.0 (Raindrop Geomagic, TrianglePark, NC) with a reverse modeling process, a fine geometric model was made (Fig. 1(a)).

FEA Analysis

Mesh and material assignment of femoral head and femur. After the Geometric model was constructed from the CT images, an operation channel with a 9 mm outer diameter at the greater tuberosity to a 5 mm diameter under the subchondral bone along the femur neck was cut in the formal head. The last step of the construction scheme was element discrete.

In HyperMesh, we used the geometric model created during the pre-step to carry out the mesh process. The whole bone structure was divided into 3 parts: the femoral head, the femur, and part in-between. The first 2 parts were meshed with 8-node 1st order hexahedron elements. Because the femoral head part was the main area of focus, the mesh with the element edge in the range of 0.28 ~0.62 mm was much finer then the femur part. The 3rd part was meshed with 4-node 1st order tetrahedron. The element numbers, element types, and support device are shown in Table 1.

The low quality (2 mm resolution) of the CT scan data prevented a clear view of the internal femoral bone microstructure and distribution of the internal trabecular bone, but it provided enough information to establish a high quality 3D geometric model of the femur. The quality of the mesh depends only on the meshing skill when the geometric model is adequate. In other words, the low quality of the CT scan has no effect on the element quality when a high quality 3D geometric model can be made.

After the 3-step model construction, we assigned a material property for each element. Because of the limitations of the Mimics auto-assignment function (it is only available when the mesh is created with 4-node elements), an assignment strategy was used.

Unable to use the Mimics auto-assignment function for the mixed-type mesh (mesh II), we generated a 4-node tetrahedron element mesh, named mesh I, and auto-assigned material in Mimics. The problem then presented is how to link Mesh I and II to each other. The detailed process for solving this problem is as follows:

Step 1: Generate an auto-assigned density for Mesh I in Mimics as N sets of elements. All of the sets are created based on the range of the apparent density which was evenly distributed and shown as the left side of each sub-graph in Fig. 2.

Step 2: Correspond Mesh II to Mesh I using the mass centroid coordination of each element. Since Mesh I is divided into N sets, Mesh II is also divided into N sets with the same apparent density as Mesh I. This can be seen in the right side of each sub-graph in Fig. 2.

Table 1. Mesh Information.

Parts	femoral head	femur	connector	umbrella	sleeve	total
Number	113680	59080	139366	11904	5412	329442
Element nodes	8	8	4	8	8	4 & 8
Element type	hexahedron	hexahedron	tetrahedron	hexahedron	hexahedron	h & t

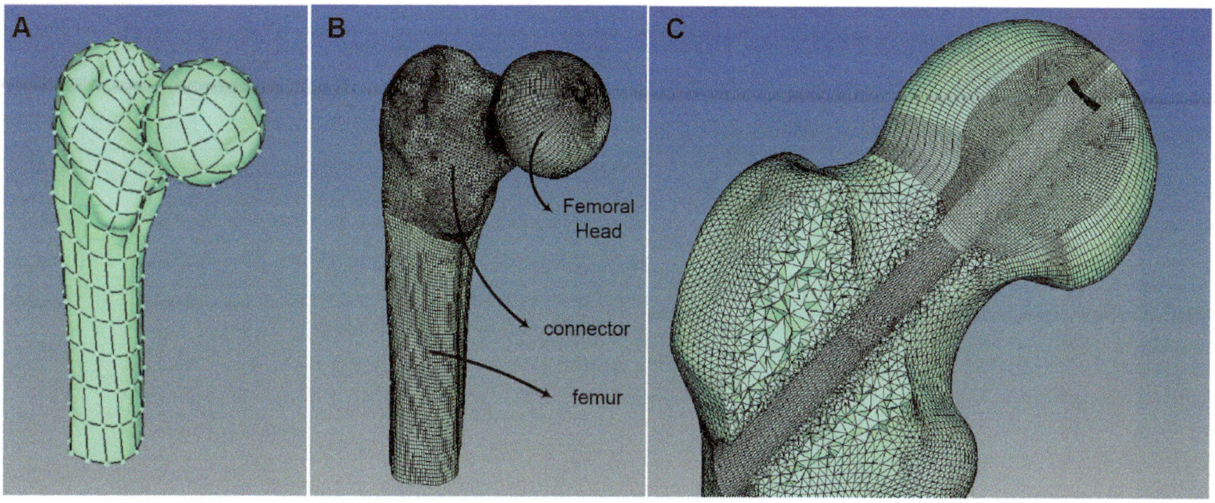

Figure 1. Digitized femur. (A) Geometric Model; (B) FE mesh model; (C) FE mesh model (local view).

Step 3: Based on the porosity-elastic module squared relation [14], E_N for set N is determined along with the failure strain for all the bone elements [15].

It's important to note that Mesh II is much finer than Mesh I. Hence, a cubic search bucket with a width 20 times the longest side of the current element E_i^{I} is created. In this bucket, we searched the corresponded element E_j^{II} that the mass centroid of E_i^{I} belonged to.

The N is set to 10, and the density, elastic module, failure strain and Poisson's ratio of each set are shown in Table 2. The corresponding elements of each set in Mesh I and II are shown with the same color, side by side. (Mesh I is show on the left side, and mesh II on the right).

In Mimics, a linear formula is used to translate the Hounsfield into the bone mass density field by the linear formula:

$$\rho = \rho_{\max} \frac{HU_j}{HU_{\max}} \qquad (1)$$

Where, j is the material property number. It is important to note that material property number and element set number are not necessarily the same, as shown in Table 2. HU_j represents the HU value of the material property j, and can be calculated with formula (2):

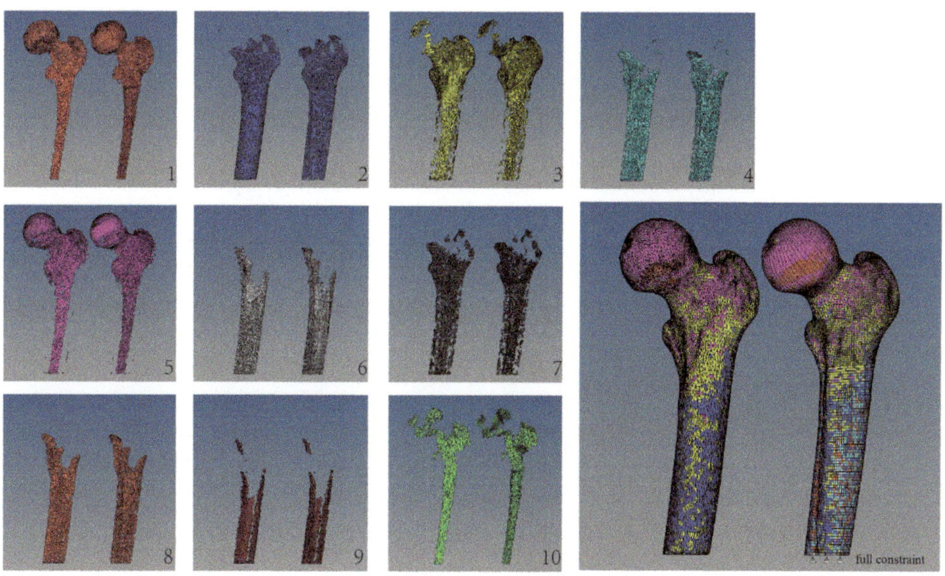

Figure 2. Bone material assignment results of 10 individual groups and the overall model. Constraint on the bone structure: In the normal step, a full constraint was applied at the bottom to eliminate rigid displacement of the whole structure.

Table 2. Material parameters for 10 different sets of bone elements.

Set | Material Property	Density (mg/mm³)	Elastic module (Gpa)	Failure strain	Poisson's ratio
1 | 2	0.63(0.53)	0.80(0.56)	0.009	0.3
2 | 5	1.57(0.31)	5.00(3.5)		
3 | 4	1.26(1.05)	3.20(2.24)		
4 | 7	2.19(1.83)	9.80(6.68)		
5 | 3	0.94(0.79)	1.80(1.26)		
6 | 9	2.83(2.37)	16.20(11.34)		
7 | 6	1.88(1.57)	7.20(5.04)		
8 | 8	2.51(2.10)	12.80(8.96)		
9 | 10	3.14(2.63)	20.00(14.00)		
10 | 1	0.32(0.27)	0.20(0.14)		

$$HU_j = \begin{cases} 168 & HU \le 252 \quad and \quad j=1 \\ j \times 168 & j*168-84 < HU \le j*168+84 \quad and \quad j=2,9 \\ 1680 & 1596 < HU \le 1680 \quad and \quad j=10 \end{cases} \qquad (2)$$

The HU value range 168~1680 was used to separate the muscle and soft tissue, while maintaining the best shape of the femur and formal head.

With $\rho_{max} = 3.14 \times 10^{-6}$ Kg/mm³, the bone mass density field is calculated. Then, the squared relation [14] is used to calculate the elastic module:

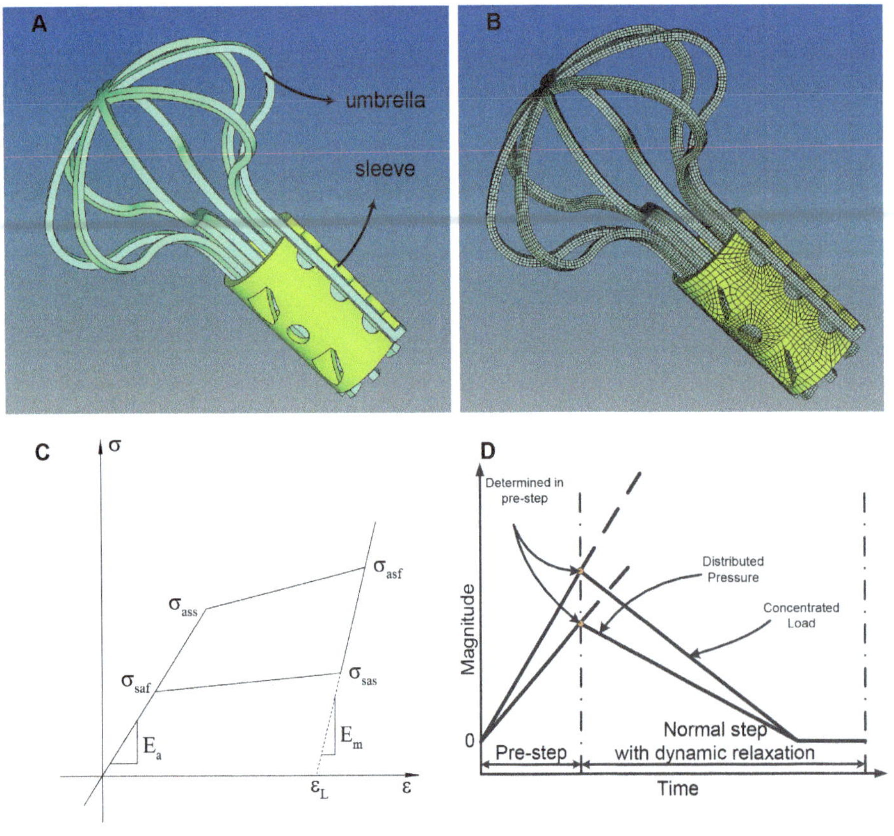

Figure 3. Implant devices and analysis setting in Lsdyna. (A) Umbrella-shaped femoral head support device geometric model; (B) Umbrella-shaped femoral head support device FE mesh model; (C) Material model in Lsdyna; (D) User-defined load curve in pre-step and normal step in: Lsdyna.

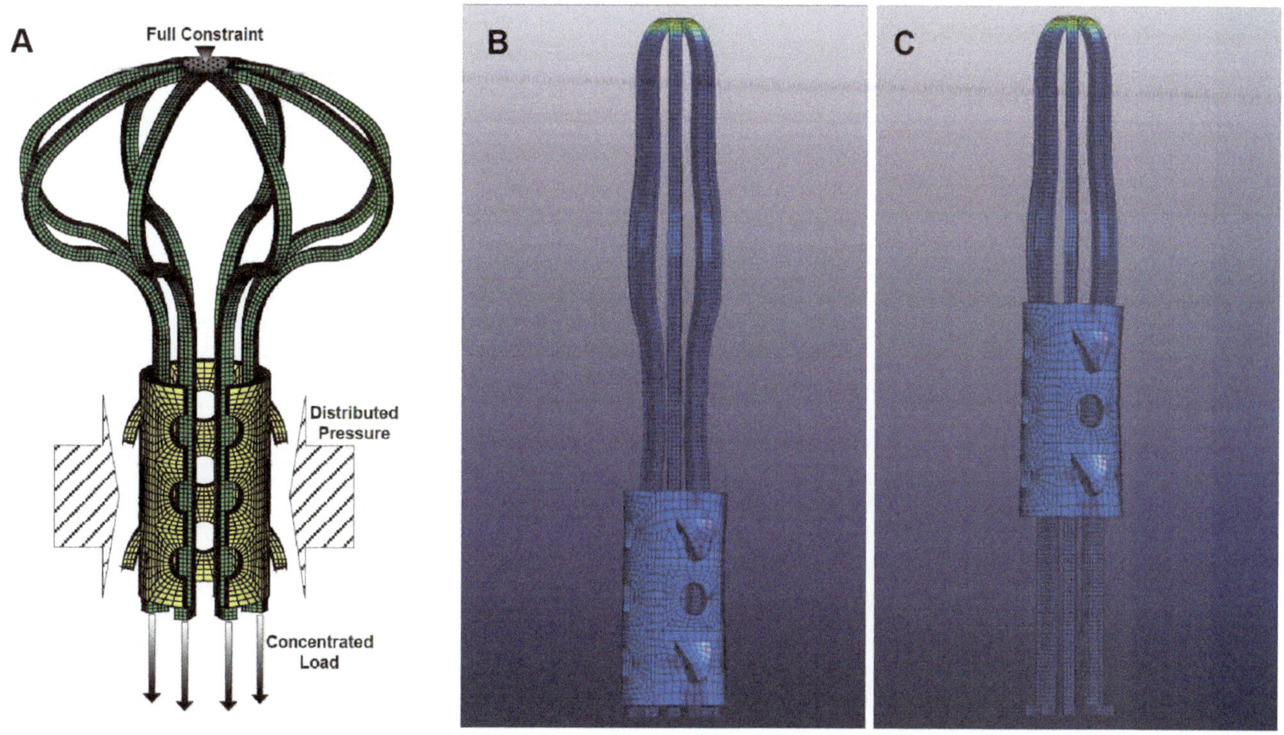

Figure 4. Constraint and load on implant devices and two different positions of the sleeve. (A) constraint and load on implant devices in pre-step and normal step:a full constraint at the top of the umbrella, concentrated load on the bottom of the umbrella, distributed pressure on the sleeve, the loads increase with time in the pre-step and decrease with time in the normal step; (B) Position I: sleeve at the bottom; (C) Position II: sleeve in the middle.

$$E = E_0\left(\frac{\rho}{\rho_0}\right)^2 \quad (3)$$

Where $\rho_0 = 3.14 \times 10^{-6}$ Kg/mm^3, $E_0 = 20.0$ Gpa. Because of a lack of previous experiments conducted on actual femoral head bone material, the approximate squared relationship is a good and relatively simple choice. Moreover, it is often used for bone structure simulations [21].

The equivalent strain failure criterion was used to judge the failure of the bone element. When the equivalent strain reached 0.009, the bone element was damaged and removed from the calculation. This element deletion will damage the original contact surface area, which forms on the bone element's surface. Thus, all the contacts involving bone are set to an eroding-type contact, in which the contact surface can be updated whenever the original contact surface was damaged.

When the patient suffered from severe osteoporosis, a 16.34% bone mass loss was assumed and the elastic module was 30% less than normal (Table 2). The values in and out of the brackets correspond respectively to the osteoporosis bone and normal bone.

Umbrella-shaped Femoral Head Support Device

The geometric model of the Ni-Ti umbrella-shaped femoral head support device at 50°C is shown in Fig. 3(a). The implant device contains two parts: the umbrella and the sleeve, marked in green and yellow, respectively. The outer diameter of the sleeve is 12 mm. The umbrella height is 50 mm; the outer diameter is 36.25 mm; and the width of the umbrella arm is 1.2 mm. The thickness is 1 mm in both parts. The umbrella and sleeve are all meshed with 8-node hexahedron elements. There are at least 3 layers of elements width-wise. The element numbers of the umbrella and sleeve are shown in Table 1.

Ni-Ti SMA Constitutive Relation

There are three kinds of constitutive relations that can be used to describe the shape of the memory alloy: a microscopic thermodynamic model, macroscopic phenomenological model [16], and multivariant micromechanical model [17]. The microscopic thermodynamic model is useful for determining the nucleation, interfacial movement, growth of martensite, and other microscopic mechanisms of a material. Using the microscopic thermodynamic model, the macroscopic constitutive relation in the Multi-scale model is determined. Although the physical meaning of these two methods is clear, they remain difficult to use in practical engineering. The macroscopic phenomenological model [18,19,20] has developed rapidly in concert with the enrichment of experimental results. However the phenomenological constitutive model equation and the phase transition thermodynamics equations are nonlinear. In other words, it's easy to not use these equations as they require a many resources and demand a great deal of time to solve.

As previously mentioned, Lsdyna provides a simplified macroscopic phenomenological model through which the phase-changing process is made linear (Fig. 4(a)). Where σ_{ass} and σ_{asf} are the start and final stress values for the forward phase transformation, respectively. σ_{sas} and σ_{saf} are the start and final stress value for the reverse phase transformation, respectively. When the ambient temperature of 50°C was higher than A_f, which is the Austenite Finish temperature (material parameter which is 37 °C), the stress-strain curve of the SMA under an isothermal environment is determined (Fig. 3(c)). The mechanical load placed upon the alloy

Table 3. SMA material parameters setting.

Density (mg/mm^3)	E_m (Gpa)	E_a (Gpa)	Poisson's Ratio	σ_{ass} (Gpa)	σ_{asf} (Gpa)	σ_{sas} (Gpa)	σ_{saf} (Gpa)	EPSL	ALPHA
6.3×10^{-6}	63.0	26.3	0.3	0.3528	0.4228	0.2856	0.1794	0.067	0.0

produces a stress on the martensite phase transformation; when the stress reaches σ_{ass} the alloy starts to transform from the austenite phase to the martensite phase. When the stress reaches σ_{asf} the forward transformation is complete. This type of phase transformation remains stable only when under a mechanical load. Even if unheated, when the mechanical load was lifted the inverse transformation occurred. When the stress decreases to σ_{sas}, the inverse transformation to austenite begins; when the stress reaches σ_{saf}, the inverse transformation occurred. When the stress decreased to 0, i.e. when the mechanical load was essentially cancelled, the SMA recovers to its original shape.

The material parameters are shown in Table 3. Temperatures M_f, M_s, A_s, A_f(representing Martensite Finish, Martensite Start, Austenite Start, and Austenite Finish, respectively) are set to 9°C, 18.4°C, 29.3°C,and 37°C. These temperatures are set in accordance with Brinskon [20] and Yu [9]. The transformation constants C_m and C_A, used to describe the relationship of the temperature and the critical stress to the induced transformation, are 0.008 $Gpa/^\circ C$ and 0.0138 $Gpa/^\circ C$, respectively. σ_s^{cr} and σ_f^{cr} which represent the critical stress value below M_s are 0.1 Gpa and 0.17 Gpa, respectively. Equations for evaluating the four stress values used in Lsdyan from the material parameters mentioned above are:

$$\sigma_{ass} = \sigma_s^{cr} + C_m(T - M_s) \tag{4}$$

$$\sigma_{asf} = \sigma_f^{cr} + C_m(T - M_s) \tag{5}$$

$$\sigma_{sas} = C_A(T - A_f) \tag{6}$$

$$\sigma_{saf} = C_A(T - A_s) \tag{7}$$

When the temperature was set to 50°C, the material parameters used in Lsdyna are obtained and shown in Table 3.

The EPSL refers to the maximum residual strain; and the ALPHA refers to the parameter measuring the differences between the material responses in for both the tension and compression.

Constraint and Load

The simplified linearized pseudo elastic model does not include permanent strain. In other words, after unloading, there is no stable deformation. This remains true even if the deformation is larger than the maximum strain set to.067, as described in more detail above. To properly maintain the shape below 0°C, the constrained boundary and a tension load are applied on the umbrella. A pressure is also applied on the sleeve in the normal step, as seen in Fig. 4(a). Note that the constrain and load shown above are the same values used to calculate the shape of the support device under 0°C in the pre-step. The magnitudes of these loads, i.e. the inflection points in Fig. 3(d), are chosen so that the device matches the shape presented in previous study [9]. More specifically, the outer diameter of the umbrella is 8 mm and the outer diameter of the sleeve is 9 mm.

After the reshape phase under 0°C (the pre-step), the bone structure with a full constraint at the bottom was added to the simulation (the normal step). When the distributed pressure and concentrated load began decreasing, the umbrella and sleeve began to recover to their original shape, leading to bone element

Table 4. Information of four different scenarios.

Scenario	Initial Position		Bone Quality		Constraint and Load	
	I	II	Normal	Osteoporosis	Yes	No
1	√		√			√
2	√		√		√	
3	√			√	√	
4		√	√		√	

failure. By the end of the simulation, the artificial load on the device has decreased to zero, and the final shape is obtained. The user-defined load curves of the distributed pressure and concentrated load are shown in Fig. 3(d). Two different phases–the reshape phase (pre-step phase) and open phase (normal step phase)–are included. The inflection points are determined in the pre-step phase with multiple computations.

Although the surgery process has been comprehensively described, the optimized initial position of the support device has not been determined. Likewise, there are problems remaining that relate to the damage inside the femoral head as well as variability of bone quality as seen in different patients. Thus, in the normal step phase, 4 different scenarios are simulated (Table 4).

Scenario 1 is the only one scenario without a constraint: the umbrella and sleeve can move freely, no load has been applied the umbrella and the sleeve, and the initial position I is used (Fig. 4(b)). In Scenario 2, we constrain the umbrella at the top; the concentrated load and distributed pressure are slowly released. Scenario 3 is almost the same as scenario 2, except that the bone material is different. Scenario 4 is the only scenario that uses the initial position II (Fig. 4(c)); otherwise, the conditions are identical to Scenario 2.

In all 4 scenarios, the contacts are set for the umbrella, the sleeve and formal head with each other. Two self-contacts are set for the umbrella and sleeve. More specifically, eroding-type contacts are implemented when formal bone is involved. When bone elements are deleted because of failure, a new contact surface is generated in the eroding-type contact.

Results

After reshaping under 0°C, the Ni-Ti alloy umbrella-shaped support device is implanted in the formal head. Hot saline (50°C) is poured into the formal head, and the support device begins to recover to its original shape. The primary focus of this research is to evaluate how the final shape of the support device functions in the human body. However, because of the resistance of the cancellous bone inside the formal head, the final shape is not the same as original shape, (Fig. 5(a)). In other words, the support device cannot totally recover its shape. Likewise, there is a compression deformation with respect to the original shape. Thus, the support device contains a potential energy expansion, and plays an active role in allowing the formal head to resist the pressure caused by normal bodily activities.

After the simulation, several conclusions were reached:

1) The top of the umbrella should be fully constrained to avoid the umbrella opening in an unexpected location (Fig. 5(c)). When the umbrella penetrates the formal head, the head suffers severe bone damage.
2) In Scenario 2, the final shape of the support device is similar to the original shape but with a decreased outer diameter. The outer diameter of the sleeve decreased, on average, from 12 mm to 11.26 mm (Fig. 5(b)). The maximum outer diameter of the umbrella decreased on average from 36.225 mm to 31.62 mm, which is quite close to previously observed data (32 mm) [9]. A typical pair of 4 opposite umbrella arm pairs for each scenario is shown in Fig. 5(a).
3) In Scenario 3, the operation failed, penetrating the femoral heads of the patients with severe osteoporosis. The failure position was near the bottom of the femoral head (marked in black circle in Fig. 5(e)). This failure was caused by the low elastic module, which itself was the result of severe osteoporosis (Table 2). The osteoporosis bone elements are much more vulnerable than normal bone elements.
4) The final shape of the umbrella is almost identical in Scenario 2 and 4, which means that the initial position of the sleeve does not affect the final shape of umbrella. However, the traces left by the sleeve are much different. In Scenario 2, when the sleeve is placed at the bottom and the temperature is rising, the sleeve expanded and dragged by the umbrella-shaped support device. A columnar hole of 20 mm diameter and 22.5 mm depth is formed along the decompression channel (Fig. 5(d)). However, in Scenario 4, the sleeve was placed in the middle and there was no additional damage done to the decompression channel (Fig. 5(f)).
5) There are stresses placed upon the support device and formal head because of the shape taken during the recovery process (Fig. 5(g) and (h)). These stresses correspond to the strains caused by the deformation of the umbrella-shaped device. The cancellous bone inside the femoral bone partially prevents the device from recovering to its original shape; thus the device squeezes the femoral head from inside to outside. The stresses and strain are helpful for the formal head to support the pressure brought upon the femoral head during daily activities. This means the umbrella-shaped support device is much more effective than other devices. The usefulness of this feature can be seen in the porous tantalum rod implant [21]: when there is almost no deformation in the implant device, additional enforcement of the femur head is only created by the implant device's stiffness.

Discussion

The implant surgery process includes opening the umbrella-shaped device. This device cuts through the cancellous bone and soft tissue inside the femoral head, thus causing element failure. The explicit integration method in Lsdyna is used to simulate the implant process.

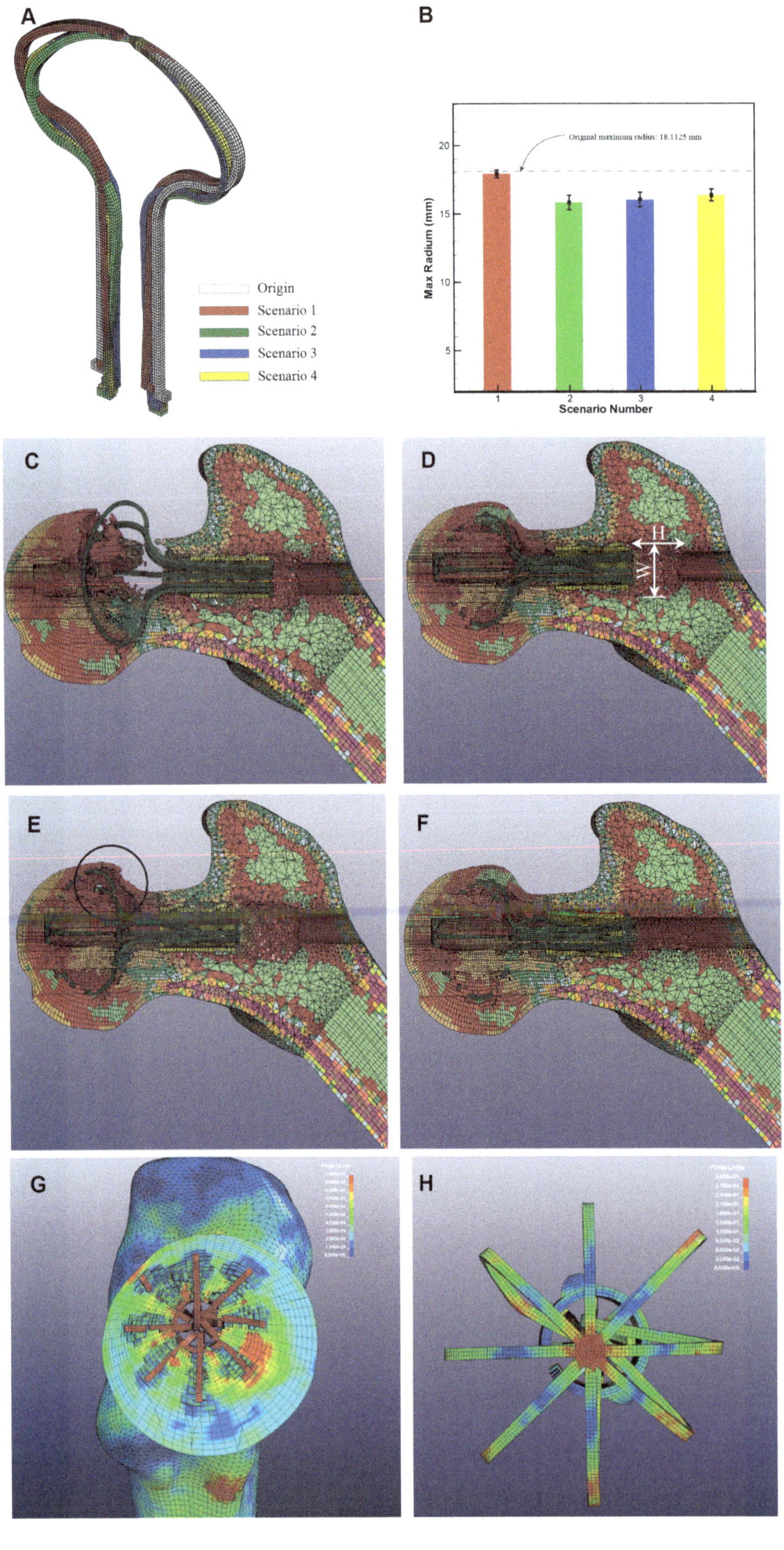
A
B
Origin
Scenario 1
Scenario 2
Scenario 3
Scenario 4
Original maximum radius: 18.1125 mm
Max Radium (mm)
Scenario Number
C
D
H
W
E
F
G
H

Figure 5. Analysis results. (A) Final shape of one typical pair of 4 opposite umbrella arm pairs in each scenario; (B) Statistical figure of maximum radius of each scenario; (C) scenario 1, without constraint; (D) scenario 2, initial position 1, Normal bone quality. H = 22.5 mm, W = 20 mm; (E) scenario 3, with osteoporosis, failure location marked with black circle line; (F) scenario 4, initial position 2; (G) Stress field distrubution inside femoral head in secnario 4; (H) Stress field distrubution of umberalle-shape device in secnario 4.

In this study, a 3-step scheme is used to construct the formal head FEA mesh model. The Correspond Method is used for assigning material to the mixed-element type mesh which is not suitable for auto-assigning material in Mimics. Finally, based on Lsdyna, an analysis is conducted with a dynamic relaxation for the stress initialization wherein the prescribed geometry is obtained from the pre-step.

The simulation revealed that inside the formal head the final shape of the umbrella-shaped device is not the same as the original shape. An outward expansion strain is formed inside the formal head because of the resistance created during the recovery process of the device. Penetration traces corresponding to the umbrella arms were formed inside the formal head. The traces were not strictly made along the radial direction, with some deflection caused by the uneven bone density.

The results of the analysis indicate that the simulation method is suitable and accurate. More specifically, the maximum radius of the simulation's umbrella-shaped device was almost identical to the observation data. Placing the sleeve in the middle (position II) is a better choice than the bottom of the umbrella (position I), because there is no additional damage caused in this position to the decompression channel.

Interestingly, during the simulation we noted that if the patient suffered from severe osteoporosis, and then the operation would fail. More specifically, the failure occurred when the umbrella arm punctured the formal head. In other words, a bone mineral density test will help a doctor determine if a patient is suitable for the implant surgery.

The proposed FEA method for a computational study on the surgery simulation is proven to be reasonable and effective. For an individual patient, different sizes of support devices, initial positions and other conditions can be simulated. In other words, an individual treatment for different patients is possible with pre-FEA for specialized treatment. Our later study will focus on the evaluation of the effect of the Ni-Ti implant treatment by comparing the bearing capacity of the formal head before and after surgery through FEA.

Acknowledgments

The authors would like to thank Kangyu Jia for his contribution to syntax correction.

Author Contributions

Conceived and designed the experiments: ZD. Performed the experiments: QT. Analyzed the data: WY XL. Contributed reagents/materials/analysis tools: WY XL. Wrote the paper: WY XL.

References

1. Zhao G, Yamamoto T, Ikemura S, Motomura G, Mawatari T, et al. (2010) Radiological outcome analysis of transtrochanteric curved varus osteotomy for osteonecrosis of the femoral head at a mean follow-up of 12.4 years. J Bone Joint Surg Br 92B: 781–786.
2. Marker DR, Seyler TM, McGrath MS, Delanois RE, Ulrich SD, et al. (2008) Treatment of early stage osteonecrosis of the femoral head. J Bone Joint Surg Am 90 (Supplement 4): 175–187.
3. Wang Y, Chai W, Wang Z, Zhou Y, Zhang G, et al. (2009) Superelastic cage implantation: a new technique for treating osteonecrosis of the femoral head with mid-term follow-ups. J Arthroplasty 24: 1006–1014.
4. Sugioka Y, HOTOKEBUCHI T, TSUTSUI H (1992) Transtrochanteric anterior rotational osteotomy for idiopathic and steroid-induced necrosis of the femoral head: indications and long-term results. Clin Orthop Relat Res 277: 111–120.
5. Koo KH, Kim R, Ko GH, Song HR, Jeong ST, et al. (1995) Preventing collapse in early osteonecrosis of the femoral head. A randomised clinical trial of core decompression. J Bone Joint Surg Br 77: 870–874.
6. Plakseychuk AY, Kim S, Park B, Varitimidis SE, Rubash HE, et al. (2003) Vascularized compared with nonvascularized fibular grafting for the treatment of osteonecrosis of the femoral head. J Bone Joint Surg Am 85: 589–596.
7. AldridgeIII JM, Berend KR, Gunneson EE, Urbaniak JR (2004) Free Vascularized Fibular Grafting for the Treatment of Postcollapse Osteonecrosis of the Femoral HeadSurgical Technique. J Bone Joint Surg Am 86: 87–101.
8. Shuler MS, Rooks MD, Roberson JR (2007) Porous tantalum implant in early osteonecrosis of the hip: preliminary report on operative, survival, and outcomes results. J Arthroplasty 22: 26–31.
9. Yu X, Jiang W, Pan Q, Wu T, Zhang Y, et al. (2013) Umbrella-shaped, memory alloy femoral head support device for treatment of avascular osteonecrosis of the femoral head. Int Orthop: 1–8.
10. Kainuma R, Matsumoto M, Honma T. The mechanism of the all-round shape memory effect in a Ni-rich TiNi alloy; 1986. 717–722.
11. Christ D, Reese S (2009) A finite element model for shape memory alloys considering thermomechanical couplings at large strains. Int J Solids Struct 46: 3694–3709.
12. Necchi S, Taschieri S, Petrini L, Migliavacca F (2008) Mechanical behaviour of nickel-titanium rotary endodontic instruments in simulated clinical conditions: a computational study. Int Endod J 41: 939–949.
13. Auricchio F, Taylor RL (1997) Shape-memory alloys: modelling and numerical simulations of the finite-strain superelastic behavior. Comput Method Appl Mech Eng 143: 175–194.
14. Gibson LJ, Ashby MF (1999) Cellular solids: structure and properties: Cambridge university press. 449 p.
15. Burgers TA, Mason J, Niebur G, Ploeg HL (2008) Compressive properties of trabecular bone in the distal femur. J Biomech 41: 1077–1085.
16. Tanaka K (1986) A thermomechanical sketch of shape memory effect: one-dimensional tensile behavior. Res Mechanica 18: 251–263.
17. Gao X, Huang M, Brinson LC (2000) A multivariant micromechanical model for SMAs Part 1. Crystallographic issues for single crystal model. Int J Plasticity 16: 1345–1369.
18. Müller I (1979) A model for a body with shape-memory. Arch Ration Mech Anal 70: 61–77.
19. Sun QP, Hwang KC (1993) Micromechanics modelling for the constitutive behavior of polycrystalline shape memory alloys–I. Derivation of general relations. J Mech Phys Solids 41: 1–17.
20. Brinson LC (1993) One-dimensional constitutive behavior of shape memory alloys: thermomechanical derivation with non-constant material functions and redefined martensite internal variable. J Intell Mater Syst Struct 4: 229–242.
21. Lutz AE, Nackenhorst U, von Lewinski G, Windhagen H, Floerkemeier T (2011) Numerical studies on alternative therapies for femoral head necrosis. Biomech Model Mechanobiol 10: 627–640.

15

Control of Bone Resorption by Semaphorin 4D Is Dependent on Ovarian Function

Romain Dacquin[1], Chantal Domenget[1], Atsushi Kumanogoh[2], Hitoshi Kikutani[2], Pierre Jurdic[1], Irma Machuca-Gayet[1]*

1 Institut de Génomique Fonctionnelle de Lyon, Université de Lyon, CNRS, Ecole Normale Supérieure de Lyon, Lyon, France, **2** Department of Immunopathology, Research Institute for Microbial Diseases, Osaka University, Suita, Osaka, Japan

Abstract

Osteoporosis is one of the most common bone pathologies, which are characterized by a decrease in bone mass. It is well established that bone mass, which results from a balanced bone formation and bone resorption, is regulated by many hormonal, environmental and genetic factors. Here we report that the immune semaphorin 4D (*Sema4D*) is a novel factor controlling bone resorption. *Sema4D*-deficient primary osteoclasts showed impaired spreading, adhesion, migration and resorption due to altered ß3 integrin sub-unit downstream signaling. In apparent accordance with these *in vitro* results, *Sema4D* deletion in sexually mature female mice led to a high bone mass phenotype due to defective bone resorption by osteoclasts. Mutant males, however, displayed normal bone mass and the female osteopetrotic phenotype was only detected at the onset of sexual maturity, indicating that, *in vivo*, this intrinsic osteoclast defect might be overcome in these mice. Using bone marrow cross transplantation, we confirmed that *Sema4D* controls bone resorption through an indirect mechanism. In addition, we show that *Sema4D* −/− mice were less fertile than their WT littermates. A decrease in Gnrh1 hypothalamic expression and a reduced number of ovarian follicles can explain this attenuated fertility. Interestingly, ovariectomy abrogated the bone resorption phenotype in *Sema4D* −/− mice, providing the evidence that the observed high bone mass phenotype is strictly dependent on ovarian function. Altogether, this study reveals that, *in vivo*, *Sema4D* is an indirect regulator of bone resorption, which acts via its effect on reproductive function.

Editor: Hector Escriva, Laboratoire Arago, France

Funding: This work was supported by a grant and a fellowship from ARC (Association pour la Recherche contre le Cancer). The funders had no role in study design, data collection and analysis, decision to publish or preparation of the manuscript.

Competing Interests: The authors have declared that no competing interests exist.

* E-mail: imachuca@ens-lyon.fr

Introduction

Osteoporosis is one of the most common bone pathology, which is characterized by a decrease in bone mass, leading to an increased fracture risk. Therefore, slowing the osteoporosis progression has become a major health issue in the aging population of the northern hemisphere. Reproductive hormones fluctuations have a well-established role in osteoporosis. In early menopause, the acute phase of estrogens deficiency is associated with an increased bone loss [1]. However, clinical studies, have provided evidence that the etiology of this disease is more complex than just a question of estrogen withdrawal and that overall bone mass is influenced by many environmental, but also genetic factors [2]. Among those factors, several studies have suggested a role for semaphorin family members in the control of bone mass. *Sema3B* expression in osteoblasts is induced by vitamin D3 and its deficiency leads to osteopenia, secondary to increased osteoclastogenesis [3]. Sema7A is also expressed in bone cells [4]. *Sema7A* as well as *Plexin A2* (Sema 3A receptor) polymorphisms have been associated with decreased bone mineral density and increased fracture risk in postmenopausal Korean woman [5,6]. Deficiency in *Plexin A1*, the *Sema6D* receptor, leads to increased bone mass due to a defect in osteoclast differentiation [7].

Sema4D is a membrane-bound class 4 semaphorin that was first identified in the immune synapse where it mediates cell-to-cell interactions and regulates the immune response [8]. *Sema4D* is in fact expressed in other tissues including platelets, ovaries and the nervous system, where it has several functions [9]. *Sema4D* stimulates both *in vitro* and *in vivo* angiogenesis [10,11]. In the nervous system, *Sema4D* is involved in neuronal migration and neurite outgrowth. For example, *Sema4D* has been shown to regulate gonadotropin hormone-releasing hormone-1 (*Gnrh1*) positive neuron migration through the *PlexinB1-Met* complex [12,13]. *Sema4D* acts on another level of the hypothalamic-hypophyseal-ovarian axis, as *ex vivo* data has shown that *Sema4D* is involved in mouse ovary follicle maturation [14]. Interestingly, structural studies have revealed strong similarities between the *Sema4D* homodimer and the αVß3 integrin heterodimer, which is the most abundant integrin receptor expressed in bone resorbing osteoclasts [15]. αVß3 integrin plays a major role in osteoclast function, both *in vitro* and *in vivo*. For instance, integrin ß3 −/− mice become progressively osteosclerotic with age due to dysfunctional osteoclasts that fail to polarize correctly and develop abnormal ruffled membranes [16]. In the present study, using the loss of function approach, we addressed the question whether *Sema4D* could also play a role in bone resorption. We first show that *Sema4D* is expressed in osteoclasts and that like *ß3integrin*-deficient osteoclasts, *Sema4D* −/− osteoclasts exhibit a resorption defect consecutive to reduced migration and spreading. We then provide evidence that *Sema4D*−/− females displayed a high bone mass phenotype associated to a bone resorption defect. Interestingly this high bone mass phenotype was not found in males and in sexually immature female. Besides this phenotype, we showed that *Sema4D*−/− females exhibited a reproductive defect. Finally, we demonstrate that the bone resorption phenotype does not result from an osteoclast-specific defect but that it is strictly dependent on *Sema4D* action on ovarian function. Thus *Sema4D* is an indirect regulator of bone resorption that acts through its effect on the reproductive system in females.

Results

Sema4D expressed in osteoclasts, delays osteoclasts differenciation and affects osteoclast function

The most abundant integrin in osteoclasts is αVß3 integrin, which plays a major role in regulating the bone resorption process [17]. Because *Sema4D* homodimers share many structural similarities with the αVß3 integrin heterodimer [15], we hypothesized that *Sema4D* could have similar functions. We found that *Sema4D* mRNA, as well as the protein, is expressed in pre- and in mature primary osteoclasts (Figs. 1A–B) [18]. In contrast, *Sema4D* was not detected in primary osteoblasts derived from mouse calvaria (Fig. 1B). Moreover, FACS analysis showed that *Sema4D* is expressed at the osteoclast cell membrane. We further localized *Sema4D* within cytoskeletal structures by specific ß3 integrin co-immunolabeling in mature osteoclasts (Figs. 1C–D). As expected, anti-β3 integrin labeled the podosome belt at the periphery of mature osteoclasts and *Sema4D* partially colocalized with ß3 integrin. These observations were compatible with a role for *Sema4D* in osteoclast mediated bone resorption. To explore the potential effect of *Sema4D* on osteoclast differentiation, we first carried out classical *in vitro* primary osteoclast differentiation assays in the presence of M-CSF and RANKL. Osteoclast differentiation assays of WT or *Sema4D*-deficient bone marrow isolated precursors revealed that differentiation was reduced in the absence of *Sema4D*, as the number of osteoclasts measured in WT cultures was higher that in *Sema4D* −/− on days 4 and 5 (Fig. 1E). In order to assess if the reduced number of osteoclasts obtained in *Sema4D*−/− cultures was due to a proliferation or a fusion defect in progenitor cells, we first performed a proliferation test on osteoclast precursors isolated from *Sema4D* −/− or WT bone marrow in the presence of M-CSF. Crystal violet proliferation tests revealed that bone-marrow derived precursors isolated from *Sema4D*-deficient mice exhibited a small but statistically significant proliferation delay at early time points, which was abrogated after 5 days in culture (Fig. 1F). This later result strongly suggested that the fusion process had decreased, as a consequence of a slightly lower proliferation of *Sema4D* −/− precursors. To definitively prove that the reduced number of *Sema4D* osteoclasts was not due to an intrinsic fusion defect, but to proliferation, we plated 20% more *Sema4D* −/− precursors than WT in the presence of MCSF and RANKL to overcome their slower proliferation rate. Under such plating conditions, the same number of mature osteoclasts was obtained. Indeed, they contained the same number of nuclei as WT, showing that under such conditions the process of differentiation was not affected by *Sema4D* deficiency (Fig. 1G). These plating conditions allowed us to really compare *Sema4D* −/− and WT osteoclasts from the same differentiation stage, and have been used all along this study.

To then test whether osteoclast function could be affected in the absence of *Sema4D*, we performed resorption tests on an apatite collagen complex (ACC) and showed that in the absence of *Sema4D*, the percentage of resorbed area per osteoclast was significantly reduced, by two fold, in the *Sema4D*-deficient osteoclasts compared to WT (Fig. 2A). As resorption by osteoclasts is a multistep process that requires adhesion, spreading, resorption per se, and migration [19], we wanted to determine which of these steps was affected in the absence of *Sema4D*. Measurements by time-lapse video microscopy of WT and *Sema4D* −/− mature osteoclasts (n≥80) revealed that mature *Sema4D*-deficient osteoclasts migrated more slowly than WT osteoclasts (Fig. 2B). Cell spreading was delayed in the absence of *Sema4D* −/− as cell area was reduced during the early stages of adhesion on vitronectin. This difference was not observed at the latest time point, indicating that *Sema4D* −/− osteoclasts were able to make up the delay (Fig. 2C). Altogether, these data indicate that *Sema4D*-deficient osteoclasts migrate more slowly than WT and subsequently resorb mineralized matrix less efficiently than WT osteoclasts.

Altered αVß3 integrin mediated adhesion dependent signaling in *Sema4D* −/− osteoclasts

Osteoclast migration, adhesion and resorption are highly linked processes. They are all promoted by dynamic cytoskeletal reorganization, which involves αVß3 integrin-dependent signaling. Having shown that spreading, migration and resorption are affected in *Sema4D* −/− osteoclasts, we asked whether downstream signaling in response to αVβ3 integrin activation could normally occur in osteoclasts lacking *Sema4D*. To address this question, we analyzed c-Src and Pyk2 phosphorylation, both molecular components of the adhesion complex triggered by αVß3 integrin engagement. Osteoclasts cultured with M-CSF and RANKL for four days were detached and either maintained in suspension or layered on vitronectin coated plates for 30 min. Hyper-phosphorylation of both kinases was observed in the *Sema4D* −/− osteoclasts, either maintained in suspension or adherent as if they were constitutively active in the mutant cells (Fig. 2E). We sought to determine whether further αVβ3 downstream signalling was also perturbed. Rac1-GTPase regulates cellular actin-dynamics, and it is the downstream target of αVß3 induced cytoskeleton reorganization in osteoclasts [20]. In accordance with c-Src and Pyk2 hyper-phosphorylation, we found that the Rac1-GTP content was higher in *Sema4D* −/− osteoclasts, regardless of the substratum (Fig. 2F), whereas the GTP-bound Rac1 level in steady-state osteoclasts was similarly low in both WT and *Sema4D* −/−. In summary, a *Sema4D* deficiency in primary osteoclasts led to reduced resorption activity, in part due to dysfunction of the adhesion properties and an unbalanced regulation of ß3 integrin sub-unit signaling.

Sema4D deficiency leads to high bone mass phenotype due to decreased bone resorption in sexually mature female mice

To determine if *Sema4D* has a function in bone, we first analyzed *Sema4D*-deficient mice using histomorphometry. In 3-month-old female vertebrae, quantification of the trabecular bone volume revealed a 33% increased bone mass in *Sema4D*-deficient mice compared to WT (Fig. 3A). Bone structure was also modified, the thickness of the trabeculae being unaffected, while the number of nodes and the trabecular spacing were significantly lower in *Sema4D*-deficient mice compared to WT, indicating that the number, but not the size, of the trabeculae was modified in the *Sema4D*-deficient mice (Fig. 3B). We then tested resorption parameters *in vivo*. Deoxypiridinoline crosslinks (DPD) were decreased in the *Sema4D*-deficient mice when compared to their WT littermates, showing that the increased bone mass resulted, at least in part, from decreased bone resorption (Fig. 3D). Neither the

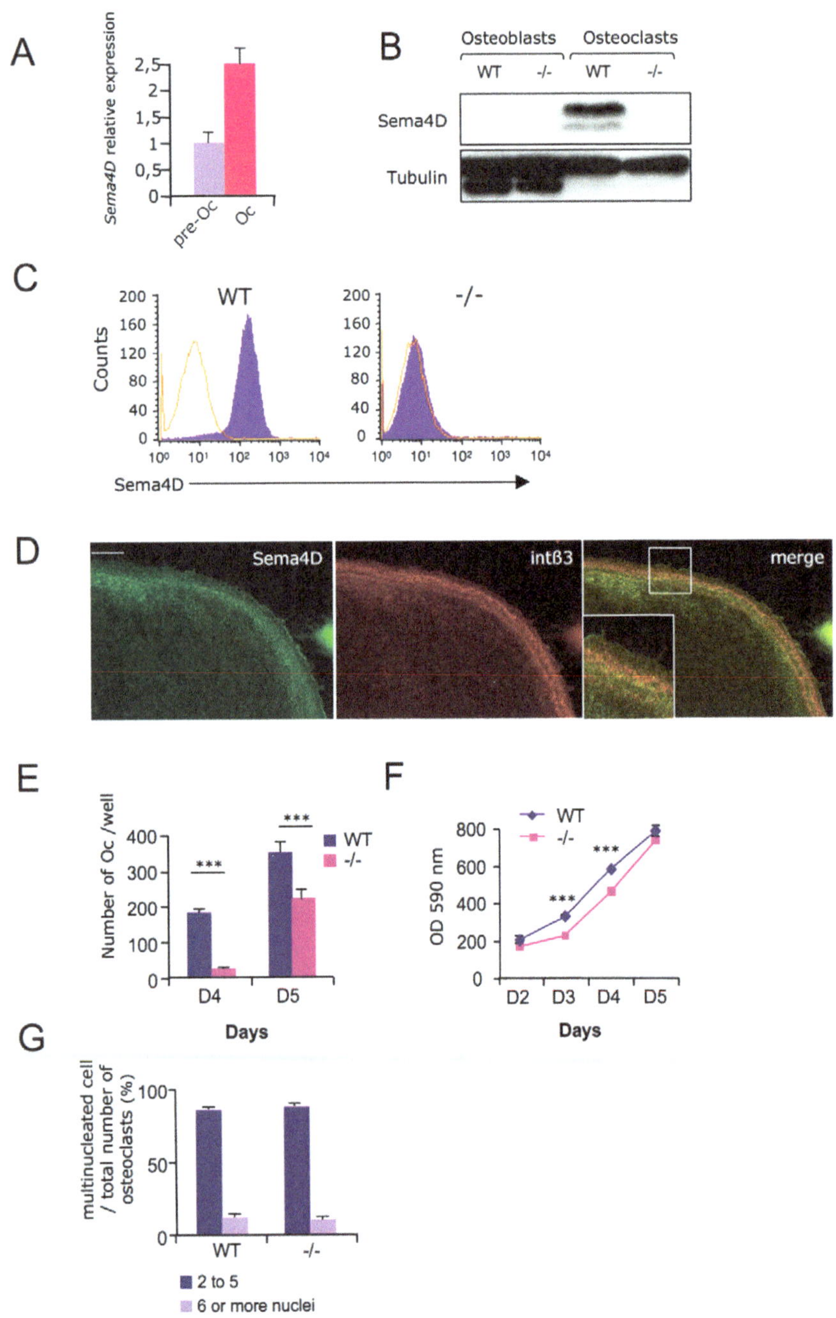

Figure 1. ***Sema4D*** **is expressed in osteoclasts and its deletion delays osteoclasts progenitors proliferation and differentiation** ***in vitro.*** A–D) *Sema4D* expression and localization. A/ QPCR analysis showing an increase of *Sema4D* expression along the osteoclast differentiation pathway, B/ Total cell extract, either from primary calvaria derived osteoblast cultures or from osteoclasts isolated from WT or *Sema4D*-deficient mice, were immunoblotted using an anti-*Sema4D* specific antibody. *Sema4D* is present in WT osteoclasts. α-tubulin was used as loading control. C/ FACS analysis on non-permeabilized pre-osteoclasts shows that *Sema4D* is expressed at the WT cell surface but not in *Sema4D* −/− cells. D/ Mature osteoclasts were fixed and immunolabeled with anti-*Sema4D* or anti-ß3 integrin chain antibodies. Merge picture and inset show that *Sema4D* partially colocalized with the ß3 integrin chain (bar: 10 μm). E–G) *Sema4D* −/− osteoclast progenitors differentiation and proliferation rate. E/ Bone marrow precursor cultured for either 4 or 5 days in the presence of MCSF and RANKL. Cultures were then stained for TRAP activity and TRAP positive multinucleated cells formed were counted. This showed that the formation of TRAP positive multinucleated osteoclasts from *Sema4D* −/− precursors was reduced compared with WT. F/ Bone marrow precursors were cultured in the presence of MCSF to assess proliferation of progenitor cells. At each time point, the cells were fixed and stained with crystal and the 590 nm OD measured, reflecting the cell number. This shows that *Sema4D* −/− precursors proliferate more slowly than their WT counterparts during the growth phase. G/ To confirm that the delay in *Sema4D* −/− osteoclast formation could be due to their impaired proliferation rate, 20% more *Sema4D* −/− bone marrow precursors (375 cells/mm^2) were seeded than WT (312 cells/mm^2) in the presence of M-CSF and RANKL. Mature multinucleated TRAP positive osteoclasts were counted on day 5. Similar osteoclast counts were obtained in both cultures and they displayed the same degree of multinucleation. Error bars represent SEM, *** indicate a p value≤0.001.

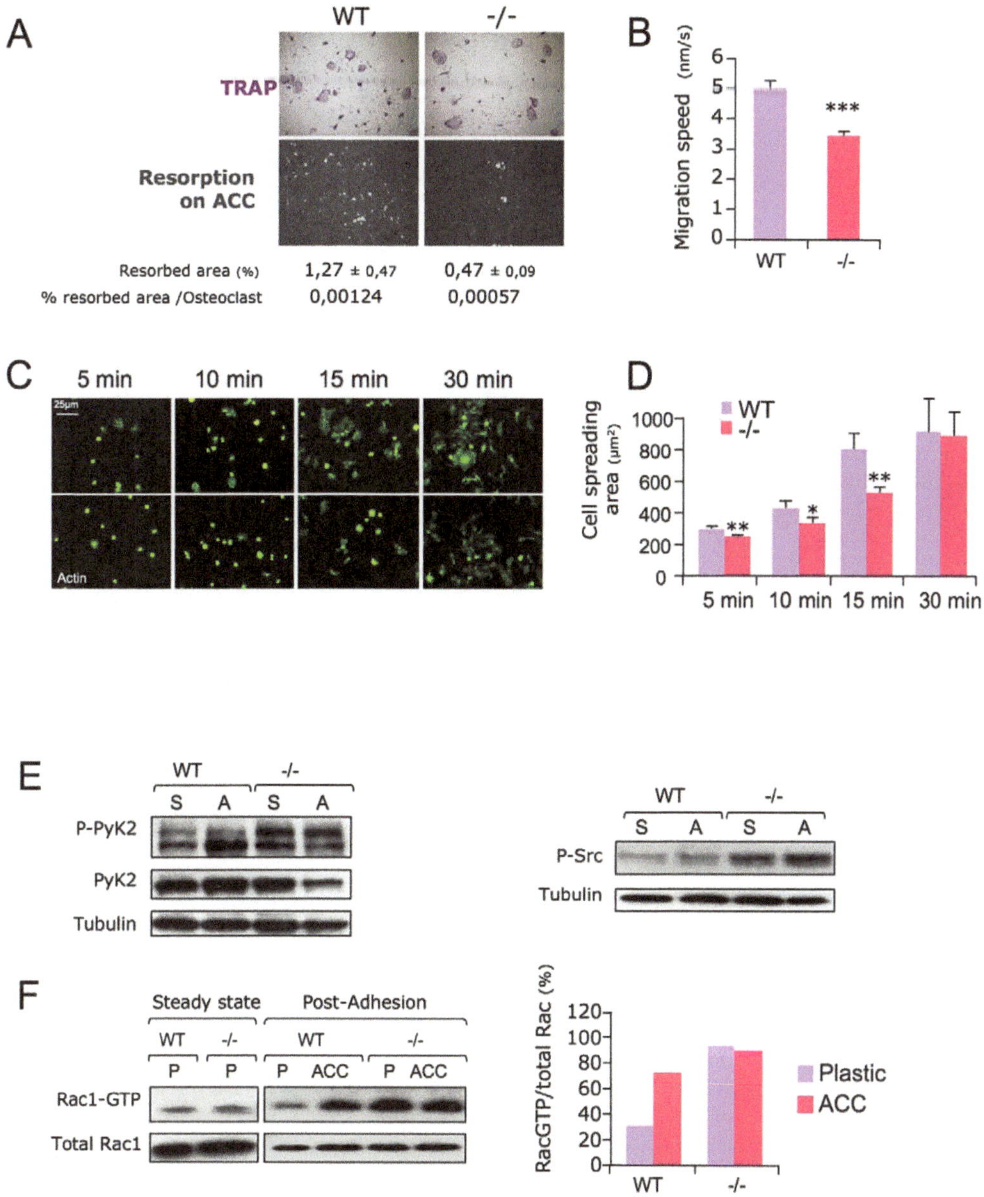

Figure 2. *Sema4D −/−* osteoclasts resorb less than WT and display an altered signaling of ß3 integrin sub-unit mediated adhesion. F/ A/ Resorption tests: osteoclasts were seeded on apatite collagen complex (ACC) coverslips or on plastic. 24 hours after seeding, TRAP staining was performed to assess the number of multinucleated osteoclasts (3 or more nuclei). ACC coverslips were then stained with silver nitrate to measure the percentage of resorbed area (white) versus the total area with ImageJ software micrographs are representaive of several independent experiments. B/ The migration speed of resorbing osteoclasts on ACC was measured by videomicroscopy, followed by software-assisted quantification. C/ Cell spreading ability was assessed by seeding WT and *Sema4D*-deficient osteoclasts on vitronectin- coated coverslips for the stated time. D/ The F-actin content was labeled with 488-Alexa-Phalloidin and the surface area measured using ImageJ software. Results are representative of 3 independent experiments, n≥150 (n = cell number per time point). Error bars represent SEM; * p≤0.01; ** p≤0.001; *** p≤0.0001. E/ Hyperphosphorylation of Pyk2 and c-Src in *Sema4D −/−* osteoclasts compared to WT. Osteoclasts were detached and either maintained in suspension (S) or plated on vitronectin for 30 min and lysed. The Pyk2 and c-Src phosporylation levels were revealed on total cell lysates by immunoblotting with anti-P-Pyk2 or anti-P-c-Src antibodies. This shows hyperphosphorylation of Pyk2 and c-Src in *Sema4D −/−* osteoclasts compared to WT. Increased Rac1 activity in *Sema4D −/−* pre-osteoclasts versus WT. F/ Four-hour-starved pre-osteoclasts were lifted and replated either on plastic (P) or Apatite Collagen Complex (ACC). 1 hour post-adhesion, cells extracts were pulled down for the GTP-bound Rac1 content. Rac1-GTP and total Rac1 were detected by immunoblotting and the corresponding signals were densitometrically quantitated, for steady state analysis, no treatment was applied to cells prior the GTP-Rac1 pull down. Results are representative of at least 3 independent experiments.

number nor the size of osteoclasts had been affected in the *Sema4D*-deficient mice, showing that the decreased bone resorption observed in *Sema4D*-deficient mice was due to a functional defect in the osteoclasts (Fig. 3C). On the other hand, the measured cellular and dynamic bone formation parameters were similar in *Sema4D*-deficient and WT mice (Fig. S1A–B). Altogether these data show that *Sema4D* is indeed a physiological regulator of bone resorption, without affecting bone formation.

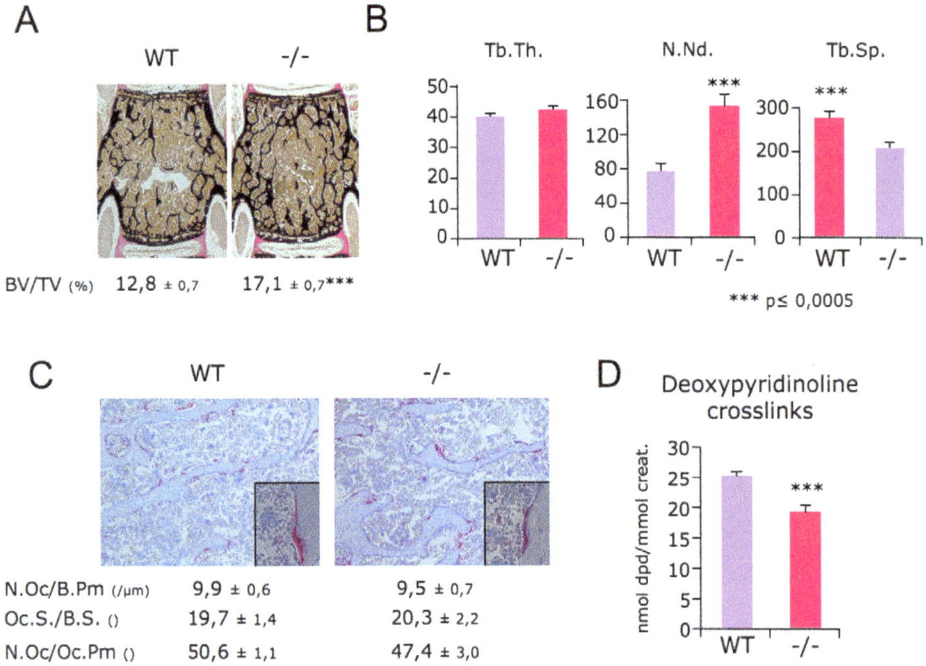

Figure 3. High bone mass and functional bone resorption defect in 3-month-old *Sema4D*-deficient females. A/ Bone volume and bone micro architecture parameters of 3-month-old WT and *Sema4D*-deficient mice were measured on vertebrae sections stained with von Kossa/Van Gieson stain. B/ B.V./T.V., bone volume/tissue volume; Tb.Th., trabecular thickness; N.Nd., number of nodes, Tb.Sp.; trabecular spacing n≥10 for both genotype. C/ *In vivo* quantification of osteoclast numbers and sizes of 3-month-old female vertebral sections stained for TRAP activity and with alcian blue, revealed that osteoclast differentiation is not affected in the absence of *Sema4D*. (N.Oc./B.Pm., number of Oc per bone perimeter; Oc.S./B.S., Oc surface per bone surface; N.Oc./Oc.Pm number of Oc per Oc perimeter) n = 8 for both genotypes. D/ Urinary deoxypyridinoline (DPD) cross-links elimination was significantly lower in *Sema4D* −/− animals compared to WT, indicating that the *Sema4D* deficiency results in a functional decrease in bone resorption n = 8 for WT and n = 14 for *Sema4D*−/− mice. Error bar represents SEM; *** indicate a p value≤0.0001 between two groups.

The bone resorption phenotype of *Sema4D*-deficient mice is gender dependent and is not osteoclast autonomous

We further analyzed the bone phenotypes of WT and *Sema4D*-deficient females at earlier and later stages (1 and 6 months). These analyses revealed that the bone resorption phenotype was only present in sexually mature females, since 6-month-old females had increased bone mass similar to the 3-month-old mice, while 1-month-old *Sema4D*-deficient females had normal bone mass (Fig. 4A). On the other hand, 3-month-old *Sema4D*-deficient males had similar bone mass than their WT littermates (Fig. 4A). Those observations questioned the assumption that the bone phenotype observed in *Sema4D* −/− animals relied on an osteoclast-related intrinsic defect. To answer this question, we performed *Sema4D* −/− or WT bone marrow cross transplants in WT and *Sema4D*-deficient mice, following lethal doses of gamma radiation leading to hematopoietic lineage depletion, including that of osteoclasts. The results of these bone marrow cross transplants revealed that the bone phenotype of the transplanted mice did not depend on the donor genotype but on genetic background of the transplanted mice. Indeed, *Sema4D*-deficient mice had a higher BV/TV than the WT mice, whether they have been grafted with *Sema4D*-deficient or WT osteoclasts (Fig. 4B). Similarly, urinary DPD levels were higher in *Sema4D* −/− recipient mice than in the WT mice regardless of the graft genotype (Fig. S2). Thus, this unexpected result showed that the *Sema4D* −/− bone resorption phenotype is not secondary to an osteoclast-specific defect. In other words, the functional defects of *Sema4D* −/− osteoclasts that we observed *in vitro* are either too mild to be detected *in vivo* or are compensated for *in vivo*. Defective activities of osteoclasts lacking *Sema4D* have revealed an altered ß3 integrin sub-unit down-stream signaling, suggesting a common pathway for both proteins and a functional cross talk. To test this latter hypothesis, we transduced BMMs derived either from WT or *Sema4D* −/− mice, with empty retroviruses (PMX) or retroviruses expressing the full-length ß3 cDNA. After antibiotic selection, mature osteoclasts were differentiated and their ability to resorb mineralized matrix assessed. Over expression of the integrin ß3 chain in *Sema4D* −/− osteoclasts rescued their deficiencies. Indeed, integrin ß3 transduced *Sema4D* −/− osteoclasts were able to resorb mineral matrix to the same extent as WT osteoclasts (Fig. 4C). These results show that the integrin ß3 chain over expression can compensate for *Sema4D* −/− osteoclast resorption defects at least *in vitro* and indicate that *Sema4D* regulates bone resorption by an indirect mechanism *in vivo*.

Reproductive defect in *Sema4D*-deficient mice

While characterizing the origin of the *Sema4D* −/− mice high bone mass phenotype, we noticed that these mice produced fewer pups than WT, suggesting that *Sema4D* −/− mice were less fertile. Quantification of both the number of pups per brood and the number of litters per breeding period confirmed the decreased reproductive ability of *Sema4D*-deficient mice (Fig. 5A–D). We then asked how the *Sema4D* deficiency influenced the decreased fertility observed in these mice. It has been reported that deletion of *Sema4D* receptor plexinB1 (PlexB1) leads to a reduced number of *Gnrh1* secreting neurons in adult mice hypothalamus. We speculated though that *Sema4D*-deficient mice might present a

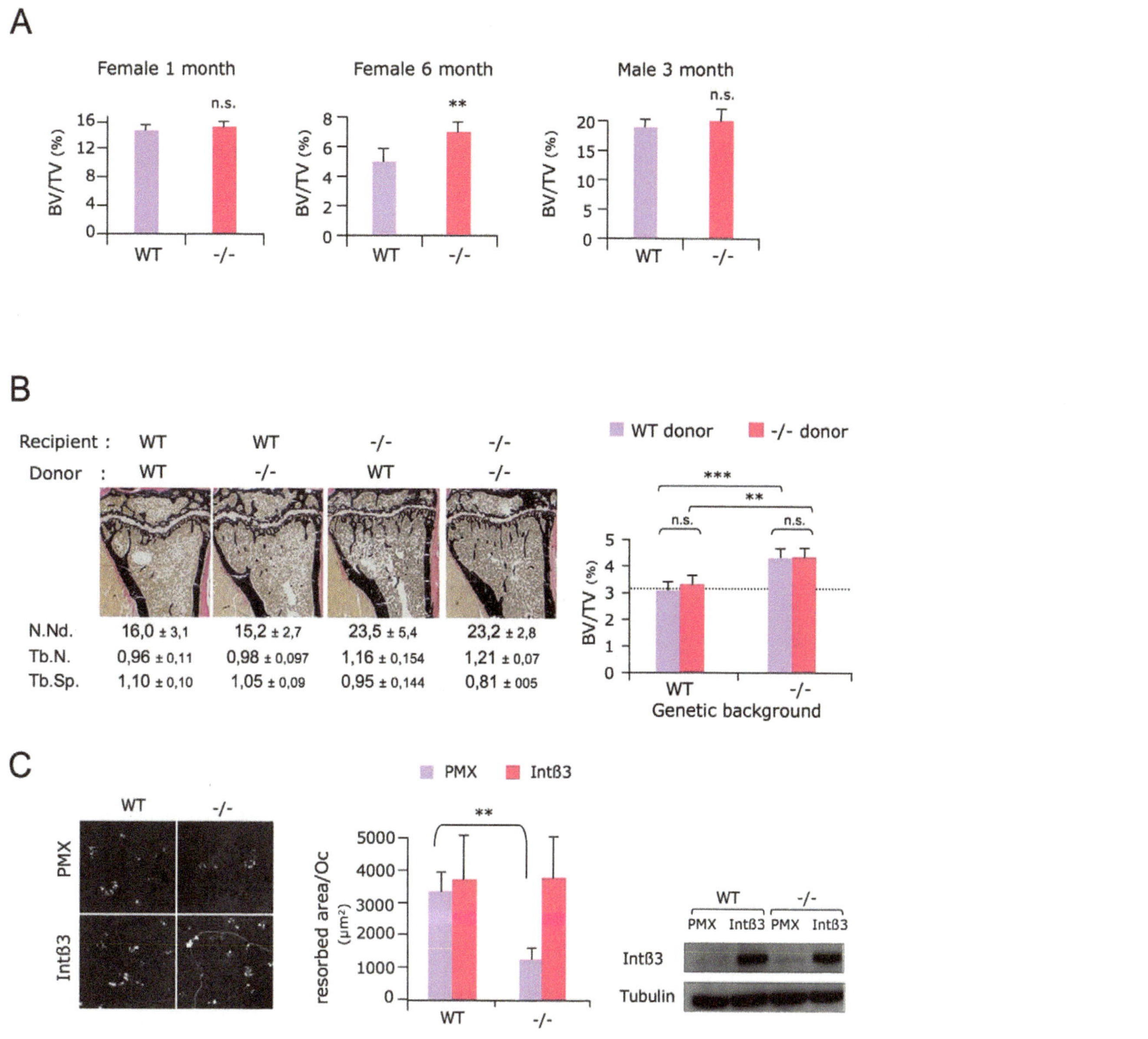

Figure 4. ***In vivo* increased bone mass in *Sema4D −/−* mice is not due to an osteoclast defect.** A/ Bone volume measurement of 1-month-old female and of 3-month-old male vertebrae by histomorphometrical analysis (respectively: n = 9 and n = 11 for WT; n = 9 and n = 12 for *Sema4D−/−* mice), and of 6-month-old femurs by microCT (n = 12 for WT and n = 9 for *Sema4D−/−* mice), revealed that the high bone mass phenotype of *Sema4D −/−* mice is only present in sexually mature females, but not in males. B/ 2-month-old *Sema4D −/−* and WT littermates received lethal doses of γ radiation and were subsequently transplanted with *Sema4D −/−* or WT bone marrow. The bone volume of female femurs was measured by histomorphometry 1 month after transplantation (i.e. in 3-month-old mice) n = 12 per group. C/ Defective resorption of *Sema4D−/−* osteoclasts is compensated by integrin ß3 chain overexpression. Micrographs of a representative experiment show the mineralized resorbed surfaces by transduced osteoclasts. The histogram shows that ß3 integrin chain over-expression in *Sema4D −/−* osteoclasts could rescue their resorption defects. Results represent the mean of two independent experiments (four ACC coverslips were used for each conditions). Total protein lysates of infected osteoclast progenitors were analyzed by western blotting for their ß3 integrin sub-unit content. It shows hß3 integrin expression in lanes Int ß3 compared to lanes corresponding to empty vector PMX transduced cell extracts. Equal loading was assessed by tubulin.

similar phenotype [12]. Indeed, quantitative PCR revealed a 40% reduction in the *Gnrh1* transcript level in the hypothalamus of *Sema4D −/−* mice, whereas no variation was observed in frontal brain used as a tissue control (Fig. 5D). As gonadotropin-hormone releasing hormone-1 (*Gnrh1*) is involved in the hypothalamic-pituitary-ovarian axis, we then wondered if the decreased expression of *Gnrh1* could result in impaired ovarian function, which could explain the decreased fertility observed in *Sema4D −/−* mice. We compared the morphological follicles organization and counted the number of classified follicles in the ovaries of mutant versus WT mice. Analysis of histological ovary sections showed a significant reduced number of secondary follicles in the *Sema4D −/−* mice (Fig. 5E). On the other hand, ovary and uterus weights were similar in three-month-old *Sema4D −/−* females, compared to their WT counterparts (Fig. S3A–B). Accordingly, we did not find any significant variations in the basal levels of estradiol (E2) (Fig. S3B). Altogether our results show that *Sema4D* deficiency is required for proper female reproductive function.

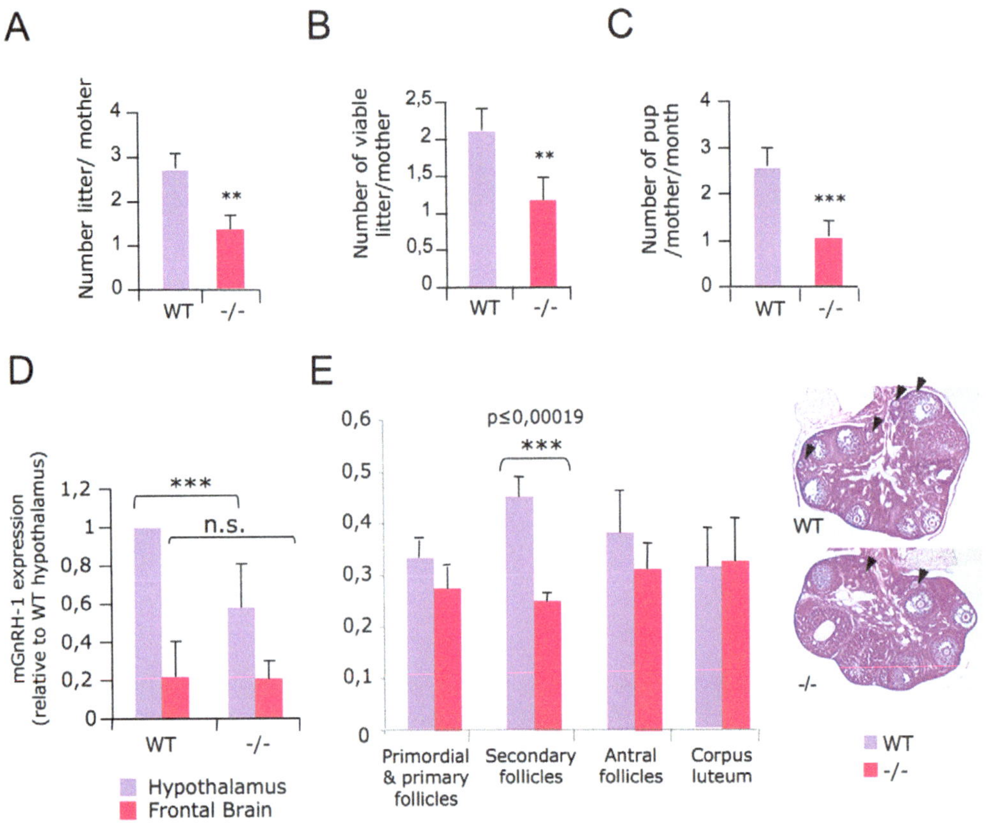

Figure 5. ***Sema4D*** **deficiency decreases fertility and modifies the hypothalamic-pituitary-ovarian axis.** A–C/ Monitoring of mating revealed a statistically significant decrease, in the number of litters per mother, of viable litters and the average number of pups per mother (number of cages n = 7 for WT and 11 for *Sema4D* −/−; performed twice). D/ *Gnrh1* expression in the *Sema4D* −/− adult female brain. Total mRNA was extracted either from total brain or hypothalamus of 3 month-old WT and mutant females. *Sema4D* −/− *Gnrh1* transcript levels were monitored by real time PCR and expressed as fold difference to the WT level, n = 4. E/ Morphological classification and quantification of follicles based on granulosa cell layers. Arrows indicate primordial or primary follicles containing an oocyte surrounded by a layer of granulosa cells. Graph shows the average number of follicles over 9 sections of each phenotype (n = 8).

Sema4D regulation of bone resorption is dependent on female reproductive function

The bone marrow transplant experiment demonstrated that the bone resorption defect observed in *Sema4D* −/− mice did not result in an intrinsic osteoclast defect (Fig. 4B). Moreover this phenotype was observed only in sexually mature *Sema4D* −/− females, but not in males and the *Sema4D* −/− reproductive function was impaired (Fig. 4A and 5A–C). Altogether these results strongly suggested that the *Sema4D* bone resorption defect was dependent on ovarian function. To confirm this assertion, we ovariectomized 2-month-old *Sema4D*-deficient females and analyzed their bone phenotype one month later. As expected, WT ovariectomized mice had a lower uterine weight and lost about 20% of their tibial trabecular bone mass as a result of an increased bone resorption (Fig. 6A–B and S2A). On the other hand, following ovariectomy, *Sema4D*-deficient mice showed a 45% increase in bone resorption than WT mice (Fig. 6B). As a result, *Sema4D* −/− ovariectomized females had similar bone volumes to those of the WT ovariectomized females (Fig. 6A). The observation that the phenotype is osteoclast independent but sex dependent, together with impaired reproductive function, strongly suggests that the *Sema4D* −/− resorption phenotype is directly linked to ovarian function.

Discussion

Although semaphorins were first identified as axon guidance cues, they have since, been shown to be important regulators of a wide variety of biological functions. The present study has uncovered new functions for semaphorin 4D as a regulator of bone resorption both *in vitro* and *in vivo*.

In vitro, *Sema4D* −/− osteoclasts are unable to resorb mineralized matrix properly and this defect is, at least in part, due to altered adhesion ability and subsequently to a migration defect. Remarkably these features are similar to those observed in *integrin β3* −/− osteoclasts, such as defective adhesion, spreading and bone resorption [16]. Together with those similarities, we found that *Sema4D* deficiency in osteoclasts leads to sustain phosphorylation of components of the adhesion complex (Pyk2 and c-Src) (Fig. 2E). This also affects the activity of the downstream effector Rac-1 (Fig. 2F). Moreover, *Sema4D* −/− defective resorption is rescued by integrin β3 chain over-expression.Thus our data show for the first time that *Sema4D* can act as a modulator of αVβ3 integrin downstream signaling in osteoclasts and suggest functional cross-talk between *β3 integrin* and *Sema4D* (Fig. 4C). This might be a general property of *Sema4D*. Notably, *Sema4D* and *β3 integrin* are co-expressed in platelets and it is conceivable that the functional crosstalk between *β3 integrin* and

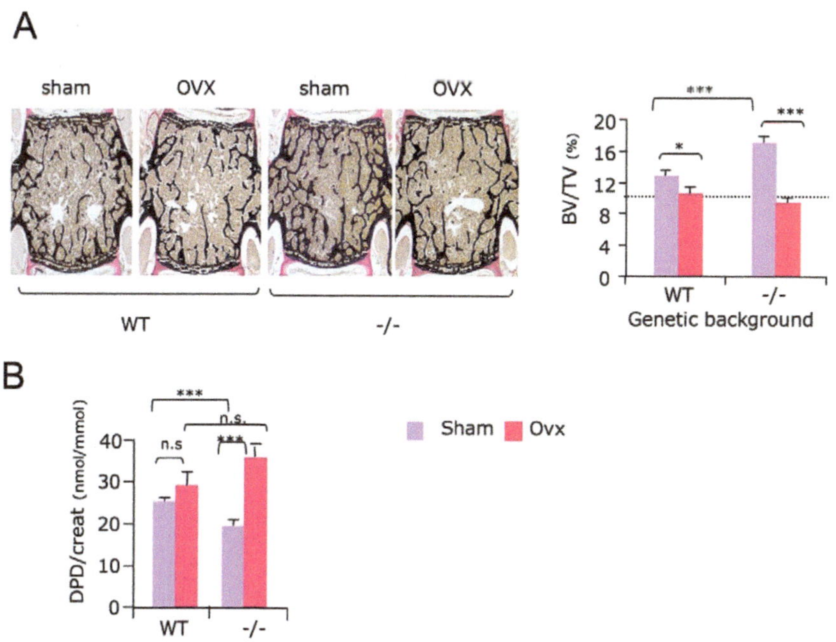

Figure 6. Increased bone mass in *Sema4D −/−* mice depends on ovarian function. A/ Bone volume quantification of 3-month-old *Sema4D −/−* and WT mice vertebrae one month after ovariectomy or sham surgery. B/ Quantification of urinary deoxypyridinoline residues from 3-month-old *Sema4D −/−* and WT mice, one month after ovariectomy or sham surgery show greater increases in bone resorption in *Sema4D −/−* than in WT, (n = 8). Error bar represents SEM; * p≤0.01; ** p≤0.001; *** p≤0.0001.

Sema4D also occurs platelets [9]. Strengthening this idea a very recent study reported that such a crosstalk between *Sema4D* and $\alpha_{IIB}\beta3$ integrin takes place for thrombus formation by platelets [21].

In apparent agreement with the *in vitro* data showing functional defects in osteoclasts, we report that *Sema4D*-deficient females present a high bone mass phenotype linked to defective bone resorption. Histomorphometrical data show a functional rather than a differentiation defect of the osteoclasts in *Sema4D*-deficient females, since their osteoclast numbers and sizes did not differ from WT (Fig. 3B–C). However, this phenotype was gender specific, and only observed in sexually mature females. In addition, bone marrow cross transplant experiments confirmed that the decreased bone resorption *in vivo* was not due to an intrinsic defect in the osteoclasts (Fig. 4A–B). The discrepancy between our *in vitro* and *in vivo* data indicates that the functional defect of *Sema4D −/−* osteoclasts might be compensated for *in vivo* and that, unexpectedly, *Sema4D* controls bone mass mostly through an indirect pathway. Two non-exclusive mechanisms could explain these differences. First, our data suggest a functional cross-talk between ß3 integrin and *Sema4D* as it modulates ß3 integrin intracellular signaling, although they do not interact directly (data not shown). It is thus conceivable, that the *Sema4D* osteoclast-specific effect could be compensated, at least partially, *in vivo*, by ß3 integrin subunit. Second, *in vivo Sema4D −/−* high bone mass phenotype is dependent on mice hormonal status that dominates over the osteoclast intrinsic resorption defect. Therefore, the bone resorption defect observed in *Sema4D*-deficient mice is the result of an indirect mechanism.

In addition to the bone phenotype, we observed that reproduction is impaired in *Sema4D*-deficient mice, revealing a new physiological function of *Sema4D*. Our data showed that the *Sema4D−/−* defective gonadal function could, at least in part, be explained by a significant decrease in *Gnrh1* hypothalamic expression and reduced ovarian follicle maturation (Fig. 5D–E). These latter results obtained from the analysis of *Sema4D−/−* mice abnormalities strengthen two recent reports showing that *Sema4D* is indeed involved in hypothalamic-hypophyseal-ovarian axis development. First, *ex vivo*, *Sema4D* is implicated in mouse ovary follicular development [14]. Second, analysis of *Sema4D receptor PlexinB1*-deficient mice phenotype revealed that *PlexinB1* depletion results in a reduction of *Gnrh1*secreting neuron in mice adult brain due to a defective *Sema4D* induced neuron migration [12].

On the other hand no change was detected in *Sema4D −/−* mice body or uterine weights, in accordance with the fact that these mice have similar E2 blood basal levels as WT mice (Fig. S3A–B). Although no hypogonadism was detected in *Sema4D −/−* mice, they presented a decreased fertility. This observation reminds of clinical cases in women, in which primary ovarian deficiencies were observed along with normal E2 blood levels [22,23]. Although we measured normal basal E2 blood level found in *Sema4D −/−* mice, we cannot also exclude a fine deregulation of E2 cycles. Alternatively, it is also possible that other hormones from the ovarian axis might explain the reproductive function defects and the secondary bone phenotype. Indeed, contribution of other than E2 hypothalamic-hypophyseal-ovarian axis hormones to bone mass regulation has largely been established [1,24,25]. For instance, it has been demonstrated that FSH directly regulate bone mass independently of E2 by activating bone resorption and therefore it might be a potential factor involved in *Sema4D −/−* bone resorption phenotype [24]. In the same way, we did not completely rule out the possibility that *Gnrh1* could act directly on osteoclasts, to promote bone resorption, although it has been shown that *Gnrh1* have no effect on osteoclastogenesis [24] and that hypogonadism is currently associated with bone loss [26]. In addition to the FSH direct effect on bone, recent studies have reported that elevated FSH levels increase bone formation, independently of E2, and that this increased bone formation is correlated to the FSH induced ovarian secretion of inhibin and androgens [27]. There are accumulating evidences showing that gonadal factors, such as inhibins, would regulate bone remodeling either acting on bone formation if their mode of exposure is continuous or bone resorption if it secreted in a cycling mode [28]. This complex endocrine regulation of bone mass by the inhibins can also be observed in woman prior to menopause [29,30]. Thus inhibins might also be good candidates to play a role in the indirect regulation of bone mass by *Sema4D*.

Nevertheless, we have shown the dependence of the *Sema4D* −/− mice bone resorption phenotype on ovarian functions. Beside the gender specificity of the bone resorption phenotype, we found that the ovariectomy of sexually mature *Sema4D* −/− females abrogates the bone phenotype. This result clearly demonstrates the absolute requirement of mature ovaries to observe the bone phenotype in *Sema4D*-deficient female mice (Fig. 6A–B). In summary, our present study demonstrates first that *in vitro* the defective resorption activity of sema4D−/− osteoclast is due to dysfunction of adhesion and migration properties reflected by an hyperphosphorylation of ß3integrin sub-unit down-stream effectors. Secondly, we provide evidence that the observed high-bone mass phenotype of *Sema4D*−/− female mice is due to a functional defective resorption. We show that this *in vivo* effect of *Sema4D* on bone resorption does not result from an osteoclast-specific defect but is rather dependent on the ovarian function by an as-yet-undefined pathway. Thus *Sema4D* is an indirect regulator of bone resorption that acts through its effect on the reproductive system in females. In conclusion, *Sema4D* is a factor involved in the cross talk between bone remodeling and gonadal function.

Materials and Methods

Kits and Reagents

LSM (Lymphocyte Separation Media) and RNA-Now were purchased from Eurobio. α-MEM and fetal calf serum were from Invitrogen and Biowest, respectively. Ascorbic acid, sodium b-glycerophosphate, culture cell BSA and Leukocyte acid phosphatase kit for TRAP staining were from SIGMA. Vitronectin was purchased from BD Biosciences. RNeasy Kit, Quantitec primer assay and Mix-Quantitect SYBR Green were from Qiagen. I-ScripTM cDNA synthesis Kit was from BioRad. Antibodies: anti-*Sema4D* antibodies were BMA12, Abm30 clones and CD16/32 (clone2.4G2) respectively from Cliniscience and BD Biosciences. Anti-P-Pyk2 was from Biosource, anti-P-cSrc (Y-416) from Cell Signaling. Anti-cSrc, , goat anti ß3 integrin, was purchased from Santa-Cruz and hamster anti ß3 integrin from BD pharmingen. Secondary antibodies, mouse and rat IgGs were from Jackson.

The RNeasy Kit, Quantitec primer assay (QT 01062600) and Mix-Quantitect SYBR Green were from Qiagen. I-ScripTM cDNA synthesis Kit was from BioRad. Pyrilinks-D immunoassay and creatinin kits were used according to the manufacturer Quidel Corporation's protocols. E2 levels we measured by EIA from 2 consecutive days collected blood samples (Cayman, Chemical). Statistical differences between groups were assessed using *t*-tests.

Mice

Sema4D-deficient mice were described in [18], were backcrossed with C57BL/6 mice. Background strain characterization by Charles Rivers genetic testing services indicated that 89,43% of the 110 tested markers were specific of the C57Bl6 background.

All mice were maintained in our animal facility and cared for in accordance with institutional guidelines for animal welfare (Approval was given by "the comité regional d'éthique pour l'expérimentation animale" on May 06 2008) with the register approval number 0265). For the induced sex hormone deficiency, 8-week-old female mice underwent ovariectomies (ovx), whereas the controls consisted of sham-operated mice (sham).

Statistical differences between groups were assessed using *t*-tests.

Primary osteoblast cultures from calvaria

Osteoblasts were isolated from enzymatically dissociated calvaria from 3-day-old mice and were plated in differentiation medium: a-MEM) containing 10% heat-inactivated serum 50 g/ml ascorbic acid and 10 mM sodium ß-glycerophosphate. After 24 h, the cells were harvested using 0.01% trypsin in PBS and the cells were plated at 20 cells/mm^2 and grown for 22 days in the same differentiation medium (replaced every two days).

Primary osteoclast cultures

Bone marrow mononuclear cells from 8-week-old WT or *Sema4D* −/− mice were cultured at 500cells/mm^2 for 5 to 6 days in the presence of a-MEM containing 10% (v/v) fetal calf serum, M-CSF (20 ng/ml) and GST-RANKL (30 ng/ml) [31]. We designated as pre-osteoclasts, cells containing 2 to 3 nuclei, obtained after 3 days of culture, whereas osteoclasts were multinucleated cells showing 5 to 10 nuclei and mature osteoclasts were large multinucleated cells with a high number of nuclei (n≥10). TRAP activity in cells was assessed after staining with leukocyte acid phosphatase kit (Sigma).

Quantification of proliferation

At each time point cells seeded on multi-well plates are fixed in 1,1% glutaraldhedyde for 15 min and washed twice in water and air dried. Prior lysis in acetic acid 10%, cells are stained in crystal violet 0,1% for 20 min, washed and air dried, plates are read at OD 590 nm for quantification.

Adhesion and spreading assay

For *in vitro* spreading assays, osteoclasts were detached with 0.02% EDTA in PBS and washed twice with a-MEM containing 10 mM Hepes and 0.1% culture cell BSA. They were kept in suspension for 2 hours at 37°C and then either maintained in suspension or plated on 5 µg/ml vitronectin-coated dishes, according to the manufacturer's instructions. At the stated time, cells were lysed, and an equal amount of protein was analyzed by Western blotting.

For the spreading assay, osteoclasts were seeded on 5 µg/ml vitronectin pre-coated cover slips for 5, 10, 15 or 30 min and fixed with 4% PFA, permeabilized and F-actin labeled with 488-Alexa-Fluor phalloidin. Cells were imaged with a planNeofluar 20× objective (NA 0.5) using a Zeiss axioplan microscope. The surface area was automatically measured with ImageJ software, using an ImageJ plug-in developed by our imaging facility (Platim IFR128).

BMMs retroviral infection

PMX derived retroviral particles were produced in Plat-E retroviral packaging cells (Cell Biolabs). In parallel PMX -IRES-GFP retrovirus (from Dr. T. Kitamura –Tokyo) was produced using the same conditions to be able to visualize and follow transfection and infection under an inverted microscope. Briefly, on day 1, PMX DNA constructs (PMX empty, or expressing human integrin ß3 chain) were transfected in Plate-E cells with Fugen 6 (Roche), on day 2 fresh media was added. The media was collected on day 4 and centrifuged to remove the cell debris. M-CSF (20 ng/ml) and 8 µg/ml of polybrene (Sigma) were added to supernatant, which was used to infect overnight bone marrow mononuclear cells prepared on day 3 in presence of MEM 10% FCS and 25 ng/ml of M-CSF. The following day, the inoculum was removed and the transduced cells were subjected to blasticidin selection (1 μg/ml) for 2 days in presence of MEM 10% FCS and 20 ng/ml of M-CSF. Then medium was replaced by classical osteoclast differentiation medium (MEM 10% FCS 20 ng/ml of M-CSF and 30 ng/ml of RANK-L for an additional 3days before lifting and seeding the mature osteoclasts on mineral for 24 h [32].

Cell transfer experiments

Two-month-old wild-type or *Sema4D* −/− mice were irradiated with lethal doses of gamma radiation (10 Gray) and reconstituted with a retro-orbital injection of 1 million bone marrow cells derived from wild-type or *Sema4D* −/− mice, un-transplanted mice died after 10 days. One month after grafting, the mice were sacrificed for bone analysis.

Histology and histomorphometric analyses

Non-decalcified bones were embedded in methyl methacrylate, before being stained for Von Kossa, TRAP staining or histological analysis. Mice were injected with 100 μl of a 5 mg/ml of a calcein solution, 6 and 2 days before sacrifice and were processed for plastic embedding, as previously described [33]. Measurements were performed with the OsteoMeasure Analysis System (Osteometrics) using a 3CCD color video DXC-390camera (Sony) coupled to a Leica microscope, according to standard procedure [34].

Morphological classification of follicles

Three-month-old females were sacrificed. Frozen ovaries were sectioned and hematoxylin stained. Results were obtained through averaging all serial sections (200 μM). Follicles were classified according to Myers [35].

RNA extraction and RT-PCR

Real-time RT-PCR was performed using the MXP-3000P PCR-system (Stratagene). Samples were run in triplicate and the cycle parameters were 95°C for 15 min, followed by 40 cycles at 95°C for 30 s, 55°C for 30 s and 72°C for 30 s. Gene expression levels were calculated using the ΔΔCt method. Expression was normalized using the mouse ribosomal gene (Rps17).

Statistical analysis

Statistical differences were analyzed with Student's t-test and error bars represent SEM. Values of $P \leq 0{,}01$ were considered significant. * p≤0.01; ** p≤0.001; *** p≤0.0001 when not otherwise specified.

Supporting Information

Figure S1 A/ Cellular and B/ Dynamic bone formation parameter measurements using alcian blue and double calcein labeling, respectively, show an absence of bone formation defects in 3-month-old *Sema4D* −/− females compared to their WT littermates. (N.Ob./B.Pm., number of Ob per bone perimeter; Ob.S./B.S. Ob surface per bone surface; BFR, bone formation rate; MAR, mineral apposition rate; M.S./B.S., mineralized surface per bone surface). Error bar represents SEM, *** indicate a p value≤0.001 between two groups (n = 12).

Figure S2 Urinary DPD measurement of 3-month-old *Sema4D* −/− and WT irradiated mice one month after transplantation (n = 10 for WT and n = 12 for *Sema4D*−/− respectively).

Figure S3 A/ Uterine weight of 3-month-old *Sema4D* −/− and WT mice: after ovariectomy or sham surgery (n = 7 and 8 respectively). B–C/ No significant differences were observed in ovary weight and estradiol levels in 3 month-old females (n = 8 and n = 20 respectively). Error bar represents SEM, *** p≤0.005.

Acknowledgments

We are grateful to Elodie Decembre for technical assistance, Christophe Chamot and Claire Lionet from the PLATIM imaging platform of SFR BioSciences Gerland (UMS3444/US8) for their help. We thank S. Teitelbaum for kindly providing us with the PMX constructs.

Author Contributions

Conceived and designed the experiments: RD IMG. Performed the experiments: RD IMG CD. Analyzed the data: RD PJ IMG. Contributed reagents/materials/analysis tools: AK HK. Wrote the paper: RD PJ IMG.

References

1. Nicks KM, Fowler TW, Gaddy D (2010) Reproductive hormones and bone. Curr Osteoporos Rep 8: 60–67.
2. Seeman E (2002) Pathogenesis of bone fragility in women and men. Lancet 359: 1841–1850.
3. Sutton AL, Zhang X, Dowd DR, Kharode YP, Komm BS, et al. (2008) Semaphorin 3B is a 1,25-Dihydroxyvitamin D3-induced gene in osteoblasts that promotes osteoclastogenesis and induces osteopenia in mice. Mol Endocrinol 22: 1370–1381.
4. Delorme G, Saltel F, Bonnelye E, Jurdic P, Machuca-Gayet I (2005) Expression and function of semaphorin 7A in bone cells. Biol Cell 97: 589–597.
5. Koh JM, Oh B, Lee JY, Lee JK, Kimm K, et al. (2006) Association study of semaphorin 7a (sema7a) polymorphisms with bone mineral density and fracture risk in postmenopausal Korean women. J Hum Genet 51: 112–117.
6. Hwang JY, Lee JY, Park MH, Kim KS, Kim KK, et al. (2006) Association of PLXNA2 polymorphisms with vertebral fracture risk and bone mineral density in postmenopausal Korean population. Osteoporos Int 17: 1592–1601.
7. Takegahara N, Takamatsu H, Toyofuku T, Tsujimura T, Okuno T, et al. (2006) Plexin-A1 and its interaction with DAP12 in immune responses and bone homeostasis. Nat Cell Biol 8: 615–622.
8. Kikutani H, Suzuki K, Kumanogoh A (2007) Immune semaphorins: increasing members and their diverse roles. Adv Immunol 93: 121–143.
9. Zhu L, Bergmeier W, Wu J, Jiang H, Stalker TJ, et al. (2007) Regulated surface expression and shedding support a dual role for semaphorin 4D in platelet responses to vascular injury. Proc Natl Acad Sci U S A 104: 1621–1626.
10. Conrotto P, Valdembri D, Corso S, Serini G, Tamagnone L, et al. (2005) Sema4D induces angiogenesis through Met recruitment by Plexin B1. Blood 105: 4321–4329.
11. Sierra JR, Corso S, Caione L, Cepero V, Conrotto P, et al. (2008) Tumor angiogenesis and progression are enhanced by Sema4D produced by tumor-associated macrophages. J Exp Med 205: 1673–1685.
12. Giacobini P, Messina A, Morello F, Ferraris N, Corso S, et al. (2008) Semaphorin 4D regulates gonadotropin hormone-releasing hormone-1 neuronal migration through PlexinB1-Met complex. J Cell Biol 183: 555–566.
13. Oinuma I, Katoh H, Negishi M (2004) Molecular dissection of the semaphorin 4D receptor plexin-B1-stimulated R-Ras GTPase-activating protein activity and neurite remodeling in hippocampal neurons. J Neurosci 24: 11473–11480.
14. Regev A, Goldman S, Shalev E (2007) Semaphorin-4D (Sema-4D), the Plexin-B1 ligand, is involved in mouse ovary follicular development. Reprod Biol Endocrinol 5: 12.
15. Love CA, Harlos K, Mavaddat N, Davis SJ, Stuart DI, et al. (2003) The ligand-binding face of the semaphorins revealed by the high-resolution crystal structure of SEMA4D. Nat Struct Biol 10: 843–848.
16. McHugh KP, Hodivala-Dilke K, Zheng MH, Namba N, Lam J, et al. (2000) Mice lacking beta3 integrins are osteosclerotic because of dysfunctional osteoclasts. J Clin Invest 105: 433–440.
17. Ross FP, Teitelbaum SL (2005) alphavbeta3 and macrophage colony-stimulating factor: partners in osteoclast biology. Immunol Rev 208: 88–105.
18. Shi W, Kumanogoh A, Watanabe C, Uchida J, Wang X, et al. (2000) The class IV semaphorin CD100 plays nonredundant roles in the immune system:

defective B and T cell activation in CD100-deficient mice. Immunity 13: 633–642.
19. Saltel F, Destaing O, Bard F, Eichert D, Jurdic P (2004) Apatite-mediated actin dynamics in resorbing osteoclasts. Mol Biol Cell 15: 5231–5241.
20. Faccio R, Teitelbaum SL, Fujikawa K, Chappel J, Zallone A, et al. (2005) Vav3 regulates osteoclast function and bone mass. Nat Med 11: 284–290.
21. Wannemacher KM, Zhu L, Jiang H, Fong KP, Stalker TJ, et al. (2010) Diminished contact-dependent reinforcement of Syk activation underlies impaired thrombus growth in mice lacking Semaphorin 4D. Blood 116: 5707–5715.
22. Katsoff B, Check JH (2008) Secondary amenorrhea with normal ovulatory cycles in a young virgin with normal follicle stimulating hormone levels–a case report. Clin Exp Obstet Gynecol 35: 147–148.
23. Touraine P (2010) [Phenotype-genotype correlation in mutations of the gonadotrophin receptor gene in women]. Ann Endocrinol (Paris) 71: 203–205.
24. Sun L, Peng Y, Sharrow AC, Iqbal J, Zhang Z, et al. (2006) FSH directly regulates bone mass. Cell 125: 247–260.
25. Li JY, Tawfeek H, Bedi B, Yang X, Adams J, et al. Ovariectomy disregulates osteoblast and osteoclast formation through the T-cell receptor CD40 ligand. Proc Natl Acad Sci U S A 108: 768–773.
26. Allan CM, Wang Y, Jimenez M, Marshan B, Spaliviero J, et al. (2006) Follicle-stimulating hormone increases primordial follicle reserve in mature female hypogonadal mice. J Endocrinol 188: 549–557.
27. Allan CM, Kalak R, Dunstan CR, McTavish KJ, Zhou H, et al. Follicle-stimulating hormone increases bone mass in female mice. Proc Natl Acad Sci U S A 107: 22629–22634.
28. Gaddy D (2008) Inhibin and the regulation of bone mass. Curr Osteoporos Rep 6: 51–56.
29. Perrien DS, Akel NS, Edwards PK, Carver AA, Bendre MS, et al. (2007) Inhibin A is an endocrine stimulator of bone mass and strength. Endocrinology 148: 1654–1665.
30. Nicks KM, Fowler TW, Akel NS, Perrien DS, Suva LJ, et al. (2010) Bone turnover across the menopause transition: The role of gonadal inhibins. Ann N Y Acad Sci 1192: 153–160.
31. Anginot A, Dacquin R, Mazzorana M, Jurdic P (2007) Lymphocytes and the Dap12 adaptor are key regulators of osteoclast activation associated with gonadal failure. PLoS ONE 2: e585.
32. Feng X, Novack DV, Faccio R, Ory DS, Aya K, et al. (2001) A Glanzmann's mutation in beta 3 integrin specifically impairs osteoclast function. J Clin Invest 107: 1137–1144.
33. Dacquin R, Davey RA, Laplace C, Levasseur R, Morris HA, et al. (2004) Amylin inhibits bone resorption while the calcitonin receptor controls bone formation in vivo. J Cell Biol 164: 509–514.
34. Parfitt AM, Drezner MK, Glorieux FH, Kanis JA, Malluche H, et al. (1987) Bone histomorphometry: standardization of nomenclature, symbols, and units. Report of the ASBMR Histomorphometry Nomenclature Committee. J Bone Miner Res 2: 595–610.
35. Myers M, Britt KL, Wreford NG, Ebling FJ, Kerr JB (2004) Methods for quantifying follicular numbers within the mouse ovary. Reproduction 127: 569–580.

The Effect of HIV-Hepatitis C Co-Infection on Bone Mineral Density and Fracture

Tyler J. O'Neill[1]*, Laura Rivera[1], Vladi Struchkov[1,3], Ahmad Zaheen[3], Hla-Hla Thein[1,2]

1 Dalla Lana School of Public Health, University of Toronto, Toronto, Ontario, Canada, **2** Ontario Institute for Cancer Research/Cancer Care Ontario, Toronto, Ontario, Canada, **3** Faculty of Medicine, University of Toronto, Toronto, Ontario, Canada

Abstract

Objective: There is a variable body of evidence on adverse bone outcomes in HIV patients co-infected with hepatitis C virus (HCV). We examined the association of HIV/HCV co-infection on osteoporosis or osteopenia (reduced bone mineral density; BMD) and fracture.

Design: Systematic review and random effects meta-analyses.

Methods: A systematic literature search was conducted for articles published in English up to 1 April 2013. All studies reporting either BMD (g/cm^2, or as a T-score) or incident fractures in HIV/HCV co-infected patients compared to either HIV mono-infected or HIV/HCV uninfected/seronegative controls were included. Random effects meta-analyses estimated the pooled odds ratio (OR) and the relative risk (RR) and associated 95% confidence intervals (CI).

Results: Thirteen eligible publications (BMD N = 6; Fracture = 7) of 2,064 identified were included with a total of 427,352 subjects. No publications reported data on HCV mono-infected controls. Meta-analysis of cross-sectional studies confirmed that low bone mineral density was increasingly prevalent among co-infected patients compared to HIV mono-infected controls (pooled OR 1.98, 95% CI 1.18, 3.31) but not those uninfected (pooled OR 1.47, 95% CI 0.78, 2.78). Significant association between co-infection and fracture was found compared to HIV mono-infected from cohort and case-control studies (pooled RR 1.57, 95% CI 1.33, 1.86) and compared to HIV/HCV uninfected from cohort (pooled RR 2.46, 95% CI 1.03, 3.88) and cross-sectional studies (pooled OR 2.30, 95% CI 2.09, 2.23).

Conclusions: The associations of co-infection with prevalent low BMD and risk of fracture are confirmed in this meta-analysis. Although the mechanisms of HIV/HCV co-infection's effect on BMD and fracture are not well understood, there is evidence to suggest that adverse outcomes among HIV/HCV co-infected patients are substantial.

Editor: Wenyu Lin, Harvard Medical School, United States of America

Funding: These authors have no support or funding to report.

Competing Interests: The authors have declared that no competing interests exist.

* Email: t.oneill@mail.utoronto.ca

Introduction

The success of antiretroviral therapy (ART) and other advanced therapeutics in reducing the mortality of human immunodeficiency virus (HIV)-infected patients has changed the clinical course of this disease. HIV infected patients are less likely to experience death as a result of 'AIDS-related' causes, but are susceptible to 'non-AIDS-related' conditions in the course of their treatment [1] including adverse metabolic outcomes of the skeletal system [2,3]. A common comorbid feature is co-infection with hepatitis C virus (HCV). Studies among HIV patients report hepatic-associated effects of chronic HCV infection, including hepatitis, fibrosis, cirrhosis, and carcinoma, are complicated by HIV co-infection [4]. The effect of non-hepatic outcomes, including mechanisms leading to low bone mineral density (BMD) and fractures associated with hepatic osteodystrophy, remains unclear due to limited evidence of the effects of co-infection [5,6,7].

Osteoporosis is a systemic skeletal disorder characterized by low bone mass. Osteopenia (BMD <1 standard deviations of the mean BMD of a sex-matched, young healthy population below normal BMD, i.e. T-score −1 to −2.5) often precedes osteoporosis (i.e. T-score <−2.5), predisposing affected patients to fracture [8,9,10]. Low BMD is prevalent in HIV patients [11]. Although the incidence of fractures among HIV patients is low, they can be debilitating and potentially life-threatening leading to lower quality of life [12,13,14,15,16,17,18,19,20]. Studies have found higher rates of osteoporotic-associated fractures in HIV patients compared to uninfected controls matched for age [21,22]. The use of ART by HIV mono-patients has also been implicated in exacerbating the severity of adverse skeletal outcomes [3,11,21]. However, it is unclear if it is HIV infection per se, ART, or both that lead to bone loss [10].

Multiple cross-sectional studies have reported an association between chronic HCV infections, reduced BMD [23,24,25,26], and increased risk of fracture [27]. HCV co-infection, compared to HIV mono-infected patients, significantly increases the risk of fractures at many sites [7,28,29]. Low BMD is a recognized complication of HIV infection [11], HIV/HCV co-infection [30], or use of ART [3]. Thus, the risk of fracture in co-infected patients may be greater than that of HIV or HCV mono-infected patients. Not only is co-infection globally prevalent [31], with osteoporotic fractures leading to $12–18 billion USD in direct health care costs annually. Loss of productivity from work because of continual pain, increased absenteeism, and psychological factors add significantly to the total cost of low BMD [32].

Conflicting evidence suggests that adverse bone outcomes are common amongst HIV [2] and HCV [29] mono-infected patients. For example, Lo Re et al. [7] did not find any significant difference in risk of hip fracture between HIV/HCV co-infected and HIV mono-infected patients. While in contrast, Lo Re et al. [30] reported a higher rate of hip fracture was found in co-infected patients compared to HCV mono-infected. However, the suspected synergistic effects of co-infection, including increased inflammation and higher risk of vitamin D deficiency [3], on these outcomes have not been reported as a primary outcome. Therefore, the objective of this systematic review and meta-analysis is to estimate the association of HIV/HCV co-infection on adverse skeletal outcomes (low BMD and risk of fracture). Furthermore, this study intends to generate an estimate for the associations of co-infection with both reduced BMD and bone fracture to stimulate investigation in this important area of growing understanding among HIV patients' comorbidities.

Methods

Search Strategy

Using MEDLINE, EMBASE, Cochrane Library (CENTRAL), and Scopus databases available to the University of Toronto, two investigators (VS and LR) performed a systematic search for relevant literature ever published up to 14 April 2013. The search strategy used MeSH terms ("human immunodeficiency virus" OR "human immunodeficiency virus infection" OR "HIV-1") and ("hepatitis co-infection" OR "hepatitis C" OR "HCV") and ("bone disease" OR "bone density" OR "bone mineral density" OR "osteoporosis" OR "osteopenia" OR "fracture" OR "bone fracture"). In addition, grey literature (e.g. government reports, theses) was searched in The NLM Gateway, The American Society for Bone and Mineral Research, and The Annual Conference on Retroviruses and Opportunistic Infections. The references of identified publications were crosschecked through review of references of relevant publications included in the review (Figure 1).

Study Selection

A Publication was considered eligible for inclusion if it: (1) evaluated the association between HIV-1/HCV co-infection and at least one skeletal outcome (BMD or fracture); (2) reported in English; (3) was a full-length, peer-reviewed observational or randomized control trial (RCTs); (4) reported controls that were either HIV or HCV mono-infected, or uninfected/seronegative; (5) had BMD measured by dual energy X-ray absorptiometry (DXA or DEXA); (6) reported the occurrence of osteoporosis or osteopenia as defined by The World Health Organization (WHO) [10]; and/or (7) reported incident pathologic fracture at any location was reported. Pathologic fractures were defined as fractures possibly due to low BMD (at least osteopenia), typically caused by low energy trauma [28]. Studies in non-human populations, individuals <18 years of age, review articles, case reports or studies that lacked relevant controls, studies on HIV-2 or other HIV strains, and those that did not clearly report the outcomes of interest were excluded from the review.

A two-step procedure was used to screen publications by title and abstract followed by full text review by two investigators (LR and AZ) independently. Any discrepancy concerning a publication's relevancy for inclusion was discussed until consensus was reached. If consensus was not reached, two investigators (HHT and TJO) adjudicated publications.

Data Abstraction

Using a standardized abstraction form, data were extracted by two reviewers (LR and TJO) applying inclusion and exclusion criteria. Information extracted from each study included: (1) study factors: publication status, year of publication, study design, duration of follow-up, inclusion and exclusion criteria, sample size; (2) host factors: age, gender, body mass index (BMI), baseline osteoporotic risk factors, fracture risk factors; (3) infection factors (HIV or HCV): HIV severity as measured by CD4 lymphocyte count and HIV RNA viral load, duration of HIV or HCV infection, clinical symptoms; (4) HCV treatment and ART duration and protocol(s); and (5) outcome factors, relating to BMD and/or fracture. The WHO (1994) criteria were used to define osteopenia (T-score −1.0 to −2.5) and osteoporosis (T-score <−2.5) at any anatomical site. Normal BMD was defined as a T-score greater than −1.0. Fracture could have occurred at any anatomical site. Ascertainments of fracture from radiological confirmation, reports of diagnosis from medical or insurance records, or by patient self-report were included.

Publications were included if they were population-based and reported co-infection as an independent variable and BMD (g/cm^2) or incident fracture as outcome measures. Furthermore, included publication were those in which summary estimates, such as odds ratio (OR) or risk ratio (RR) with 95% confidence interval (CI), were reported or if the publication allowed for the estimation of the summary estimates based on reported data.

Statistical analysis

For case-control and cross-sectional designs, if the adjusted OR of osteopenia or osteoporosis were reported, it was extracted along with covariates controlled for in the model. An unadjusted OR was extracted if an adjusted estimate was not reported. Where necessary, risk was estimated from reported odds according to King and Zeng [33]. The measure of association for cohort studies was summarized using the adjusted RR and 95% CI along with covariates.

Unadjusted measures were estimated where appropriate. For BMD, the mean and its standard deviation (SD) of BMD (g/cm^2) at any location for cases and controls were extracted. The T-score was then calculated comparing to a healthy 30-year old Caucasian female [10] and unadjusted odds were estimated. The odds of having a T-score consistent with osteopenia or osteoporosis were pooled to estimate a dichotomous outcome of low BMD. For publications reporting fracture data (e.g. number of fractures in each group), odds or risk and exact 95% CI were estimated using the reported number of individuals with incident fractures compared to controls.

Pooled analyses, comparing co-infected patients with mono- or uninfected controls, were estimated using random effects models to account for both within- and between-study variability [34]. An inverse variance method was used to weight each estimate. If BMD was measured with more than one control group (e.g. study reported both HIV negative and mono-infected controls) and an average was not reported, data were reported as separate studies within a single publication. If a study evaluated BMD at multiple time points, the value from the first measurement (most reflective of baseline) was selected to avoid dependence. Similarly, only

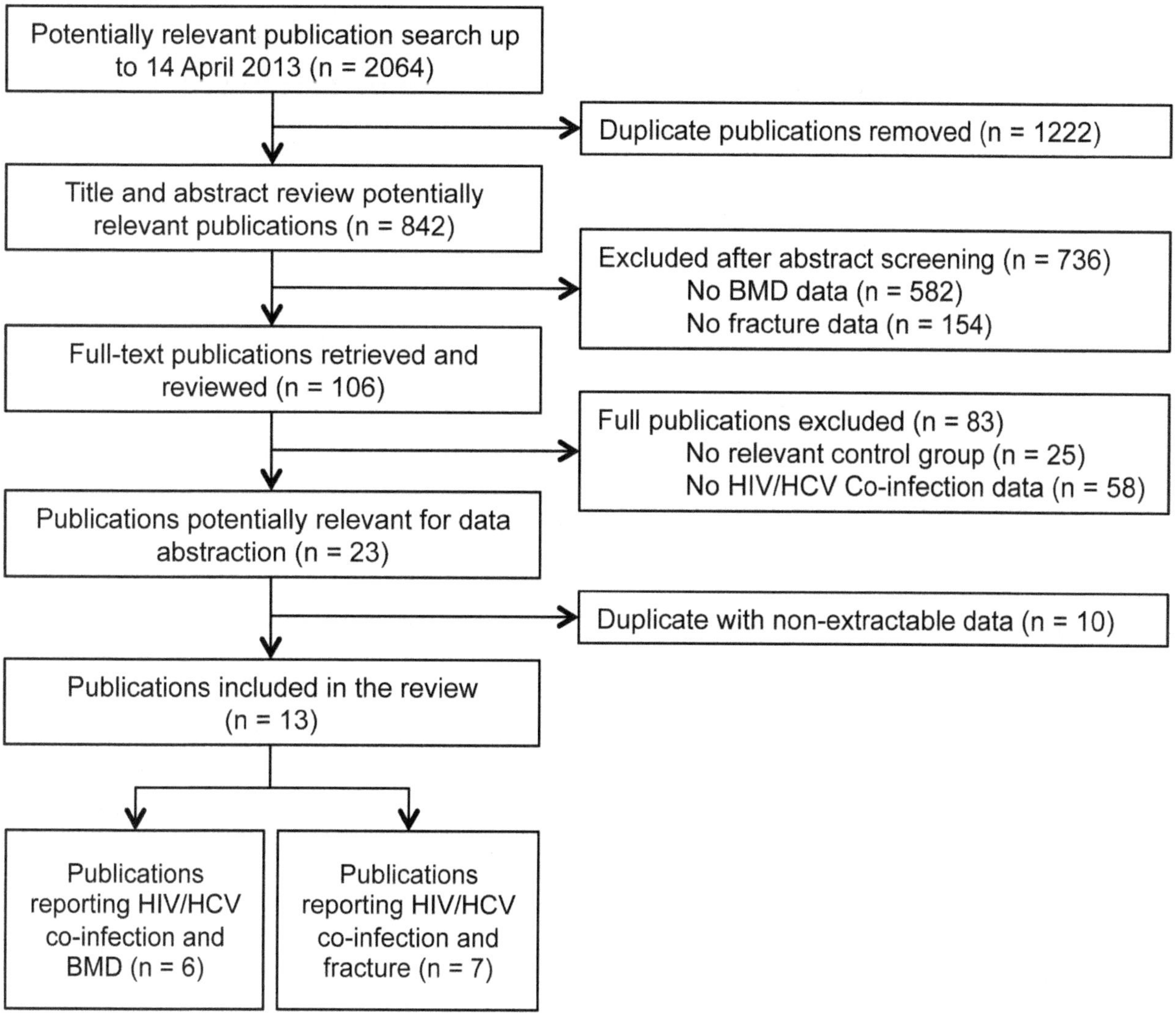

Figure 1. Identification of relevant literature on HIV/HCV co-infection and outcomes of (i) low bone mineral density (BMD) and (ii) fracture. BMD, bone mineral density; HCV, hepatitis C virus; HIV, human immunodeficiency virus.

incident fractures were considered. When sufficient information was provided to stratify data for multiple groups (e.g. gender, age), separate estimates were calculated for each group; again, treating the data as separate studies from a single publication.

The I^2 statistic was estimated as a measure of the total variation in point estimates attributable to between-study heterogeneity [35,36]. The magnitude was interpreted as low ($I^2 \leq 25\%$), medium ($I^2 = 50\%$) and high heterogeneity ($I^2 \geq 75\%$). A χ^2 test was used to assess statistical significance of heterogeneity within each analysis ($\alpha = 0.05$). Sensitivity analyses were employed to determine the causes of heterogeneity by evaluating whether BMD or fracture risk varied significantly based on demographic differences amongst publications. Furthermore, the included publications were selected for step-wise analysis of heterogeneity. Studies were systematically removed and replaced to estimate individual effects on pooled analyses. We evaluated publication bias using Egger regression asymmetry test and Begg's t. The analysis was conducted using Review Manager (RevMan, version 5.2, The Cochrane Collaboration, Copenhagen) and STATA (version 12, StataCorp, College Station, Tx). PRISMA reporting guidelines were adhered to in this publication (Checklist S1).

Results

Selection of Studies

The systematic search identified 2,064 potentially relevant publications (Figure 1). After exclusion of duplicates, and titles and abstracts were screened, 106 independent full-text publications were further evaluated. Studies were subsequently excluded due to lack of relevant control group (n = 25) or no co-infection data reported (n = 58), leaving 23 studies for data abstraction. Ten publications were excluded from abstraction because they did not report BMD or fractures in a co-infected population compared to controls. A total of 13 publications (n = 472,352 subjects) met all inclusion criteria and reported outcome(s) of interest. Manual review of included publication references did not yield any additional articles.

Only one publication required author contact [19] to clarify an adjusted OR point estimate and associated 95% CI due to a clerical error in the original publication. All reported adjusted measures of association were abstracted except one comparison of co- to mono-infected patients from Anastos et al. [19] that required unadjusted estimation of the OR based on reported data.

Demographic and Clinical Characteristics of Included Publications

Published between 2005 and 2012, all included publications reported observational study designs: 7 cohort, 5 cross-sectional, and a single matched case-control (Table 1). Publications were conducted in the United States (n = 7) [7,19,29,38,39,40,41] or Italy (n = 3) [30,37,42], with single publications reporting data from Iran [44], Denmark [28], and Australia [43]. Only effective sample sizes (those used to calculate the measure(s) of interest) were extracted, and ranged from 25 adults from a national multiyear, multicenter cohort [39] to 462,656 individuals in a retrospective cohort analysis of US Medicaid patients [7]. The majority of individuals included were male except for two publications [19,40] with an all-female population. Similar distribution of mean or median ages, BMI, and race was found across publications with no significant differences reported in included publications between cases and controls (Table 1). Lo Re et al. [30] stratified outcomes on gender; Lo Re et al. [7,30] stratified on both age and gender. In the analysis, these were treated as separate studies within each publication.

All studies reported control groups of either HIV mono- [7,19,29,30,39,41,42,43] or uninfected populations [7,19,28,40,44]. Lo Re et al. [7] did not find any significant difference in risk of hip fracture between HIV/HCV co-infected and HIV mono-infected patients. Thus, no data were reported in the publication and were not included in the analysis. In a single publication [30] evaluating rates of incident fracture among co-infected patients and HCV mono-infected controls, a higher rate of hip fracture was found in co-infected patients (HR 1.38, 95% CI 1.25, 1.53). In this study, there were insufficient data for pooled estimates using HCV mono-infection as a comparator.

Details of control selection were reported in all publications selected for pooled analyses. Five studies selected controls from within established cohorts: Lo Re et al. [7,30] used HIV mono- or uninfected controls from the US Medicaid recipients; the ANRS CO8 APROCOC-COPILOTE cohort [39] included HIV mono-infected controls on combination PI-ART; Bedimo et al. [29] used HIV mono-infected patients in the Veterans' Health Administration Clinical Case Registry data; and Anastos et al. [19] and Yin et al. [40] had HIV mono-infected (HAART naïve, non-PI HAART, PI HAART groups) and uninfected female controls, respectively, both from the Women's Interagency HIV Study. ART amongst co-infected patients was also reported in Lo Re et al. [7] compared to antiretroviral treated HIV mono-infected patients. Four publications used population-based controls. The NHANES III cohort in Fausto et al. [42] and Badie et al. [44], described hospital-based controls, matched on age, gender, HBV/HCV infection status, and injecting drug use. The NHAMCS-OPDs cohort in Young et al. [41] obtained controls matched on age and gender. Hansen et al. [28] linked the Danish HIV Cohort study to the Danish Civil Registration System and Danish National Hospital Registry. Hospital-based cohorts were included in three publications with age, gender, and duration of HIV infection individually matched by Yong et al. [43] to mono-infected controls, and HIV mono-infected controls at a single hospital included in Lo Re et al. [7,30].

Individuals on ART at the time of assessment were reported in all publications but one [38] (Table 2). Six publications had an outcome of BMD [19,30,37,38,42,44] whereas 8 reported fracture risk [7,28,29,30,39,40,41,43]. The wrist, hip, and lumbar spine were common locations for assessment of outcomes. All publications used DXA to evaluate BMD. T-scores and Z-scores equivalent to osteopenia or osteoporosis were reported by three [19,42,44] and one [30] publications, respectively. In contrast, less than half of the publications identified incident fracture events by means of International Classification of Disease (ICD) version 9 (ICD-9) [29,43] or 10 (ICD-10) [28]. Diagnosis of fracture was included in the analysis of residents in multiple US states receiving Medicaid [7,30]. Cohort members from the HIV Outpatient Study (HOPS) [43] treated at non-HOPS sites self-reported incident fracture as did Yin et al. [40] and Young et al. [41], who abstracted incident fractures from patient charts similar to Collin et al. [39]. In the meta-analysis of 4 cross-sectional studies, low BMD was increasingly prevalent among co-infected patients compared to those HIV mono-infected (pooled OR 1.98, 95% CI 1.18, 3.31) despite substantial and significant heterogeneity ($I^2 = 83\%$, $p<0.001$) (Figure 2). In contrast, no significant changes in BMD odds or heterogeneity were found by pooling data from two cross-sectional that compared co-infected to uninfected individuals (pooled OR 1.47, 95% CI 0.78, 2.78) ($I^2 = 0\%$, $p = 0.54$). All publications reported adjusted measures.

In the meta-analysis of 5 cohort and 1 case-control study, significant associations between co-infected patients and fracture was estimated compared to HIV mono-infected patients (pooled RR 1.57, 95% CI 1.33, 1.86) with moderate, non-significant heterogeneity ($I^2 = 52\%$, $p = 0.06$) (Figure 3). An increased association with fracture among co-infected individuals compared to those uninfected with HIV or HCV was found from both cohorts (pooled RR 2.46, 95% CI 1.03, 3.88), despite substantial and significant heterogeneity ($I^2 = 94\%$, $p<0.001$), and cross-sectional studies (pooled OR 2.3, 95% CI 2.09, 2.53) with no heterogeneity identified ($I^2 = 1.0\%$, $p = 0.41$). All publications but one [28] reported adjusted measures. There was no evidence of publication bias as indicated by a non-significant Egger test (all $p>0.05$) and Begg's test (all $p>0.05$) in all analyses.

Sensitivity analysis

Moderately attenuated heterogeneity and odds of low BMD (co-infected compared to HIV mono-infected) were found using step-wise publication of a single publication [19] (OR 1.58, 95% CI 1.02, 2.45; $I^2 = 44\%$, $p = 0.17$). Risk of fracture and heterogeneity were substantially attenuated using step-wise publication exclusion of Collin et al. [39] (co-infected compared to HIV mono-infected) (RR 1.51, 95% CI 1.22, 1.71; $I^2 = 31\%$, $p = 0.22$). No significant changes were observed when either analyses were repeated with omission of the total female populations reported in Yin et al. [40] or Anastos et al. [19], or by individual removal of publications from all comparisons.

Discussion

In this meta-analysis, low BMD and fracture was increasingly associated with HIV/HCV co-infection compared to HIV mono-infected and HIV/HCV uninfected or seronegative individuals, suggesting that HCV contributes to a burden a disease greater than HIV infection alone. Despite heterogeneity present in the analysis, the visual trends of the forest plots are suggestive of a positive clinical effect in the population. These findings confirm that co-infection is a risk factor for adverse bone health outcomes. This meta-analysis also confirmed the association between HIV mono-infection and low BMD or fracture as reported in previous studies [2,3]. This is the first attempt to synthesize data across publications to estimate the odds of low BMD or risk of fracture amongst HIV/HCV co-infected patients. Despite significant outcomes, the pooled associations of low BMD or risk of fracture among co-infected patients varied across publications, possibly due to differences in demographics of the study populations.

Table 1. Descriptive characteristics of studies meeting inclusion criteria for low BMD and fracture risk amongst HIV/HCV co-infected patients.

Author	Study Design	Country	N, Total	N, Co-infected (HIV+/HCV+)	Control group(s)		Sex (% Male)		Age (years)	
					N, Monoinfected (HIV+)	N, Uninfected		Ethnicity (% HIV+)		Body Mass Index (kg/m^2, SD)
Anastos 2007	Cross-sectional	USA	387	112	152	123	0	Black (61.3)	36.7 (HIV–)	29.9, 6.72 (HIV–)
									42.1 (HIV+ ART−)	28.9, 6.24 (HIV+ ART−)
								Caucasian (19.7)	40.5 (HIV+ non-PI ART+)	26.8, 5.81 (HIV+ non-PI ART+)
								Hispanic (18.9)	43.8 (HIV+ PI ART+) (median)	28.4, 6.87 (HIV+ PI ART+)
Badie 2011	Cross-sectional	Iran	101	61	40	-	79.2	Middle Eastern (100.0)	39.4, 7.7 (HIV+ ART+)	22.7, 3.40 (HIV+ ART–)
									34.9, 7.3 (HIV+ ART−)	22.7, 3.30 (HIV+ ART−)
									36.6, 10.5 (HIV–) (mean, SD)	22.8, 3.40 (HIV–)
Bedimo 2012	Cohort	USA	951	485	-	466	98.0	Black (56.0)	46 (median)	Not reported
								Caucasian (18.0)		
								Hispanic (23.0)		
								Other (2.0)		
Collin 2009	Cohort	USA	25	13	-	12	77.2	Not reported	36.2 (median)	22.0 (Not reported) (HIV+)
El-Maouche 2011	Cross-sectional	USA	338	Not reported	Not reported	Not reported	55.0	Black (93.8)	42.5, 8 (mean, SD)	23.9, 2.90 (HIV+)*
Fausto 2006	Cross-sectional	Italy	161	55	-	106	64.0	Caucasian (100.0)	38.6, 4.18 (mean, SD)	22.9, 3.16 (HIV+ ART−)
										23.1, 3.47 (HIV+ ART+)
Hansen 2012	Cohort	Denmark	5306	851	Not reported	-	76.0	Caucasian (80.0)	36.7, 30.5–44.5 (mean, 95% CI)	Not reported
Lo Re 2009	Cross-sectional	Italy	1237	625	-	612	62.0	Not reported	43, 10–18 (median, IQR)	23.5, 3.44 (HIV+)*
										23.1, 4.10 (HIV+ HCV+)*
Lo Re 2012	Cohort	USA	462656		366829	95827	63.0	Black (43.1)	39, 33–46 (mean, IQR)	Not reported
								Caucasian (27.4)		
								Hispanic (8.3)		
								Other (21.1)		
Li Vecchi 2012	Cohort	Italy	188	41	76	71	55.9	Caucasian (100.0)	47, 9.7 (HIV+)	22.9, 3.62 (HIV+)*

Table 1. Cont.

Author	Study Design	Country	N, Total	N, Co-infected (HIV+/HCV+)	Control group(s)		Sex (% Male)		Age (years)	
					N, Monoinfected (HIV+)	N, Uninfected		Ethnicity (% HIV+)		Body Mass Index (kg/m^2, SD)
									49, 49, 11.3 (HIV–) (mean, SD)	23.4, 3.81 (HIV–)*
Yin 2010	Cohort	USA	1101	438	663	-	0	Black (56.3)	40.4, 8.8 (HIV+)	28.5, 7.50 (HIV+)
								Caucasian (13.3)		
								Hispanic (27.7)	36.1, 9.9 (HIV–) (mean, SD)	30.0, 8.20 (HIV–)
								Other (3.2)		
Yong 2011	Case-control	Australia	46	16	-	30	88.5	Black (3.0)	49.8 (Case)	24.2, 2.91 (Case)*
								Caucasian (92.0)	49.5 (Control) (mean)	25.6, 3.47 (Control)*
								Asian (5.0)		
Young 2011	Cohort	USA	193	51	-	142	79.0	Black (33.0)	40, 34–46 (median, IQR)	26.7, 4.83 (HIV+)
								Caucasian (51.8)		
								Hispanic (11.7)		
								Other (3.5)		

HIV, Human Immunodeficiency Virus; HCV, Hepatitis C Virus; ART, antiretroviral therapy; CI, confidence interval; IQR, interquartile range; PI, protease inhibitor; SD, standard deviation.
*Mean (SD) estimated from descriptive categorical data reported in publication.

Table 2. Clinical characteristics and reported outcomes of publications included in the HIV/HCV co-infection review.

Author	ART exposure (%)	Reported outcome(s) (classification method)	Location	Co-variates adjusted
Anastos 2007	46.5	BMD (DXA)	Lumbar spine	White, Race, Nadir BMI, HIV+ ART naïve, HIV+ non-PI ART, HIV+ PI ART, post-menopausal
			Femoral neck	
Badie 2011	30.0	BMD (DXA)	Hip	Age, Gender, BMI, Smoking, Alcohol, Exercise, HBV infection, IV drug use, Prison
			Lumbar spine	
Bedimo 2012	69.4	Incident osteoporotic fracture (ICD-9 codes)	Wrist	ART+, CKD, Race, Age, Tobacco use, Diabetes, BMI
			Vertebra	
			Hip	
Collin 2009	100.0	Incident non-stress fracture (patient charts)	Any location	Age, HIV+, HIV-RNA, BMI, Location of birth, PI used first, Alcohol, CD4+ count,
El-Maouche 2011	Not reported	BMD (DXA)	Hip	Gender, Age, BMI, Race, Smoking, Alcohol, IV drug use, Hypogonadal/menopausal, HIV+, Methadone use, ART+, Hormone exposure, Vitamin D
			Femoral neck	
			Lumbar spine	
Fausto 2006	70.2	BMD (DXA)	Hip	Gender, Age, CDC Stage, IV drug use, Lypodistrophy, BMI, CD4+ count, HIV–RNA, HAART+, Length of HIV infection, Bone resorption, Bone formation, Vitamin D
			Lumbar spine	
Hansen 2012	78.0	Incident low energy fracture (ICD-10 codes)	Any location	
Lo Re 2009	79.0	BMD (DXA)	Lumbar spine	Age, Gender, BMI, Length of HIV infection, CD4+ count, ART+, Smoking, Alcohol, Exercise, Amenorrhea, eGFR
			Femoral neck	
Lo Re 2012	100	Incident low energy fracture (Medicaid claim codes)	Hip	Age, Gender, State (location), Propensity score
		BMD (DXA)		
Li Vecchi 2012	93.0	BMD (DXA)	Lumbar spine	Age, Yogurt intake, CD4+, Drug addiction
			Femoral neck	
Yin 2010	65.6	Incident low energy fracture (self-reported)	Hip	HIV+, Age, Race, BMI, Post-menopausal, Fracture before index, Serum creatinine
			Wrist	
			Spine	
Yong 2011	83.6	Incident non-stress fracture (ICD-9 codes)	Any location	HBV status, Previous opportunistic infection, CD4+ count, BMI, HIV-RNA, Duration of viral suppression, Type of DXA performed
Young 2011	72.7	Incident low energy fracture (patient charts; self-reported)	Wrist	Gender, Age, CD4+ count,
			Vertebra	
			Femoral neck	

ART, antiretroviral therapy; BMI, body mass index; CKD, chronic kidney disease; DXA, Dual energy x-ray absorbiometry; eGFR, estimated glomerular filtration rate; HAART, highly active antiretroviral therapy; HBV, hepatitis B virus; ICD, International Classification of Diseases; PI, protease inhibitor.

The inclusion of a co-infected state without regard for the estimated duration of HCV infection relative to HIV infection (and thus, the stage of dynamic fibrosis progression) limits our understanding of infection and its role on either outcome. Although a single study [7] reported significantly greater fracture risk among HCV patients compared to HIV mono-infected patients, we were unable to compare HCV alone to explore the relative contributions of either infection to fractures or BMD. Recent cross-sectional studies have suggested that HCV infected patients with hepatic decompensation have lower BMD than HCV-infected patients with healthy liver function [23,24,30]. The non-hepatic outcomes of HCV remain unclear, including mechanisms leading to low BMD and fractures associated with hepatic osteodystrophy [5,6,7].

Co-infection may have a compounded negative impact on bone strength due to reduced osteoclastic activity and hepatic osteodystrophy leading to increased fractures. This is consistent with findings in this analysis and Lo Re et al. [30], who reported both high odds of low BMD and risk of fracture compared to mono- and uninfected individuals. Unfortunately, no study in this analysis

[A]

Study or Subgroup	Weight	Odds Ratio IV, Random, 95% CI
Anastos, 2007	31.5%	2.93 [2.55, 3.36]
Fausto, 2005	25.0%	1.39 [0.85, 2.27]
Lo Re, 2009 (F)	18.5%	2.99 [1.37, 6.55]
Lo Re, 2009 (M)	25.0%	1.26 [0.77, 2.06]
Total (95% CI)	**100.0%**	**1.98 [1.18, 3.31]**

Heterogeneity: $Tau^2 = 0.21$; $Chi^2 = 17.65$, df = 3 (P = 0.0005); $I^2 = 83\%$
Test for overall effect: Z = 2.59 (P = 0.010)

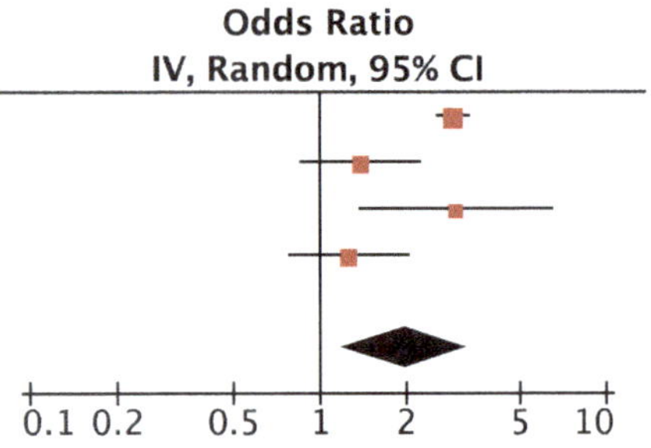

[B]

Study or Subgroup	Weight	Odds Ratio IV, Random, 95% CI
Anastos, 2007	85.5%	1.60 [0.81, 3.18]
Badie, 2011	14.5%	0.91 [0.17, 4.81]
Total (95% CI)	**100.0%**	**1.47 [0.78, 2.78]**

Heterogeneity: $Tau^2 = 0.00$; $Chi^2 = 0.38$, df = 1 (P = 0.54); $I^2 = 0\%$
Test for overall effect: Z = 1.20 (P = 0.23)

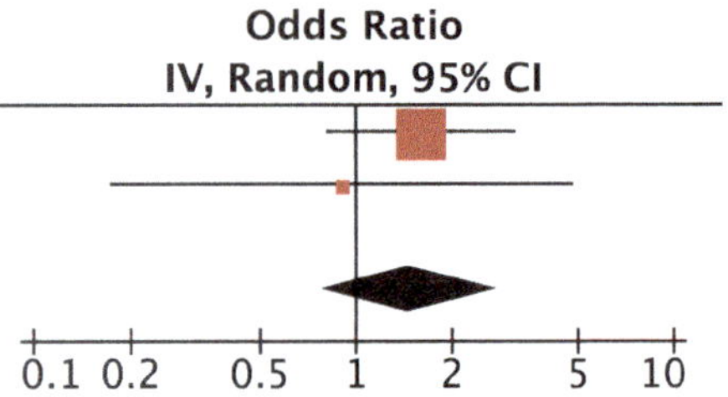

Figure 2. Odds of low bone mineral density between individuals co-infected with HIV and hepatitis C virus compared to HIV mono- (A) or uninfected (B) individuals. HIV, human immunodeficiency virus; HCV, hepatitis C virus.

reported low BMD and risk of fracture as independent outcomes. Therefore, no association between low BMD and fracture risk could be estimated. The theories explaining the causal associations between co-infection and negative skeletal outcomes are reasonable, but require further research into clinical and pathological mechanisms for further clarification.

Risk factors and mechanisms that underlie the increased association between co-infection and low BMD or fracture have not been fully explained. It is likely to be multifactorial, representing complex interactions between infection, traditional osteoporotic risk factors, and ART. It is estimated that up to 9% of all HIV mono-infected patients have low BMD, irrespective of treatment modality [5,54,55] due to chronic inflammation leading to bone resorption [56]. HIV itself may also have direct effects on osteoclastic activity leading to osteoporosis, with the incidence greatly increased among those on ART [56]. Initiation of ART has been associated with 2–6% decrease in BMD over the first two years on therapy [11]. This magnitude in BMD reduction is similar to the first two years of a woman in early menopause. With increased duration of therapy, however, the BMD stabilizes or even improves thereafter. Large subsets of the HIV infected populations (both mono- and co-infected) were on ART of some variation. Insufficient data in the publications on ART duration precluded stratification or adjustment of this potential confounding variable. It is possible that ART patients may have biased the estimates towards a stronger association.

Comparisons between publications are only valid in so far as the groups were demographically similar in other respects. Several studies have reported the prevalence of low BMD in HIV infected patients compared to controls [3,16,50] but few have adjusted for potential confounding variables and heterogeneity of included study groups (e.g. including individuals who acquired HIV through different modes of transmission). No difference of low BMD was estimated between co-infected patients and HIV/HCV uninfected individuals. This may be attributed to the small number of studies included in this analysis of co-infected individuals where the baseline risk of low BMD may have been greater in controls, which lead to conservative estimates.

No association was found when all female populations [19,40] were excluded. It is unlikely that the low BMD was entirely attributed to accelerated bone loss during the menopausal transition given that the reported mean ages were less than the average menopausal woman [52,53] in the United States, where the studies were conducted. Inflammation, leading to bone resorption, and higher risks of vitamin D deficiency have also been reported among mono- and co-infected patients [3,7,8]. Most publications reported a primarily middle-aged (40–55 years) male, Caucasian population. However, non-black race is a known risk factor for osteoporosis as noted in a recent meta-analysis by Shiau et al [2]. It was found that race modified the relationship between HIV infection and fracture, but co-infection was not reported. Although matching was reported in one case control study [43], some publications reported notable differences between HIV-infected individuals that may affect BMD, such as advancing age, menopausal status (estrogen deficiency), smoking history, and alcohol consumption. It is unclear if these potentially modifiable risk factors or other potentially important variables, such as dietary calcium intake, use of medications inducing bone loss (e.g. glucocorticoids), use of antidepressants (e.g. serotonin re-uptake inhibitors), or level of physical activity influenced the results [11,32]. Few publications adequately reported important potential confounding variables (e.g. gender; age; BMI; substance and alcohol consumption; sedentary lifestyle; digestive, renal, and endocrine disorders including diabetes; nadir CD4+ cell count; viral load) that could have potentially biased the measures

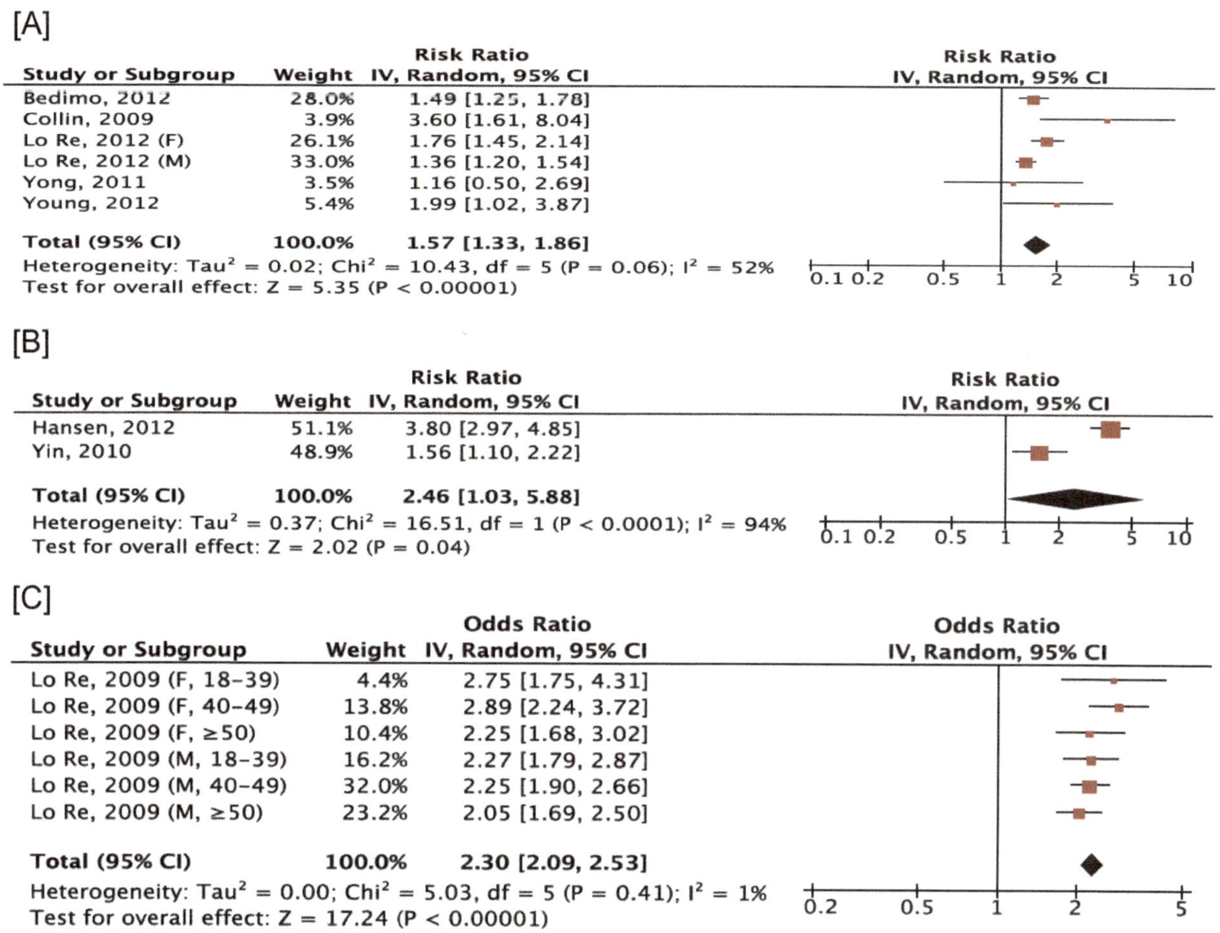

Figure 3. Risk of fracture between individuals co-infected with HIV and hepatitis C virus compared to HIV mono- (A) or uninfected individuals (B), with odds of fracture estimated from cross-sectional studies comparing HIV/HCV co-infected patients to HIV or HCV uninfected individuals (C). HIV, human immunodeficiency virus; HCV, hepatitis C virus.

estimated. Unfortunately, we were unable to adequately adjust in the analysis for this limitation due to inadequate reporting.

Osteopenia is not as sensitive as osteoporosis as a designation of reduced BMD [9]. Developed for post-menopausal women, the T-score has been applied to other adult populations despite controversy around its utility as a metric to quantify bone loss in men and pre-menopausal women [9,48,49]. Thus, age and T-scores are the key predictive factors in determining the BMD testing for screening purposes. The utility of estimating the association of low BMD in co-infected patients relates to the risk of future pathologic fracture. There is a continuous non-linear relationship between BMD and fracture risk [8,46], and measurement of BMD is regarded as the single best predictor of fractures [46,47]. The sensitivity of BMD for fracture prediction is low over most reasonable assumptions, but the specificity is high. Thus, many fractures will occur in individuals with BMD values in the normal range, but fracture risk is quite low. By contrast, fracture risk is very high in individuals with low BMD.

Reporting of fracture diagnosis varied among publications. Studies comparing results of questionnaires and information obtained by medical charts or ICD databases have been inconsistent with both over-reporting and underreporting [51]. The level of misclassification of incident fractures could not be estimated in the included publications and is a limitation of the present study. However, diagnosis of fractures from ICD databases, insurance claims, and charted data for fractures has been reported to be highly valid [45].

This study had several limitations. First, the potential biases of the original studies, methodological issues, and different strategies for adjusting for confounders could affect the results of this meta-analysis. The cross-sectional association may have been confounded by other unadjusted factors or selection bias. Selection bias may also exist in studies using data from electronic records, claims-based, or primary care databases. Second, the number of cohort studies available was limited and the follow-up durations may not be sufficiently long to be able to detect associations. Third, different publications reported different definitions of incident fracture events that would affect the estimates of prevalence/incidence. However, all reported that pathologic fractures were likely due to low BMD [7,28,29,30,40,41,43] or lead to limited activity post-fracture possibly due to osteoporosis [39]. These differences could have also contributed to the observed high heterogeneity seen within some studies [57,58,59]. Last, publication bias may be of concern because studies that report statistically significant results are more likely to be published than studies reporting non-significant results, and this could have distorted the findings in this meta-analysis. Although the Egger's test and Begg's test indicated limited evidence of publication bias, the estimation may not be accurate enough as the number of studies may be insufficient.

The findings in this study add evidence to the importance of monitoring for and informing co-infected patients on the negative outcomes affecting the skeletal system. Increasing studies of multiple morbidities are necessary, as the incidence of co-infection with HIV and viral hepatitis increases and patients live longer. Outcomes will also directly benefit patient health through improved care guidelines (e.g. recommendations to improve physical activity to reduce bone loss once infected). Although the clinical validity of *a priori* chosen measures of association (relative effects) compared to absolute effects (important for interpretation) should be considered, the majority of publications reported adjusted odds or rates with insufficient data to estimate absolute risks. Thus, consideration should be made when interpreting the data as doubling of risk (i.e. 100% greater risk) may only mean an absolute difference of 1% (i.e. from 1 to 2% increase in risk).

In conclusion, this meta-analysis suggests that HIV/HCV co-infection is associated with significantly increased association between HIV/HCV co-infection and low BMD and fractures compared to an uninfected or HIV mono-infected population. The estimated significant cross-sectional and longitudinal associations in the analysis could suggest that there may be an increased risk for adverse bone health outcomes, including pathologic fractures, among co-infected patients. However, the impact of other factors on the estimated outcomes, such as HIV or HCV disease severity and duration, could not be determined. Further controlled, longitudinal studies are necessary to clarify the causal nature of HIV/HCV co-infection according to severity of disease, ART (type or duration), and demographic differences on reduced BMD and risk of fracture. This is especially warranted as the risk of skeletal disease is expected to increase in the future as both HIV and HCV-infected population continue to age. Better understanding of this will provide insight and improvement in screening and early treatment of targeted populations to mitigate fracture risk among aging HIV-infected patients.

Supporting Information

Checklist S1 PRISMA checklist.

Author Contributions

Conceived and designed the experiments: TJO LR HHT. Performed the experiments: TJO LR VS AZ HHT. Analyzed the data: TJO LR HHT. Contributed reagents/materials/analysis tools: TJO LR AZ HHT. Wrote the paper: TJO LR HHT.

References

1. Sackoff JE, Hanna DB, Pfeiffer MR, Torian LV (2006) Causes of death among persons with AIDS in the era of highly active antiretroviral therapy: New York City. Ann Intern Med 145: 397–406.
2. Shiau S, Broun EC, Arpadi SM, Yin MT (2013) Incident fractures in HIV-infected individuals. AIDS 27(12): 1949–57.
3. Brown TT, Qaqish RB (2006) Antiretroviral therapy and the prevalence of osteopenia and osteoporosis: a meta-analytic review. AIDS 20(17): 2165–74.
4. Seef LB (2002) Natural history of chronic hepatitis. Hepatology 36(S1): S35–46.
5. Tebas P, Powderly W, Yarasheski K (2000) Response to 'accelerate bone mineral loss in HIV-infected patients receiving potent antiretroviral therapy' by Drs Weil and Lenhard. AIDS 14(15): 2417.
6. Negredo E, Martinex E, Cinquegrana D, Estany C, Clotet B (2007) Therapeutic management of bone demineralization in the HIV-infected population. AIDS 21(6): 657–63.
7. Lo Re V, Volk J, Newcomb CW, Yang YX, Freeman CP, et al. (2012) Risk of hip fracture associated with hepatitis C virus infection and hepatitis C/human immunodeficiency virus coinfection. Hepatology 56(6): 1699–98.
8. Cummings SR, Nevitt MC, Haber RJ (1985) Prevention of osteoporosis and osteoporotic fractures. West J Med 143(5): 684–7.
9. Kanis JA (1994) Assessment of fracture risk and its application to screening for postmenopausal osteoporosis: synopsis of a WHO report. WHO Study Group. Osteoporosis Int 4(6): 368–81.
10. WHO (World Health Organization) (2000) Prevention and management of osteoporosis: report of the WHO scientific group. WHO Scientific Group on the Prevention and Management of Osteoporosis. Available: http://www.whqlibdoc.who.int/trs/WHO_TRS_921.pdf: Accessed 8 September 2013.
11. McComsey GA, Tebas P, Shane E, Yin MT, Turner Overton E, et al. (2010) Bone disease in HIV infection: a practical review and recommendations for HIV care providers. Clin Infect Dis 51(8): 937–46.
12. Tebas P (2001) Editorial comment: re-emerging infections – implicating the immune reconstitution syndrome. AIDS Read 11(12): 610.
13. Grinspoon SK, Bilesikian JP (1992) HIV disease and endocrine system. N Engl J Med 327(19): 1360–5.
14. Meyer D, Behrens G, Schmidt RE, Stoll M (1999) Osteonecrosis of the femoral head in patients receiving HIV protease inhibitors. AIDS 13(9): 1147–8.
15. Stephens EA, Das R, Madge S, Barter J, Johnson MA (1999) Symptomatic osteoporosis in two young HIV-positive African women. AIDS 13(18): 2605–6.
16. Moore AL, Vashisht A, Sabin CA, Mocroft A, Madge S, et al. (2001) Reduced bone mineral density in HIV-positive individuals. AIDS 15(13): 1731–3.
17. Knobel H, Guelar A, Vallecillo G, Nogues X, Diez A (2001) Osteopenia in HIV-infected patients: is it disease or is it treatment? AIDS 15: 807–8.
18. Thomas J, Doherty SM (2003) HIV infection – a risk factor for osteoporosis. JAIDS 33(3): 281–91.
19. Anastos K, Lu D, Shi O, Mulligan K, Tien PC, et al. (2007) The association of bone mineral density with HIV infection and antiretroviral treatment in women. Antiviral Therapy 12: 1049–58.
20. Paton NIJ, Macallan DC, Griffin GE, Pazianas M (1997) Bone mineral density in patients with Human Immunodeficiency Virus infection. Calcified Tissue Int 61(1): 30–2.
21. Triant VA, Brown TD, Lee H, Grinspoon SK (2008) Fracture prevalence among Human Immunodeficiency Virus (HIV)-infected versus non-HIV-infected patients in a large U.S. healthcare system. Endocrine Care 93(9): 3499.
22. Womack JA, Goulet JL, Gibert C, Brandt C, Chang CC, et al. (2011) Increased risk of fragility fractures among HIV infected compared to uninfected male vetrans. PLoS One 6(2): e17217, doi:10.1371/journal.pone.0017217.
23. Gallego-Rojo FJ, Gonzalez-Calvin JL, Munoz-Torres M, Mundi JL, Fernandez-Perez R, et al. (1998) Bone mineral density, serum insulin-like growth factor I, and bone turnover markers in viral cirrhosis. Hepatology 28(3): 695–9.
24. Gonzalez-Calvin JL, Gallego-Rojo F, Fernandez-Perez R, Casado-Caballero F, Ruiz-Escolano E, et al. (2004) Osteoporosis, mineral metabolism, and serum tumor necrosis factor receptor p55 in viral cirrhosis. J Clin Endocrinol Metab 89: 4325.
25. Leslie WD, Bernstein CN, Leboff MS (2003) AGA technical review on osteoporosis in hepatic disorders. Gastroenterology; 125: 941–66.
26. Rouillard S, Lane NE (2001) Hepatic osteodystrophy. Hepatology 33: 301–7.
27. Cummings SR, Black DM, Nevitt MC (1993) Bone density at various sites for prediction of hip fractures. Lancet 341: 72–5.
28. Hansen ABE, Gerstoft J, Kronborg G, Larsen CS, Pedersen G, et al. (2012) Incidence of low and high-energy fractures in persons with and without HIV infection: a Danish population-based cohort study. AIDS 26(3): 285–93.
29. Bedimo R, Maalouf NM, Zhang S, Drechsler H, Tebas P (2012) Osteoporotic fracture risk associated with cumulative exposure in tenofovir and other antiretroviral agents. AIDS 26(7): 825–31.
30. Lo Re V, Volk J, Newcomb CW, Yang YX, Freeman CP, et al. (2009) Viral hepatitis is associated with reduced bone mineral density in HIV-infected women but not men. AIDS 23: 2191–8.
31. Thein HH, Ti Q, Dore GJ, Krahn MD (2008) Estimation of stage-specific fibrosis progression rates in chronic hepatitis C virus infection: a meta-analysis and meta-regression. Hepatology 48(2): 418–31.
32. USPSTF (U.S. Preventive Services Task Force) (2011) Screening for osteoporosis: U.S. Preventive Services Task Force recommendation statement. Ann Intern Med 154: 356–64.
33. King G, Langche Z (2002) Estimating risk and rate levels, ratios, and difference in case-control studies. Stats Med 21: 1409–27.
34. Hedges LV, Pigott TD (2004) The power of statistical tests for moderators in meta-analysis. Psych Methods 9(4): 426–55.
35. Higgins JPT, Thompson SG (2002) Quantifying heterogeneity in meta-analysis. Stat Med 21(11): 1539–58.
36. Higgins JPT, Thompson SG, Deeks JJ, Altman DG (2003) Measuring inconsistency in meta-analyses. BMJ 327(7414): 557–60.
37. Li Vecchi V, Soresi M, Giannitrapani L, Mazzola G, La Sala S, et al. (2012) Dairy calcium intake and lifestyle risk factors for bone loss in HIV-infected and uninfected Mediterranean subjects. BMC Infect Dis 12: 192.
38. El-Maouche D, Mehta SH, Sutcliffe CG, Higgins Y, Torbenson MS, et al. (2013) Vitamin D deficiency and its relation to bone mineral density and liver fibrosis in HIV-HCV co-infection. Antivir Ther 18(2): 237–42.
39. Collin F, Duval X, Moing VL, Piroth L, Al Kaied F, et al. (2009) Ten year incidence and risk factors of bone fractures in a cohort of treated HIV1-infected adults. AIDS 23: 1021–6.

40. Yin MT, Shi Q, Hoover DR, Anastos K, Young M, et al. (2010) Fracture incidence in HIV-infected women: results from the Women's Interagency HIV Study. AIDS 24: 2678–86.
41. Young B, Dao CN, Baker R, Brooks JT (2011) Increased rates of bone fracture among HIV-infected persons in the HIV Outpatient Study (HOPS) compared with the US general population, 2000–2006. Clin Infect Dis 52: 1061–8.
42. Fausto A, Bongiovanni M, Cicconi P, Menicagli L, Ligabo EV, et al. (2006) Potential predictive factors of osteoporosis in HIV-positive subjects. Bone 38: 893–7.
43. Yong MK, Elliott JH, Woolley IJ, Hoy JF (2011). Low CD4 count is associated with an increased risk in fragility fracture in HIV fracture in HIV-infected patients. JAIDS 57: 205–10.
44. Badie BM, Soori T, Kheirandish P, Izadyar S (2011) Evaluation of bone mineral density in Iranian HIV/AIDS patients. Acta Medica Iranica 49(7): 460–7.
45. Ray WA, Griffin MR, Fought RL, Adams ML (1992) Identification of fractures from computerized medicare files. J Clin Epidemiol 45(7): 703–14.
46. Lofman O, Hallberg I, Berglund K, Wahsltrom O, Kartous L, et al. (2007) Women with low-energy fracture should be investigated for osteoporosis. Acta Orthop 78(6): 813–21.
47. Kanis JA, Melton LJ, Christiansen C, Johnston CC, Khaltaev N (1994) The diagnosis of osteoporosis. J Bone Miner Res 9: 1137–41.
48. Lewiecki EM (2004) Low bone mineral density in premenopausal women. South Med J 97(6): 544–50.
49. Lewiecki EM, Miller PD, Leib ES, Bilezikian JP (2005) Response to "The perspective of the International Osteoporosis Foundation on the Official Positions of the International Society for Clinical Densitometry," by John A. Kanis, et al. J Clin Densitom 8(2): 143–4.
50. Binkley N, Buehring B (2009) Beyond FRAX: It's time to consider "sarco-osteopenia". J Clin Densitom 12(4): 413–6.
51. Siggeirsdottir K, Aspelund T, Sigurdsson G, Mogensen B, Chang M, et al. (2007) Inaccuracy in self-report of fractures may underestimate association with health outcomes when compared with medical record based fracture registry. Eur J Epidemiol 22: 631–9.
52. Hernandez CJ, Beaupre GS, Carter DR (2003) A theoretical analysis of the relative influences of peak BMD age-related bone loss and menopause on the development of osteoporosis. Osteoporos Int 14: 843–47.
53. Palacios S, Henderson VW, Siseles N, Tan D, Villaseca P (2010) Age of menopause and impact of climacteric symptoms by geographical region. Climacentric 13(5): 419–28.
54. Amiel C, Ostertag A, Slama L, Baudoin C, N'Guyen T, et al. (2004). BMD is reduced in HIV-infected men irrespective of treatment. J Bone Min Res 19(3): 402–9.
55. Carr A, Miller J, Eisman J, Cooper D (2001) Osteopenia in HIV-infected men: association with asymptomatic lactic academia and lower weight preantiretroviral therapy. AIDS 15(6): 703.
56. Aukrust P, Haug C, Ueland T, Lien E, Muller F, et al. (1999) Decreased bone formative and enhanced resorptive markers in Human Immunodeficiency Virus infection: indication of normalization of the bone-remodeling process during highly active antiretroviral therapy. J Clinc Endocrin Metab 84(1): 145–50.
57. Egger M (1998) Meta-analysis bias in location and selection of studies. BMJ 316: 61.
58. Stroup DF, Berlin JA, Morton SC, Olkin I, Williamson GD, et al. (2000) Meta-analsysis of observational studies in epidemiology: a proposal for reporting. JAMA 283(15): 2008–12.
59. Huedo-Medina T, Sanchez-Meca J, Marin-Martinez F, Botella J (2006) Assessing heterogeneity in meta-analysis: Q statistic or I2 index? Psychol Methods 11(2): 193–206.

17

Isolation and Characterization of Novel Murine Epiphysis Derived Mesenchymal Stem Cells

Chun-Chun Cheng[1], Wei-Shiung Lian[2,3], Felix Shih-Hsiang Hsiao[1], I-Hsuan Liu[4,5], Shau-Ping Lin[1], Yen-Hua Lee[4], Chia-Chun Chang[4], Guan-Yu Xiao[4], Hsin-Yi Huang[4], Ching-Feng Cheng[2,3], Winston Teng-Kuei Cheng[4,6], Shinn-Chih Wu[1,4]*

1 Institute of Biotechnology, National Taiwan University, Taipei, Taiwan, **2** Department of Medical Research, Tzu Chi General Hospital and Department of Pediatrics, Tzu Chi University, Hualien, Taiwan, **3** Institute of Biomedical Sciences, Academia Sinica, Taipei, Taiwan, **4** Department of Animal Science and Technology, National Taiwan University, Taipei, Taiwan, **5** Research Center for Developmental Biology and Regenerative Medicine, National Taiwan University, Taipei, Taiwan, **6** Department of Animal Science and Biotechnology, Tunghai University, Taichung, Taiwan

Abstract

Background: While bone marrow (BM) is a rich source of mesenchymal stem cells (MSCs), previous studies have shown that MSCs derived from mouse BM (BMMSCs) were difficult to manipulate as compared to MSCs derived from other species. The objective of this study was to find an alternative murine MSCs source that could provide sufficient MSCs.

Methodology/Principal Findings: In this study, we described a novel type of MSCs that migrates directly from the mouse epiphysis in culture. Epiphysis-derived MSCs (EMSCs) could be extensively expanded in plastic adherent culture, and they had a greater ability for clonogenic formation and cell proliferation than BMMSCs. Under specific induction conditions, EMSCs demonstrated multipotency through their ability to differentiate into adipocytes, osteocytes and chondrocytes. Immunophenotypic analysis demonstrated that EMSCs were positive for CD29, CD44, CD73, CD105, CD166, Sca-1 and SSEA-4, while negative for CD11b, CD31, CD34 and CD45. Notably, EMSCs did not express major histocompatibility complex class I (MHC I) or MHC II under our culture system. EMSCs also successfully suppressed the proliferation of splenocytes triggered by concanavalin A (Con A) or allogeneic splenocytes, and decreased the expression of IL-1, IL-6 and TNF-α in Con A-stimulated splenocytes suggesting their anti-inflammatory properties. Moreover, EMSCs enhanced fracture repair, ameliorated necrosis in ischemic skin flap, and improved blood perfusion in hindlimb ischemia in the *in vivo* experiments.

Conclusions/Significances: These results indicate that EMSCs, a new type of MSCs established by our simple isolation method, are a preferable alternative for mice MSCs due to their better growth and differentiation potentialities.

Editor: Giovanni Camussi, University of Torino, Italy

Funding: This work was supported by grants from National Taiwan University (97~99R0066-41) and Council of Agriculture (99AS-1.2.3-ST-aM). The funders had no role in study design, data collection and analysis, decision to publish, or preparation of the manuscript.

Competing Interests: The authors have declared that no competing interests exist.

* E-mail: scw01@ntu.edu.tw

Introduction

Friedenstein and colleagues first defined mesenchymal stem cells (MSCs) in the 1970s as cells that are capable of self-renewal and possess multipotency [1]. Over decades MSCs have been shown to not only be able to differentiate into three mesodermal lineages, including adipocytes, osteocytes and chondrocytes [2,3,4], but also into cells types with non-mesenchymal lineages, such as hepatocytes [5,6], pancreatic-like cells [7,8,9] and neuron-like cells [10,11]. Hence, MSCs have become an attractive cell source for use in regenerative medicine. In addition, the low immunogenicity of MSCs makes them suitable for use in transplantation [12,13,14], and their immunomodulatory properties make them suitable for use in the treatment of many immune disorders [15,16,17].

MSCs were initially obtained from bone marrow [1,4], but they can also be derived from other sources, such as skeletal muscle [18], umbilical cord blood [19,20], dental pulp [21], adipose tissue [22,23] and amniotic fluid [24,25]. MSCs have been successfully isolated and expanded from human [4], rat [26], rabbit [27], canine [26], pig [28] and mouse [29]. Mouse is the most widely used species in laboratory research because they are easy to manipulate and their genetic information is readily available. However, murine is the most difficult species to establish MSCs from BM [30]. Murine BM is composed of heterogeneous cell populations that contain few MSCs (10^{-5}–10^{-6} cells) [31]. In addition, BMMSCs are located near the inner surface of the bone, making it difficult to flush them out [32]. Another problem in establishing mouse BMMSCs is contamination with large amount of hematopoietic cells [33]. Therefore, it is necessary to expand MSCs *ex vivo*. Such manipulation could cause cellular senescence by the loss of proliferation, differentiation and therapeutic potentials [34,35]. This prompted us to look for an alternative source for MSCs with better *ex vivo* expansion capability.

Endochondral ossification occurs during the process of long bone formation in foetal development. Primary ossification occurs at the bone centre for forming marrow cavity, while secondary ossification is formed in the bone epiphysis, followed by the formation of uncalcified cartilage, perichondrium and epiphyseal blood vessel penetration [36,37,38]. Hence, we hypothesized the possibility of a biological niche for mesenchymal progenitors in the epiphysis. In this study, we derived novel MSCs from murine epiphysis without enzymatic digestion. We characterized the morphology, proliferation and functional properties of EMSCs and compared these results with those of BMMSCs under the same cell culture conditions. We also evaluated the therapeutic effects of EMSCs on bone fracture and two types of ischemia mouse animal models. To our knowledge, this is a novel approach for the isolation of MSCs from murine bone.

Results

Establishment of EMSCs

Because surface antigens specific to MSCs have not been identified, MSCs are mainly isolated using their characteristic of plastic adherence. We obtained BMMSCs using a BM flush-out method and EMSCs using our newly developed method for acquiring MSCs (Figure 1A). Epiphysis was dissected out and directly cultured in culture dishes without enzymatic digestion. After seven days of culturing, EMSCs can be observed as triangle, spindle-shaped (Figure 1B), while BMMSCs had a flat, spindle-shaped morphology (Figure 1C). Since both methods had the same problem of hematopoietic cells contamination, we purified the primary culture of EMSCs migrating from epiphysis and BMMSCs from bone marrow by the transient lower-density plastic adherence (tLDA) method [39] to avoid hematopoietic cells contamination. In subsequent passages, EMSCs maintained their characteristic spindle-shape (Figure 1D), whereas BMMSCs changed their morphology and displayed enlarged and flattened phenotypic appearances (Figure 1E).

Characterization of EMSCs

To verify the cells derived from the epiphysis are MSCs, a panel of antibodies against stem cells markers was chosen to evaluate whether the phenotypes of EMSCs are similar to MSCs. EMSCs were positive for most positive BMMSCs markers, such as CD29, CD44, CD73, CD105 (Figure 2A) and with stronger Sca-1 signal than BMMSCs (Figure 2A, 2B), while negative for hematopoietic cells markers, CD11b, CD45 and CD34, and for endothelial cell marker, CD31 (Figure 2A) as BMMSCs (Figure 2B). In addition, EMSCs were positive for markers, CD106, CD166 and SSEA-4 (Figure 2A), while BMMSCs were negative (Figure 2B).

MSCs have reportedly low immunogenicity, because MHC II is not expressed. We found that EMSCs were also negative for MHC II (Figure 2A). Interestingly, EMSCs were negative for MHC I (Figure 2A), whereas BMMSCs were positive (Figure 2B). To test whether the EMSCs are able to express MHC I, we treated EMSCs with 10 ng and 200 ng IFN-γ (Figure 3A, 3B, respectively) and detected the MHC molecules expressions. Although MHC class I and II molecules were not expressed by EMSCs under our isolation method and culture conditions, their expression could be induced by IFN-γ treatment.

Furthermore, we monitored immunophenotype changes that occurred during serial passages. Among the antibody panel used, four surface markers gradually decreased with increased serial passage, including CD73, CD166, SSEA-4 and Sca-1 (Figure 3C), which became more similar to BMMSCs (Figure 2B) but the MHC I expression was still negative even with additional passages (data not shown).

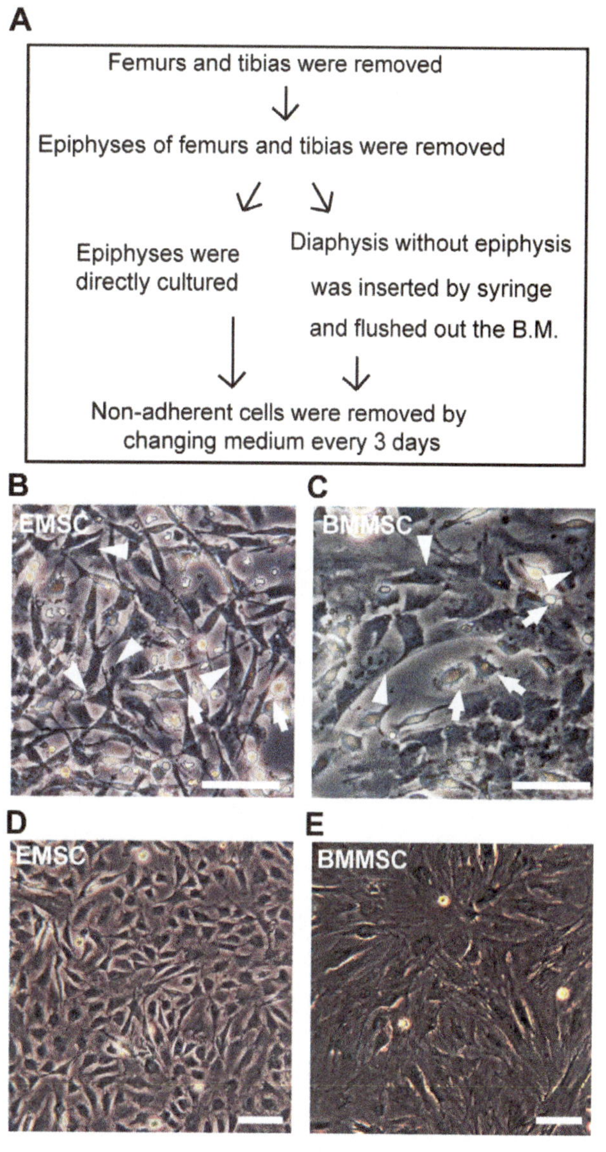

Figure 1. Establishment of EMSCs and BMMSCs. (A) Schematic protocol for the establishment of cultures of EMSCs and BMMSCs. (B) Phase-contrast micrograph of EMSCs in primary culture after seven days. Arrow heads indicate triangle, spindle-shaped, fibroblast-like EMSCs. Lymphohematopoietic cells are indicated by arrows. (C) Phase-contrast micrograph of BMMSCs in primary culture after seven days. Arrow heads indicate flat, fibroblast-like BMMSCs and arrows indicate lymphohematopoietic cells. (D) Phase contrast micrograph of EMSCs at the fifth passage showing that EMSCs maintained their shape during propagating. (E) Phase contrast micrograph of BMMSCs upon the fifth passage showing that BMMSCs became flatted with increasing passages. All the scale bars represent 100 μm.

EMSCs Have Better Proliferation Potential

We evaluated EMSCs proliferation potential using a colony-forming assay. EMSCs formed 23.17±2.92 CFUs, showing significantly higher clonogenic ability than BMMSCs (5.83±1.60 CFUs) (Figure 4A). EMSCs also contained more CFUs that grow into large colonies than BMMSCs (Figure 4B).

The population doubling time (PDT) assay was performed to evaluate the proliferation ability of EMSCs. The curves of both EMSCs at the third and the fifth passages were higher than

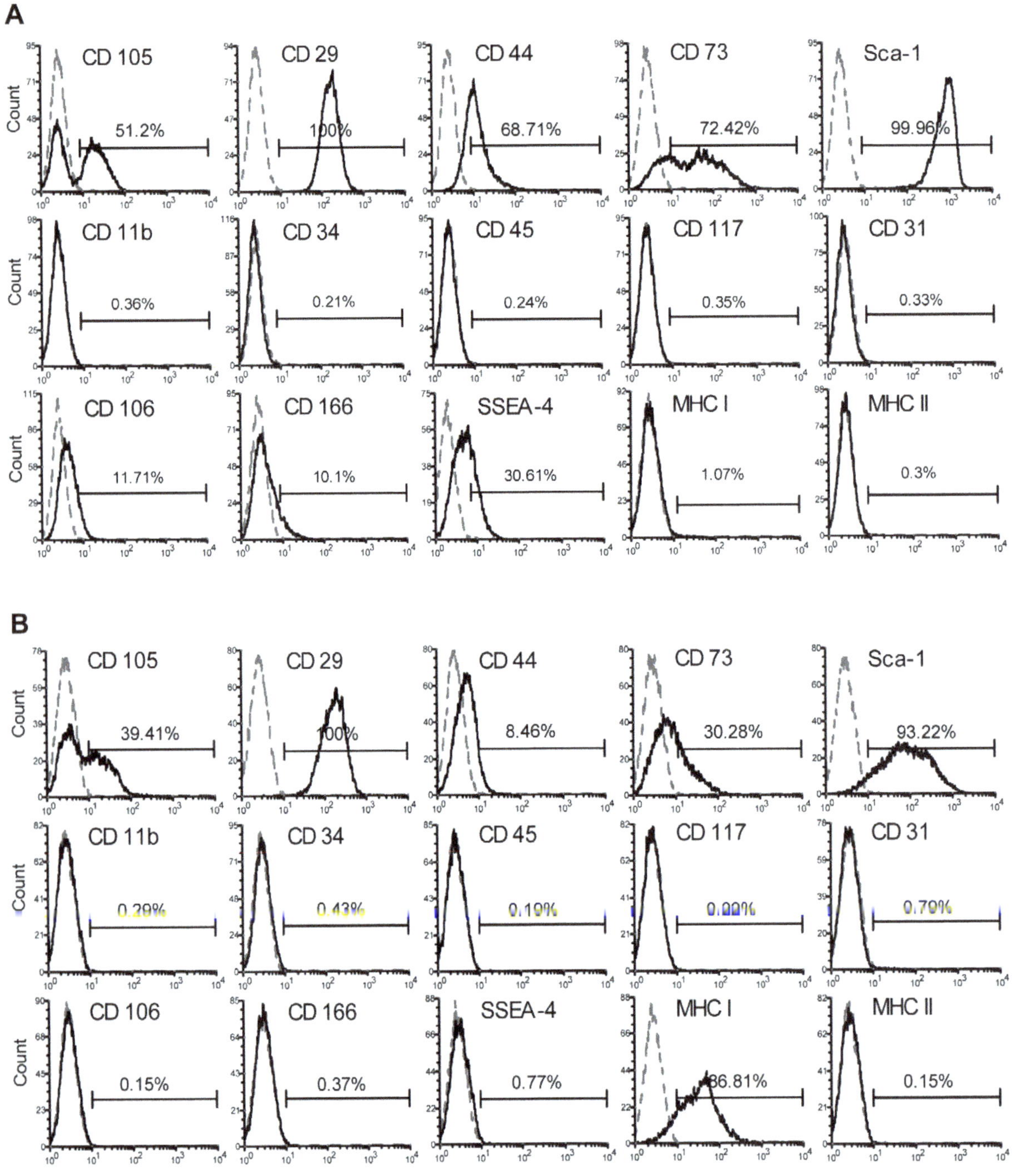

Figure 2. Immunophenotypes of EMSCs and BMMSCs. (A) Flow cytometric analysis of markers related to stem cells, mesenchymal stem cells, hematopoietic cells, endothelial cells and immune cells on EMSCs and (B) BMMSCs at the first passage. The dotted line indicates the respective isotype control.

BMMSCs (Figure 4C), and the PDTs for EMSCs (27.99±2.34 hours at the third passage and 29.51±0.70 hours at the fifth passage) were less than that for BMMSCs (46.63±3.11 and 70.78±5.18 hours) (Figure 4C). Hence, EMSCs showed higher proliferation capability than BMMSCs. We further investigated the propagating ability of EMSCs, and the data showed that EMSCs could be significantly propagated until passage nine in which the cell number was not significantly increased in next passage (Figure 4D). In contrast, BMMSCs could only be propagated until passage five (Figure 4D). Thus, EMSCs can reach to a higher propagating passage than BMMSCs and have higher proliferative potential.

Since telomere length and telomerase activity are in relation to cell proliferation and aging, we further evaluated these properties in EMSCs and BMMSCs, and according by both telomere length and telomerase activity were greater in EMSCs than in BMMSCs (Figure 4E, 4F). Hence, EMSCs derived by our protocol showed higher proliferation potential.

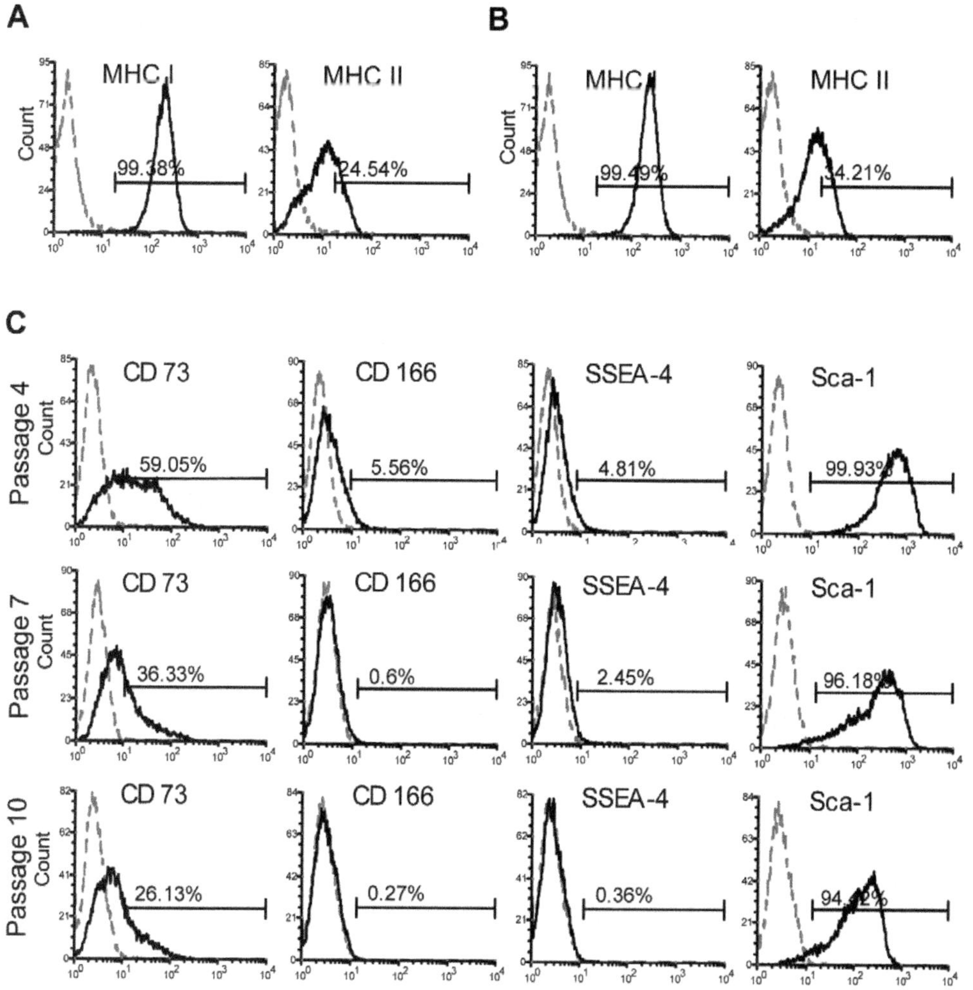

Figure 3. Surface markers analysis of EMSCs after IFN-γ treatment and during increased serial passages. (A) MHC I and MHC II expression profiles for EMSCs (passage five) were analysed under 10 ng or (B) 100 ng IFN-γ treatment. EMSCs were positive for MHC I and MHC II after IFN-γ treatment. (C) EMSCs surface antigen profiles were detected via flow cytometric analysis during increasing passages. The markers of CD73, CD166, SSEA-4 and Sca-1 were decreased with propagating. Respective isotype control is indicated by the dotted line.

EMSCs Show Higher Multipotent Potentials than BMMSCs

Previous studies have demonstrated that MSCs are capable of differentiation into osteocytes, adipocytes and chondrocytes. Firstly, we investigated and compared the *in vitro* adipogenic differentiation capability by culturing EMSCs and BMMSCs in adipogenic induction medium and performing histochemical staining with Oil Red O. EMSCs formed more intracellular lipid droplets upon staining (Figure 5A-i, 5A-ii) compared to BMMSCs (Figure 5A-iii, 5A-iv). Lipid droplets observed in EMSCs were also larger and more apparent. Quantitative analysis of Oil Red O staining showed that EMSCs had significantly better adipogenic differentiation capability than BMMSCs (Figure 5B). Accordingly, quantification of the adipogenic gene expression also showed that EMSCs had stronger expression both in early adipogenesis marker PPARγ (Figure 5C) and late adipogenesis marker LPL (Figure 5D). Furthermore, EMSCs maintained negative expression of MHC I during adipogenesis (Figure 5E).

Secondly, after a seven-day culture period in osteogenic induction medium, EMSCs formed calcium deposition and mature nodules structures, which were stained with Alizarin red S (ARS) (Figure 5F-i, 5F-ii). Compared to BMMSCs (Figure 5F-iii, 5F-iv), EMSCs formed relatively more nodules. Quantitative results from ARS staining showed that EMSCs had better osteogenic differentiation capability than BMMSCs (Figure 5G). The qPCR data showed greater expression of early osteogenic marker Runx2 (Figure 5H) and late osteogenic marker Colla1 (Figure 5I) in EMSCs than in BMMSCs. Furthermore, EMSCs maintained negative expression of MHC I during osteogenesis (Figure 5J).

Finally, the chondrogenic differentiation capability of EMSCs and BMMSCs were analyzed using a pelleted micromass culture system. After 21 days of chondrogenic induction culture, EMSCs differentiated into chondrocytes. The formation of chondrocytes was confirmed with toluidine blue staining, shown as a purple-colour stained matrix (Figure 5K-i). EMSCs showed more toluidine blue positive staining, whereas BMMSCs were only faintly stained (Figure 5K-ii) suggesting that EMSCs were more efficient in chondrogenesis.

Although both EMSCs and BMMSCs were able to differentiate into mesodermal cell lineages including adipocytes, osteocytes and chondrocytes, EMSCs showed higher potential to differentiate into these lineages.

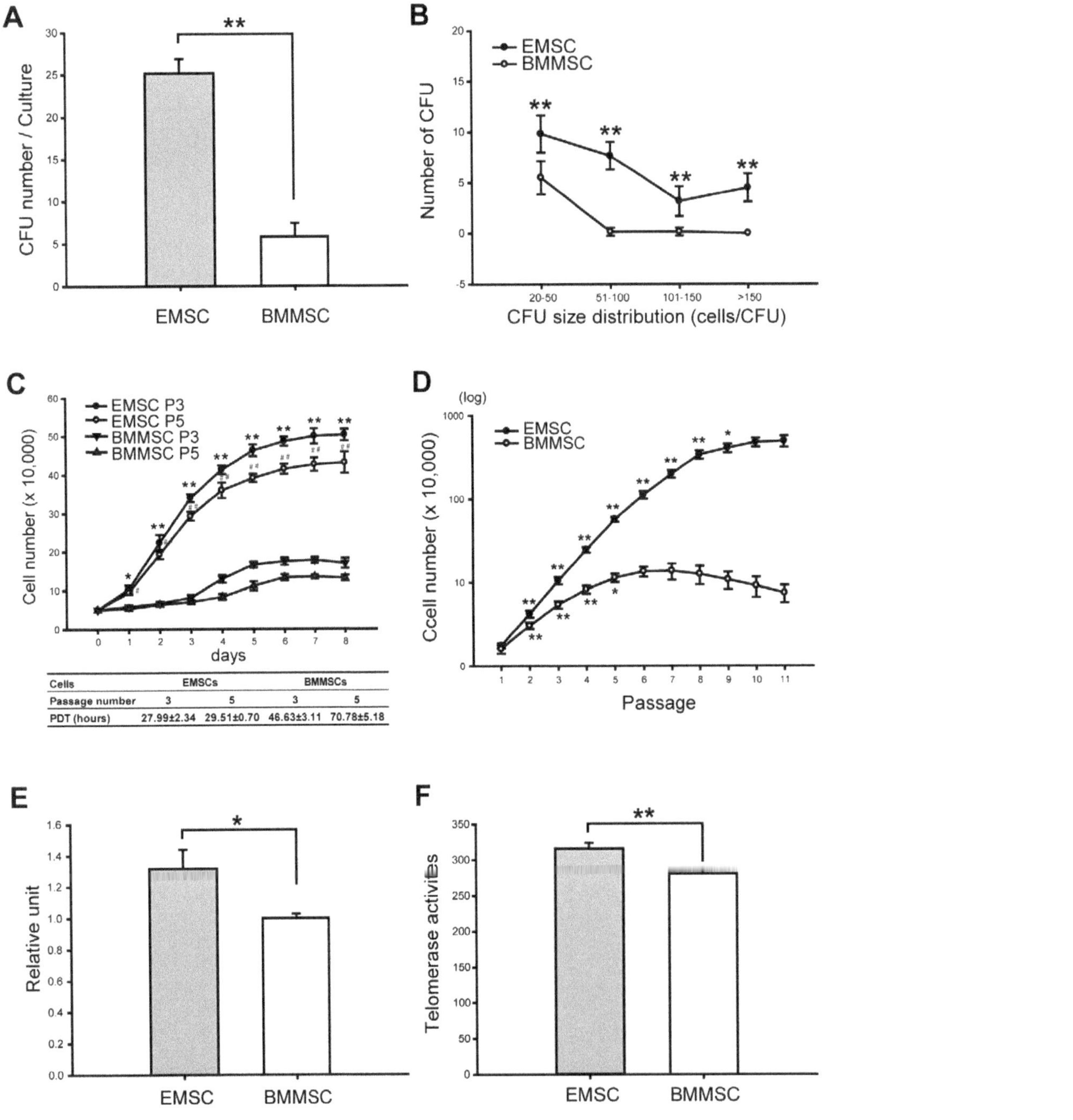

Cells	EMSCs		BMMSCs	
Passage number	3	5	3	5
PDT (hours)	27.99±2.34	29.51±0.70	46.63±3.11	70.78±5.18

Figure 4. Cell proliferation profiles of EMSCs and BMMSCs. (A) Colony-forming activity of EMSCs and BMMSCs at the first passage. EMSCs formed 23.17±2.92 CFUs whereas BMMSCs formed 5.83±1.60 CFUs (n = 6). (B) CFUs size distribution for EMSCs and BMMSCs. EMSCs formed more and larger CFUs than BMMSCs. ** represents $P<0.01$ (n = 6). (C) PDTs for EMSCs were compared to BMMSCs at the third (P3) and the fifth (P5) passages. The curves of EMSCs are higher than the ones of BMMSCs (n = 3). * represents $P<0.05$, ** represents $P<0.01$, which was compared at the third passage. # represents $P<0.05$, ## represents $P<0.01$, which was compared at the fifth passage. (D) Propagating abilities of EMSCs and BMMSCs. Cells were propagated for 2 days at each passage and cell numbers were calculated. EMSCs could be propagated for more passages that cells still retained proliferation ability than BMMSCs (n = 5). * represents $P<0.05$, ** represents $P<0.01$, as compared to previous passage. (E) Telomere length and (F) telomerase activity of EMSCs and BMMSCs (at the first passage) were detected and compared. EMSCs expressed significantly longer telomere length and higher telomerase activity than BMMSCs (n = 3). * represents $P<0.05$, ** represents $P<0.01$. Data are presented as mean ± s.d. and analyzed with Student's *t*-test.

Senescence of EMSCs during Culture

Senescence can be identified not only by morphological evaluation but also by the expression of senescence-associated β-galactosidase (SA-β-gal). Blue SA-β-gal-positive cells could be found in both EMSCs (Figure 6A) and BMMSCs cultures (Figure 6B). Quantified data showed that there were more SA-β-gal-positive cells in BMMSCs than in EMSCs (Figure 6C).

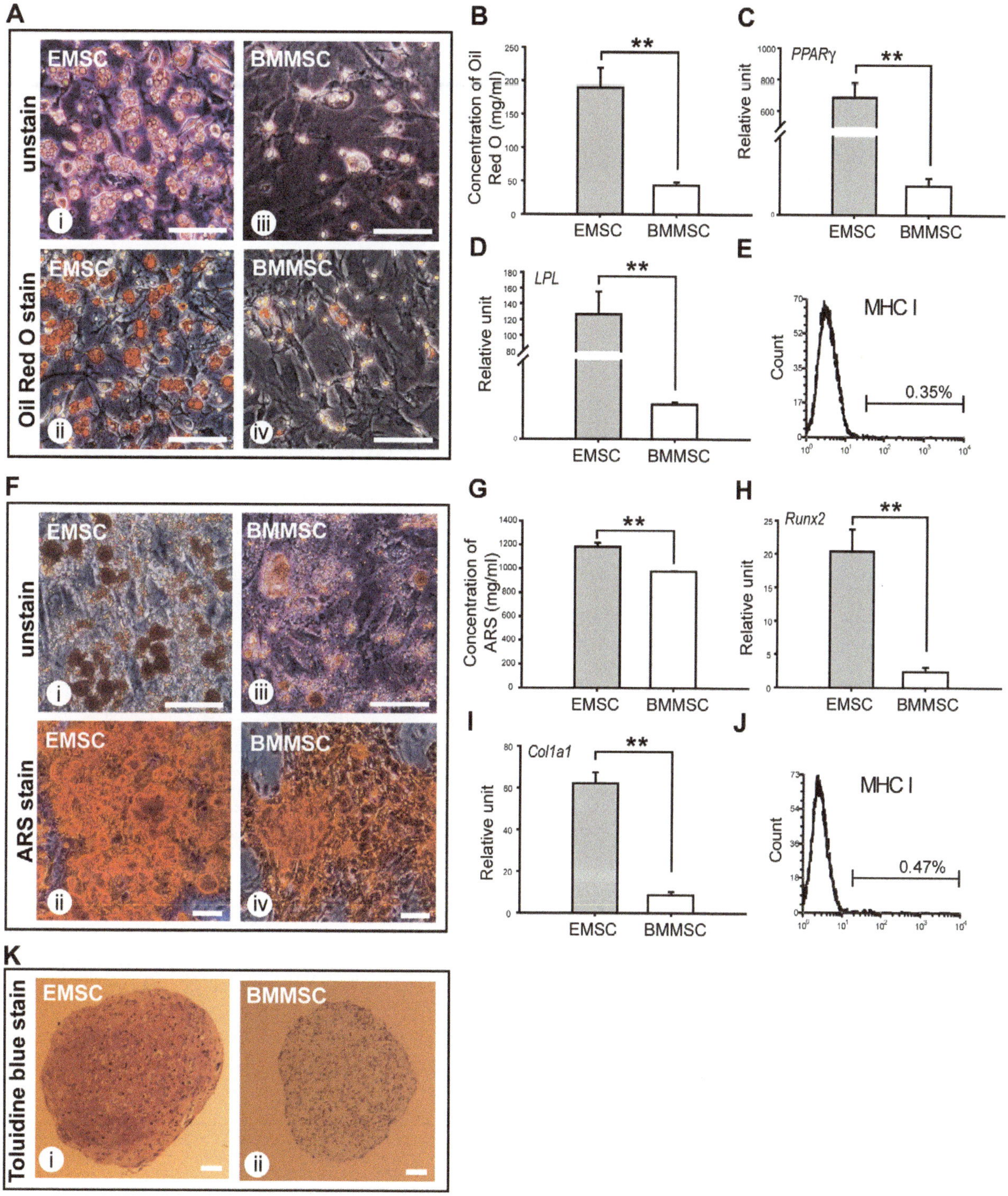

Figure 5. Differentiation potential of EMSCs and BMMSCs. (A) Adipogenic differentiation of EMSCs and BMMSCs at the fifth passage. Adipogenic capability was characterized by Oil Red O staining after seven days induction. EMSCs showed larger and more lipid drops than BMMSCs. (B) Oil Red O staining of EMSCs and BMMSCs were quantified for comparison (n = 3). (C, D) Expression level of adipogenic related genes were assessed by qPCR. EMSCs showed higher adipogenic gene expression level after seven days induction (n = 3). (E) MHC I expression profile of EMSCs was analysed by flow cytometry after seven days adipogenic induction. After adipogenesis, EMSCs were still negative for MHC I expression. (F) Osteogenic differentiation of EMSCs and BMMSCs at the fifth passage. Osteogenic capability was characterized by ARS staining after seven days induction. EMSCs showed higher calcium deposition than BMMSCs. (G) Quantitative results of ARS were performed to compare the osteogenic capacity of EMSCs and BMMSCs (n = 3). (H, I) Expression level of osteogenic related genes were assessed by qPCR. EMSCs showed higher osteogenic gene expression level after seven days induction (n = 3). (J) MHC I expression profile of EMSCs was analysed by flow cytometry after seven days osteogenic induction. After osteogenesis, EMSCs were still negative for MHC I expression. (K) Chondrogenic differentiation of EMSCs and BMMSCs at the fifth passage. Chondrogenic capability was evaluated by histological section of micromass pellet cultures after 21 days induction. Glycosaminoglycan content of the pellet was characterized by toluidine blue staining. EMSCs showed deeper purple stained matrix than BMMSCs. All the scale bars represent 100 μm. ** represents $P<0.01$. Data are presented as mean ± s.d. and analyzed with Student's *t*-test.

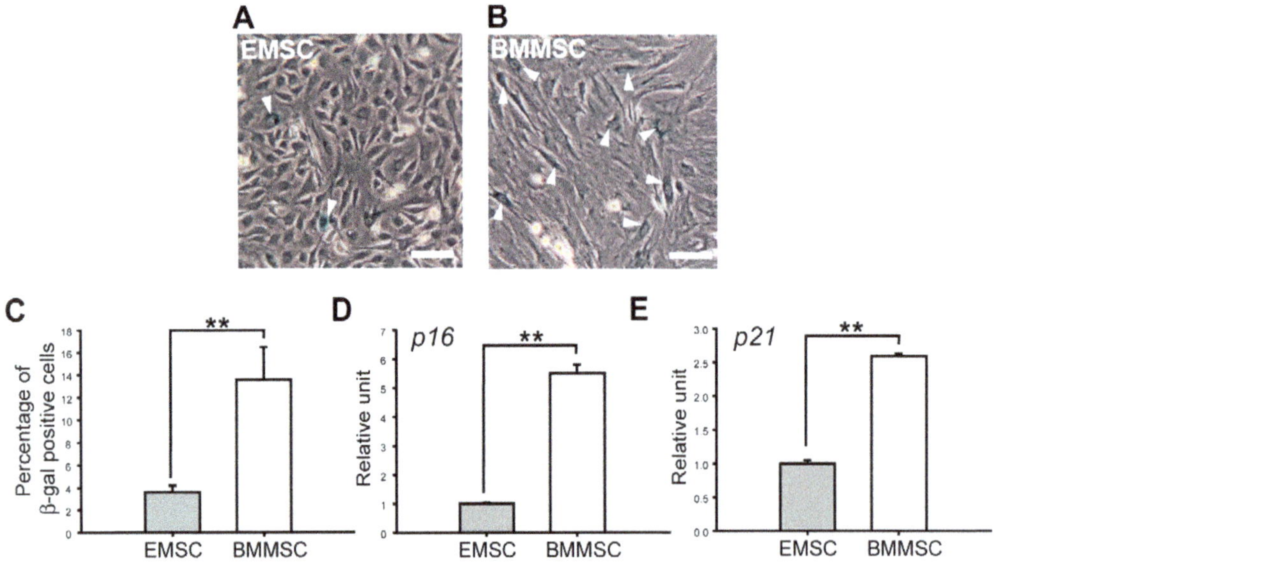

Figure 6. Analysis of cellular aging related markers of EMSCs and BMMSCs. (A) Determination of senescence marker, SA-β-gal, upon the fifth passage of EMSCs and (B) BMMSCs. SA-β-gal positive cells were showed as blue color and indicated by arrow heads. (C) The number of SA-β-gal positive cells was calculated from EMSCs or BMMSCs cultures. EMSCs showed lower SA-β-gal positive cells than BMMSCs (n = 4). (D) mRNA levels of cyclin-dependent kinase inhibitors p16 and (E) p21 were evaluated by qPCR. Both p16 and p21 expression levels were lower in EMSCs than BMMSCs (n = 3). All the scale bars represent 100 μm. ** represents $P<0.01$. Data are presented as mean ± s.d. and analyzed with Student's *t*-test.

We further examined the cell cycle regulators (cyclin-dependent kinase inhibitors) and senescence markers, p16 and p21. The transcript expression level of both *p16* and *p21* (Figure 6D, 6E) were lower in EMSCs than in BMMSCs.

EMSCs are Immunosuppressive and Anti-inflammatory

MSCs show low immunogenicity and exhibit the ability to suppress T-cell proliferation stimulated by either non-specific lymphocyte mitogens or mix lymphocyte reaction. We speculated that EMSCs have similar features. EMSCs co-cultured with autologous C57/BL/6 splenocytes in the presence of Con A significantly inhibited Con A-induced splenocyte proliferation in a dose-dependent manner (Figure 7A). For EMSCs co-cultured with allologous BALB/c splenocytes stimulated by Con A, the same effects could be observed (Figure 7B). In addition, EMSCs also repressed the allogeneic-induced splenocyte proliferation when co-cultured with allogeneic-stimulated splenocytes. Similarly, EMSCs exhibited dose-dependent suppression with allogeneic T-cell response (Figure 7C). These results indicated that EMSCs were able to suppress splenocyte proliferation *in vitro* and suggested EMSCs' role in immunosuppression.

To determine if anti-inflammatory actions of EMSCs could be induced through a paracrine effect, EMSCs and splenocytes were separated using the trans-well culture system, and IL-1, IL-6 and TNF-α of splenocytes were quantified. We found that IL-1, IL-6 and TNF-α were enhanced when splenocytes were stimulated by Con A and the surge of these pro-inflammatory signals could be repressed with the presence of EMSCs (Figure 7D–F). Hence, EMSCs are immunosuppressive via suppressing T-cell proliferation and inhibiting the release of pro-inflammatory signals.

Therapeutic Potentials of EMSCs

EMSCs showed greater potentials of proliferation and differentiation than BMMSCs, and also demonstrated paracrine anti-inflammation ability by which derived various therapeutic effects of MSCs [40,41]. To further confirm the potential of clinical application of EMSCs, we first investigated the osteogenesis potential of EMSCs using bone fracture model. EMSCs were seeded on a collagen-based gelatin sponge (SPONGOSTAN) and implanted into the fracture site. 14 days after surgery, osteocalcification of the injured sites was evaluated by X-ray image, and significantly higher bone density was observed in the EMSCs treated group indicating that EMSCs can improve bone repair response (Figure 8A, 8B). Histological examination of fracture sites revealed that newly formed bone tissue and capillaries were formed in the EMSCs implanted group while the control group showed the presence of disorganized tissue accompanied with more leukocytes infiltration (Figure 8C).

Recent studies showed MSCs could enhance angiogenesis and that play a pivotal role in repairing ischemic tissue damage and wound healing [42,43]. Therefore, we used mouse dorsal skin flap to investigate the potential therapeutic effects of EMSCs in ischemic chronic wound. In consistent with the results of other sources of MSCs [44], EMSCs improved wound healing at incisions (Figure 9A) and significantly reduced necrotic area (6.95±1.6%) as compared with the control group (29.9±3.94%) (Figure 9B). Skin thickness in the EMSCs injected group was decreased and the mucinous layer was enriched below the platysma muscle when compared to the control group (Figure 9C). More severe hemorrhages and erythrocyte extravasations in the dermis could be observed in the control group than in the EMSCs injected group (Figure 9D). Immunostaining of von Willebrand factor (vWF) indicated a significantly increased capillary density in the EMSCs injected group (Figure 9E, 9F), and suggested that EMSCs have beneficial effects on chronic ischemic wound healing probably by promoting angiogenesis.

A mouse hindlimb ischemia was also used to further confirm the effect of EMSCs on angiogenesis *in vivo*. Seven days after the onset of ischemia, laser Doppler perfusion imaging showed significant recovery of perfusion in the EMSCs injected group (0.71±0.12, relative to the non-ischemic limb) as compared to the control group (0.21±0.09) (Figure 10A, 10B). H&E staining showed

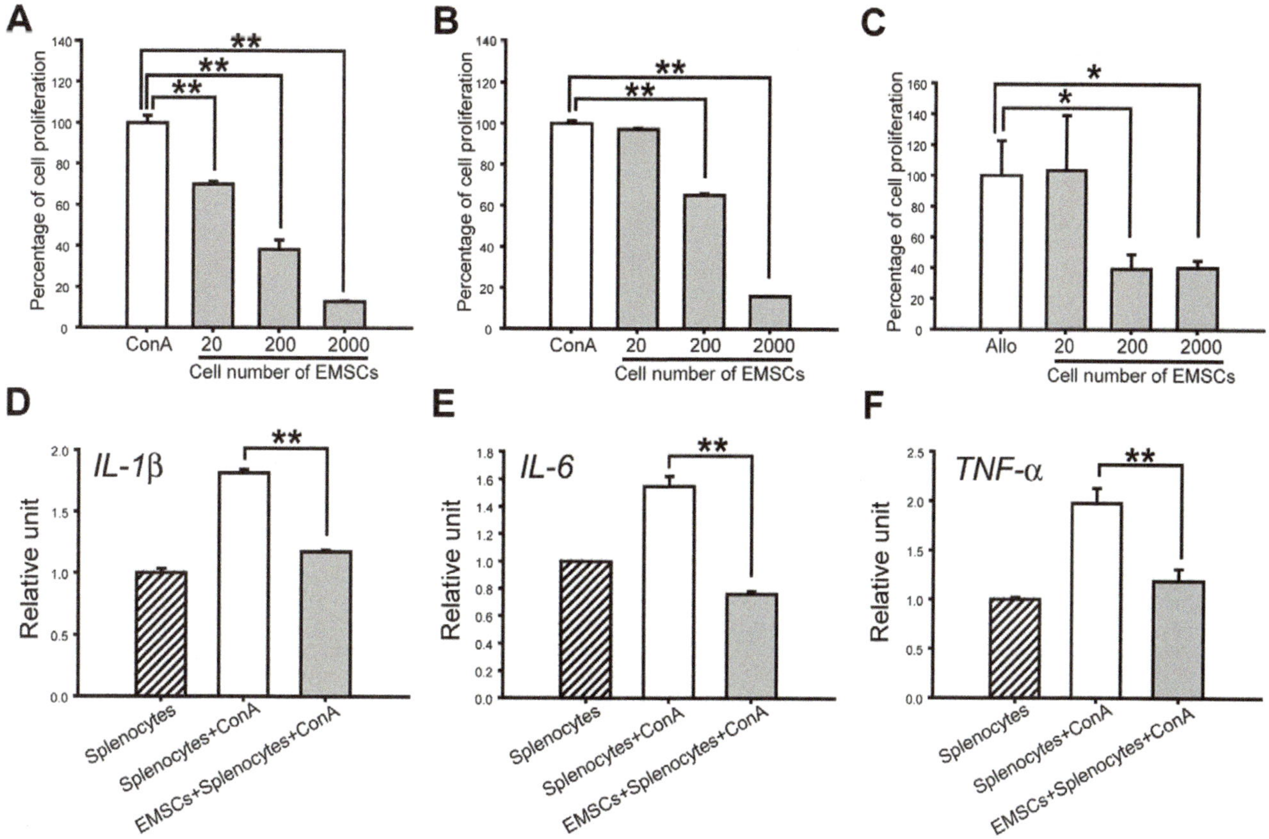

Figure 7. Immunomodulatory properties of EMSCs. (A) Responding splenocytes from C57BL/6 or (B) BALB/c mice were stimulated with Con A in the presence or absence of graded numbers of C57BL/6 EMSCs. The results are shown as percentage of cell proliferation in comparison with control cell proliferation. Splenocytes proliferation was inhibited by culture with EMSCs (at the fifth passage) in a dose dependent manner (n = 3). (C) Responding splenocytes from C57BL/6 mice were cultured with an equal number of mitomycin C-treated BALB/c splenocytes and with or without graded number of C57BL/6 EMSCs (n = 3). Allo indicates allogeneic splenocytes culture. EMSCs inhibited the splenocyte proliferation stimulated by allogeneic cells in a dose dependent manner. (D–F) Analysis of inflammatory cytokine production of splenocyte stimulated by Con A. Inflammatory cytokines expression level of splenocytes were decreased when co-cultured with EMSCs (at the fifth passage) (n=3). * represents $P<0.05$, **represents $P<0.01$. Data are presented as mean ± s.d. and analyzed with Student's *t*-test.

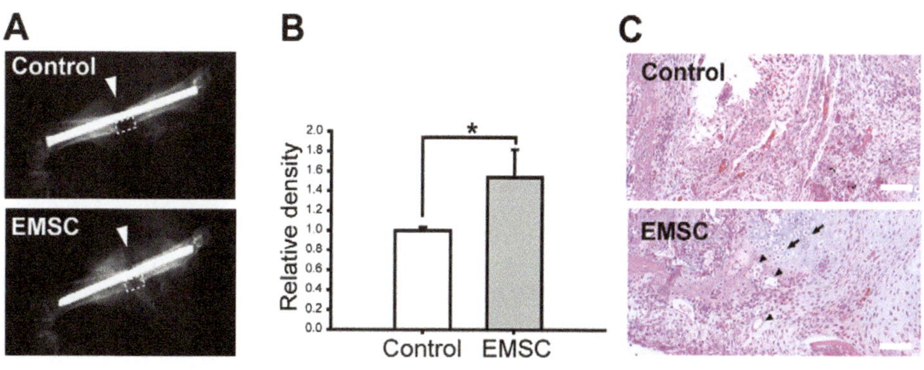

Figure 8. Repair of bone fracture in mice after transplantation of EMSCs. (A) Fracture healing was assessed by X-ray after 14 days with or without EMSCs (at the fifth passage) transplantation. Arrowheads indicate the site of fracture. (B) The bone density of fracture site (dotted box in Figure 8A) was quantified (n = 4). EMSCs transplantation significantly improved osteocalcification as compared to the control group. (C) The morphology of fracture sites were examined by H&E staining. Tissue disorganization was showed in the control group while the EMSCs transplanted group newly formed bone tissue (arrow) and capillaries (arrowhead). * represents $P<0.05$. Scale bars represent 100 μm. Data are presented as mean ± s.d. and analyzed with Student's *t*-test. Control: SPONGOSTAN carried with complete medium-transplantation group; EMSC: SPONGOSTAN carried with EMSCs-transplantation group.

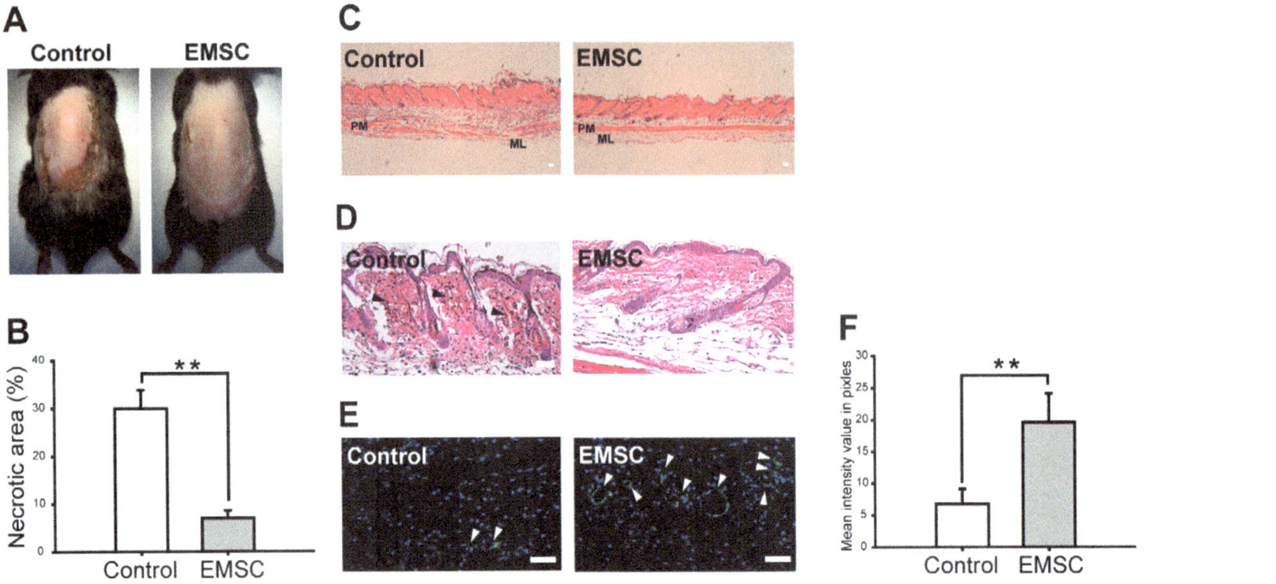

Figure 9. Prevention of skin flap necrosis in mice by EMSCs injection. (A) Ischemic flap showed necrosis in the control mice and near complete healing in the EMSCs (at the fifth passage) injected mice after 6 days of surgery. (B) Percentage of necrosis was quantified by planimetry. Percentage of necrotic area is significantly larger in the control group than in the EMSCs injected group (n = 4). (C) The skin structure was evaluated by H&E staining. Skin thickness is decreased and mucinous layer is preserved in the EMSCs injected group as compared to the control group. (D) In higher magnification, extra vascular erythrocytes and hemorrhage (arrowhead) can be observed in the control group. (E) Immunostaining of von Willebrand factor (vWF) of skin flap, and (F) its quantification showed significantly more vWF expressed cells (arrowhead) in the EMSCs injected group than the control group. **represents $P<0.01$. Scale bars represent 100 μm. Data are presented as mean ± s.d. and analyzed with Student's *t*-test. PM: platysma muscle; ML: mucinous layer; Control: complete medium injection-group; EMSC: EMSCs-injection group.

muscle degeneration, and Masson's Trichrome staining showed severe fibrosis in the ischemic region in the control group. On the other hand, significantly reduced muscle degeneration and minimal fibrosis were observed in the EMSCs treated group (Figure 10C–10E). In consistent with the results from skin flap model, immunostaining of vWF of ischemic muscle indicated an increase in capillary density in the EMSCs injected group (Figure 10F, 10G), and supported that EMSCs could promote angiogenesis to improve in blood perfusion and muscle recovery in ischemic hindlimbs.

Discussion

MSCs can serve as progenitors for bone, cartilage, adipose, muscle and other tissues [45,46,47]. Despite the use of BMMSCs as a common adult stem cell source, murine BM cells are more difficult to isolate and culture than those of other species due to low frequency and mixed cell contamination [48,49,50]. Therefore the use of BMMSCs requires *ex vivo* cell expansion, and usually results in more senescent cells. In addition to bone marrow, researchers also tried to isolate MSCs from compact bone [51] or trabecular bone [52,53] to overcome this limitation. The purpose of this study was to find alternative murine MSCs sources that provide sufficient MSCs in earlier passages. In this study, we demonstrated that the epiphysis serves as an easy-access and rich stem cell reservoir, resolving difficulties that arise from isolating and expanding murine BMMSCs. To verify MSCs establishment, EMSCs were analysed for general MSCs features and their key capabilities were compared with those of BMMSCs.

The minimum criteria for defining MSCs includes three parameters: clonogenic capabilities, specific surface antigens identification and differentiation potentials [54]. Experimental results revealed that EMSCs exhibited significantly stronger colony- forming ability, not only in numbers but also in size, when compared with BMMSCs. In addition, proliferation capability was determined by PDT assay. We found that BMMSCs growth decreased after few passages, whereas EMSCs continued to grow rapidly. Hence, EMSCs might have an advantage over BMMSCs in providing a large quantity of cells in a short culture period.

We demonstrated through differentiation studies that EMSCs have the potentials to differentiate into adipogenic, osteogenic and chondrogenic cell lineages. EMSCs showed significantly better differentiation capabilities than BMMSCs, especially in adipogenesis and chondrogenesis. In adipogenesis, EMSCs formed lipid droplets more readily, and the number and size of lipid droplets in EMSCs were more than in BMMSCs. Accordingly, EMSCs expressed higher level of early (PPARγ) and late (LPL) adipogenesis markers than BMMSCs. In chondrogenesis, EMSCs showed deeper coloured and larger mast cell accumulation on toluidine blue staining. These results suggest that EMSCs exhibit higher differentiation potentials than BMMSCs.

We examined the expression of EMSCs markers and found that some differed from those of BMMSCs. The data confirmed that EMSCs cultured in our system gave rise to a population of cells with MSCs characteristics. In consistent with general MSCs profiles, EMSCs were positive for CD29, CD44 and CD73, and negative for CD11b, CD45 and CD31, suggesting that the established EMSCs were not from hematopoietic and endothelial lineages. EMSCs exhibited higher and more homogeneous Sca-1 expression might be related to their high proliferation capabilities [55,56]. In accordance of previous studies, CD105 and CD166 were demonstrated to relate to chondrogenic potential [57,58] and our data also indicated that EMSCs, with CD166 positive, were superior in chondrogenic potential. Notably, EMSCs were negative for MHC I expression under our culture condition,

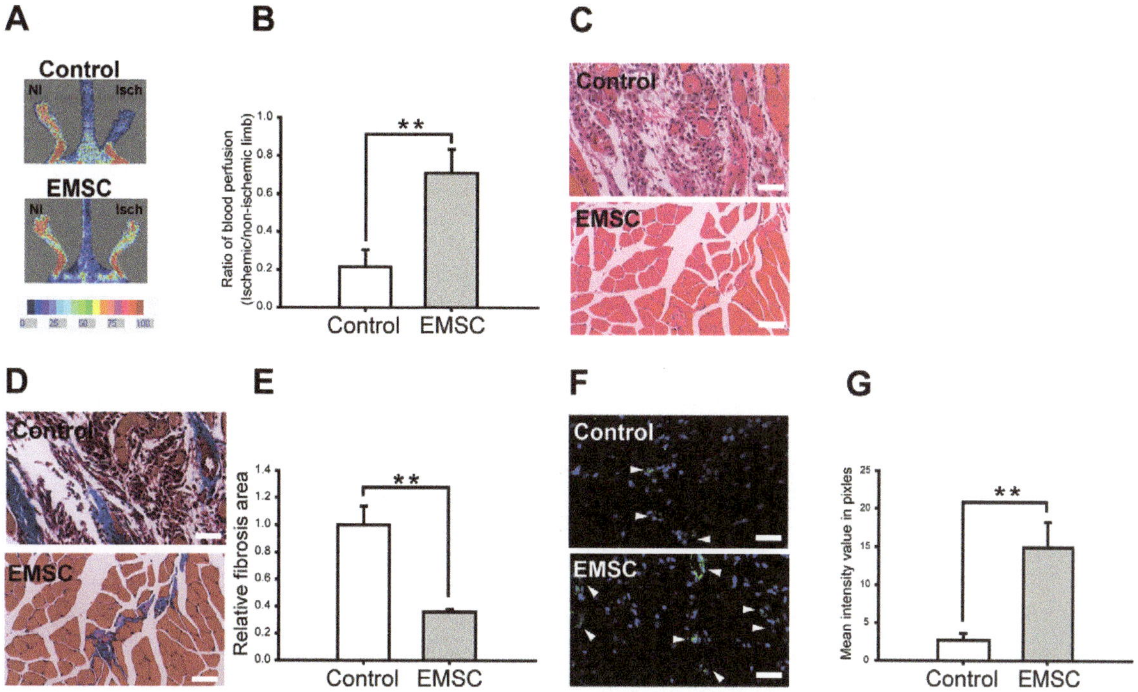

Figure 10. Transplanted EMSCs improved blood perfusion in ischemic limb. (A) Foot perfusion was evaluated by laser Doppler blood perfusion analysis at day 7 post ischemia. In color-coded images, red represents normal perfusion, while dark blue represents low or absent perfusion. (B) Quantification of the foot perfusion showed that EMSCs (at the fifth passage) transplantation significantly improved blood perfusion (n = 3). (C) H&E staining showed massive muscle degeneration in ischemic regions in the control group compared to the markedly reduced muscle degeneration in the EMSCs group. (D) Masson's Trichrome staining and (E) its quantification showed significantly larger fibrotic area in the control group than the EMSCs injected group. (F) Immunostaining of von Willebrand factor (vWF) of ischemic limb muscle and (G) its quantification showed significantly more vWF expressed cells (arrowhead) in the EMSCs injected group than the control group. Scale bars represent 100 μm. **represents $P<0.01$. Data are presented as mean ± s.d. and analyzed with Student's *t*-test. Isch: ischemic limb; NI: non-ischemic limb; Control: complete medium injection-group; EMSC: EMSCs-injection group.

whereas BMMSCs were positive. When treated with IFN-γ, a cytokine known to enhance the MHC molecules expression, EMSCs were found to be positive for MHC I, implying that MHC I molecules exist in the cytoplasm, but not on the cell surface. Following changes in phenotype that occured over several passages revealed that CD73, CD166, SSEA-4 and Sca-1 decreased with increased propagation, and grew in similarity to BMMSCs while the MHC I expression was still negative for EMSCs. In conclusion, our established EMSCs can be classified as mesenchymal stem cells and were distinct from BMMSCs.

In principle, cellular aging can be accelerated with increased propagating and can affect amplified differentiation potential [59,60]. Our results showed that cultured EMSCs showed less SA-β-gal positive cells than BMMSCs over several passages. Cyclin-dependent kinase markers, p16 and p21, were important for terminal growth arrest, and EMSCs showed lower p16 and p21 expression than BMMSCs regardless of primary or longer passages.

Due to the potentials of multilineage differentiation and low immunogenicity, MSCs draw attention for the use in regenerative medicine. Recent researches also demonstrated that some therapeutic effects of MSCs may derive from their paracrine effects [61,62]. In our study, EMSCs not only showed great proliferation and differentiation potentials but also demonstrated immunosuppressive and anti-inflammation capacities through a paracrine effect. Thus, it is reasonable to expect that EMSCs are at least as potential as other MSCs for cell therapy. We evaluated the therapeutic effects of EMSCs in three animal models, including bone fracture, skin flap and hindlimb ischemia models. Our study showed that transplanted EMSCs accelerated the fracture healing process and enhanced osteocalcification indicating that EMSCs can promote fracture repair. It has been shown that MSCs contribute to angiogenesis directly by participating in new vessel formation, or indirectly by secreting angiogenic factors [63,64,65]. Therefore, we used dorsal skin flap model, in which an oxygen tension gradient occurs in the ischemic tissue [66], to investigate the effects of EMSCs on the neovascularization *in vivo*. Transplanted EMSCs obviously reduced necrosis and almost fully protected the edge of the flap. In addition, EMSCs effectively preserved skin structures including the mucinous layer which is important for skin water content and tissue structural integrity [67]. In hindlimb ischemia model, EMSCs improved blood perfusion and reduced muscle degeneration and tissue fibrosis. Moreover, EMSCs treatment significantly increased vWF positive capillary cells in both skin flap and hindlimb ischemia models, suggesting that EMSCs enhance neovascularization and might play a beneficial role in ischemic/hypoxia environment.

Collectively, EMSCs were characterized as MSCs due to their capacities for differentiation into multiple lineages and cell surface marker expression profiles, while EMSCs were found to have greater abilities to proliferate and differentiate than BMMSCs. Our data demonstrates that EMSCs provide an efficient and reproducible method for obtaining MSCs with high proliferating potential, and hence EMSCs can be used as an alternative to MSCs for cell therapy. We provide a novel and reliable method for preparing an improved population of murine MSCs.

Materials and Methods

Animals and Ethics Statement

C57BL/6 and BALB/c mice of 6–8 weeks were purchased from the Laboratory Animal Center of Medical College in National Taiwan University (Taipei, Taiwan). Mice were kept under standard conditions, and all experimental procedures were approved by the Institutional Animal Care and Use Committee (IACUC) of National Taiwan University (approval number 96-EL-22-NTU).

Isolation and Culture of EMSCs

C57BL/6 mice were sacrificed by cervical dislocation. The femurs and tibias were isolated and the adherent soft tissues on femurs and tibias were removed thoroughly. The epiphyses were then removed by a shears and transferred to 22.1 cm^2 culture dish (TPP, Trasadingen, Switzerland) and cultured in complete medium composed of MEM alpha (Sigma-Aldrich, St. Louis, MO) supplemented with 20% fetal bovine serum (FBS; ECS tested; Hyclone, Logan, UT), 2 mM L-glutamine (Invitrogen, Carlsbad, CA), 100 U/ml penicillin, and 100 µg/ml streptomycin (Invitrogen). The cells were incubated in a humidified atmosphere containing 95% air and 5% CO_2 at 37°C. The non-adherent cells were removed by changing the medium every 3 days. After 11 days, the primary culture reached approximately 70% confluence, and the cells were detached by 0.25% trypsin/0.1 mM ethylenediaminetetraacetic acid (trypsin/EDTA; Invitrogen) for 1 min at 37°C. After that, the reaction was stopped by adding complete medium. The cells that cannot be lifted within 1 min were discarded. The detached cells were centrifuged at 400 *g* for 5 min and resuspended in the complete medium and were ready for the transient lower-density plastic adherence (tLDA) purification as described below.

Isolation and Culture of BMMSCs

BMMSCs were obtained as previously described [39,68]. In brief, the femurs and tibias were isolated from cervical dislocated C57BL/6 mice and the adherent soft tissues were cleaned thoroughly. Then the epiphyses were removed by a rongeur. The marrow cells were harvested from diaphysis by inserting a syringe needle (23-gauge and 26-gauge for femurs and tibias, respectively) and flushing with complete medium consisting of MEM alpha (Sigma-Aldrich) supplemented with 20% FBS (Hyclone), 2 mM L-glutamine (Invitrogen), 100 U/ml penicillin, and 100 µg/ml streptomycin (Invitrogen). We plated the cells onto 60 cm^2 culture dishes (TPP) at a density of 2×10^5 cells/cm^2. The cells were incubated in a humidified atmosphere containing 95% air and 5% CO_2 at 37°C. The non-adherent cells were removed by changing medium every 3 days. When these primary cultures reached 70% confluence, the cells were lifted by incubating with 0.25% trypsin/EDTA (Invitrogen) for 1 min at 37°C. These cells were ready for tLDA purification as described below.

tLDA Approach

The tLDA approach has been described previously [39]. Briefly, the lifted cells from the primary culture were passed through a 40 µm mesh (BD Biosciences, San Jose, CA) and then the filtered single cells were replated onto 60 cm^2 culture dishes at a density of 1.25×10^4 cells/cm^2. These cells were allowed to adhere for 2–3 h at 37°C in a humidified atmosphere containing 95% air and 5% CO_2. Afterwards, the cells were lifted by incubating with 0.025% trypsin/EDTA (Invitrogen) for 5 min at 37°C and were seeded at a density of 5×10^4 cells/cm^2 for subsequent analysis.

Population Doubling Time (PDT)

The mean PDT was calculated according to the equation: $TD = t_p \log 2/(\log Nt - \log No)$, where Nt is the number of cells harvested, No is the number of cells inoculated, and t is the time of the culture (in hour). The trypan blue exclusion test was used to count the cells with the hemocytometer [69].

Colony Formation Assay

For determination of colony forming units (CFUs), cells were plated at a density of 150 cells/9.01 cm^2 culture dish (TPP). After incubation for 9 days, the colonies formed were fixed by methanol (Sigma-Aldrich) and stained with Geimsa solution (Sigma-Aldrich). A cluster of at least 20 cells was defined as a CFU. CFU sizes and CFU number were enumerated by a light microscope. To determine the relationship between CFU size and cell number, CFU was categorized depending on cell number per CFU: 20–50 cells/CFU, 51–100 cells/CFU, 101–150 cells/CFU and >151 cells/CFU.

In Vitro Differentiation

To induce adipogenic differentiation, cells were cultured to near confluence and cultured in adipogenic induction medium consisting of MEM alpha (Sigma-Aldrich) supplemented with 10% FBS (Hyclone), 10 µg/ml insulin (Sigma-Aldrich), 1 µM dexamethasone (Sigma-Aldrich), 0.5 mM isobutyl-methylxanthine (Sigma-Aldrich), and 100 µM indomethacin (Sigma-Aldrich) for 7 days. The induction medium was changed every 3 days [29]. At the end of the differentiation period, cells were fixed with 10% formalin for 10 min and lipid droplets were stained by Oil Red O (Sigma-Aldrich) staining. To quantify the Oil Red O staining results, we extracted the Oil Red O from lipid droplets by DMSO (Sigma-Aldrich) and measured the absorbance by SpectraMax 190 ELISA plate reader (Molecular Devices, Sunnyvale, CA) at 550 nm.

To induce osteogenic differentiation, the confluent cells were incubated in osteogenic induction medium consisting of MEM alpha (Sigma-Aldrich) supplemented with 10% FBS (Hyclone), 0.1 µM dexamethasone (Sigma-Aldrich), 10 mM β-glycerolphosphate (Sigma-Aldrich) and 50 µM ascorbic acid (Sigma-Aldrich) for 7 days [29]. The induction medium was changed every 3 days. The bone matrix mineralization was evaluated by Alizarin red S (ARS; Sigma-Aldrich) staining. The ARS was extracted by adding 10% cetylpyridinium chloride (Sigma) in 8 mM Na_2HPO_4 (Merck, Darmstadt, Germany) and 1.5 mM KH_2PO_4 (Merck) and the absorbance was measured by SpectraMax 190 ELISA plate reader (Molecular Devices) at 550 nm.

To induce chondrogenic differentiation, a pellet culture system was used to differentiate. Chondrogenic induction medium consisted of MEM alpha supplemented with 1% FBS (Hyclone), 6.25 µg/ml insulin (Sigma-Aldrich), 50 µM ascorbic acid (Sigma-Aldrich), and 10 ng/ml TGF-β1 (R&D Systems, Minneapolis, MN). The induction medium was changed twice per week. The production of proteoglycan was characterized by toluidine blue (Sigma-Aldrich) staining [70].

Flow Cytometric Analysis

Cells were stained with fluorescent isothiocyanate (FITC) or PE-conjugate monoclonal antibodies (Table 1) for 30 min at 4°C in dark according to the product instructions. Ten thousand events were acquired on a FACSCalibur (BD Biosciences, Franklin Lakes, NJ), and analyzed by FCS Express software (Version 4.0; Denovo software, Los Angeles, CA). All experiments included

Table 1. List of Antibodies Used in Flow Cytometry Analysis.

Antibody	Clone	Ref. No.	Conjugated	Isotype	Supplier
CD11b	M1/70	12-0112	PE	Rat IgG2b	eBioscience
CD29	HMb1-1	12-0291	PE	Armenian Hamster IgG	eBioscience
CD31	390	12-0311	PE	Rat IgG2a	eBioscience
CD34	RAM34	560238	FITC	RatIgG2a	BD Pharmingen
CD44	IM7	12-0441	PE	Rat IgG2b	eBioscience
CD45	30-F11	12-0451	PE	Rat IgG2b	eBioscience
CD73	TY/11.8	12-0731	PE	Rat IgG1	eBioscience
CD105	MJ7/18	12-1051	PE	Rat IgG2a	eBioscience
CD106	429	11-1061	FITC	Rat IgG2a	eBioscience
CD117	2B8	12-1171	PE	Rat IgG2b	eBioscience
CD166	eBioALC-48	12-1661	PE	Rat IgG2a	eBioscience
Sca-1	D7	12-5981	PE	Rat IgG2a	eBioscience
SSEA-4	MC-813-70	12-8843	PE	Mouse IgG3	eBioscience
MHC class I	34-1-2S	12-5998	PE	Mouse IgG2a	eBioscience
MHC class II	M5/114.15.2	12-5321	PE	Rat IgG2b	eBioscience

negative controls without antibodies or with isotype controls (eBioscience, San Diego, CA).

Quantitative Real Time Reverse Transcription-Polymerase Chain Reaction (qPCR)

Total cellular RNA was extracted using TRIzol reagent (Invitrogen) and then treated with RNase free DNase Set (Promega, Madison, MI) according to manufacturer's instructions. Reverse transcription reactions were performed with 5 μg total RNA using the SuperScript First-Strand Synthesis System (Invitrogen), according to the manufacturer's instructions. Real-time PCR (ABI PRISM 7000; Applied Biosystems; Foster City, CA) was performed with 1 μL of the single-stranded cDNA sample with SYBR Green PCR master mix (Applied Biosystems). The sequences of primers used were as follows: forward 5′-CATGGCCTTCCGTGTTCCTA-3′, reverse 5′-GCGGCACG-TCAGATCCA-3′ for *Glyceraldehyde-3-phosphate dehydrogenase* (*GAPDH*); forward 5′-ACATAAAGTCCTTCCCGCTGACCA-3′, reverse 5′-AAATTCGGATGGCCACCTCTTTGC-3′ for *peroxisome proliferator activated receptor gamma* (*PPARγ*); forward 5′-ACGAGCGCTCCATTCATCTCTTCA-3′, reverse 5′-TCT-TGCTGCTTCTCTTGGCTCTGA-3′ for *lipoprotein lipase* (*LPL*); forward 5′-GCTTTCATTAGGCAGGGCCAACAA-3′, reverse 5′- AGGGCTGGATCTCAAACTCACACA-3′ for *runt related transcription factor 2* (*Runx2*); forward 5′-TTCTCCTGGCAAA-GACGGACTCAA-3′, reverse 5′- AGGAAGCTGAAGTCA-TAACCGCCA-3′ for *collagen, type I, alpha 1* (*Col1a1*); forward 5′-GAACTCTTTCGGTCGTACCC-3′, reverse 5′-CGAATCTG-CACCGTAGTTGA-3′ for *p16*; forward 5′- CCAGGCCAA-GATGGTGTCTT-3′, reverse 5′-TGAGAAAGGATCAGC-CATTGC-3′ for *p21*. Annealing temperature was 60°C. Each amplification reaction was checked to confirm the absence of nonspecific PCR product by melting curve analysis. The relative gene expression level was calculated and presented with the $2^{-\Delta\Delta Ct}$ method. *GAPDH* was used as a reference gene to normalize specific gene expression in each sample.

Quantification of Telomere Length

Average telomere length (ATL) was measured by real-time PCR from total genomic mouse DNA as previous study [71]. In brief, total genomic DNA was extracted using Dneasy Blood and Tissue Kit (Qiagen, Hilden, Germany) according to manufacturer's instructions. 20 ng samples of each DNA were performed by real-time PCR (ABI PRISM 7000; Applied Biosystems) with SYBR Green PCR master mix (Applied Biosystems). The average telomere length ratio was determined by the level of telomeric DNA normalized to the quantity of a single copy gene, the *acidic ribosomal phosphoprotein PO* (*36B4*). Forward and reverse telomeric primers were 5′-CGGTTTGTTTGGGTTTGGGTTTGGGTT-TGGGTTTGGGTT-3′ and 5′-GGCTTGCCTTACCCTTA-CCCTTACCCTTACCCTTACCCT-3′ respectively. Forward and reverse primers of *36B4* gene were 5′-ACTGGTCTAG-GACCCGAGAAG-3′ and 5′-TCAATGGTGCCTCTGGA-GATT -3′, respectively.

Telomerase Activity

Telomerase activity was performed in triplicates with the TRAPeze® XL Telomerase Detection kit (Millipore, Billerica, MA) as the manufacturer's instructions. Briefly, cells were lysed by CHAPS lysis buffer and incubated on ice for 30 min. Then, cells were centrifuged at 12,000 *g* at 4°C, and the supernatant was assayed for telomerase. For PCR amplification, each reaction volume is 50 μl, containing 10 μl of the 5× TRAPeze® XL Reaction Mix, 0.4 μl of Tag Polymerase (5 U/ml; Invitrogen), 37.6 μl of ddH_2O, and 2 μl of the sample extracted. In a themocycler (ABI 2700; Applied Biosystems), performed a 4-step PCR at 94°C for 30 s, 59°C for 30 s, 72°C for 1 min for 36 cycles, followed by a 72°C for 3 min extension step and then 55°C for 25 min, concluding with a 4°C incubation. The fluorescence of each reaction was detected with a Fluoroskan Ascent FL fluorescent plate reader (Labsystems; Farnborough, UK). The telomerase activity was determined by calculating the log of the relative ratio net fluorescence increase (Δ fluorescein absorbance/ Δ sulforhodamine absorbance) for each reaction described detail in the manufacturer's instructions

SA-β-Gal Staining

Cells were grown to 50% confluence and stained by senescence cells histochemical staining kit (Sigma-Aldrich) as manual described. Briefly, cells were fixed in fixation buffer, washed with PBS and stained the cells by incubating in freshly prepared staining mixture at 37°C without O_2 overnight.

Mitogen Proliferation Assays and Allogeneic Mixed Lymphocyte Reaction (MLR)

The splenocytes from C57BL/6 and BALB/c mice were prepared using Ficoll-Paque density centrifugation (1.077 g/ml; Amersham Pharmacia Biotech, NJ) followed by two washes in RPMI 1640 (Invitrogen) supplemented with 50 μM 2-mercapto-ethanol (Sigma-Aldrich), 10% FBS (Hyclone), 100 U/ml penicillin, and 100 μg/ml streptomycin (Invitrogen). A graded number of mitomycin C (Sigma-Aldrich)-treated EMSCs or BMMSCs were seeded in triplicate in flat-bottom 96-well plates and maintained at 37°C for 6 h. In mitogen proliferation assays, splenocytes (2×10^5 cells/well) from C57BL/6 or BALB/c mice treated with 5 μg/ml Con A (Sigma-Aldrich) were cultured with or without EMSCs or BMMSCs from C57BL/6 mice. In MLR, responding splenocytes (2×10^5 cells/well) from C57BL/6 mice and an equal number of mitomycin C-treated allogeneic stimulating splenocytes from BALB/c mice were added into the EMSCs or BMMSCs culture. Proliferation assays were performed after 4 or 5 days using the CellTiter 96 Aqueous Nonradioactive Cell Proliferation Assay kit (Promega, Madison, WI), according to the manufacturer's instructions. The absorbance was measured by SpectraMax 190 ELISA plate reader (Molecular Devices) at 490 nm.

Transwell and Coculture Assay

EMSCs (2×10^4 cells/ml) were cultured in an upper chamber of the Transwell insert (Millipore) with or without splenocytes (2×10^6 cells/ml) cultured in a lower chamber. The transwell membrane was semipermeable with a pore size of 0.4 μm. After three days of culture, splenocytes were collected for mRNA analysis.

Bone Fracture Model

Eight-week-old female C57BL/6 mice were subjected to a bone fracture model as previously described [72,73]. Briefly, a closed transverse fracture was performed in the midsection of the femur by a motorized drill (2 mm in diameter) and fractured femurs were reconnected by a pin (25-gauge needle). EMSCs (5×10^5 cells/mouse) were plated on 2 mm×2 mm SPONGOSTAN (Johnson & Johnson, New Jersey, USA) at 37°C for 2 h and then transplanted by covering on the fracture site. Experimented mice were examined by X-ray (SkyScan 1076; SkyScan, Belgium) 14 days post-transplantation and the bone density of the fracture site was assessed using ImageJ software (NIH). Femurs were collected for hematoxylin and eosin (H&E) staining.

Skin Flap Model

Eight-week-old female C57BL/6 mice underwent skin flap surgery at their back as previously described [74,75]. In brief, a peninsular-shaped flap (3 cm×2 cm) was elevated on mouse dorsal skin and two vascular pedicles from the lateral thoracic arteries were sectioned. Following surgery, the flap was injected with 200 μl of EMSCs (5×10^5 cells/mouse) or complete medium intradermally using 29-guage needle. The injected solution was separated at four sites near the vascular cutting sites. Mice were photographed for six days after the surgery and then sacrificed to collect flap tissues for H&E staining and immunostaining. The necrotic area was quantified using the ImageJ software (NIH).

Hindlimb Ischemia Model

Eight-week-old female C57BL/6 mice were subjected to surgical ligature at the proximal end of the left femoral artery as previously described [76,77]. Seven days after surgery, 100 μl of EMSCs (2×10^6 cells/mouse) or complete medium was injected intramuscularly into 5 sites of the gracilis muscle in the medial thigh immediately. Laser Doppler perfusion imaging (moorLDI2; Moor Instruments Ltd., Devon, UK) was performed seven days after the surgery and ischemic limb muscles were then harvested for immunohistochemistry analysis. H&E staining and Masson's Trichrome (Sigma-Aldrich) staining were performed, and fibrosis area was calculated with ImageJ software (NIH).

Immunohistochemical Staining

Samples were embedded in paraffin blocks. Tissue slides were deparaffinized, treated with epitope retrieval buffer (Thermal scientific, Inc., Odessa, TX) at 95°C for 25 min, and then incubated with a primary antibody, rabbit anti-von Willebrand factor (vWF; 1:400; Abcam, Cambridge, UK), at 4°C overnight. Goat anti-rabbit conjugated Alexa-488 antibody (1:200; Invitrogen) was used as the secondary antibody. For nuclear staining, sections were incubated in 0.1 μg/ml 4,6 diamidino-2-phenylindole (DAPI; Invitrogen) for 3 min. Fluorescence was observed microscopically and fluorescence intensity of immunostaining was evaluated with ImageJ software (NIH).

Statistical Analysis

All experiments have more than 3 biological repeats and all values were presented as mean ± standard deviation. Statistical comparisons were analyzed with the Student's *t* test and a *p* value less than 0.05 was considered statistically significant.

Acknowledgments

We would like to thank Prof. Osamu Ohneda (Department of Regenerative Medicine and Stem Cell Biology, University of Tsukuba) and Dr. Kenichi Kimura (Department of Regenerative Medicine and Stem Cell Biology, University of Tsukuba) for their invaluable advice and technical assistance, Dr. Georgina To'a Salazar (Department of Regenerative Medicine and Stem Cell Biology, University of Tsukuba) for discussions and comments on the manuscript, and Taiwan Mouse Clinic which is funded by National Research Program for Biopharmaceuticals (NRPB) at the National Science Council (NSC) of Taiwan for technical support in experiment.

Author Contributions

Conceived and designed the experiments: CC. Cheng WSL FSHH SCW. Performed the experiments: CC. Cheng WSL YHL CC. Chang GYX. Analyzed the data: CC. Cheng WSL IHL. Contributed reagents/materials/analysis tools: SPL HYH CFC WTKC SCW. Wrote the paper: CC. Cheng.

References

1. Friedenstein AJ, Chailakhjan RK, Lalykina KS (1970) The development of fibroblast colonies in monolayer cultures of guinea-pig bone marrow and spleen cells. Cell Tissue Kinet 3: 393–403.
2. Bianco P, Robey PG, Simmons PJ (2008) Mesenchymal stem cells: revisiting history, concepts, and assays. Cell Stem Cell 2: 313–319.
3. Chamberlain G, Fox J, Ashton B, Middleton J (2007) Concise review: mesenchymal stem cells: their phenotype, differentiation capacity, immunological features, and potential for homing. Stem Cells 25: 2739–2749.

4. Pittenger MF, Mackay AM, Beck SC, Jaiswal RK, Douglas R, et al. (1999) Multilineage potential of adult human mesenchymal stem cells. Science 284: 143–147.
5. Lee KD, Kuo TK, Whang-Peng J, Chung YF, Lin CT, et al. (2004) In vitro hepatic differentiation of human mesenchymal stem cells. Hepatology 40: 1275–1284.
6. Talens-Visconti R, Bonora A, Jover R, Mirabet V, Carbonell F, et al. (2006) Hepatogenic differentiation of human mesenchymal stem cells from adipose tissue in comparison with bone marrow mesenchymal stem cells. World J Gastroenterol 12: 5834–5845.
7. Hisanaga E, Park KY, Yamada S, Hashimoto H, Takeuchi T, et al. (2008) A simple method to induce differentiation of murine bone marrow mesenchymal cells to insulin-producing cells using conophylline and betacellulin-delta4. Endocr J 55: 535–543.
8. Chao KC, Chao KF, Fu YS, Liu SH (2008) Islet-like clusters derived from mesenchymal stem cells in Wharton's Jelly of the human umbilical cord for transplantation to control type 1 diabetes. PLoS One 3: e1451.
9. Zanini C, Bruno S, Mandili G, Baci D, Cerutti F, et al. (2011) Differentiation of mesenchymal stem cells derived from pancreatic islets and bone marrow into islet-like cell phenotype. PLoS One 6: e28175.
10. Lu P, Blesch A, Tuszynski MH (2004) Induction of bone marrow stromal cells to neurons: differentiation, transdifferentiation, or artifact? J Neurosci Res 77: 174–191.
11. Greco SJ, Zhou C, Ye JH, Rameshwar P (2007) An interdisciplinary approach and characterization of neuronal cells transdifferentiated from human mesenchymal stem cells. Stem Cells Dev 16: 811–826.
12. Nauta AJ, Fibbe WE (2007) Immunomodulatory properties of mesenchymal stromal cells. Blood 110: 3499–3506.
13. Castillo MD, Trzaska KA, Greco SJ, Ponzio NM, Rameshwar P (2008) Immunostimulatory effects of mesenchymal stem cell-derived neurons: implications for stem cell therapy in allogeneic transplantations. Clin Transl Sci 1: 27–34.
14. Patel SA, Sherman L, Munoz J, Rameshwar P (2008) Immunological properties of mesenchymal stem cells and clinical implications. Arch Immunol Ther Exp (Warsz) 56: 1–8.
15. Zhao S, Wehner R, Bornhauser M, Wassmuth R, Bachmann M, et al. (2010) Immunomodulatory properties of mesenchymal stromal cells and their therapeutic consequences for immune-mediated disorders. Stem Cells Dev 19: 607–614.
16. Uccelli A, Laroni A, Freedman MS (2011) Mesenchymal stem cells for the treatment of multiple sclerosis and other neurological diseases. Lancet Neurol 10: 649–656.
17. Ben-Ami E, Berrih-Aknin S, Miller A (2011) Mesenchymal stem cells as an immunomodulatory therapeutic strategy for autoimmune diseases. Autoimmun Rev 10: 410–415.
18. Williams JT, Southerland SS, Souza J, Calcutt AF, Cartledge RG (1999) Cells isolated from adult human skeletal muscle capable of differentiating into multiple mesodermal phenotypes. Am Surg 65: 22–26.
19. Erices A, Conget P, Minguell JJ (2000) Mesenchymal progenitor cells in human umbilical cord blood. Br J Haematol 109: 235–242.
20. Peters R, Wolf MJ, van den Broek M, Nuvolone M, Dannenmann S, et al. (2010) Efficient generation of multipotent mesenchymal stem cells from umbilical cord blood in stroma-free liquid culture. PLoS One 5: e15689.
21. Gronthos S, Mankani M, Brahim J, Robey PG, Shi S (2000) Postnatal human dental pulp stem cells (DPSCs) in vitro and in vivo. Proc Natl Acad Sci U S A 97: 13625–13630.
22. Zuk PA, Zhu M, Mizuno H, Huang J, Futrell JW, et al. (2001) Multilineage cells from human adipose tissue: implications for cell-based therapies. Tissue Eng 7: 211–228.
23. Lopatina T, Kalinina N, Karagyaur M, Stambolsky D, Rubina K, et al. (2011) Adipose-derived stem cells stimulate regeneration of peripheral nerves: BDNF secreted by these cells promotes nerve healing and axon growth de novo. PLoS One 6: e17899.
24. In 't Anker PS, Scherjon SA, Kleijburg-van der Keur C, Noort WA, Claas FH, et al. (2003) Amniotic fluid as a novel source of mesenchymal stem cells for therapeutic transplantation. Blood 102: 1548–1549.
25. Moorefield EC, McKee EE, Solchaga L, Orlando G, Yoo JJ, et al. (2011) Cloned, CD117 Selected Human Amniotic Fluid Stem Cells Are Capable of Modulating the Immune Response. PLoS One 6: e26535.
26. Yoshimura H, Muneta T, Nimura A, Yokoyama A, Koga H, et al. (2007) Comparison of rat mesenchymal stem cells derived from bone marrow, synovium, periosteum, adipose tissue, and muscle. Cell Tissue Res 327: 449–462.
27. Lapi S, Nocchi F, Lamanna R, Passeri S, Iorio M, et al. (2008) Different media and supplements modulate the clonogenic and expansion properties of rabbit bone marrow mesenchymal stem cells. BMC Res Notes 1: 53.
28. Zeng L, Rahrmann E, Hu Q, Lund T, Sandquist L, et al. (2006) Multipotent adult progenitor cells from swine bone marrow. Stem Cells 24: 2355–2366.
29. Peister A, Mellad JA, Larson BL, Hall BM, Gibson LF, et al. (2004) Adult stem cells from bone marrow (MSCs) isolated from different strains of inbred mice vary in surface epitopes, rates of proliferation, and differentiation potential. Blood 103: 1662–1668.
30. Sun S, Guo Z, Xiao X, Liu B, Liu X, et al. (2003) Isolation of mouse marrow mesenchymal progenitors by a novel and reliable method. Stem Cells 21: 527–535.
31. Phinney DG (2008) Isolation of mesenchymal stem cells from murine bone marrow by immunodepletion. Methods Mol Biol 449: 171–186.
32. Nakamura Y, Arai F, Iwasaki H, Hosokawa K, Kobayashi I, et al. (2010) Isolation and characterization of endosteal niche cell populations that regulate hematopoietic stem cells. Blood 116: 1422–1432.
33. Kitano Y, Radu A, Shaaban A, Flake AW (2000) Selection, enrichment, and culture expansion of murine mesenchymal progenitor cells by retroviral transduction of cycling adherent bone marrow cells. Exp Hematol 28: 1460–1469.
34. Baxter MA, Wynn RF, Jowitt SN, Wraith JE, Fairbairn LJ, et al. (2004) Study of telomere length reveals rapid aging of human marrow stromal cells following in vitro expansion. Stem Cells 22: 675–682.
35. Digirolamo CM, Stokes D, Colter D, Phinney DG, Class R, et al. (1999) Propagation and senescence of human marrow stromal cells in culture: a simple colony-forming assay identifies samples with the greatest potential to propagate and differentiate. Br J Haematol 107: 275–281.
36. Ornitz DM, Marie PJ (2002) FGF signaling pathways in endochondral and intramembranous bone development and human genetic disease. Genes Dev 16: 1446–1465.
37. Olsen BR, Reginato AM, Wang W (2000) Bone development. Annu Rev Cell Dev Biol 16: 191–220.
38. Shapiro F (2008) Bone development and its relation to fracture repair. The role of mesenchymal osteoblasts and surface osteoblasts. Eur Cell Mater 15: 53–76.
39. Hsiao FS, Cheng CC, Peng SY, Huang HY, Lian WS, et al. (2010) Isolation of therapeutically functional mouse bone marrow mesenchymal stem cells within 3 h by an effective single-step plastic-adherent method. Cell Prolif 43: 235–248.
40. da Silva Meirelles L, Caplan AI, Nardi NB (2008) In search of the in vivo identity of mesenchymal stem cells. Stem Cells 26: 2287–2299.
41. Caplan AI (2007) Adult mesenchymal stem cells for tissue engineering versus regenerative medicine. J Cell Physiol 213: 341–347.
42. Wu Y, Chen L, Scott PG, Tredget EE (2007) Mesenchymal stem cells enhance wound healing through differentiation and angiogenesis. Stem Cells 25: 2648–2659.
43. Chen L, Tredget EE, Wu PY, Wu Y (2008) Paracrine factors of mesenchymal stem cells recruit macrophages and endothelial lineage cells and enhance wound healing. PLoS One 3: e1886.
44. Uysal AC, Mizuno H, Tobita M, Ogawa R, Hyakusoku H (2009) The effect of adipose-derived stem cells on ischemia-reperfusion injury: immunohistochemical and ultrastructural evaluation. Plast Reconstr Surg 124: 804–815.
45. Bianco P, Gehron Robey P (2000) Marrow stromal stem cells. J Clin Invest 105: 1663–1668.
46. Gronthos S, Simmons PJ (1996) The biology and application of human bone marrow stromal cell precursors. J Hematother 5: 15–23.
47. Prockop DJ (1997) Marrow stromal cells as stem cells for nonhematopoietic tissues. Science 276: 71–74.
48. Meirelles Lda S, Nardi NB (2003) Murine marrow-derived mesenchymal stem cell: isolation, in vitro expansion, and characterization. Br J Haematol 123: 702–711.
49. Phinney DG, Kopen G, Isaacson RL, Prockop DJ (1999) Plastic adherent stromal cells from the bone marrow of commonly used strains of inbred mice: variations in yield, growth, and differentiation. J Cell Biochem 72: 570–585.
50. Eslaminejad MB, Nikmahzar A, Taghiyar L, Nadri S, Massumi M (2006) Murine mesenchymal stem cells isolated by low density primary culture system. Dev Growth Differ 48: 361–370.
51. Zhu H, Guo ZK, Jiang XX, Li H, Wang XY, et al. (2010) A protocol for isolation and culture of mesenchymal stem cells from mouse compact bone. Nat Protoc 5: 550–560.
52. Sakaguchi Y, Sekiya I, Yagishita K, Ichinose S, Shinomiya K, et al. (2004) Suspended cells from trabecular bone by collagenase digestion become virtually identical to mesenchymal stem cells obtained from marrow aspirates. Blood 104: 2728–2735.
53. Tuli R, Tuli S, Nandi S, Wang ML, Alexander PG, et al. (2003) Characterization of multipotential mesenchymal progenitor cells derived from human trabecular bone. Stem Cells 21: 681–693.
54. Horwitz EM, Le Blanc K, Dominici M, Mueller I, Slaper-Cortenbach I, et al. (2005) Clarification of the nomenclature for MSC: The International Society for Cellular Therapy position statement. Cytotherapy 7: 393–395.
55. Epting CL, King FW, Pedersen A, Zaman J, Ritner C, et al. (2008) Stem cell antigen-1 localizes to lipid microdomains and associates with insulin degrading enzyme in skeletal myoblasts. J Cell Physiol 217: 250–260.
56. Holmes C, Stanford WL (2007) Concise review: stem cell antigen-1: expression, function, and enigma. Stem Cells 25: 1339–1347.
57. Ozbey O, Sahin Z, Acar N, Ustunel I (2010) Distribution of CD105 and CD166 positive cells in the proximal epiphysis of developing rat humerus. Histol Histopathol 25: 1437–1445.
58. Alsalameh S, Amin R, Gemba T, Lotz M (2004) Identification of mesenchymal progenitor cells in normal and osteoarthritic human articular cartilage. Arthritis Rheum 50: 1522–1532.
59. Li Z, Liu C, Xie Z, Song P, Zhao RC, et al. (2011) Epigenetic dysregulation in mesenchymal stem cell aging and spontaneous differentiation. PLoS One 6: e20526.

60. Wilson A, Shehadeh LA, Yu H, Webster KA (2010) Age-related molecular genetic changes of murine bone marrow mesenchymal stem cells. BMC Genomics 11: 229.
61. Granero-Molto F, Myers TJ, Weis JA, Longobardi L, Li T, et al. (2011) Mesenchymal stem cells expressing insulin-like growth factor-I (MSCIGF) promote fracture healing and restore new bone formation in Irs1 knockout mice: analyses of MSCIGF autocrine and paracrine regenerative effects. Stem Cells 29: 1537–1548.
62. Granero-Molto F, Weis JA, Miga MI, Landis B, Myers TJ, et al. (2009) Regenerative effects of transplanted mesenchymal stem cells in fracture healing. Stem Cells 27: 1887–1898.
63. Cho SW, Moon SH, Lee SH, Kang SW, Kim J, et al. (2007) Improvement of postnatal neovascularization by human embryonic stem cell derived endothelial-like cell transplantation in a mouse model of hindlimb ischemia. Circulation 116: 2409–2419.
64. Kinnaird T, Stabile E, Burnett MS, Lee CW, Barr S, et al. (2004) Marrow-derived stromal cells express genes encoding a broad spectrum of arteriogenic cytokines and promote in vitro and in vivo arteriogenesis through paracrine mechanisms. Circ Res 94: 678–685.
65. Lian WS, Cheng WT, Cheng CC, Hsiao FS, Chen JJ, et al. (2011) In vivo therapy of myocardial infarction with mesenchymal stem cells modified with prostaglandin I synthase gene improves cardiac performance in mice. Life Sci 88: 455–464.
66. Ceradini DJ, Kulkarni AR, Callaghan MJ, Tepper OM, Bastidas N, et al. (2004) Progenitor cell trafficking is regulated by hypoxic gradients through HIF-1 induction of SDF-1. Nat Med 10: 858–864.
67. Uzuka M, Nakajima K, Ohta S, Mori Y (1981) Induction of hyaluronic acid synthetase by estrogen in the mouse skin. Biochim Biophys Acta 673: 387–393.
68. Krampera M, Glennie S, Dyson J, Scott D, Laylor R, et al. (2003) Bone marrow mesenchymal stem cells inhibit the response of naive and memory antigen-specific T cells to their cognate peptide. Blood 101: 3722–3729.
69. Nadri S, Soleimani M, Hosseni RH, Massumi M, Atashi A, et al. (2007) An efficient method for isolation of murine bone marrow mesenchymal stem cells. Int J Dev Biol 51: 723–729.
70. Johnstone B, Hering TM, Caplan AI, Goldberg VM, Yoo JU (1998) In vitro chondrogenesis of bone marrow-derived mesenchymal progenitor cells. Exp Cell Res 238: 265–272.
71. Callicott RJ, Womack JE (2006) Real-time PCR assay for measurement of mouse telomeres. Comp Med 56: 17–22.
72. Nagano M, Kimura K, Yamashita T, Ohneda K, Nozawa D, et al. (2010) Hypoxia responsive mesenchymal stem cells derived from human umbilical cord blood are effective for bone repair. Stem Cells Dev 19: 1195–1210.
73. Taguchi K, Ogawa R, Migita M, Hanawa H, Ito H, et al. (2005) The role of bone marrow-derived cells in bone fracture repair in a green fluorescent protein chimeric mouse model. Biochem Biophys Res Commun 331: 31–36.
74. Nagano M, Yamashita T, Hamada H, Ohneda K, Kimura K, et al. (2007) Identification of functional endothelial progenitor cells suitable for the treatment of ischemic tissue using human umbilical cord blood. Blood 110: 151–160.
75. Toutain CE, Brouchet L, Raymond-Letron I, Vicendo P, Berges H, et al. (2009) Prevention of skin flap necrosis by estradiol involves reperfusion of a protected vascular network. Circ Res 104: 245–254, 212p following 254.
76. Zhang Y, Zhang R, Li Y, He G, Zhang D, et al. (2012) Simvastatin augments the efficacy of therapeutic angiogenesis induced by bone marrow-derived mesenchymal stem cells in a murine model of hindlimb ischemia. Mol Biol Rep 39: 285–293.
77. Dar A, Domev H, Ben-Yosef O, Tzukerman M, Zeevi-Levin N, et al. (2012) Multipotent vasculogenic pericytes from human pluripotent stem cells promote recovery of murine ischemic limb. Circulation 125: 87–99.

Protection by Salidroside against Bone Loss via Inhibition of Oxidative Stress and Bone-Resorbing Mediators

Jin-Kang Zhang[1], Liu Yang[1], Guo-Lin Meng[1], Zhi Yuan[1], Jing Fan[1], Dan Li[1], Jian-Zong Chen[2], Tian-Yao Shi[3], Hui-Min Hu[1], Bo-Yuan Wei[1], Zhuo-Jing Luo[1*], Jian Liu[1*]

1 Institute of Orthopedic Surgery, Xijing Hospital, Fourth Military Medical University, Xi'an, People's Republic of China, **2** Research Center of Traditional Chinese Medicine, Xijing Hospital, Fourth Military Medical University, Xi'an, People's Republic of China, **3** Department of Pharmacology, School of Pharmacy, Fourth Military Medical University, Xi'an, People's Republic of China

Abstract

Oxidative stress is a pivotal pathogenic factor for bone loss in mouse model. Salidroside, a phenylpropanoid glycoside extracted from Rhodiola rosea L, exhibits potent antioxidative effects. In the present study, we used an in vitro oxidative stress model induced by hydrogen peroxide (H_2O_2) in MC3T3-E1 cells and a murine ovariectomized (OVX) osteoporosis model to investigate the protective effects of salidroside on bone loss and the related mechanisms. We demonstrated that salidroside caused a significant ($P<0.05$) elevation of cell survival, alkaline phosphatase (ALP) staining and activity, calcium deposition, and the transcriptional expression of *Alp*, *Col1a1* and *Osteocalcin* (*Ocn*) in the presence of H_2O_2. Moreover, salidroside decreased the production of intracellular reactive oxygen species (ROS), and osteoclast differentiation inducing factors such as receptor activator of nuclear factor-kB ligand (RANKL) and IL-6 induced by H_2O_2. In vivo studies further demonstrated that salidroside supplementation for 3 months caused a decrease in malondialdehyde (MDA) and an increase in reduced glutathione (GSH) concentration in blood of ovariectomized mouse ($P<0.05$), it also improved trabecular bone microarchitecture and bone mineral density in the fourth lumbar vertebra and distal femur. Our study indicated that the protection provided by salidroside in alleviating bone loss was mediated, at least in part, via inhibition of the release of bone-resorbing mediators and oxidative damage to bone-forming cells, suggesting that salidroside can be used as an effective remedy in the treatment or prevention of osteoporosis.

Editor: Zhongjun Zhou, The University of Hong Kong, Hong Kong

Funding: This work was supported by Ministry of Science and Technology of China (2011CB964703), National High Technology Research and Development Program 863 (2012AA020502), China Postdoctoral Science Foundation (20100480093) and National Natural Science Foundation of China (30901504). The funders had no role in study design, data collection and analysis, decision to publish, or preparation of the manuscript.

Competing Interests: The authors have declared that no competing interests exist.

* E-mail: zjk1271984@21cn.com (JL); zjluo@fmmu.edu.cn (ZJL)

These authors contributed equally to this work.

Introduction

Osteoporosis is a degenerative bone disease characterized by low bone mass and structural deterioration of bone tissue, leading to bone fragility [1]. Oxidative stress, resulting from excessive generation of reactive oxygen species, can damage all components of the cell. At present, numerous studies have shown the positive correlation between oxidative stress and osteoporotic status. For instance, in osteoporotic postmenopausal women, decreased bone mineral density was shown to be associated with higher plasma lipid oxidation [2], and catalase and glutathione peroxidase activity were found to be lowered [3,4]. Ovariectomy induces oxidative stress in rat femurs together with a decreased activity of antioxidant systems [5]. Evidence mainly obtained from the studies in mouse model provides a paradigm shift from the 'estrogen-centric' account of the pathogenesis of involutional osteoporosis to one in which age-related mechanisms intrinsic to bone and oxidative stress are protagonists, and moreover, age-related changes in other organs and tissues, such as ovaries, accentuate them [6].

Bone mass is maintained through a dynamic balance between osteoblastic bone formation and osteoclastic bone resorption [7]. Evolving evidence suggests that reactive oxygen species can enhance bone resorption by directly or indirectly promoting osteoclasts formation and activity [8]. However, it can induce apoptosis of osteoblasts and decrease their activity leading to reduced osteoblastic bone formation [9]. As a result, the imbalance between these two types of cell leads to bone metabolic diseases, such as osteoporosis. Postmenopausal osteoporosis is associated with significant changes in bone turnover: bone formation decreases and bone resorption increases or remains unchanged, leading to a net bone loss [10]. Therefore, therapeutic strategies aimed at preventing or delaying reactive oxygen species might be a reasonable choice for the treatment of osteoporosis. Recently, attention has been focused on searching for natural substances with antioxidative potential that can scavenge free radicals and protect cells from oxidative damage.

Salidroside (structure shown in Fig. 1) is an active constituent extracted from the root of Rhodiola rosea L, which has been used as a medicinal herb for a long time. Reports have existed in the literature that salidroside possesses anti-aging, anti-cancer, anti-inflammatory, anti-hypoxia and antioxidative properties [11,12,13,14]. Moreover, recent studies have shown that salidroside protects human erythrocytes against hydrogen peroxide (H_2O_2) -induced apoptosis and protects against H_2O_2-induced injury in cardiac H9c2 cells via PI3K-Akt dependent pathway [15,16]. Our previous studies revealed that salidroside protects against 1-methyl-4-phenylpyridinium (MPP+)-induced apoptosis in PC12 cells by inhibiting the NO pathway, it can also provide neuroprotective effects against focal cerebral ischemia in vivo and H_2O_2-induced neurotoxicity in vitro [17,18].

However, whether salidroside can provide protection against bone loss associated with oxidative stress remains unknown. Therefore, in this study, we used an in vitro oxidative stress model induced by H_2O_2 in MC3T3-E1 cells, which are preosteoblastic cells from mouse calvariae commonly used in studying osteogenic development [19], and an in vivo ovariectomized (OVX) osteoporosis model in mouse to investigate the protective effects of salidroside on bone loss as well as the underlying mechanisms.

Materials and Methods

Materials

Salidroside extracted from Rhodiola rosea L (purity>99%) was obtained from National Institute for the Control of Pharmaceutical and Biological Products (Beijing, China). Fetal bovine serum (FBS) and α-Modified minimal essential medium (α-MEM) were purchased from Gibco Life Technologies (Grand Island, USA). ALP activity assay kit was purchased from GENMED scientific Inc. (USA). RANKL and IL-6 ELISA kit were purchased from R&D system Inc. (Minneapolis, MN, USA). PrimeScript RT reagent kit and SYBR Premix Ex Taq were obtained from TaKaRa Biotechnology (Dalian, China). Oligonucleotide primers were synthesized by Sangon Biological Engineering Technology Co. (Shanghai, China). BCIP/NBT Alkaline Phosphatase Color Development Kit,RIPA Lysis Buffer, Reactive Oxygen Species Assay Kit, GSH and MDA Assay kit were purchased from the Beyotime Institute of Biotechnology (Shanghai, China). All other chemicals and reagents were of analytical grade.

Cell culture

Murine osteoblastic MC3T3-E1 cells were obtained from the Center Laboratory for Tissue Engineering, College of Stomatology, Fourth Military Medical University, Xi'an, China [20,21]. MC3T3-E1 cells were maintained in a-MEM with 10% heat-inactivated FBS and 100 U/ml penicillin and 100μg/ml streptomycin under conditions of 5% CO_2 and 37°C. H_2O_2 was used as the exogenous ROS source, and N-acetyl-L-cysteine (NAC) was used as an ROS scavenger. When reaching confluence, MC3T3-E1 cells were treated with culture medium containing 10 mM β-glycerophosphate and 50μg/ml ascorbic acid to initiate differentiation. After 6 or 14 days, the cells were pre-incubated with serum-free regular culture medium containing salidroside for 24 h before treatment with 300μM H_2O_2 for another 24 h. In all the experiments, salidroside treatment continued after the pretreatment. Each experiment was performed in duplicate wells and repeated three times.

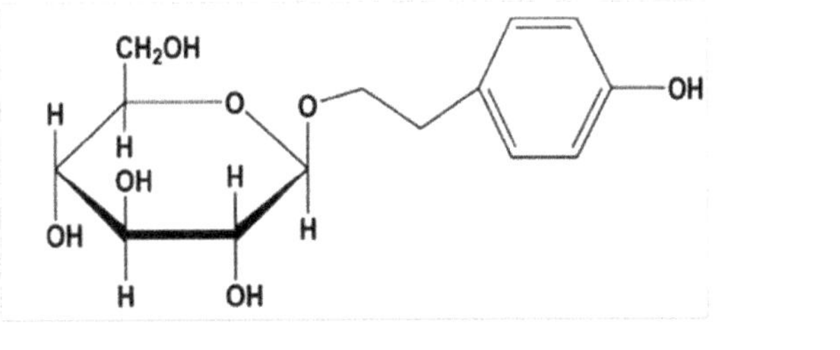

Figure 1. Chemical structure of salidroside.

Assays of cell viability

In the experiments, cells were treated with different concentrations of H_2O_2 (0, 100, 200, 300, 400μM) for 2, 6, 12, 24h or salidroside (0, 0.1, 1, 10μM) for 24, 72h to investigate the toxicity of H_2O_2 and salidroside. Then, cells were cultured with serum-free regular culture medium containing salidroside (0, 0.1, 1, 10μM) for 24 h followed by treatment with 300μM H_2O_2 for 24 h. Cell viability was measured by MTT assay. In brief, 0.02 ml MTT solution was added to each well and the plates were incubated at 37 °C for 4 h. Then DMSO was added and the plates were shaken for 5 min to dissolve formazan products. The absorbance of each well was recorded on a microplate reader at a wavelength of 492 nm. Cell viability of the control group not exposed to either H_2O_2 or salidroside was defined as 100%.

Alkaline phosphatase (ALP) staining and activity assay

After 6 days, the cells were cultured with serum-free medium containing salidroside and/or H_2O_2 for 2 days. At harvesting, cells were washed twice with phosphate-buffered saline (PBS), fixed with 10% formalin in PBS for 30 s, rinsed with deionized water, and stained with BCIP/NBT Alkaline Phosphatase Color Development Kit under protection from direct light. To measure ALP activity, the cell monolayer was lysed with RIPA. The lysate was centrifuged at 10,000×g for 5 min. The clear supernatant was used to measure the ALP activity, which was determined using an ALP activity assay kit. Total protein concentrations were determined by Bradford protein assay method. ALP activity was normalized to total protein measured with the Bradford protein assay method.

Calcium deposition assay

After 14 days, the cells were cultured with serum-free medium containing salidroside and/or H_2O_2 for 2 days. At harvesting, the cells were fixed in ice-cold 10% formalin for 20 min and stained with 40 mM Alizarin Red S (pH 4.4, Sigma) for 45 min at room temperature. For matrix calcification estimate, the stain was solubilized with 10% cetylpyridinum chloride by shaking for 15 min. The absorbance of the released Alizarin red S was measured at the wave length of 562 nm [22].

Quantitative real-time PCR

After 6 days, the cells were cultured with serum-free medium containing salidroside and/or H_2O_2 for 2 days. Total cellular RNA was extracted using the Trizol reagent according to the manufacturer's instructions (OMEGA). Single strand cDNA synthesis was performed by using PrimeScript RT reagent kit (TaKaRa). Real-time quantitative RT-PCR was performed using the CFX96 (BIO-RAD) instrument and individual PCRs were carried out in 96-well optical reaction plates with SYBR Green-I (TaKaRa) in accordance with the manufacturer's instructions. Briefly, PCR was carried out in a 25-μl final volume containing the following reagents: 12.5 μl of 2× SYBR Green-I master mix, 1 μl of 10 μM each primer, 2.5 μl of 1 μg/μl cDNA template, and 8 μl of double deionized water. PCR conditions were as follows: initial denaturation at 95°C for 30 s, followed by 40 cycles of denaturation at 95°C for 5 s, and annealing at 58°C for 15 s. Fluorescent product was measured by a single acquisition mode at 58°C after each cycle. Target genes (*Alp*, *Col1a1*, *Osteocalcin* (*Ocn*)) expression was normalized to the reference gene β-actin. The $2^{-\Delta\Delta Ct}$ method was applied to calculate relative gene expression. The PCR products were subjected to melting curve analysis and standard curve to confirm the correct amplification. All the RT-PCRs were performed in triplicates and the primers used for PCR are listed in Table 1.

Measurement of RANKL and IL-6

After 6 days, the cells were cultured with serum-free medium containing salidroside and/or H_2O_2 for 2 days. RANKL and IL-6 contents in culture medium were measured using sandwich ELISA assay kit, according to the manufacturer's recommendation. Total protein concentrations were determined by Bradford protein assay method.

Measurement of intracellular ROS

The level of intracellular ROS was quantified using Reactive Oxygen Species Assay Kit. DCFH-DA is oxidized by ROS in viable cells to 2′,7′-dichlorofluorescein (DCF) which is highly fluorescent at 530 nm. The cells were washed three times with PBS. DCFH-DA, diluted to a final concentration of 10 μM, was added and incubated for 30 min at 37°C in the dark. After being washed three times with PBS, the relative levels of fluorescence were quantified using a multi-detection microplate reader (485 nm excitation and 535 nm emission).

Animals and salidroside treatments

Thirty-two 9-week-old and weighing 20.3 ±1.34 g BALB/c female mice were purchased from the Experimental Animal Center of The Fourth Military Medical University (Xi'an, China) and were acclimated to laboratory conditions for 1 week before the experiment. The initial body weight of the mice was no significant difference among the four groups in this study. They were maintained in a well-ventilated controlled room at 20°C on a 12-h light/dark cycle with free access to water and food. Mice underwent sham-operation (n = 8) or were surgically ovariectomized (OVX; n = 24) under anesthesia by pentobarbital sodium (50 mg/kg body weight, i.p.). OVX was performed by removing the bilateral ovaries through a dorsal approach and sham surgery was performed by identifying the bilateral ovaries. The mice were randomly divided into four groups: (1) untreated (Sham: sham-operated controls); (2) untreated (OVX controls); (3) OVX administered intraperitoneally with salidroside (5 mg/kg body weight) daily; (4) OVX administered intraperitoneally with salidroside (20 mg/kg body weight) daily. Salidroside were dissolved in distilled water and distilled water alone was administered to untreated mice. The treatments started 1week after the surgery and lasted for 15 weeks. Blood samples were taken from the heart in anesthetized mice and serum was then prepared by centrifugation. The left femur and the 4 th lumbar vertebra (L4) from each mouse were removed and cleaned of adherent tissue. All experimental procedures in animals were approved by the Ethics in Animal Research Committee of the Fourth Military Medical University (permission code 2010C00843).

Table 1. Real-time PCR primers for amplification of specific MC3T3-E1 mRNA.

Gene	Forward (5′-3′)	Reverse (5′-3′)
Alp	aacccagacacaagcattcc	ccagcaagaagaagcctttg
Col1a1	gcatggccaagaagacatcc	cctcgggtttccacgtctc
Ocn	ctgacaaagccttcatgtccaa	gcgccggagtctgttcacta
β-actin	ctggcaccacaccttctaca	ggtacgaccagaggcataca

Measurements of serum reduced glutathione (GSH) and malondialdehyde (MDA)

The GSH in whole blood samples were determined using a GSH Assay kit following the manufacturer's instructions. Determination of GSH is based on the reaction of GSH with 5.50-dithiobis-2-nitrobenzoic acid (DTNB) to form a product that can be detected by a spectrophotometer at 412 nm. The MDA in whole blood samples were determined using a Lipid peroxidation MDA Assay Kit following the manufacturer's instructions. The binding of thiobarbituric acid to MDA which was formed during lipid peroxidation results in a chromogenic complex.

Bone microarchitecture assessment by micro-computed tomography

Bone microarchitecture in the 4 th lumbar vertebra (L4) and distal femur was scanned using explore Locus SP Pre-Clinical Specimen micro-computed tomography (GE Healthcare, USA) with 8-μm resolution, tube voltage of 50 kV and tube current of 0.1 mA. The reconstruction and 3D quantitative analyses were performed by using software provided by a desktop micro-CT system (GE Healthcare, USA). The same settings for scan and analysis were used for all samples. In the femora, scanning regions were confined to the distal metaphysis, extending proximally 2.0 mm from the proximal tip of the primary spongiosa. Trabecular bone region from the vertebral body was outlined for each micro-CT slice, excluding both the cranial and caudal endplate regions. Within these regions, trabecular bone was separated from cortical bone with boundaries defined by the endocortical bone surfaces. The following 3D indices in the defined region of interest (ROI) were analyzed: relative bone volume over total volume (BV/TV, %), trabecular number (Tb.N), trabecular separation (Tb.Sp), trabecular thickness (Tb.Th), connectivity density (Conn.D), structure model index (SMI) and bone mineral density (BMD).The operator conducting the scan analysis was blinded to the treatments associated with the specimens.

Undecalcified histological examination

The left femur of each mouse was collected and fixed in 4% paraformaldehyde for 48 hours. All samples were dehydrated in graded alcohols and embedded in polymethyl-methacrylate (PMMA). The distal femurs were cut into sections of 5 and 240μm in thickness in the coronal plane on a rotation microtome. The 5μm sections were stained with Von kossa staining to visualize calcium deposition and 240μm sections were hand grounded to a thickness of 20μm for Van Gieson staining, which is used to stain collagen fiber.

Statistical analysis

Data were expressed as means ± S.D. of multiple repeats of the same experiment (n = 5). The data for these measurements were analyzed with one-way analysis of variance (ANOVA) with subsequent post hoc multiple comparison by Dunnett's test. Statistically significant values defined as $P<0.05$.

Results

Protective effect of salidroside on H_2O_2 induced cytotoxicity in MC3T3-E1 cells

Cell viability was analyzed to determine the protective effect of salidroside on the response of MC3T3-E1 cells to oxidative stress induced by H_2O_2. As shown in Fig.2A, 100 to 400μM of H_2O_2 induced significant decrease in cell survival in a dose- and time-dependent manner. In the group treated with 300 μM H_2O_2 for 24 h, cell viability was significantly decreased by approximately 50% as compared with the control group($P<0.01$). Therefore, the treatment of 300 μM H_2O_2 for 24 h was used to induce MC3T3-E1 cell injury in subsequent experiments. As shown in Fig. 2B, salidroside alone was non-toxic to cells at the concentrations used in this study ($P>0.05$). When the cells were pretreated with salidroside for 24 h before the addition of H_2O_2 (300μM) for 24 h, salidroside (0.1~10μM) significantly increased the survival of MC3T3-E1 cells as compared to H_2O_2 alone treated cells ($P<0.05$), suggesting that salidroside suppressed H_2O_2 induced cytotoxicity (Fig. 2C). NAC, which significantly inhibited H_2O_2-induced cytotoxicity at 1mM as a potent antioxidant, was used here serving as a positive control.

Protective effect of salidroside on osteoblast dysfunction induced by H_2O_2

In order to assess the effect of salidroside on osteoblast dysfunction induced by H_2O_2, ALP staining and activity, calcium deposition and osteogenic differentiation genes (*Alp*, *Col1a1*, *Ocn*) were determined. Compared with the control cells, the presence of H_2O_2 significantly decreased cellular ALP activity, mineralization and expression of osteogenic differentiation genes (Fig.3). When osteoblasts were pretreated with salidroside in the presence of H_2O_2, salidroside (0.1-10μM) significantly increased cellular ALP activity, which is one of the major osteoblast differentiation markers (Fig. 3B). We further investigated the effect of salidroside on mineralization in the presence of H_2O_2 by measuring calcium deposition by Alizarin Red staining. As shown in Fig. 3C, salidroside (0.1–1μM) showed significant recovery effect on mineralization inhibited by H_2O_2. Moreover, salidroside supplementation significantly enhanced the expression of osteogenic differentiation genes (*Alp*, *Col1a1*, *Ocn*) compared with the group treated with H_2O_2 alone (Fig. 3D). Our results demonstrated that salidroside attenuates osteoblast dysfunction induced by H_2O_2.

Inhibition of salidroside on RANKL and IL-6 production of MC3T3-E1 cells in the presence of H_2O_2

In order to determine the possible regulation of osteoclast differentiation by osteoblasts, we examined the production of RANKL and IL-6, which are primarily released from osteoblast cells. Osteoblast-derived RANKL binds to RANK on osteoclasts, resulting in osteoclast activation, and IL-6 have also been demonstrated to increase osteoclastic activity. When 0.3 mM H_2O_2 was added to the cells, the production of RANKL and IL-6 increased significantly. However, H_2O_2-induced RANKL and IL-6 production was significantly inhibited by pretreatment of salidroside at concentrations of 0.1–10μM and 0.1–1μM, respectively (Fig.4).

Salidroside reduces the production of ROS induced by H_2O_2

To investigate whether cell-protective action of salidroside is related to its antioxidant activity, the production of ROS detected by fluorescent probe DCFH-DA was assessed. As shown in Fig. 5, the production of ROS was increased significantly by treatment of 0.3 mM H_2O_2. These results suggest that H_2O_2 enhanced oxidant generation and may cause damage to osteoblastic MC3T3-E1 cells. However, the production of ROS was significantly inhibited when pretreated with salidroside at concentrations of 0.1–10μM (Fig.5). These data support the hypothesis that the cytoprotective effect offered by salidroside may be associated with its antioxidant capacity.

Inhibition of salidroside on oxidative status in serum

Serum MDA and GSH levels are potential biomarkers for measurement of oxidative stress. As shown in Fig. 6, serum MDA level was increased and GSH level was decreased in OVX mice when compared with sham groups ($P<0.05$). Salidroside supplementation (20 mg/kg) significantly decreased serum MDA concentrations and increased GSH level ($P<0.05$). No differences in MDA and GSH levels were observed in OVX mice treated with different concentrations of salidroside ($P>0.05$).

Protective effect of salidroside against bone loss in OVX mice

We administered salidroside as early as 7 days after ovariectomy to evaluate its effects on trabecular bone microarchitecture. We sacrificed all the animals 16 weeks after the operation. No significant difference in body weight of the mice in four groups was noted. The analysis of the properties of trabecular bone in distal femoral metaphyses and lumber vertebrate (L4) indicated that ovariectomy induced deterioration of the trabecular bone microarchitecture in mice, as demonstrated by the reduction in BV/TV, Conn.D, Tb.N, Tb.Th and BMD when compared with the sham group mice ($P<0.01$) (Table 2). In contrast, as shown in Table 2, SMI and Tb.Sp were significantly increased in response to OVX ($P<0.05$ for both). However, treating OVX mice with a high dose of salidroside at 20 mg/kg could significantly ($P<0.05$) reverse the changes in these parameters induced by ovariectomy and could maintain the microarchitecture of trabecular bone in distal femoral metaphyses and lumber vertebrate (L4).These increments in trabecular bone parameters were readily observable in micro-CT images of the distal femur (Fig. 7). Salidroside at 5 mg/kg improved the trabecular bone mass loss and microarchitecture deterioration, but no significant difference was noticed (P>0.05) when compared with the OVX group. Van Gieson and Von Kossa staining also showed similar results (Fig. 8). Compared with the sham group, the trabecular number was reduced and spaces between trabecules were broader in the OVX groups. Salidroside supplementation inhibited these deleterious effects, as demonstrated by an increase in the trabecular number and a decrease in the trabecular space in the OVX+salidroside groups (Fig. 8).

Discussion

Oxidative stress is characterized by an increased level of reactive oxygen species (ROS) that disrupts the intracellular reduction–oxidation (redox) balance. Numerous studies have suggested that increased oxidative stress is involved in the pathogenesis of osteoporosis, caused by aging and estrogen deficiency [23,24]. H_2O_2 is generated from nearly all sources of oxidative stress and has been demonstrated to play a crucial role in estrogen deficiency osteoporosis [25]. Therefore, we used H_2O_2-induced oxidative

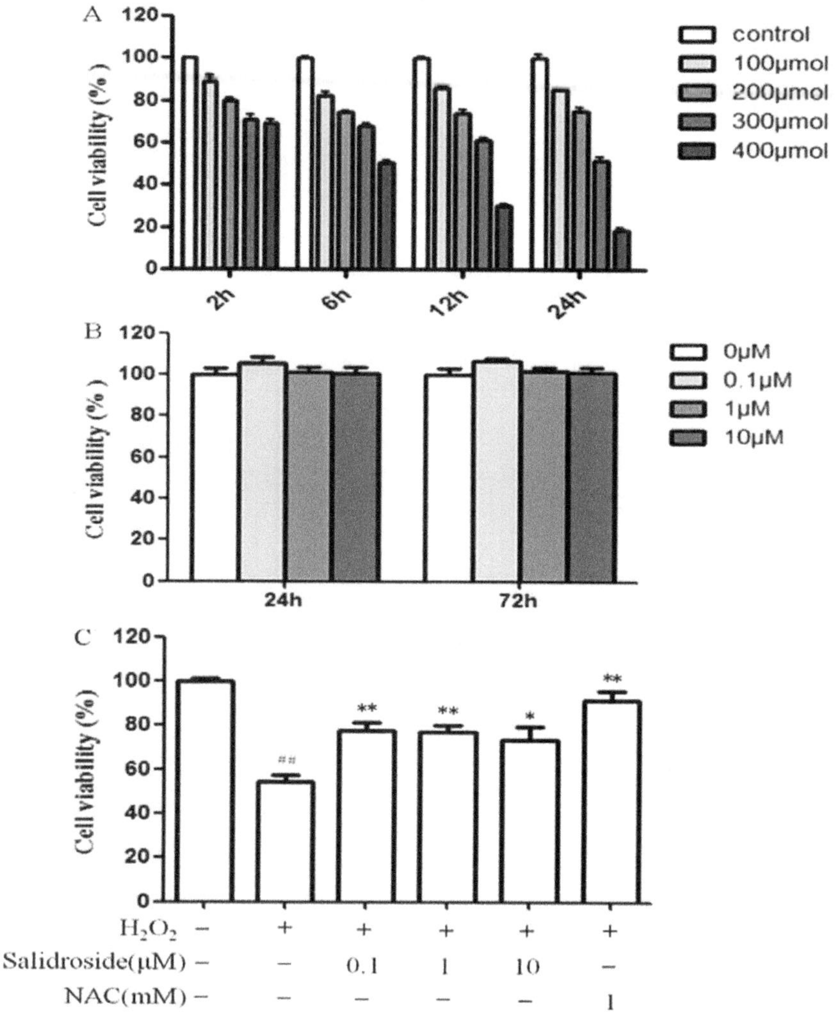

Figure 2. Protective effect of salidroside on H_2O_2 induced cytotoxicity in MC3T3-E1 cells. A: Concentration- and time-dependent effects of H_2O_2 on cell viability. B: Cells were incubated in different concentrations of salidroside alone. C: Cells were pretreated with salidroside for 24 h before treatment with 0.3 mM H_2O_2 for 24 h. NAC was used as positive control. The control value for cell viability was 0.431±0.05 OD. $^{##}P<0.01$ versus untreated control cells; $^{*}P<0.05$ and $^{**}P<0.01$ compared with the group treated with H_2O_2 alone.

stress model in the present study. Fatokun reported that exposure of MC3T3-E1 cells to a concentration of at least 0.2 mM H_2O_2 for 1 h was required to produce significant lethality involving both apoptosis and necrosis [26].Our results showed that H_2O_2 substantially reduced cell viability in a dose-dependent manner, but the toxic effect was reversed to some degree when pretreated with different concentrations of salidroside for 24 h. Our previous studies revealed that salidroside protects against (MPP+)-induced apoptosis in PC12 cells, it can provide neuroprotective effects against focal cerebral ischemia in vivo and H_2O_2-induced neurotoxicity in vitro [17,18]. The present study indicated that salidroside reduced the cytotoxicity induced by H_2O_2 in osteoblastic MC3T3-E1 cells.

Apart from affecting cell viability, oxidative stress also influences osteoblast differentiation. Liu et al. showed that H_2O_2 induced oxidative stress and suppressed the osteoblastic differentiation in primary mouse BMSCs [27]. This inhibition of cell differentiation was characterized by a reduction in ALP activity, which is an early differentiation marker and is important to regulate mineralization of bone matrix [28]. Subsequently, Bai et al. reported that H_2O_2-treated osteoblasts exhibited a reduction in levels of differentiation markers including *Alp*, *Col a1*, colony-forming unit-osteoprogenitor (CFU-O) formation, and nuclear phosphorylation of the transcription factor *Runx2* [29]. More recently, it was indicated that H_2O_2 diminished mineralization and decreased the expression of osteogenic genes *Runx2*, *Alp* and bone sialoprotein in MC3T3-E1cells [30]. The present study has demonstrated that H_2O_2 significantly decreased cellular ALP activity, mineralization and expression of osteogenic differentiation genes *Alp*, *Col1a1* and *Ocn*, which confirms the previous observations that H_2O_2 toxicity leads to dysfunction of osteoblasts. Meanwhile, we found that the inhibition induced by H_2O_2 of osteogenic differentiation can be reversed by salidroside. According to our unpublished date, salidroside alone could not improve the proliferation and osteogenic differentiation of MC3T3-E1 cells significantly within the observed concentration. Therefore, we deduced that the protection of salidroside may mainly contribute to its antioxidant ability, suggesting that salidroside may be a beneficial agent in preventing osteoporosis associated with oxidative stress by enhancing osteoblast function.

Osteoblasts are coupled with osteoclasts in terms of the release of various bone-resorbing cytokines, such as receptor activator of

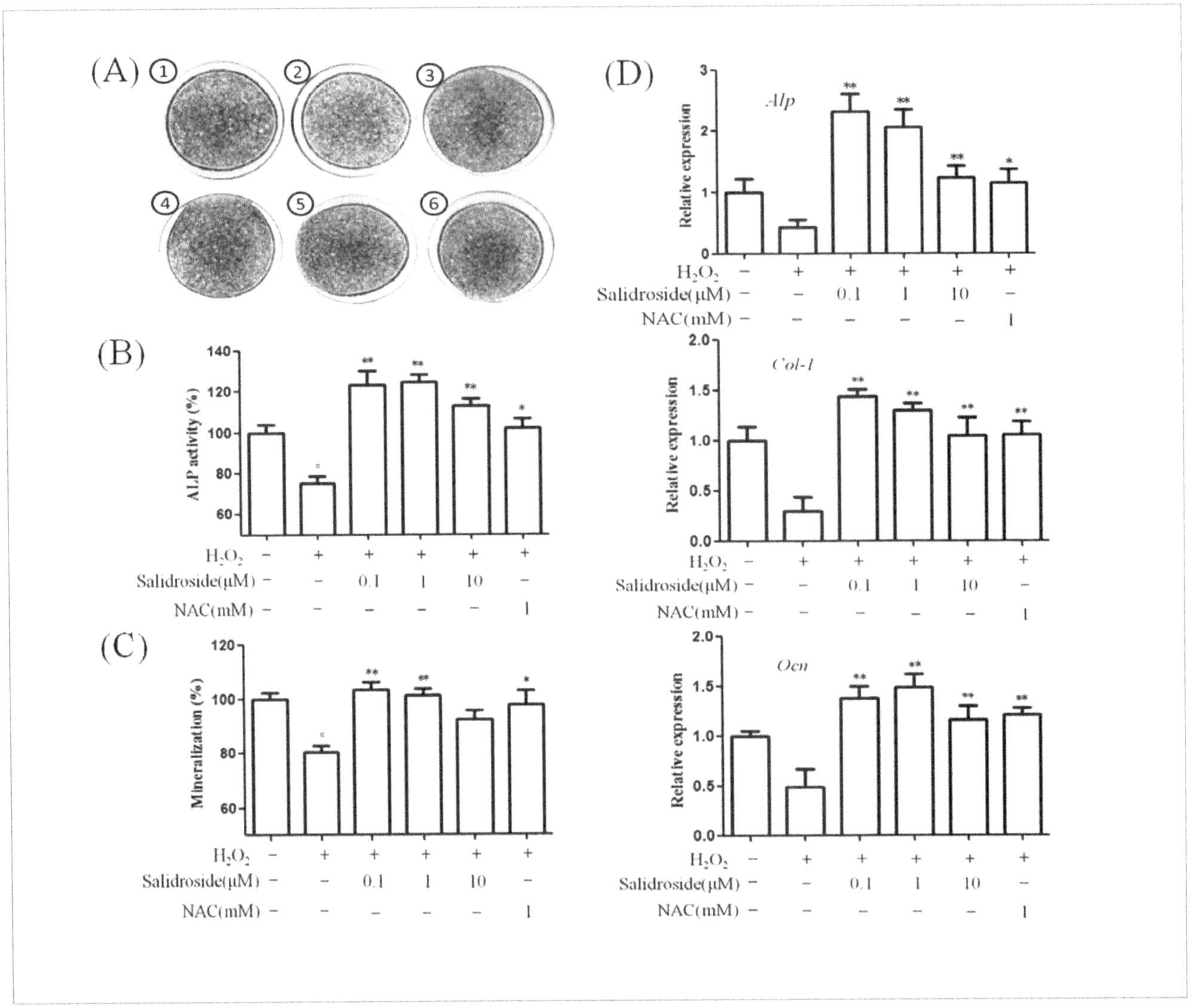

Figure 3. Protective effect of salidroside on H_2O_2 induced osteoblast dysfunction. After differentiation induction of 6 or 14 days, MC3T3-E1 cells were pretreated with salidroside for 24 h before treatment with 0.3 mM H_2O_2 for 24 h. NAC was used as positive control. A: Effect of salidroside on the ALP staining of MC3T3-E1 cells in the presence of H_2O_2. ① the control group; ② H_2O_2; ③ H_2O_2+ salidroside (0.1μM); ④ H_2O_2+ salidroside (1μM); ⑤ H_2O_2+ salidroside (10μM); ⑥ H_2O_2+NAC(1 mM). B: Effect of salidroside on the ALP activity of MC3T3-E1 cells in the presence of H_2O_2. The control value for ALP activity was 0.682 ± 0.021 unit /μg protein. C: Effect of salidroside on the mineralization of MC3T3-E1 cells in the presence of H_2O_2. The control value for mineralization was 1.392±0.31 OD. D: Effect of salidroside on the mRNA expression of *Alp*, *Col-1* and *Ocn* in the presence of H_2O_2. $^{\#}P<0.05$ versus untreated control cells;$^{*}P<0.05$ and $^{**}P<0.01$ compared with the group treated with H_2O_2 alone.

nuclear factor (NFκB) ligand (RANKL) and IL-6. RANKL, highly expressed on osteoblasts, marrow stromal cells and T cells, is an essential cytokine involved in osteoclastogenesis. RANKL acts by binding to the RANK receptor on osteoclast progenitor cells, leading to expression of osteoclast differentiation genes, prolonged survival of osteoclasts and increased bone resorption [31]. RANKL is prevented by osteoprotegerin (OPG), a soluble decoy receptor that competes with RANK for binding to RANKL and is also expressed by osteoblasts [32]. Bai et al. reported that ROS stimulates RANKL expression in mouse osteoblasts and human MG63 cells [33]. IL-6 was also reported to be produced by osteoblasts [34] and can induce RANKL mRNA expression, promote the differentiation of osteoclasts from its precursor and play an important role in the pathogenesis of osteoporosis due to estrogen deficiency [35,36]. ROS might indirectly stimulate osteoclasts by augmenting expression of resorptive cytokines such as RANKL, TNF-α and IL-6 that have been strongly implicated in estrogen deficiency bone loss [37]. In this study, salidroside inhibited the production of RANKL and IL-6 induced by H_2O_2 in osteoblastic cells. The inhibitory effect on RANKL and IL-6 production may contribute to bone anti-resorbing effect of salidroside, and may play a role in the reduction of bone loss.

Reactive oxygen species (ROS) such as superoxides anions, hydroxyl radicals, and H_2O_2 can cause severe damage to DNA, protein, and lipids [38]. High levels of oxidant produced during normal cellular metabolism or from environmental stimuli perturb the normal redox balance and shift cells into a state of oxidative stress. Accumulating evidence suggests that ROS may play its role in bone loss-related diseases in two ways: suppression of bone formation and stimulation of bone resorption. Salidroside is extracted from Rhodiola rosea L, which is one of Chinese traditional medicine, has been reported to possess antioxidative

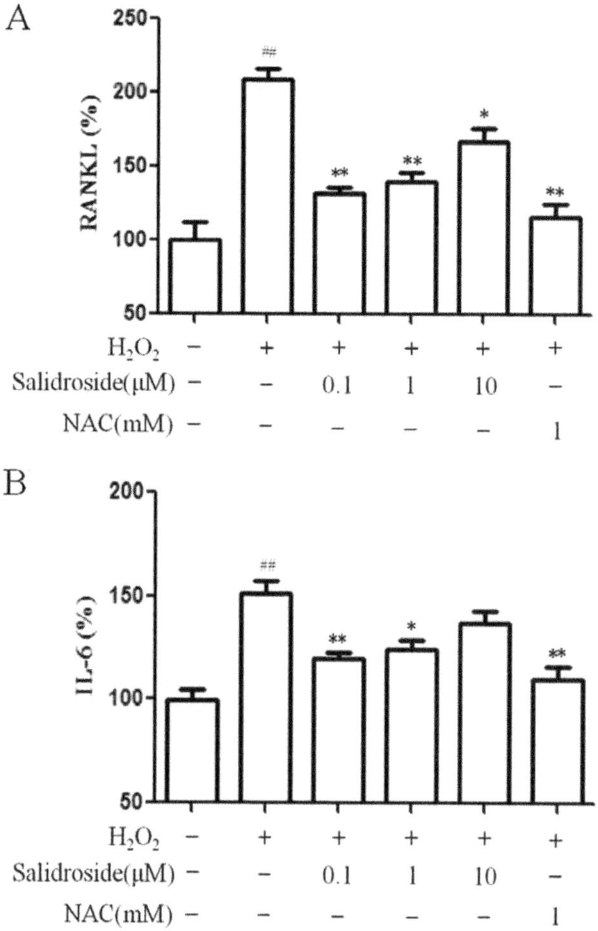

Figure 4. Inhibition of salidroside on RANKL and IL-6 production of MC3T3-E1 cells in the presence of H_2O_2. After differentiation induction of 6 days, MC3T3-E1 cells were pretreated with salidroside for 24 h before treatment with 0.3 mM H_2O_2 for 24 h. NAC was used as positive control. A: The production of RANKL in the presence of salidroside and/or H_2O_2. The control value for RANKL was 3.792±0.271ng/mg. B: The production of IL-6 in the presence of salidroside and/or H_2O_2. The control value for IL-6 was 0.429±0.391 ng/mg. $^{\#\#}P<0.01$ versus untreated control cells;$^{*}P<0.05$ and $^{**}P<0.01$ compared with the group treated with H_2O_2 alone.

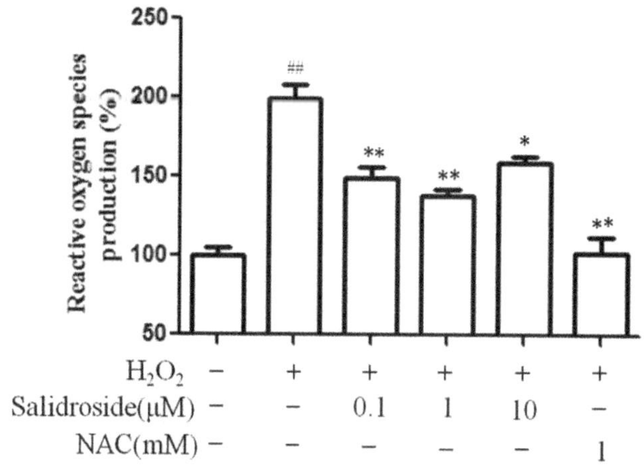

Figure 5. Inhibition of salidroside on reactive oxygen species generation induced by H_2O_2 in MC3T3-E1 cells. After differentiation induction of 6 days, MC3T3-E1 cells were pretreated with salidroside for 24 h before treatment with 0.3 mM H_2O_2 for 24 h. NAC was used as positive control. The data shows changes in levels of ROS, which was measured by DCF fluorescence method. $^{\#\#}$ $P<0.01$ versus untreated control cells;$^{*}P<0.05$ and $^{**}P<0.01$ compared with the group treated with H_2O_2 alone.

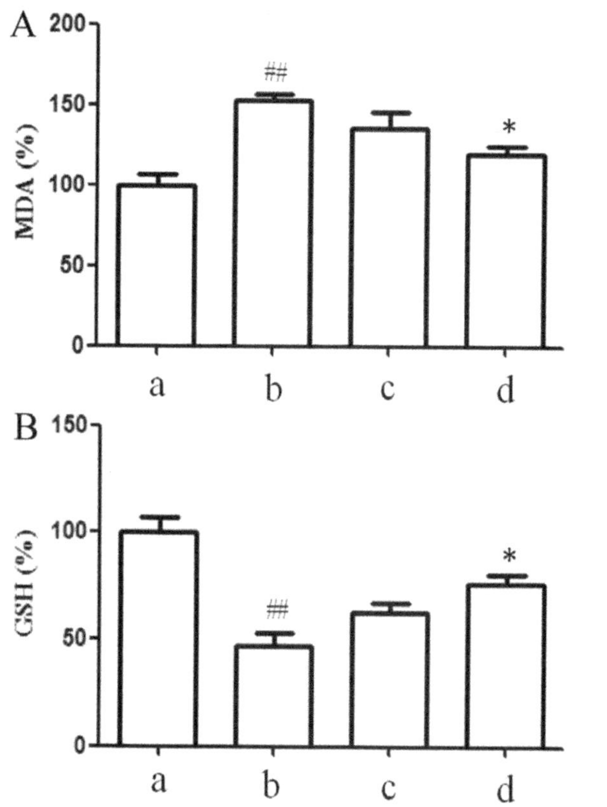

Figure 6. Inhibition of salidroside on oxidative status in serum of ovariectomized mice. A: Serum MDA concentrations in ovariectomized mice supplemented with different concentration of salidroside. B: Serum GSH concentrations in ovariectomized mice supplemented with different concentration of salidroside. a: sham; b: OVX; c: OVX+salidroside (5 mg/kg); d: OVX+salidroside (20 mg/kg). The control value for MDA and GSH was 7.692±0.928 nM/mg and 13.24±1.391 nM/mg.$^{\#\#}P<0.01$ versus sham group;$^{*}P<0.05$ compared with OVX group.

properties [14]. In the present study, pretreatment with salidroside for 24 h could reverse the production of ROS induced by H_2O_2 to some degree. Therefore, the results of the present study demonstrated that salidroside can act as a biological antioxidant and protect cells from oxidative stress-induced toxicity. Accordingly, the protective effect provided by salidroside to osteoblastic MC3T3-E1 cells might be mediated, at least in part, via its antioxidant ability.

Protection against oxidative stress is a possible mechanism explaining salidroside's beneficial effects. However, there is a paucity of knowledge regarding its molecular mode of action. We speculated that it may degrade H_2O_2 directly, elevate the endogenous antioxidant defenses or through ROS-irrelevant mechanisms. Wiegant et al. reported that Rhodiola rosea L. could increase expression of hemeoxygenase-1 (HO-1), a protein that can be activated by the antioxidant-response element (ARE) in response to oxidative challenge [39]. ARE is a *cis*-acting enhancer element in the 5′flanking region of the cytoprotective enzymes.

Table 2. Effect of salidroside on bone microarchitecture indices in mice measured by Micro-CT.

Indices	Sham	OVX	OVX+salidroside(5)	OVX+salidroside(20)
Distal femur				
BV/TV (%)	0.107±0.029	0.031±0.004$^{\#\#}$	0.041±0.002*	0.073±0.011**
Tb.Th. (mm)	0.032±0.003	0.021±0.002$^{\#\#}$	0.025±0.002	0.028±0.004*
Tb.N. (1/mm)	3.59±0.331	1.441±0.111$^{\#\#}$	1.762±0.136	2.96±0.433**
Tb.Sp. (mm)	0.250±0.024	0.676±0.053$^{\#\#}$	0.579±0.048*	0.317±0.047**
Conn.D (1/mm^3)	107.004±15.928	32.739±9.391$^{\#\#}$	45.551±7.697	66.516±10.429**
SMI	2.346±0.079	3.299±0.249$^{\#\#}$	2.925±0.187**	2.658±0.143**
BMD (mg/cm^3)	213.043±22.29	120.028±14.94$^{\#\#}$	139.135±20.283	161.576±27.259**
Lumbar vertebra				
BV/TV (%)	0.189±0.562	0.093±0.031$^{\#\#}$	0.128±0.007**	0.145±0.081**
Tb.Th. (mm)	0.049±0.015	0.028±0.007$^{\#\#}$	0.036±0.011	0.043±0.009*
Tb.N. (1/mm)	4.753±1.427	2.897±0.678$^{\#}$	3.745±1.087	4.054±0.873
Tb.Sp. (mm)	0.184±0.065	0.365±0.083$^{\#\#}$	0.277±0.088	0.218±0.053*
Conn.D (1/mm^3)	154.732±17.973	68.537±12.338$^{\#\#}$	85.447±13.46	119.781±15.749**
SMI	1.649±0.183	2.524±0.12$^{\#\#}$	2.171±0.21**	1.867±0.159**
BMD (mg/cm^3)	183.984±20.14	92.661±15.592$^{\#\#}$	121.059±26.827	143.759±22.349*

Data were expressed as means ± S.D., n = 8 in each group.
$^{\#}P<0.05$ and $^{\#\#}P<0.01$vs. the sham group.
$^{*}P<0.05$ and $^{**}P<0.01$vs. the OVX group.

This element regulates many antioxidant enzymes including the glutathione *S*-transferases, HO-1 and NQO1, and its activation by transcription factor nuclear erythroid-2 related factor-2 (Nrf-2) confers a resistance to oxidative damage. Salidroside is an active constituent extracted from Rhodiola rosea L. Therefore, we speculate that salidroside provided protection effects against H_2O_2-induced cytotoxicity and osteoblast dysfunction in MC3T3-E1 cells may through the HO-1 and Nrf-2 signaling pathways. We will confirm this molecular mechanism in the further study.

The mechanisms through which estrogen deficiency stimulates bone loss remain controversial. Recently, oxidative stress has been suggested to be responsible for the development of postmenopausal osteoporosis. Serum MDA levels is one of the potential

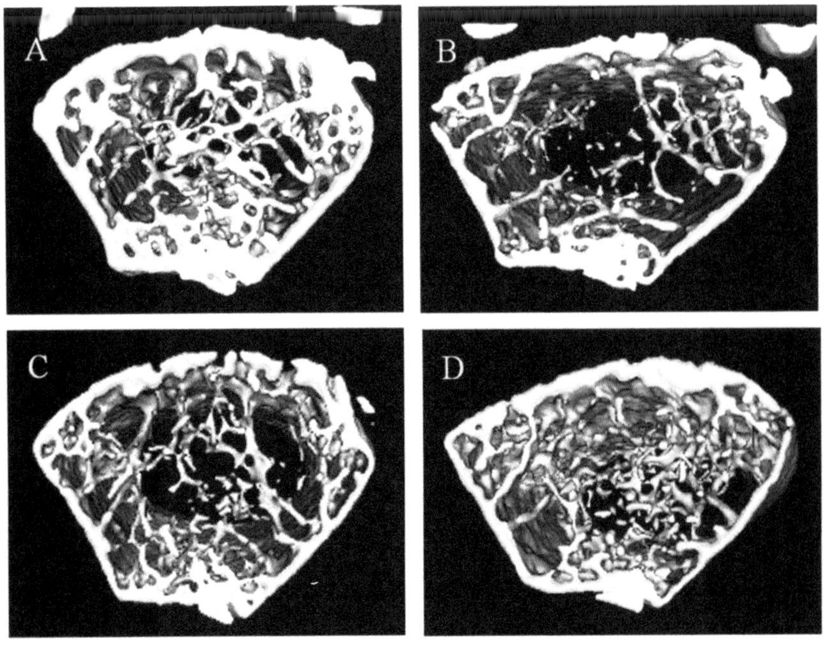

Figure 7. Analysis of micro-computed tomography within the distal metaphyseal femur region. A: sham, B: OVX, C: OVX+salidroside(5 mg/kg), D: OVX+salidroside(20 mg/kg).

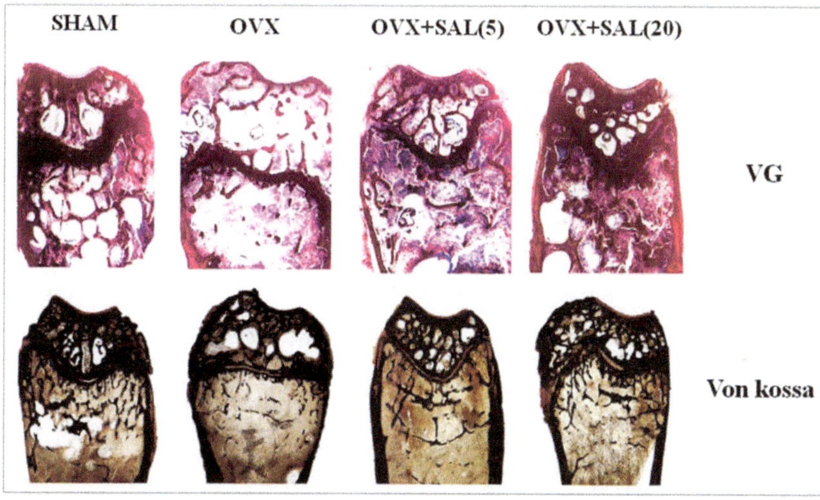

Figure 8. Van Gieson (VG) and Von Kossa (Silver nitrate) staining of the distal femur. The figure was 40× of the original section.

biomarkers for oxidative stress [40]. Lipid peroxides (MDA) is the end product of lipid peroxidation caused by ROS. It can cause increased cell membrane permeability [41]. Reduced glutathione is one of the most important reducer agents which maintain the intracellular redox balance [42]. Decrease of GSH level is also a marker for oxidative stress [43]. In our study, salidroside treatment for 3 months prevented the increased serum MDA level and decreased GSH level resulting from OVX. Our results indicated that salidroside could improve the oxidative status in estrogen deficient osteoporosis model. Bone quality is determined by microarchitecture, geometry and material properties of the bone. Measuring such microarchitectural parameters as BV/TV, Tb.N, Tb.Sp, Tb.Th, Conn.D, SMI and BMD may improve our ability to estimate bone strength [44,45]. The effects of ovariectomy on bone are smaller in cortical compartments than in trabecular compartments [46].Therefore, we observed the effect of salidroside on trabecular microarchitecture by scanning with Micro-CT. All parameters, such as BMD, BV/TV, Tb.N, and Tb.Sp, showed that salidroside treatment with 20 mg/kg for 3 months improved bone structural indices, bone mineral density and trabecular thickness compromised by OVX. Meanwhile, histological examination also showed that ovariectomy had negative effects on the microarchitecture of the trabecular bone. However, this effect could be reversed by supplementation of salidroside to some degree. These data implied that salidroside may significantly increase trabecular bone mass in ovariectomized mouse model and salidroside has a therapeutic effect in prevention of estrogen-deficient osteoporosis.

In conclusion, our studies demonstrated that salidroside protects MC3T3-E1 cells from H_2O_2-induced cell damage and dysfunction of osteoblasts via inhibition of oxidative stress and bone-resorbing mediators. Moreover, salidroside reduces the oxidative status in serum and prevents bone loss and deterioration of trabecular microarchitecture in OVX-induced osteoporosis mouse model. Our results suggest that salidroside could be used as a good candidate for preventing and treating osteoporosis. Further investigation is required in order to clarify the detailed molecular mechanisms of action of salidroside in bone.

Acknowledgments

We would like to thank Jun Wang from the institute of orthopedic surgery in Xijing hospital for Micro-CT scanning and analysis.

Author Contributions

Conceived and designed the experiments: JZ ZJL JL. Performed the experiments: JKZ LY GLM ZY JF. Analyzed the data: JZC HMH BYW. Contributed reagents/materials/analysis tools: TYS DL. Wrote the paper: JKZ LY.

References

1. (2001) Osteoporosis prevention, diagnosis, and therapy. JAMA 285: 785–795.
2. Sendur OF, Turan Y, Tastaban E, Serter M (2009) Antioxidant status in patients with osteoporosis: a controlled study. Joint Bone Spine 76: 514–518.
3. Ozgocmen S, Kaya H, Fadillioglu E, Aydogan R, Yilmaz Z (2007) Role of antioxidant systems, lipid peroxidation, and nitric oxide in postmenopausal osteoporosis. Mol Cell Biochem 295: 45–52.
4. Ozgocmen S, Kaya H, Fadillioglu E, Yilmaz Z (2007) Effects of calcitonin, risedronate, and raloxifene on erythrocyte antioxidant enzyme activity, lipid peroxidation, and nitric oxide in postmenopausal osteoporosis. Arch Med Res 38: 196–205.
5. Muthusami S, Ramachandran I, Muthusamy B, Vasudevan G, Prabhu V, et al. (2005) Ovariectomy induces oxidative stress and impairs bone antioxidant system in adult rats. Clin Chim Acta 360: 81–86.
6. Manolagas SC (2010) From estrogen-centric to aging and oxidative stress: a revised perspective of the pathogenesis of osteoporosis. Endocr Rev 31: 266–300.
7. Seeman E, Delmas PD (2006) Bone quality--the material and structural basis of bone strength and fragility. N Engl J Med 354: 2250–2261.
8. Lee NK, Choi YG, Baik JY, Han SY, Jeong DW, et al. (2005) A crucial role for reactive oxygen species in RANKL-induced osteoclast differentiation. Blood 106: 852–859.
9. Arai M, Shibata Y, Pugdee K, Abiko Y, Ogata Y (2007) Effects of reactive oxygen species (ROS) on antioxidant system and osteoblastic differentiation in MC3T3-E1 cells. IUBMB Life 59: 27–33.
10. Isomura H, Fujie K, Shibata K, Inoue N, Iizuka T, et al. (2004) Bone metabolism and oxidative stress in postmenopausal rats with iron overload. Toxicology 197: 93–100.
11. Mao GX, Deng HB, Yuan LG, Li DD, Li YY, et al. (2010) Protective role of salidroside against aging in a mouse model induced by D-galactose. Biomed Environ Sci 23: 161–166.
12. Skopinska-Rozewska E, Malinowski M, Wasiutynski A, Sommer E, Furmanowa M, et al. (2008) The influence of Rhodiola quadrifida 50% hydro-alcoholic extract and salidroside on tumor-induced angiogenesis in mice. Pol J Vet Sci 11: 97–104.
13. Yu S, Liu M, Gu X, Ding F (2008) Neuroprotective effects of salidroside in the PC12 cell model exposed to hypoglycemia and serum limitation. Cell Mol Neurobiol 28: 1067–1078.

14. Yu P, Hu C, Meehan EJ, Chen L (2007) X-ray crystal structure and antioxidant activity of salidroside, a phenylethanoid glycoside. Chem Biodivers 4: 508–513.
15. Qian EW, Ge DT, Kong SK (2012) Salidroside Protects Human Erythrocytes against Hydrogen Peroxide-Induced Apoptosis. J Nat Prod 75: 531–537.
16. Zhu Y, Shi YP, Wu D, Ji YJ, Wang X, et al. (2011) Salidroside protects against hydrogen peroxide-induced injury in cardiac H9c2 cells via PI3K-Akt dependent pathway. DNA Cell Biol 30: 809–819.
17. Li X, Ye X, Li X, Sun X, Liang Q, et al. (2011) Salidroside protects against MPP(+)-induced apoptosis in PC12 cells by inhibiting the NO pathway. Brain Res 1382: 9-18.
18. Shi TY, Feng SF, Xing JH, Wu YM, Li XQ, et al. (2012) Neuroprotective effects of Salidroside and its analogue tyrosol galactoside against focal cerebral ischemia in vivo and H2O2-induced neurotoxicity in vitro. Neurotox Res 21: 358–367.
19. Fatokun AA, Stone TW, Smith RA (2008) Responses of differentiated MC3T3-E1 osteoblast-like cells to reactive oxygen species. Eur J Pharmacol 587: 35–41.
20. Li Y, Tang L, Duan Y, Ding Y (2010) Upregulation of MMP-13 and TIMP-1 expression in response to mechanical strain in MC3T3-E1 osteoblastic cells. BMC Res Notes 3: 309.
21. Li Y, Ma W, Feng Z, Wang Z, Zha N, et al. (2012) Effects of irradiation on osteoblast-like cells on different titanium surfaces in vitro. J Biomed Mater Res B Appl Biomater.
22. Stanford CM, Jacobson PA, Eanes ED, Lembke LA, Midura RJ (1995) Rapidly forming apatitic mineral in an osteoblastic cell line (UMR 106-01 BSP). J Biol Chem 270: 9420–9428.
23. Baek KH, Oh KW, Lee WY, Lee SS, Kim MK, et al. (2010) Association of oxidative stress with postmenopausal osteoporosis and the effects of hydrogen peroxide on osteoclast formation in human bone marrow cell cultures. Calcif Tissue Int 87: 226–235.
24. Maggio D, Barabani M, Pierandrei M, Polidori MC, Catani M, et al. (2003) Marked decrease in plasma antioxidants in aged osteoporotic women: results of a cross-sectional study. J Clin Endocrinol Metab 88: 1523–1527.
25. Lean JM, Jagger CJ, Kirstein B, Fuller K, Chambers TJ (2005) Hydrogen peroxide is essential for estrogen-deficiency bone loss and osteoclast formation. Endocrinology 146: 728–735.
26. Fatokun AA, Stone TW, Smith RA (2006) Hydrogen peroxide-induced oxidative stress in MC3T3-E1 cells: The effects of glutamate and protection by purines. Bone 39: 542–551.
27. Liu AL, Zhang ZM, Zhu BF, Liao ZH, Liu Z (2004) Metallothionein protects bone marrow stromal cells against hydrogen peroxide-induced inhibition of osteoblastic differentiation. Cell Biol Int 28: 905–911.
28. Hessle L, Johnson KA, Anderson HC, Narisawa S, Sali A, et al. (2002) Tissue-nonspecific alkaline phosphatase and plasma cell membrane glycoprotein-1 are central antagonistic regulators of bone mineralization. Proc Natl Acad Sci U S A 99: 9445–9449.
29. Bai XC, Lu D, Bai J, Zheng H, Ke ZY, et al. (2004) Oxidative stress inhibits osteoblastic differentiation of bone cells by ERK and NF-kappaB. Biochem Biophys Res Commun 314: 197–207.
30. Arai M, Shibata Y, Pugdee K, Abiko Y, Ogata Y (2007) Effects of reactive oxygen species (ROS) on antioxidant system and osteoblastic differentiation in MC3T3-E1 cells. IUBMB Life 59: 27–33.
31. Boyle WJ, Simonet WS, Lacey DL (2003) Osteoclast differentiation and activation. Nature 423: 337–342.
32. Li J, Sarosi I, Yan XQ, Morony S, Capparelli C, et al. (2000) RANK is the intrinsic hematopoietic cell surface receptor that controls osteoclastogenesis and regulation of bone mass and calcium metabolism. Proc Natl Acad Sci U S A 97: 1566–1571.
33. Bai XC, Lu D, Liu AL, Zhang ZM, Li XM, et al. (2005) Reactive oxygen species stimulates receptor activator of NF-kappaB ligand expression in osteoblast. J Biol Chem 280: 17497–17506.
34. Girasole G, Jilka RL, Passeri G, Boswell S, Boder G, et al. (1992) 17 beta-estradiol inhibits interleukin-6 production by bone marrow-derived stromal cells and osteoblasts in vitro: a potential mechanism for the antiosteoporotic effect of estrogens. J Clin Invest 89: 883–891.
35. Kurihara N, Bertolini D, Suda T, Akiyama Y, Roodman GD (1990) IL-6 stimulates osteoclast-like multinucleated cell formation in long term human marrow cultures by inducing IL-1 release. J Immunol 144: 4226–4230.
36. Papanicolaou DA, Vgontzas AN (2000) Interleukin-6: the endocrine cytokine. J Clin Endocrinol Metab 85: 1331–1333.
37. Kitazawa R, Kimble RB, Vannice JL, Kung VT, Pacifici R (1994) Interleukin-1 receptor antagonist and tumor necrosis factor binding protein decrease osteoclast formation and bone resorption in ovariectomized mice. J Clin Invest 94: 2397–2406.
38. Naka K, Muraguchi T, Hoshii T, Hirao A (2008) Regulation of reactive oxygen species and genomic stability in hematopoietic stem cells. Antioxid Redox Signal 10: 1883–1894.
39. Wiegant FA, Surinova S, Ytsma E, Langelaar-Makkinje M, Wikman G, et al. (2009) Plant adaptogens increase lifespan and stress resistance in C. elegans. Biogerontology 10: 27–42.
40. Nielsen F, Mikkelsen BB, Nielsen JB, Andersen HR, Grandjean P (1997) Plasma malondialdehyde as biomarker for oxidative stress: reference interval and effects of life-style factors. Clin Chem 43: 1209–1214.
41. Yang P, He XQ, Peng L, Li AP, Wang XR, et al. (2007) The role of oxidative stress in hormesis induced by sodium arsenite in human embryo lung fibroblast (HELF) cellular proliferation model. J Toxicol Environ Health A 70: 976–983.
42. Ning J, Grant MH (2000) The role of reduced glutathione and glutathione reductase in the cytotoxicity of chromium (VI) in osteoblasts. Toxicol In Vitro 14: 329–335.
43. Kinov P, Leithner A, Radl R, Bodo K, Khoschsorur GA, et al. (2006) Role of free radicals in aseptic loosening of hip arthroplasty. J Orthop Res 24: 55–62.
44. Kazakia GJ, Majumdar S (2006) New imaging technologies in the diagnosis of osteoporosis. Rev Endocr Metab Disord 7: 67–74.
45. Teo JC, Si-Hoe KM, Keh JE, Teoh SH (2006) Relationship between CT intensity, micro-architecture and mechanical properties of porcine vertebral cancellous bone. Clin Biomech (Bristol, Avon) 21: 235–244.
46. Peng ZQ, Vaananen HK, Zhang HX, Tuukkanen J (1997) Long-term effects of ovariectomy on the mechanical properties and chemical composition of rat bone. Bone 20: 207–212.

Time of Progression to Osteopenia/Osteoporosis in Chronically HIV-Infected Patients: Screening DXA Scan

Eugenia Negredo[1]*, Anna Bonjoch[1], Moisés Gómez-Mateu[2], Carla Estany[1], Jordi Puig[1], Nuria Perez-Alvarez[1,2], Joaquin Rosales[3], Silvana di Gregorio[3], Luis del Rio[3], Guadalupe Gómez[2], Bonaventura Clotet[1,4]

1 Lluita contra la SIDA Foundation, Hospital Universitari Germans Trias i Pujol, Universitat Autònoma de Barcelona, Barcelona, Spain, **2** Statistics and Operations Research Department, Universitat Politècnica de Catalunya, Barcelona, Spain, **3** CETIR Centre Mèdic, Barcelona, Spain, **4** Irsicaixa Foundation, Barcelona, Spain

Abstract

Background: Algorithms for bone mineral density (BMD) management in HIV-infected patients are lacking. Our objective was to assess how often a dual-energy x-ray absorptiometry (DXA) scan should be performed by assessing time of progression to osteopenia/osteoporosis.

Methods: All DXA scans performed between 2000 and 2009 from HIV-infected patients with at least two DXA were included. Time to an event (osteopenia and osteoporosis) was assessed using the Kaplan–Meier method. Strata (tertiles) were defined using baseline minimum T scores. Differences between strata in time to an event were compared with the log-rank test.

Results: Of 391 patients (1,639 DXAs), 49.6% had osteopenia and 21.7% osteoporosis at their first DXA scan. Of the 112 (28.6%) with normal BMD, 35.7% progressed to osteopenia; median progression time was 6.7 years. These patients were stratified: "low-risk" (baseline minimum T score >-0.2 SD), "middle-risk" (between -0.2 and -0.6 SD), and "high-risk" (from -0.6 to -1 SD); median progression time to osteopenia was 8.7, >7.2, and 1.7 years, respectively ($p<0.0001$). Of patients with osteopenia, 23.7% progressed to osteoporosis; median progression time was >8.5 years. Progression time was >8.2 years in "low-risk" tertile (T score between -1.1 and -1.6 SD), >8.5 years in "middle-risk" (between -1.6 and -2), and 3.2 years in "high-risk" (from -2 to -2.4) ($p<0.0001$).

Conclusions: Our results may help to define the BMD testing interval. The lowest T score tertiles would suggest recommending a subsequent DXA in 1–2 years; in the highest tertiles, ≥6 years. Early intervention in patients with bone demineralization could reduce fracture–related morbidity/mortality.

Editor: Songtao Shi, University of Southern California, United States of America

Funding: This work was supported in part by a grant from the Spanish Ministry of Education and Science [Grant number MTM2008-06747-C02-00]. The funders had no role in study design, data collection and analysis, decision to publish, or preparation of the manuscript. No additional external funding was received for this study.

Competing Interests: The authors have declared that no competing interests exist.

* E-mail: enegredo@flsida.org

Introduction

Bone strength is the result of bone mineral density (BMD) and bone microarchitecture. A decrease in BMD leads to deterioration of microarchitecture, and is determined by the intensity of bone remodeling. These changes lead to critical damage and porosity that weaken bone and increase the probability of fractures.[1]

Many factors lead to accelerated bone loss, and HIV infection is one of the most recently identified [2,3,4]. The results of several studies confirm a higher incidence of osteopenia and osteoporosis in HIV-infected patients than in HIV-negative individuals. In fact, up to 25% of infected patients fulfill the criteria for osteoporosis and up to 50% fulfill those of osteopenia [2,3,4,5]. Accelerated bone demineralization in this population is due to an additional number of factors such as the HIV infection itself and the chronic inflammatory status, by increasing apoptosis of osteoblast cells and promotion of osteoclastic activity [6,7,8,9,10,11,12,13,14,15], the exposure to specific antiretroviral agents [2,13,16,17,18] and the immune reconstitution [14,19,20], together with traditional risk factors, such as vitamin D insufficiency, a secondary cause of osteoporosis that is very prevalent among HIV-infected patients. [21]

In addition, the first available longitudinal studies revealed that HIV-infected patients experience more rapid bone loss [5,19,20] and more frequent fractures than HIV-negative individuals. [20,22,23,24]

The high associated morbidity and mortality of bone fractures [25] means that optimal monitoring of bone mineralization should be offered to patients at high risk of low BMD, such as the HIV-infected population.

Dual-energy X-ray absorptiometry (DXA) is the method of choice for the assessment of BMD. Most clinicians attending HIV-infected patients agree that this group should undergo DXA screening, especially those patients with traditional risk factors for bone loss. [26,27] However, the optimal BMD testing intervals remains undetermined.

This study aims to determine how often a DXA scan should be performed in chronically HIV-infected patients by assessing the time of progression to osteopenia or osteoporosis in a large cohort.

Methods

Study design, population, and objective

We performed a retrospective longitudinal observational study of all DXA scans from HIV-infected patients who attended our HIV Unit between January 2000 and December 2009.

Of a total of 671 patients with at least one DXA scan, 391 had at least two DXA scans performed during the study period. These scans were included in the present analysis. The study was performed according to the stipulations of the Declaration of Helsinki, and all patients gave their written informed consent for their medical information to be used for purposes of scientific research in accordance with the ethical committee of the participating site. A more detailed description of the methodology applied has been described elsewhere. [2]

The objective of the study was to determine the time of progression to bone loss defined as time from normal BMD to osteopenia and from osteopenia to osteoporosis.

Osteopenia and osteoporosis were defined following the World Health Organization (WHO) criteria, as follows: normal, when the T score by DXA was higher than -1.0 SD, osteopenia when the T score was between -1.0 SD and -2.5 SD, and osteoporosis when the T score was less than -2.5 SD. [28]

Assessments

A total of 1,639 DXA scans from 391 patients were included in the present analysis.

The mean BMD and T score (comparison with normal reference values for young adults expressed as standard deviation units) for the lumbar spine and femoral neck were measured using the same DXA device (Lunar Prodigy, GE Healthcare, Belgium) at an external center (CETIR Grup Mèdic, Barcelona, Spain).

Epidemiological and HIV-related data (time since diagnosis of HIV infection, time on antiretroviral treatment, viral load, CD4 T-cell count, nadir CD4 T-cell count, total time on treatment, total time on protease inhibitors, total time on tenofovir, baseline antiretroviral treatment, time with viral suppression, and hepatitis B or C coinfection) were collected from the database of our HIV Unit at time of the first DXA scan.

Statistical analysis

A descriptive analysis of the main quantitative and categorical variables was performed.

We calculated time of progression in weeks from normal BMD to osteopenia. The calculation was based on those individuals whose BMD was considered normal according to a first DXA scan and who fulfilled the criteria for osteopenia in a subsequent scan. The same procedure was followed to compute time from osteopenia to osteoporosis (ie, patients with osteopenia in a first DXA scan who progressed to osteoporosis).

Patients with normal BMD at baseline and at least 3 DXA scans who progressed from normal BMD status to osteopenia and later to osteoporosis were considered for both time from normal BMD status to osteopenia and time from osteopenia to osteoporosis.

The time to an event, namely, change of category (normal to osteopenia, osteopenia to osteoporosis), was known only for those patients who presented the event before the last DXA scan. For the remaining patients, the only known data were that the time to the event was greater than the observation time. This approach is known as administrative censoring, and the incomplete data are termed right-censored. [29]

Additionally, data were stratified by tertiles of the baseline T score. These distinct groups represent the BMD baseline status. The initial value is related to the time to an event, assuming that the T score is a monotone and decreases over time.

Survival was analyzed using the Kaplan-Meier estimator; the log-rank test was used to compare strata. If the last time of observation is not censored, then the curve fall to zero and an exact value of time is provided while, if the last observed time is censored, the survival remains constant from the last time value and result is provided as ">than" this value.

All analyses were performed using the R software, and all reported *p* values are two-tailed.

Results

Epidemiological and clinical data are summarized in Table 1.

At the first DXA scan, 112 patients of 391 (28.6%) had normal BMD, 194 (49.6%) fulfilled the criteria for osteopenia, and 85 (21.7%) fulfilled the criteria for osteoporosis.

The mean (SD) number of DXA scans per patient (DXA scans/patient) was 4 (2); 100% of patients had 2 DXA scans, 67% had 3 DXA scans, 48% had 4 DXA scans, and 35% had 5 or more. No differences were observed in mean (SD) DXA scans/patient after stratification taking the first DXA as normal (5 (3) DXA/patient), osteopenia (4 (3) DXA/patient), and osteoporosis (4 (2) DXA/patient) ($p = 0.111$).

Table 1. Epidemiological and clinical data at first DXA scan.

Gender, male, n (%)	284 (73%)
Menopause, n (%)	10 (9.5%)
Age, years	39.4 (34.9; 44.2)
BMI, kg/m^2	22.5 (20.9; 24.6)
Calcium intake, g/d	16 (4%)
Hepatitis B/C coinfection, n (%)	93 (29%)
Concomitant therapy, n (%)	
Hormone treatment, n (%)	3 (1%)
Alendronate, n (%)	7 (2%)
Time since HIV diagnosis, years	7.9 (3.7; 12.1)
Current CD4+, absolute value, cells/μL	514 (348.5; 746.5)
Nadir CD4+, cells/μL	219.5 (106.8; 318.3)
Suppressed viral load, n (%)	268 (68.5%)
Proportion of time with suppressed viral load, n (%)	30.6 (11.7; 49.3)
Naïve, n (%)	48 (12%)
Time on antiretroviral therapy, years	4.8 (1.5; 8.5)
Current use of protease inhibitors, n (%)	171 (50%)
Time on protease inhibitors, years	2.4 (1.2; 4.1)
Current use of tenofovir, n (%)	173 (51%)
Time on tenofovir, years	1 (0.3; 2.3)
Creatinine, μmol/L	87 (76; 97.5)

Values are expressed as median (IQR) or number (%).

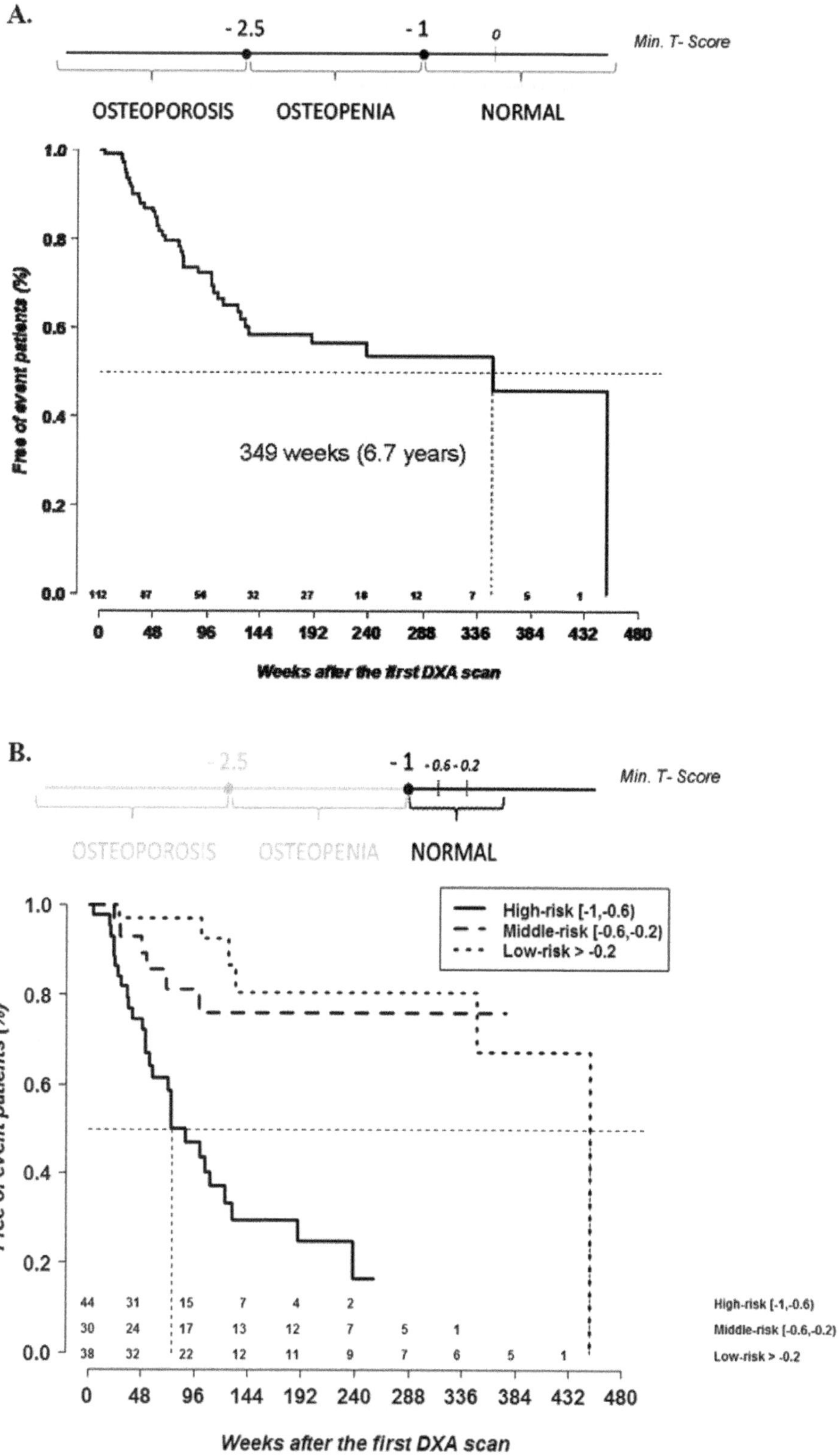

HIGH-RISK [−1, −0.6)	88 weeks
MIDDLE-RISK [−0.6,−0.2)	>375 weeks
LOW-RISK ≥−0.2	451 weeks

Figure 1. Time of progression. Time of progression from normal bone mineral density to osteopenia overall (n = 112 patients) (A) and after stratification according to minimum baseline T score ("low-risk", "middle-risk", and "high-risk") (B).

Table 2. Patients (n = 112) who progressed from normal bone mineral density to osteopenia/osteoporosis.

Follow-up (weeks)	HIGH-RISK	MIDDLE-RISK	LOW-RISK
48	25%	11%	3%
96	53%	19%	3%
144	70%	24%	20%
192	75%	24%	20%
240	84%	24%	20%
288		24%	20%
336		24%	20%
384			33%
432			33%
480			100%

Median (IQR) time between DXA scans was 33.71 weeks (25.1; 56) (0.65 years); median (IQR) time between the first and the last DXA scans was 133.1 weeks (62.7; 276.4) (2.6 years). No differences were detected in median (IQR) time between the first and the last DXA scans after stratification according to the first DXA scan (data not shown).

Change from normal BMD at baseline to osteopenia

Median follow-up for the 112 patients from this group was 152 weeks (59.1; 258) (2.9 years). Forty of these 112 patients (35.7%) progressed to osteopenia/osteoporosis.

The survival analysis showed a median (IQR) time of progression to osteopenia of 349 weeks (74; 451) (6.7 years) (Figure 1.A).

Patients with normal BMD at baseline were stratified in tertiles according to the minimum T score of their first DXA, as follows: "low-risk" tertile when the minimum T score was >−0.2 SD (38 patients, 33.9%), "middle-risk" tertile when the minimum T score was between −0.2 and −0.6 SD (30 patients, 26.8%) and "high-risk" tertile when the minimum T score was between −0.6 and −1 SD (44 patients, 39.3%) (Figure 1.B).

The three groups were similar with respect to age (p = 0.95), gender (p = 0.72), time with infection (p = 0.064), percentage of patients with viral suppression (p = 0.81), and CD4 T-cell count (p = 0.359).

The survival analysis revealed significant differences in time of progression after stratification by tertiles. Median (IQR) time of progression overall was 451 weeks (349; 451) (8.7 years) in patients from the "low-risk" tertile, >375 weeks (>375; >375) (>7.2 years) in those who were in the "middle-risk" tertile, and 88 weeks (39; 190) (1.7 years) in those who were in the "high-risk" tertile (p<0.0001) (Figure 1.B).

Table 2 shows those of the 112 patients whose status progressed from normal to osteopenia/osteoporosis after stratification by baseline minimum T score ("low-risk", "middle-risk", and "high-risk").

When patients were stratified by age tertiles in the same group, differences in time of progression were observed when we applied the following tertiles: those aged <30 years (20 patients, 17.9%), those aged 30–50 years (85 patients, 75.9%), and those aged >50 years (7 patients, 6.3%) (p = 0.016), but not when we applied the tertiles <33, 33–39, and >39 years (p = 0.418) (Figure 2.A and 2.B).

When patients were stratified by both the minimum T score of baseline DXA scan and by age, the median time of progression was significantly shorter in tertiles with a T score <−0.4, independently of age, than in those with a T score ≥−0.4 (p = 0.0003) (Figure 2.C).

No statistically significant differences were observed when patients were classified according to gender: time of progression was >392 weeks (130; >392) (>7.5 years) in women (n = 35) and 238 weeks (72; 451) (4.6 years) in men (n = 77) (p = 0.136).

Change from osteopenia at baseline to osteoporosis

A total of 211 patients had osteopenia at baseline; of these, 194 presented osteopenia at their first DXA scan and the remaining 17 had a normal DXA result at baseline, progressed to osteopenia in a subsequent DXA, and underwent additional DXA scans.

Median follow-up for the 211 patients from this group was 128 weeks (60.4; 279) (2.7 years). Fifty of these 211 patients (23.7%) progressed to osteoporosis.

Survival analysis showed a median (IQR) time of progression to osteoporosis of >443 weeks (186; >443) (>8.5 years) (Figure 3.A).

When the 211 patients were stratified according to the minimum T score of the first DXA scan, 73 (34.6%) were classed as "low-risk" (between −1.6 and −1.1 SD), 63 (29.9%) as "middle-risk" (between −2 and −1.6 SD and 75 (35.5%) as "high-risk" (between −2.4 and −2 SD) (Figure 3).

The 3 groups were similar with respect to age (p = 0.106), gender (p = 0.103), percentage of patients with viral suppression (p = 0.602), and CD4 T-cell count (p = 0.739), but not by time with infection, which was higher in patients from the "high-risk" tertile with respect to the "low-risk" tertile (9.4 years vs 7.8 years, p = 0.043).

The survival analysis showed significant differences in time of progression to osteoporosis between the 3 groups, as follows: median (IQR) time of progression of >425 weeks (359; >425), (>8.2 years) in the "low-risk" tertile, >443 weeks (347; >443) (>8.5 years) in the "middle-risk" tertile, and 161 weeks (59; 301) (3.2 years) in the "high-risk" tertile (p<0.0001) (Figure 3.B)

Table 3 shows those of the 211 patients who progressed from osteopenia to osteoporosis stratified by minimum T score ("low-risk", "middle-risk", and "high-risk").

When patients were stratified by age tertiles, no significant differences were seen for <37 years (74 patients, 35%), 37–43 years (74 patients, 35%), or >43 years of age (63 patients, 30%) (p = 0.214) (Figure 4.A).

When patients were stratified by both the minimum values of the T score of the DXA scan and age, median time of progression was significantly shorter in the group with a T score <−1.8 and age >40 years (p<0.0001) (Figure 4.B).

No differences were seen when patients were classified according to gender: median time of progression (IQR) was 359 (234; >443) weeks (6.9 years) in women (n = 60) and >428 weeks (179; >428) (>8.2 years) in men (n = 151) (p = 0.465).

As for patients with osteoporosis in the first DXA scan, 24.7% improved (osteoporosis to osteopenia or normal BMD), while 75.3% remained unchanged.

Discussion

Among our chronically HIV-infected patients, nearly one-third of those whose first DXA scan showed normal BMD progressed to osteopenia. Median time of progression to osteopenia was almost 7 years, but in those patients with normal BMD but whose baseline

A.

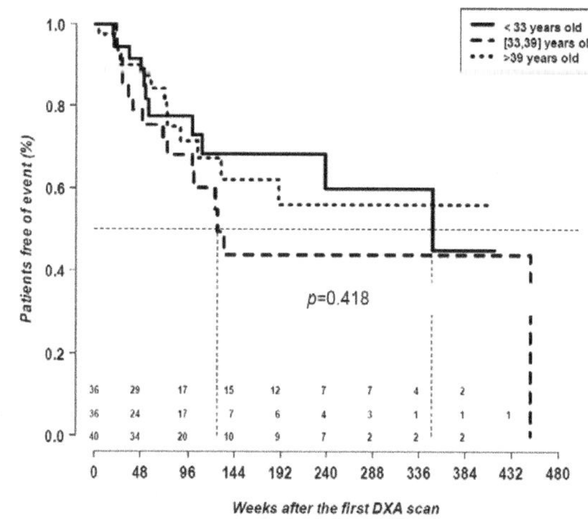

<33 years old	349 weeks
33-39 years old	126 weeks
>39 years old	>407 weeks

B.

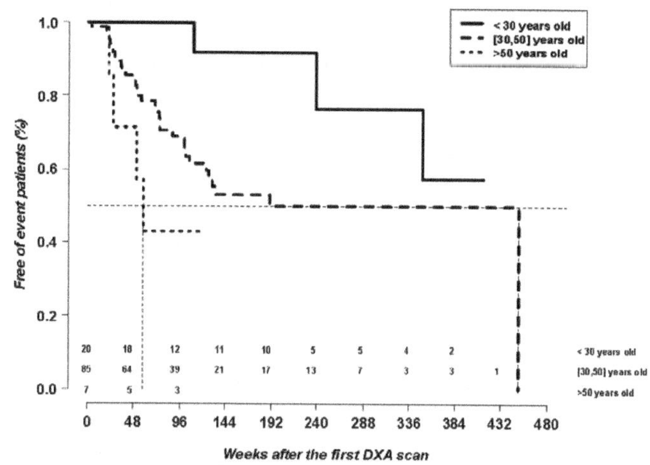

<30 years old	>414 weeks
30-50 years old	451 weeks
>50 years old	57 weeks

C.

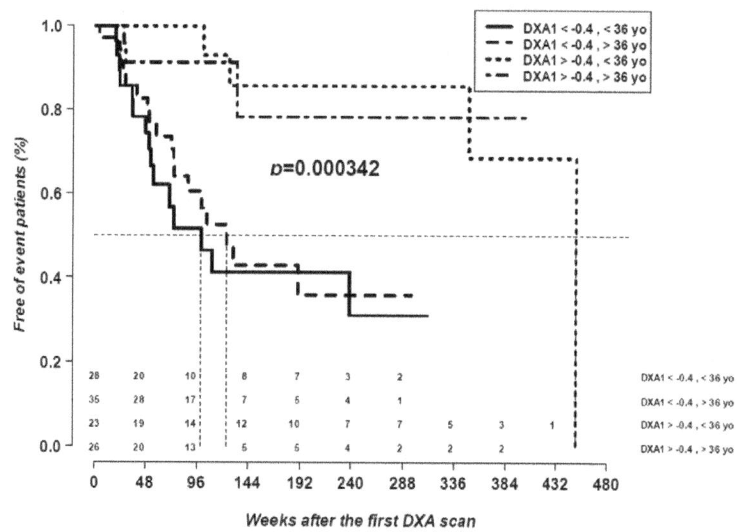

T score <–0.4 , age < 36	100 weeks
T score <–0.4 , age ≥36	124 weeks
T score ≥–0.4 , age < 36	451 weeks
T score ≥–0.4 , age ≥36	>407 weeks

Figure 2. Survival analysis by age. Survival analysis in patients with normal bone mineral density at baseline stratified by age (<33 years, 33–38 years and >38 years [A] and <30 years, 30–50 years, and >50 years [B]) and by both age and T score (less or higher than −0.4 and less or higher than 36 years [C]).

minimum T score was in the "high-risk" tertile, this progression was much faster (<2 years). Similarly, osteopenia progressed to osteoporosis in a quarter of patients. Although time of progression was more than 8 years, for patients with a minimum baseline T score <−2 SD (lower tertile) it was 3 years.

Alterations in bone strength predispose to fragility fractures, which are associated with increased morbidity and mortality in the HIV-negative population. [1,24,25,30]

Prevention of osteoporotic fractures, then, is of major interest from a public health perspective. In HIV-infected patients, osteoporosis is probably underdiagnosed. Adequate tools should be designed to identify patients at high risk for low BMD, who would be candidates for BMD screening by DXA. In the last few years, many efforts have been made to identify risk factors for bone loss—other than traditional factors—among HIV-infected patients. [2,27,31] Age (>50 years), the menopause, other secondary

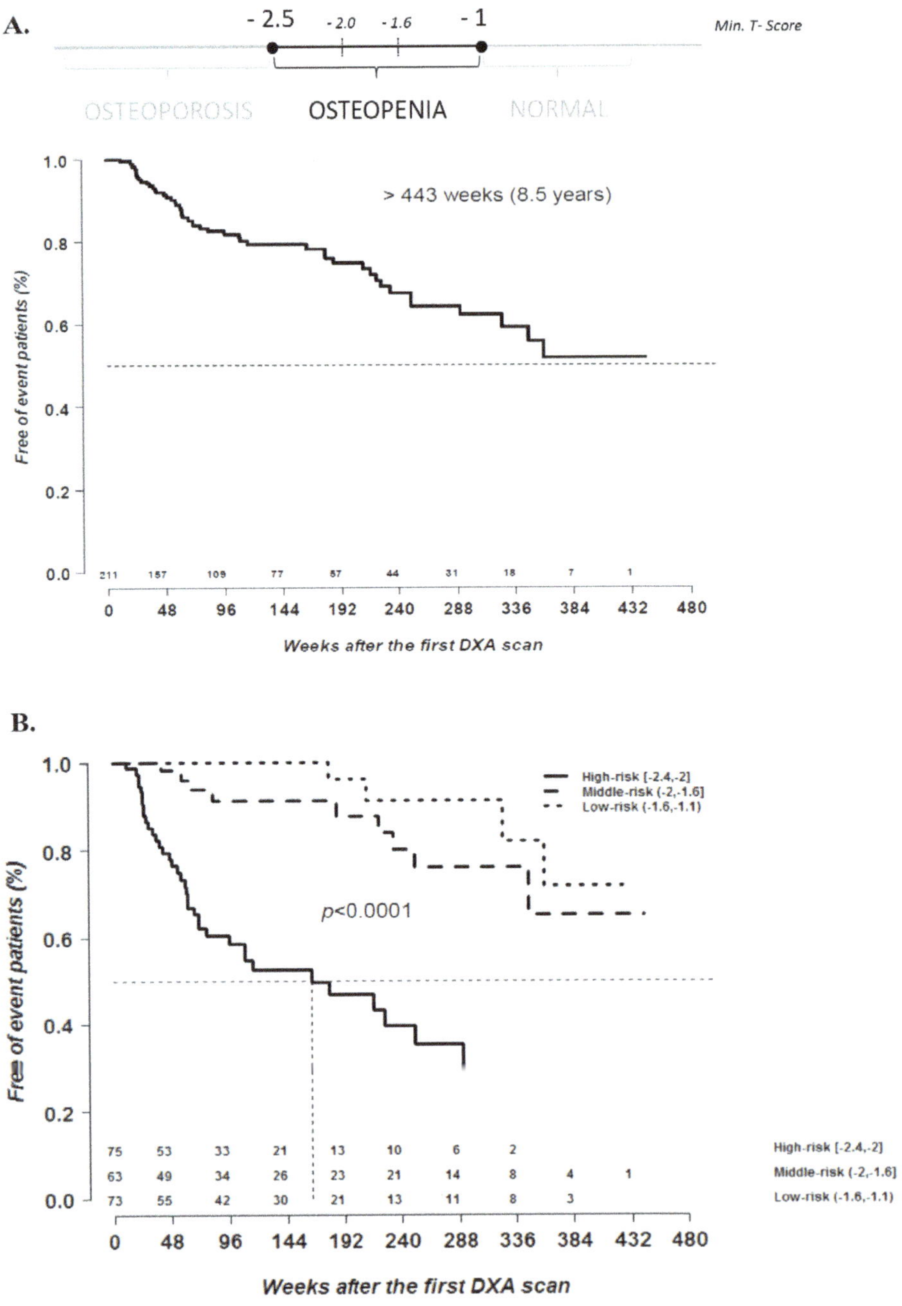

HIGH-RISK [−2.4, −2]	164 weeks
MIDDLE-RISK (−2, −1.6]	>443 weeks
LOW-RISK (−1.6, −1.1)	>425 weeks

Figure 3. Time of progression to osteoporosis. Time of progression from osteopenia to osteoporosis overall (n = 211 patients) (A) and after stratification by baseline minimum T score ("low-risk", "middle-risk", and "high-risk") (B).

causes of low BMD, and a personal or family (parents) history of fragility fractures, together with exposure to some antiretroviral drugs (tenofovir and boosted protease inhibitors), are relevant risk factors that speak in favor of screening with DXA. [31] The optimal BMD testing intervals using DXA scans, however, has not been established.

Data have been published on the rate of progression to bone loss [32,33,34], although our results are the first to show the time of progression to osteopenia/osteoporosis, information that is essential for monitoring. We observed that baseline T score, divided into tertiles, enabled us to establish time of progression of bone loss more accurately than the simple classification according to the WHO criteria (normal, osteopenia, and osteoporosis). According

Table 3. Patients (n = 211) who progressed from osteopenia to osteoporosis (B) after stratification according to minimum T score ("low-risk", "middle-risk" and "high-risk").

Follow-up (weeks)	HIGH-RISK	MIDDLE-RISK	LOW-RISK
48	22%	2%	0%
96	40%	9%	0%
144	60%	9%	0%
192	71%	13%	4%
240	71%	20%	9%
288	71%	24%	9%
336	71%	24%	18%
384		36%	28%
432		36%	
480			

to our results, time of progression to osteopenia in patients with normal BMD at the first DXA scan was enormously different depending on the tertile in which the patient was classified at baseline: from more than 8 years to less than 2 years according to whether the T score was in the low-risk tertile (>−0.2 SD) or if it was in the lowest tertile (from −0.6 to −1 SD), respectively. Similarly, the time of progression to osteoporosis varied widely among patients with osteopenia in the first DXA scan according to the tertile: 8 years for those whose minimum T score was in the higher tertile (between −1.1 and 1.6 SD), but only 3 years for those whose minimum T score was in the lowest tertile (from −2 to −2.4 SD). Ourt results are consistent with recent published data in older HIV-negative women. In this analysis of data from 4,957 women, baseline T score was the most determinant of a BMD testing interval; osteoporosis developed in 15 years for women with normal BMD or mild osteopenia (T score, greater than −1.5), 5 years for women with moderate osteopenia (T score from −1.5 to −1.99) and 1 year for women with advanced osteopenia (T score from −2.0 to −2.49) [35].

Current recommendations on the study of bone disease for HIV care providers mainly include information on candidates for BMD monitoring by DXA, [22,29] but provide very little information on the optimal frequency of subsequent DXA scans, based on the WHO categories of BMD. [31] According to our data, a reasonable proposal would be to set the frequency of DXA according to the tertile: patients in the lowest T score tertiles (defined as a T score from −0.6 to −1 in patients with normal BMD according to the WHO criteria, and from −2 to −2.4 among those with osteopenia) should undergo another DXA scan more frequently than those in the other 2 tertiles. A subsequent DXA scan should be recommended as soon as 1–2 years later for those in the lower tertiles, even when baseline BMD had been classified as normal; this frequency will help to diagnose early changes in BMD status (from normal BMD to osteopenia or from osteopenia to osteoporosis) and, in the case of progression, enable appropriate measures to be taken. Patients in the other 2 tertiles (T score from −0.6 to >−0.2 in patients with normal BMD and from −1.1 to −2 among those with osteopenia) could be assessed by a DXA scan after at least 6–7 years, even in those whose baseline BMD fulfilled the criteria for osteopenia. Since it is unlikely that a patient would progress in less than 7–8 years, more frequent DXA scanning would not affect management, although it would increase costs and inconvenience to patients.

Given our results, similar recommendations on the frequency of DXA scan should be implemented according to age, providing that the decision is based on the T score. Although age affected bone loss, when patients were classified according to their initial T score (tertiles), BMD status gave more information on the progression of bone loss. In clinical terms, however, the negative effect of age on risk of osteoporotic fracture, independently of BMD, has been reported, suggesting that both age and BMD should be taken into consideration [36] The lack of elderly patients prevents us from assessing this issue in greater depth.

As for gender, although no statistically significant differences were detected between men and women, variations in the time of progression to osteopenia/osteoporosis could be clinically relevant: those men with a normal baseline BMD, included in the high-risk tertile, progressed more rapidly to osteopenia than women (median of progression of 4.6 years in men and >7.5 years in women). This finding could suggest the need for special care and more rigorous monitoring of men from this group. These data are consistent with other published results showing the higher prevalence of low BMD and fragility fractures in men than in premenopausal women. [25]

As a retrospective observational study, our analysis presents some limitations. Variables were recorded using clinical documents as the source. Consequently, the first DXA scan for each patient did not correspond to a defined baseline; however, since at that time DXA scan was only performed when patients were seen for first time in our unit or in the context of clinical assays (metabolic studies, new antiretroviral strategies, antiretroviral-naive patients...), subjects included in the analysis seem to be a good representation of our population. Additionally, the time from normal BMD to osteopenia is only known to lie within the time interval between the first DXA with a value <−1 SD and the time immediately before this scan; the time from osteopenia to osteoporosis is only known to lie within the time interval between the first DXA with a value <−2.5 SD and the time immediately before this scan. Our analysis imputed the right end of this interval, that is the time with the first DXA <−1 SD as the time to osteopenia and <−2.5 SD as the time to osteoporosis. A statistical analysis taking into account the random nature of the intervals, where the change of status occurs, could diminish the bias due to this finding. [37] However, it is our belief that the effect of these limitations on the conclusions would be negligible. Finally, the retrospective nature of the analysis avoids knowing the presence of some clinical factors that may contribute to a different bone loss progression or bone recovery (steroid use, menopause, hypogonadism, bisphosphonate use, vitamin D or calcium supplementation, etc).

To conclude, in HIV-infected patients, the use of screening thresholds based on the minimum T scores (tertiles) provided by DXA is more efficient for predicting time of progression to osteopenia/osteoporosis and deciding on BMD testing intervals than the WHO criteria. The lowest minimum T-score tertiles indicate the recommendation of a subsequent DXA scan in 1–2 years, while in the highest tertiles, this interval could be 6 years or more. Since management algorithms are lacking, ours and other data are necessary to facilitate the design of suitable guidelines for this population. Early intervention in patients with bone demineralization could reduce the high morbidity and mortality associated with osteoporotic fractures.

A.

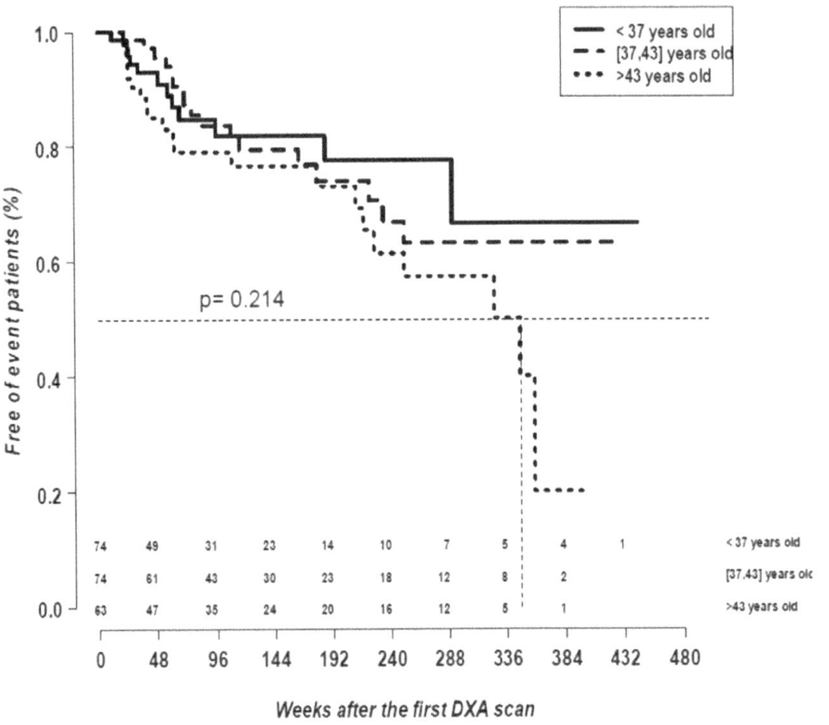

<37 years old	>443 weeks
37-43 years old	>428 weeks
>43 years old	347 weeks

B.

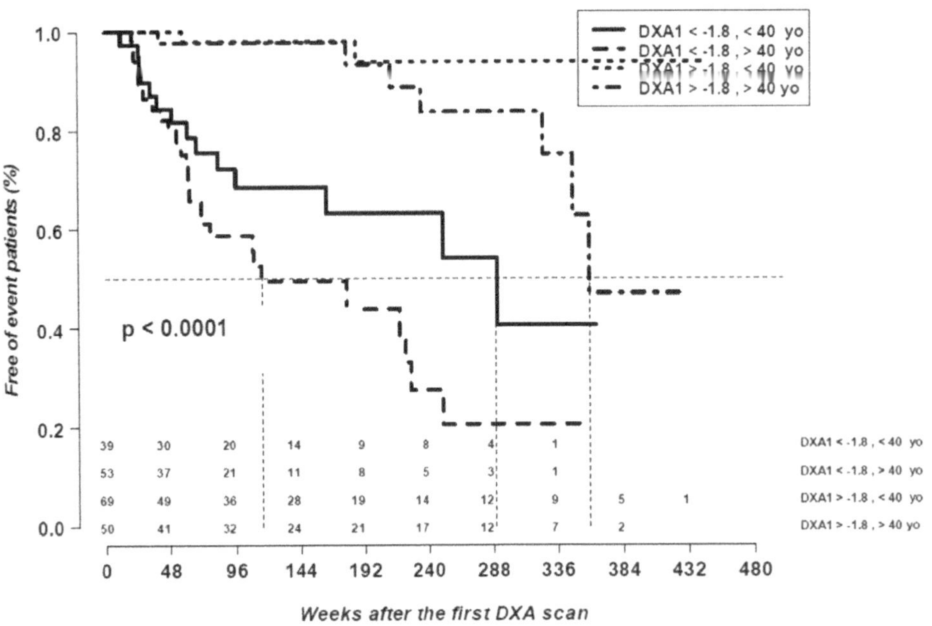

T score <-1.8, <40 years old	290 weeks
T score <-1.8, ≥40 years old	115 weeks
T score ≥-1.8, <40 years old	>443 weeks
T score ≥-1.8, ≥40 years old	359 weeks

Figure 4. Time of progression stratified by age and T score. Time of progression stratified by age: <37 years, 37–43 years and >43 years (A) and by both the minimum values of the T score and age (B).

Acknowledgments

We are grateful to Thomas O'Boyle for editorial assistance.

Author Contributions

Conceived and designed the experiments: EN AB BC. Performed the experiments: JP CE JR SdG LR. Analyzed the data: MG-M NP-A GG. Contributed reagents/materials/analysis tools: JP CE JR SdG LR. Wrote the paper: EN AB BC.

References

1. NIH Consensus Development Panel on Osteoporosis Prevention D, and Therapy, Conference CD (2001) Osteoporosis prevention, diagnosis, and therapy. JAMA 285: 785–795.
2. Bonjoch A, Figueras M, Estany C, Perez-Alvarez N, Rosales J, et al. (2010) High prevalence of and progression to low bone mineral density in HIV-infected patients: a longitudinal cohort study. AIDS 24: 2827–2833.
3. Brown TT, Qaqish RB (2006) Antiretroviral therapy and the prevalence of osteopenia and osteoporosis: a meta-analytic review. AIDS 20: 2165–2174.
4. Bruera D, Luna N, David DO, Bergoglio LM, Zamudio J (2003) Decreased bone mineral density in HIV-infected patients is independent of antiretroviral therapy. AIDS 17: 1917–1923.
5. Knobel H, Guelar A, Vallecillo G, Nogues X, Diez A (2001) Osteopenia in HIV-infected patients: is it the disease or is it the treatment? AIDS 15: 807–808.
6. Cotter EJ, Malizia AP, Chew N, Powderly WG, Doran PP (2007) HIV proteins regulate bone marker secretion and transcription factor activity in cultured human osteoblasts with consequent potential implications for osteoblast function and development. AIDS Res Hum Retroviruses 23: 1521–1530.
7. Fakruddin JM, Laurence J (2003) HIV envelope gp120-mediated regulation of osteoclastogenesis via receptor activator of nuclear factor kappa B ligand (RANKL) secretion and its modulation by certain HIV protease inhibitors through interferon-gamma/RANKL cross-talk. J Biol Chem 278: 48251–48258.
8. Gibellini D, De Crignis E, Ponti C, Borderi M, Clo A, et al. (2010) HIV-1 Tat protein enhances RANKL/M-CSF-mediated osteoclast differentiation. Biochem Biophys Res Commun 401: 429–434.
9. Gibellini D, De Crignis E, Ponti C, Cimatti L, Borderi M, et al. (2008) HIV-1 triggers apoptosis in primary osteoblasts and HOBIT cells through TNFalpha activation. J Med Virol 80: 1507–1514.
10. Grijsen ML, Vrouenraets SM, Steingrover R, Lips P, Reiss P, et al. (2010) High prevalence of reduced bone mineral density in primary HIV-1-infected men. AIDS 24: 2233–2238.
11. Gutierrez F, Masia M (2011) The role of HIV and antiretroviral therapy in bone disease. AIDS Rev 13: 109–118.
12. Hoy J (2011) Bone, fracture and frailty. Curr Opin HIV AIDS 6: 309–314.
13. Ofotokun I, Weitzmann MN (2010) HIV-1 infection and antiretroviral therapies: risk factors for osteoporosis and bone fracture. Curr Opin Endocrinol Diabetes Obes 17: 523–529.
14. Ofotokun I, Weitzmann MN (2011) HIV and bone metabolism. Discov Med 11: 385–393.
15. Wei S, Kitaura H, Zhou P, Ross FP, Teitelbaum SL (2005) IL-1 mediates TNF-induced osteoclastogenesis. J Clin Invest 115: 282–290.
16. Gallant JE, Staszewski S, Pozniak AL, DeJesus E, Suleiman JM, et al. (2004) Efficacy and safety of tenofovir DF vs stavudine in combination therapy in antiretroviral-naive patients: a 3-year randomized trial. JAMA 292: 191–201.
17. Gibellini D, Borderi M, de Crignis E, Clo A, Miserocchi A, et al. (2010) Analysis of the effects of specific protease inhibitors on OPG/RANKL regulation in an osteoblast-like cell line. New Microbiol 33: 109–115.
18. McComsey GA, Kitch D, Daar ES, Tierney C, Jahed NC, et al. (2011) Bone mineral density and fractures in antiretroviral-naive persons randomized to receive abacavir-lamivudine or tenofovir disoproxil fumarate-emtricitabine along with efavirenz or atazanavir-ritonavir: Aids Clinical Trials Group A5224s, a substudy of ACTG A5202. J Infect Dis 203: 1791–1801.
19. Ofotokun I WN, Vunnava A, Sheth A, Villinger F, Zhou J, Williams E, Sanford S, Rivas M, Lennox J, (2011) HAART-induced Immune Reconstitution: A Driving Force Behind Bone Resorption in HIV/AIDS CROI 2011.
20. Yong MK, Elliott JH, Woolley IJ, Hoy JF (2011) Low CD4 Count Is Associated With an Increased Risk of Fragility Fracture in HIV-Infected Patients. J Acquir Immune Defic Syndr 57: 205–210.
21. Dao CN, Patel P, Overton ET, Rhame F, Pals SL, et al. (2011) Low vitamin D among HIV-infected adults: prevalence of and risk factors for low vitamin D Levels in a cohort of HIV-infected adults and comparison to prevalence among adults in the US general population. Clin Infect Dis 52: 396–405.
22. Arnsten JH, Freeman R, Howard AA, Floris-Moore M, Santoro N, et al. (2006) HIV infection and bone mineral density in middle-aged women. Clin Infect Dis 42: 1014–1020.
23. Bedimo R ZS, Drechsler H, Tebas P, Maalouf N (2011) Risk of Osteoporotic Fractures Associated with Cumulative Exposure to Tenofovir and Other Antiretroviral Agents. 6th IAS Conference on HIV Pathogenesis, Treatment and Prevention, July 17–20, 2011, Rome.
24. Triant VA, Brown TT, Lee H, Grinspoon SK (2008) Fracture prevalence among human immunodeficiency virus (HIV)-infected versus non-HIV-infected patients in a large U.S. healthcare system. J Clin Endocrinol Metab 93: 3499–3504.
25. Trombetti A, Herrmann F, Hoffmeyer P, Schurch MA, Bonjour JP, et al. (2002) Survival and potential years of life lost after hip fracture in men and age-matched women. Osteoporos Int 13: 731–737.
26. Aberg JA, Kaplan JE, Libman H, Emmanuel P, Anderson JR, et al. (2009) Primary care guidelines for the management of persons infected with human immunodeficiency virus: 2009 update by the HIV medicine Association of the Infectious Diseases Society of America. Clin Infect Dis 49: 651–681.
27. Watts NB, Lewiecki EM, Miller PD, Baim S (2008) National Osteoporosis Foundation 2008 Clinician's Guide to Prevention and Treatment of Osteoporosis and the World Health Organization Fracture Risk Assessment Tool (FRAX): what they mean to the bone densitometrist and bone technologist. J Clin Densitom 11: 473–477.
28. Kanis JA (1994) Assessment of fracture risk and its application to screening for postmenopausal osteoporosis: synopsis of a WHO report. WHO Study Group. Osteoporos Int 4: 368–381.
29. Marubini EV, MG editor (2004) Analysing Survival Data from Clinical Trials and Observational Studies.
30. Cooper C (1997) The crippling consequences of fractures and their impact on quality of life. Am J Med 103: 12S–17S; discussion 17S–19S.
31. McComsey GA, Tebas P, Shane E, Yin MT, Overton ET, et al. (2010) Bone disease in HIV infection: a practical review and recommendations for HIV care providers. Clin Infect Dis 51: 937–946.
32. Cazanave C (2010) Changes in Bone Mineral Density: 2-Years of follow up of the ANRS CO3 Aquitaine Cohort. CROI 2010.
33. Dolan SE, Kanter JR, Grinspoon S (2006) Longitudinal analysis of bone density in human immunodeficiency virus-infected women. J Clin Endocrinol Metab 91: 2938–2945.
34. Sharma (2010) Longitudinal Analysis of Bone Mineral Density in Aging Men with or at Risk for HIV Infection. CROI 2010.
35. Gourlay ML, Fine JP, Preisser JS, May RC, Li C, et al. (2012) Bone-density testing interval and transition to osteoporosis in older women. N Engl J Med 366: 225–233.
36. Kanis JA, Johnell O, Oden A, Dawson A, De Laet C, et al. (2001) Ten year probabilities of osteoporotic fractures according to BMD and diagnostic thresholds. Osteoporos Int 12: 989–995.
37. Gómez G, Calle M., Oller R., Langohr K. (2009) Tutorial on methods for interval-censored data and their implementation in R. Statistical Modelling 9: 259–297.

Coating with a Modular Bone Morphogenetic Peptide Promotes Healing of a Bone-Implant Gap in an Ovine Model

Yan Lu[1,4]*, Jae Sung Lee[2], Brett Nemke[1], Ben K. Graf[4], Kevin Royalty[2], Richard Illgen III[4], Ray Vanderby Jr.[2], Mark D. Markel[1,4], William L. Murphy[2,3,4]*

1 Comparative Orthopaedic Research Laboratory, School of Veterinary Medicine, University of Wisconsin-Madison, Madison, Wisconson, United States of America, **2** Departments of Biomedical Engineering, University of Wisconsin, Madison, Wisconson, United States of America, **3** Pharmacology, University of Wisconsin, Madison, Wisconson, United States of America, **4** Orthopedics and Rehabilitation, University of Wisconsin, Madison, Wisconson, United States of America

Abstract

Despite the potential for growth factor delivery strategies to promote orthopedic implant healing, there is a need for growth factor delivery methods that are controllable and amenable to clinical translation. We have developed a modular bone growth factor, herein termed "modular bone morphogenetic peptide (mBMP)", which was designed to efficiently bind to the surface of orthopedic implants and also stimulate new bone formation. The purpose of this study was to coat a hydroxyapatite-titanium implant with mBMP and evaluate bone healing across a bone-implant gap in the sheep femoral condyle. The mBMP molecules efficiently bound to a hydroxyapatite-titanium implant and 64% of the initially bound mBMP molecules were released in a sustained manner over 28 days. The results demonstrated that the mBMP-coated implant group had significantly more mineralized bone filling in the implant-bone gap than the control group in C-arm computed tomography (DynaCT) scanning (25% more), histological (35% more) and microradiographic images (50% more). Push-out stiffness of the mBMP group was nearly 40% greater than that of control group whereas peak force did not show a significant difference. The results of this study demonstrated that mBMP coated on a hydroxyapatite-titanium implant stimulates new bone formation and may be useful to improve implant fixation in total joint arthroplasty applications.

Editor: Kent Leach, University of California Davis, United States of America

Funding: This study was funded by the Wallace H. Coulter Foundation and by the Wisconsin Alumni Research Foundation: "A Translational Research Partnership Grant from the Wallace H. Coulter Foundation" and "A Technology Accelerator Grant from the Wisconsin Alumni Research Foundation". There is no grant number from either. Smith & Nephew, Inc., provided implants for this study. The funders had no role in study design, data collection and analysis, decision to publish, or preparation of the manuscript.

Competing Interests: Smith&Nephew, Inc., provided titanium implants for this study. There are no further patents, products in development or marketed products to declare.

* E-mail: luy@svm.vetmed.wisc.edu (YL); wlmurphy@wisc.edu (WLM)

Introduction

Total joint replacement surgeries have been performed popularly because these surgeries can successfully relieve pain and improve functional outcomes. However, the failure rate of revision joint replacements is also dramatically higher than primary replacements due primarily to a challenging environment for new bone formation [1]. Therefore, there is a need to develop novel biomaterials to increase replacement success rate and reduce revision rate, and to promote successful bone healing after revision surgery. Besides improving surgery techniques [2], the key factor for successfully improving implant-bone healing in joint replacement is the ability to encourage new bone formation at the implant-native bone interface [3]. Therefore, several groups have begun to explore the use of pro-osteogenic growth factors to induce new bone formation on implant surfaces. For example, Sachse et al recently reported that the recombinant protein bone morphogenetic protein-2 (BMP-2) may foster bone healing on a titanium surface in a sheep model [4]. Further, Lamberg et al stated that transforming growth factor-β1 (TGF-β1) and insulin-like growth factor-1 (IGF-1) enhanced the mechanical fixation and osseointegration of titanium implants in cancellous bone in a dog model [5].

Collectively, previous studies demonstrate the potential for growth factor delivery strategies to promote orthopedic implant healing. However, translation of growth factor delivery to clinical applications is plagued by significant challenges [6]. First, growth factor delivery strategies typically do not use carriers with optimal physical properties. The common strategy instead involves designing a growth factor "carrier", then combining it with a standard orthopedic device with appropriate physical properties. Notable examples include recombinant protein-loaded collagen carriers combined with titanium cages [7,8] or other metallic hardware [9]. Innovative biomaterials for controlled growth factor release [10], ranging from polymer scaffolds to injectable micro- and nano-particles, also typically require combination with a structural device. In addition, existing growth factor carriers contain supraphysiologic doses delivered over relatively short timescales, which has recently led to well-documented side effects including edema [11,12], heterotopic bone formation [13], retrograde ejaculation [14], and potentially increased cancer risk [15].

Bone morphogenetic proteins (BMPs) are the key cytokines in bone formation and repair. A possible strategy to utilize BMPs' activity in clinical applications is to enhance the activity of autologous BMPs. BMP-2 incorporated into biomimetic calcium phosphate coatings has been demonstrated to be capable of inducing bone formation at an ectopic site and sustaining osteogenic activity for a considerable period of time [16,17].

We hypothesized that a modular bone morphogenetic peptide (mBMP) could be used to "dip-coat" the surface of an orthopedic implant, which in turn would be capable of promoting implant-native bone healing. Specifically, we synthesized a peptide with two functional units: i) an osteocalcin-inspired hydroxyapatite (HAP)-binding sequence; and ii) a peptide sequence previously shown to mimic some of the pro-osteogenic properties of the protein BMP-2 [18,19]. We then would perform experiments to determine whether this peptide could "dip-coat" the surface of an orthopedic implant and, in turn, promote bone healing across a well-defined bone gap in a sheep model. The bone-implant gap in the current study was designed into the implant to more effectively mimic the challenging environment that is typically present during revision joint arthroplasty. We hypothesized that an HAP-titanium implant dip-coated with mBMP inserted in cancellous bone would result in improved mechanical implant fixation and induce more bone ingrowth across the defined gap zone.

Materials and Methods

HAP-titanium Implants

Custom implants (diameter: 8 mm, HAP coated length: 14 mm. Smith and Nephew Corp. Andover, MA) were "porous coated", meaning that they incorporate a porous titanium surface that is plasma spray bound with hydroxyapatite. In addition, the implants were designed to include a 1 mm gap all around the perimeter of the cylindrical implants, so that there was a well-defined gap between the native bone and the implant surface (Fig. 1).

Peptide Binding and Release from HAP-titanium Implant

Modular bone morphogenetic peptide (Amino acid sequence of mBMP; KIPKASSVPTELSAISTLYLAAAAγEPRRγEVAγEL) was synthesized using standard Fmoc solid phase peptide synthesis, as reported previously [20,21]. Carboxyfluorescein (Molecular Probes Inc., Eugene, OR) was used to label mBMP to monitor its release from the implants into simulated body fluid (SBF; 136.8 mM NaCl, 3 mM KCl, 0.5 mM Na_2SO_4, 1.5 mM $MgCl_2$, 4.2 mM $NaHCO_3$, 2.5 mM $CaCl_2$, 1.0 mM K_2HPO_4, 50 mM Tris base). First, fluorescently labeled mBMP was bound on implants by incubating each implant in peptide solution (4 mL, 1.9 mM) for 4 hours at 37°C. The mBMP-bound implant was then incubated in 3 mL of SBF solution at 37°C in a static condition to examine the release behavior of peptide. At each time point (day 1, 2, 3, 6, 9, 13, 18, 22 and 28), the fluorescence intensity of release medium was measured and the release medium was replaced with a fresh one. After 4-week release, the mBMP remaining on implant was retrieved by incubating in 0.5 N hydrochloric acid solution overnight. The amount of mBMP was quantified using microBCA (Thermo Fisher Scientific Inc., Rockford, IL) after neutralizing with sodium hydroxide solution, and the amount of initial binding was calculated by adding to that of released peptide.

mBMP Coating of Implants for in vivo Studies

Each experimental HAP-titanium implant was incubated in 4 mL of mBMP solution (1.9 mM) 4 hours at 37°C. The mBMP solution was sterilized by passage through sterile 0.22 μm filters. All incubation procedures were performed in aseptic conditions.

In vivo Experimental Design

Twelve mature female sheep, ranging in age from 3.5 to 5 years and weighing between 70 to 110 kg (82.4±5.6 kg: mean±SD) were utilized in the study. All experimental protocols were approved by the Institutional Animal Use and Care Committee of University of Wisconsin-Madison.

In each of the 12 sheep, one of the stifles was randomized (block design) to receive an mBMP-coated HAP-titanium implant and the other (contralateral) received an un-treated implant (n = 12/ treatment). The sheep were euthanized at 4 weeks after surgery. 8 sheep (16 stifles, 8/group) were subjected to C-arm computed tomography (DynaCT) and biomechanical testing, 4 sheep (8 stifles, 4/group) were used for histologic analysis.

Surgical Procedure

Surgery was carried out under general anesthesia with isoflurane and oxygen inhalation via endotracheal intubation. Procaine Penicillin G (5 mls) was administered via muscle pre-operatively and an additional dose (5 mls) post-operatively. An 8 cm medial incision was made along the anterior edge of medial collateral ligament in one randomly selected stifle. The medial portion of medial condyle was exposed. An 8 mm diameter hole (14 mm deep) was drilled from the medial surface of the condyle near to collateral ligament origin by an 8 mm cannulated drill bit 5 mm proximal to the joint line taking care to avoid the joint. An mBMP-coated HAP-titanium implant was inserted in the hole (Fig. 1). Then the surrounding soft tissue was sutured and the implant was covered. In the contralateral stifle, the identical procedure of exposure was performed with the un-treated implant in the medial condyle. The incision was lavaged by sterile saline. The deep fascia, subcutaneous tissue and skin incision were closed as routine.

After 4 weeks, all sheep were euthanized for biomechanical, DynaCT and histological analyses.

Dyna CT Scan

At the same day of sacrifice, the medial femoral condyles were cut into uniform bone blocks (3.0×3.0×2.0 cm^3) and imaged using a Siemens Artis Zeego (Siemens Healthcare, Erlangen, Germany) C-arm computed tomography (DynaCT), which has a wide angle cone-beam x-ray tube and 40 cm × 30 cm flat-panel detector integrated with a robotic C-arm gantry. The acquisition parameters for DynaCT were as follows: 86 kV tube voltage, automatic tube current ranging from 70 to 125 mA, a 20 s rotation time (total of 496 projections over 200 degree sweep angle). The projection images were acquired in a 2 × 2 binning mode, providing a 154 μm detector element resolution. Acquired images were then transferred to a dedicated post-processing workstation (*syngo* X-Workplace, Siemens Healthcare, Erlangen, Germany) where a volume data set was reconstructed to a 512×512 matrix and 306–328 slices with an isotropic voxel size of 140 μm using a sharp bone kernel for visualization of the bony structure.

The Dyna CT image of each specimen was analyzed with Image J software (National Institutes of Health, Bethesda, MA). The area of bone ingrowth in the gap between the implant and hosting bone was calculated and compared between mBMP-coated and control groups.

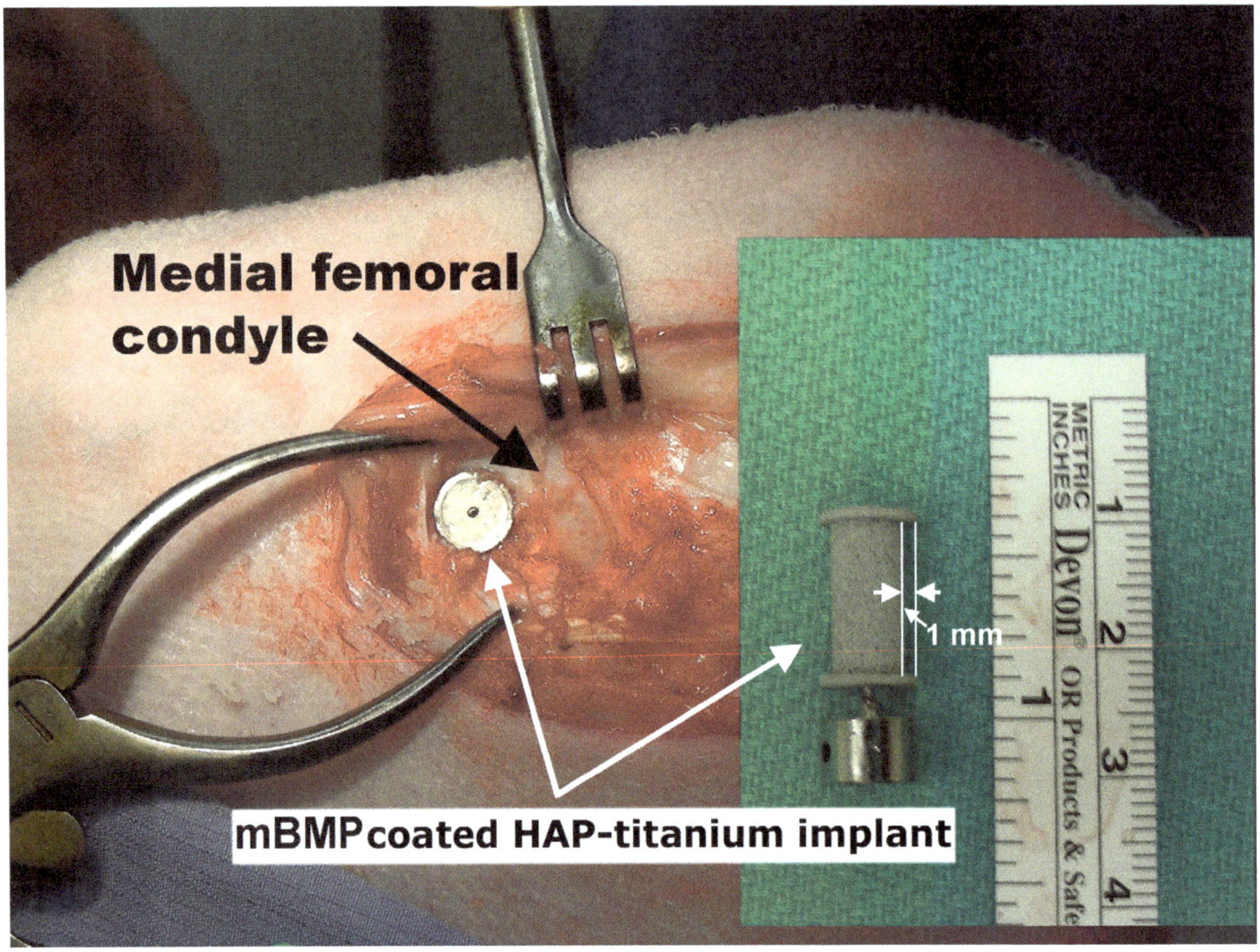

Figure 1. Image of mBMP coated HAP-titanium implant and surgical implantation in sheep medial femoral condyle.

Biomechanical Testing

After DynaCT scan, the femoral condylar bone blocks were used for push out mechanical testing. The specimen was placed in a MTS 858 BIONIX Test System (MTS Systems Corp., Eden Prairie, MN) with a 1500 lb load cell. The titanium implant in the specimen was precisely aligned with a pushing shaft. A linear extensometer was attached to measure the displacement of the implant. The displacement rate was 5.0 mm/min as previously described [22]. A 50 N preload was applied. Peak force at failure (N) and stiffness (N/mm) were measured and recorded. Peak force was determined from the load-displacement curve. Stiffness was calculated by measuring the slope from the linear portion of the curve.

Histological Analysis

The remaining 8 condyles in 4 sheep were used for histological analysis. The specimens were fixed in neutral buffered 10% formalin for 1 week. The medial condyle was sectioned sagitally into 3 equal sections crossing the implant axis. The undecalcified specimens were embedded in polymethylmethacrylate (PMMA), sectioned (100 μm) and stained with Goldner's Trichrome for the evaluation of implant to bone healing. The sections from each specimen were examined by three senior researchers blinded to group assignments. Fine detail contact microradiography (Hewlett-Packard Faxitron, McMinnville, OR. USA) combined with vacuum technique was also performed on 3 sections of each specimen as previously described. [23] The 3 sections were defined as "outer" (near to cortex), "middle", and "inner" (farther to cortex). Bone density in the implant-bone gap region of each 3 section levels and total bone density of 3 sections [(sum of bone-occupied area of "inner", "middle" and "outer" groups)/(sum of area of interest of "inner", "middle" and "outer" groups)*100] were quantified using Image J software for both histological and microradiographical images.

Statistical Analysis

The Shapiro-Wilk Test was first used to determine the normal distribution (Gaussian distribution) of histological, microradiographic, DynaCT and mechanical testing data sets. If the data sets were normally distributed, the Student's Paired t-test was used for statistical analysis for histology, microradiography, DynaCT and mechanical testing data between the two treatment groups. If the data sets were detected to be not normally distributed, the Mann-whitney U test was used to compare these differences. Differences were considered to be significant at a probability level of 95% ($p<0.05$). All statistical analyses were performed with a commercially available software program (SAS Version 8e, SAS Institute Inc., Cary, NC).

Results

In Vitro

The amount of mBMP initially bound to a HAP-titanium implant was 414.4±22.8 μg. The release profile of mBMP in SBF showed large initial release 51.1±2.9% of initially bound mBMP during first two days (Fig. 2A). Afterwards, the mBMP was released in a nearly linear fashion for 4 weeks with total release of 263.1±20.7 μg (63.4±1.8% of initially bound mBMP). As evidenced in Figure 2B, a significant amount of mBMP molecules still resides on HAP-implant surface after 28-day release.

In Vivo

No postoperative complications were seen and all sheep were fully weight-bearing at the same day after surgery. No signs of infection were observed at the time of euthanasia.

CT Results

DynaCT analysis demonstrated that the mBMP-treated group (4.7±2.0 mm^2) had a significantly higher density of mineralized bone tissue filling the 1 millimeter bone-implant gap than the control group (3.7±2.0 mm^2) ($p<0.05$) (Fig. 3).

Histological Results

Microradiographical data analyses showed the mBMP-coated HAP-titanium implants had significantly greater area of higher bone density in the bone-implant gaps compared to the controls ($p<0.05$) (Fig. 4). This increased bone formation was observed throughout the bone-implant interface - at outer, middle, and inner section levels. Microradiographical images also demonstrated that the control group had significantly less new bone formation in the bone-implant gap than the mBMP-coated implant group (Fig. 5 A and B). Histological analysis further demonstrated significantly greater new bone formation in the bone-implant gap in the mBMP-coated implant conditions (Fig. 5 C and D). Specifically, calculation of new bone formation in Goldner's trichrome stained images demonstrated a significant increase in new bone formation in the middle section and in the inner/middle/outer section levels combined for mBMP coated implants when compared to controls ($p<0.05$) (Fig. 6).

Mechanical Testing Results

The results of mechanical push-out testing demonstrated that the stiffness of the mBMP-treated group (2157±651.9 N/mm) was significantly greater than that of control group (1545±480.5 N/mm) ($p<0.05$), whereas there was no significant difference in peak force between the mBMP-treated group (1022±371.4 N) and the control group (682.2±269.3 N) groups ($p>0.05$).

Discussion

The mBMP peptides were efficiently bound to a HAP-titanium implant and released over 28 days in simulated body fluid. *In vivo* results of this study demonstrated that mBMP-coated HAP-titanium implant increased implant fixation and stimulated bone formation in the gap between implant and surrounding host cancellous bone after 4 weeks post-surgery compared to the control.

mBMP release kinetics showed a substantial initial release of over 50% during the initial 2 days, followed by minimal release kinetics over more than 28 days. These distinct regimes of mBMP release can be attributed to an initial release of poorly bound peptide due to surface saturation, followed by slower release of mBMP that was strongly bound to the hydroxyapatite surface. In particular, the solution concentration used for mBMP binding here (1.9 mM) was much higher than the concentration previously shown to saturate binding to a hydroxyapatite surface [20,24], which likely explains the rapid initial release kinetics. The minimal mBMP release after the first two days is indicative of the high mBMP-implant binding affinity, as demonstrated previously [20]. The observation that nearly 40% of the initially bound mBMP remained on the implant surface after 4 week incubation is potentially interesting in the context of contemporary growth factor delivery strategies. Rapid and poorly-localized bone growth factor delivery can lead to significant clinical side effects, as demonstrated by recent clinical analyses of BMP-2-releasing implants [13,14,25]. Although further studies will be needed to demonstrate control over mBMP dosage on the implant surface, our previous studies have demonstrated that mBMP dosage can be controlled by simply varying the mBMP concentration in solution during implant dip-coating [20,21,24].

Sheep were selected for this study because they provide similar bone density and weight to humans, and they have been widely used for evaluation implant-bone healing in previous studies [4,26–29]. The sheep femoral condyle was particularly used as a model in this study because it is rich in high quality cancellous bone with ample blood supply, which is suitable for an evaluation of early implant bone healing [22]. In addition, it is also

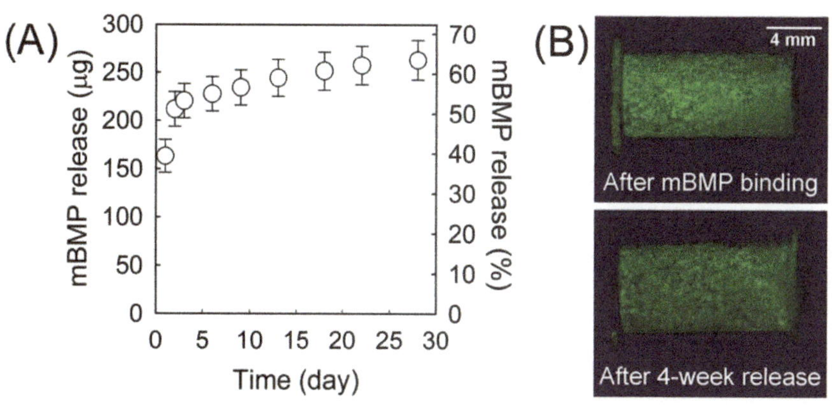

Figure 2. Images of release profile of mBMP in vitro. (A) Cumulative release of mBMP from HAP-titanium implant in SBF is over 60% at 4 weeks. (B) Fluorescent images of an implant after incorporation with fluorescently labeled mBMP (top) and after 4-week incubation in simulated body fluid (SBF) (bottom).

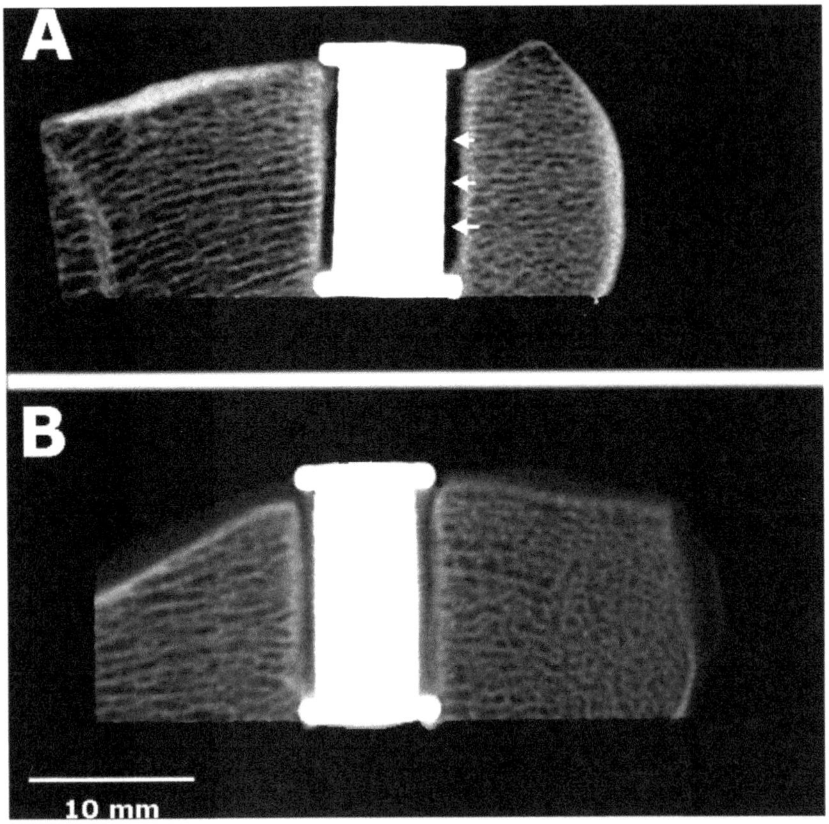

Figure 3. Images of Dyna CT results between control and mBMP coated implants. A: Control, DynaCT demonstrating that gap between the implant and host bone was still visible (white arrows). B: The gap between mBMP coated HAP-implant and host bone was filled with high density mineralized tissue.

representative of the bony fixation regions, such as proximal femoral prostheses in humans. The gap size (1.0 mm) selected for this study was defined as critical size under non-loading condition based on a previous study [22]. The sacrifice time at 4 weeks post-surgery was selected for monitoring early stage of bone ingrowth in the gap between the titanium implant and host bone. Several previous studies have used the same time point to evaluate bone ingrowth in bone-implant gaps in animal models [22,30,31].

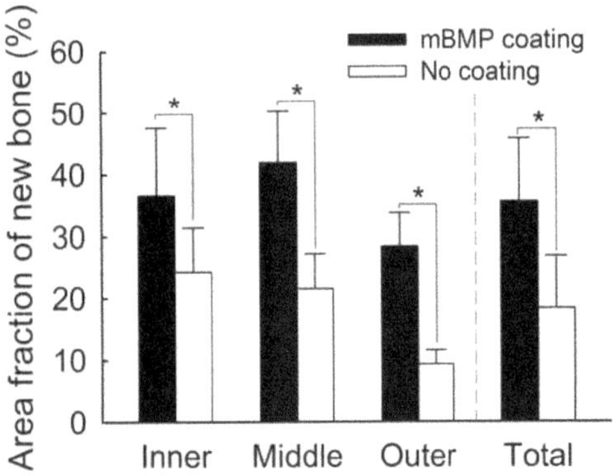

Figure 4. Microradiographic calculation of new bone formation in the gap demonstrating mBMP group had significantly more new bone ingrowth than non-mBMP group at 3 levels of the implant and in total amount. "*" means significant difference between treatments ($p<0.05$).

DynaCT, histological and microradiographical results of this study demonstrated that significantly higher density tissue and new bone formation was present in the gap between mBMP-coated HAP-titanium implant and condylar bone compared to control. An interesting observation here was that endochondral ossification with the formation of cartilaginous tissues was not observed at 4 weeks post-surgery. Instead, it appeared that direct ossification of mesenchymal tissue as intramembraneous ossification was taking place, as reported in a previous study [4].

New bone formation in the gap between the implant and native host bone can also increase rigidity and fixation of an implant, which has been validated in the current study. The push-out stiffness of mBMP coated HAP-titanium implant group was significantly greater than that of control although the peak force did not reveal a statistically significant difference. Few studies to date have performed mechanical push-out testing on HAP-titanium implants treated with biologic molecules. Elmengaard et al evaluated the effects of an Arg-Gly-Asp (RGD) peptide coating on tissue integration and titanium implant fixation across a bone-implant gap in dogs [22]. At 4 weeks post-surgery, it was reported that RGD-coated implants had significantly greater push-out stiffness compared to controls, whereas the peak strength was not significant different [22]. Sachse et al performed a study to evaluate HAP-titanium implants in sheep and reported that implants treated with BMP-2 displayed 50% higher pull-out force than controls at 20 weeks post-surgery [4]. Relative to these

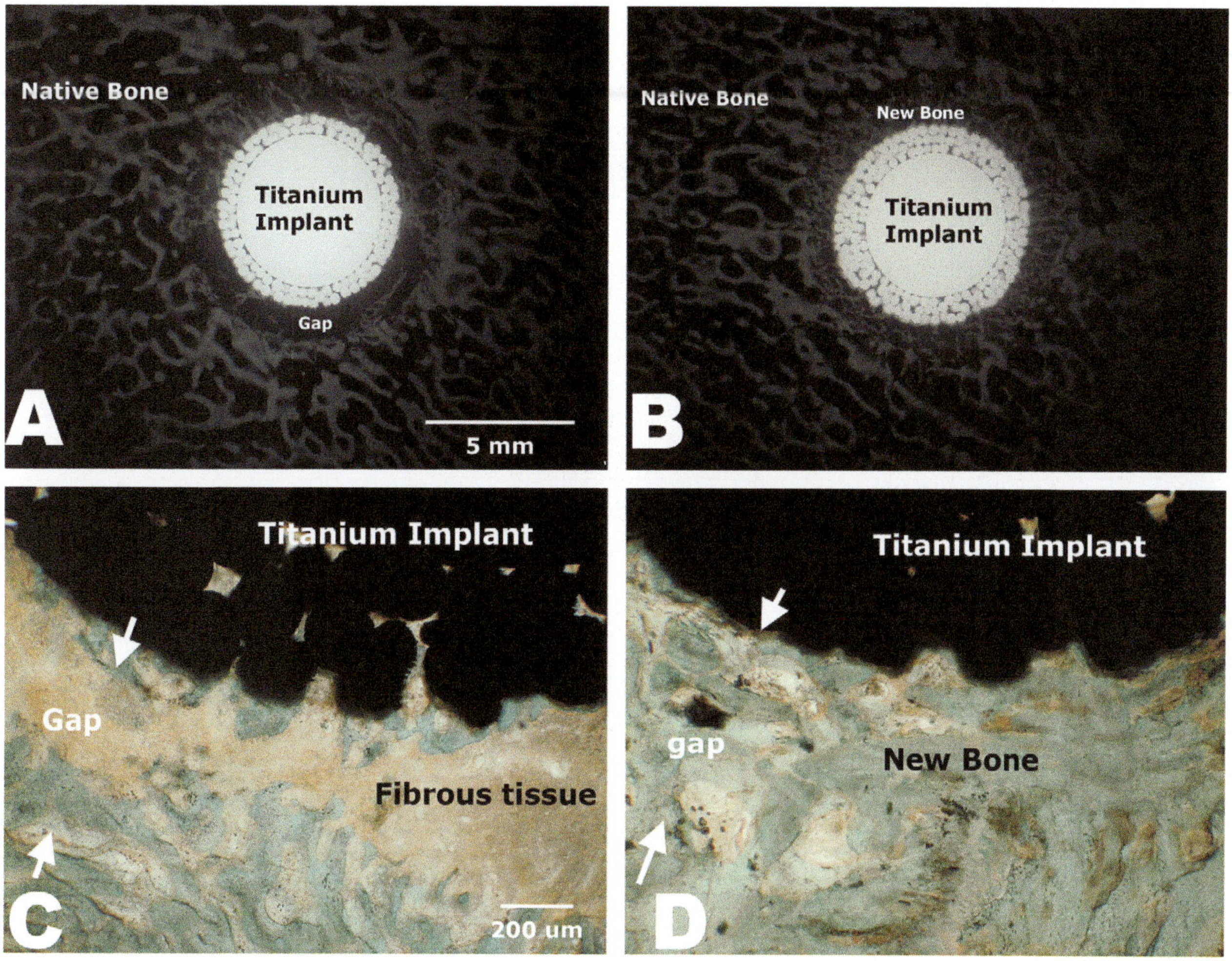

Figure 5. High detailed radiograph (A, B) and histologic section (C, D) of non-mBMP coated HAP-implants (A, C) and mBMP-coated implants (B, D). In C and D, areas between white arrows highlighted original 1-mm gap between the implant and host bone.

previous studies, the current study indicates that the modular peptide mBMP may also be useful in total joint arthoplasty, and other orthopedic implant applications. In addition, the ability of mBMP to bind with high efficiency to hydroxyapatite-containing implants may be particularly advantageous, as our previous studies have shown that efficient binding results in controllable dosages and localized release [20,21,24,32]. In addition, we have recently shown that mBMP can be modified to control the release rate from hydroxyapatite substrates [20,21,32]. Finally, recent studies indicate that the approach described here can be applied to other biologically active molecules, such as vascular endothelial growth factor (VEGF) [33]. Collectively, these studies suggest that the current approach may be useful in a range of orthopedic implant applications.

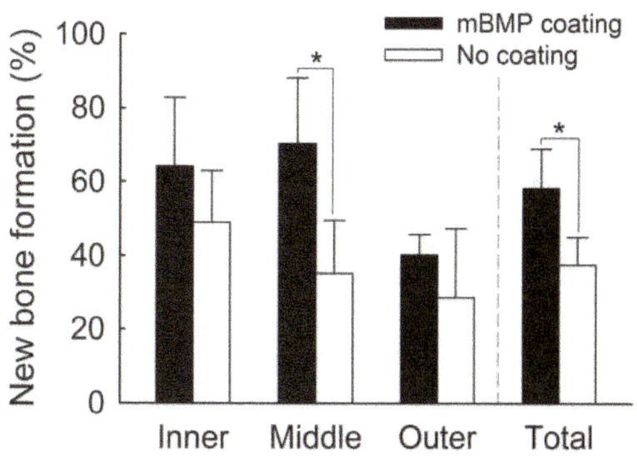

Figure 6. Histologic calculation of new bone formation in the implant-bone gap on the Goldner's trichrome staining slides demonstrated that middle section and total 3 sections of mBMP coated implant had significantly more new bone formation compared to control. "*" means significant difference between treatments ($p<0.05$).

It is noteworthy that specific aspects of this study were designed for relevance to potential clinical applications of these biomaterials. First, the bone-implant gap size of implant selected for this study (1 mm) was a critical size, which may be larger than the gap in actual human clinical applications, but may represent a challenging scenario for bone-implant healing in revision joint arthroplasty. Second, the four week evaluation time is a relatively early time point to characterize new bone formation, and may provide particular insights into the degree of accelerated bone formation. A later time point could provide insight into the ability of mBMP to promote stable long-term implant fixation, but would not indicate an ability to promote the rapid fixation that is needed. The purpose of this study was to characterize a challenging bone-implant gap and an early time point, to more directly represent the challenging environment present during revision arthroplasty, and the need to accelerate fixation and avoid development of fibrous tissue that can lead to pain and implant instability.

Conclusions

The mBMP peptides were efficiently bound to a HAP-titanium implant and released over 28 days in a sustained manner *in vitro*. *In vivo* results demonstrated that mBMP-coated HAP-titanium implants increased implant fixation and stimulated bone formation in a well-defined, critical gap between the implant and surrounding host cancellous bone after 4 weeks post-surgery compared to untreated HAP-titanium implants. This technique may be beneficial for human clinical applications, such as mBMP-coating on the stem of prosthesis, to enhance new bone formation at early stages.

Acknowledgments

The authors thank Vicki Kalscheur and Kari A. Pulfer for their technical support and Smith&Nephew Corp. for its providing HAP-titanium implants.

Author Contributions

Conceived and designed the experiments: YL JSL BKG RI RV MDM WLM. Performed the experiments: YL JSL BN. Analyzed the data: YL JSL KR RV MDM WLM. Contributed reagents/materials/analysis tools: JSL KR MDM WLM. Wrote the paper: YL. Proofread the manuscript: MDM, WLM.

References

1. Bozic KJ, Kurtz SM, Lau E, Ong K, Chiu V et al. (2010) The epidemiology of revision total knee arthroplasty in the United States. Clin Orthop Relat Res 468: 45–51.
2. Elmengaard B, Bechtold JE, Chen X, Soballe K (2009) Fixation of hydroxyapatite-coated revision implants is improved by the surgical technique of cracking the sclerotic bone rim. J Orthop Res 27: 996–1001.
3. Daugaard H, Elmengaard B, Bechtold JE, Soballe K (2008) Bone growth enhancement in vivo on press-fit titanium alloy implants with acid etched microtexture. J Biomed Mater Res A 87: 434–440.
4. Sachse A, Wagner A, Keller M, Wagner O, Wetzel WD et al. (2005) Osteointegration of hydroxyapatite-titanium implants coated with nonglycosylated recombinant human bone morphogenetic protein-2 (BMP-2) in aged sheep. Bone 37: 699–710.
5. Lamberg A, Schmidmaier G, Soballe K, Elmengaard B (2006) Locally delivered TGF-beta1 and IGF-1 enhance the fixation of titanium implants: a study in dogs. Acta Orthop 77: 799–805.
6. Hollister SJ, Murphy WL (2011) Scaffold translation: barriers between concept and clinic. Tissue Eng Part B Rev 17: 459–474.
7. Peng S, Zhou G, Luk KD, Cheung KM, Li Z et al. (2009) Strontium promotes osteogenic differentiation of mesenchymal stem cells through the Ras/MAPK signaling pathway. Cell Physiol Biochem 23: 165–174.
8. Boden SD, Zdeblick TA, Sandhu HS, Heim SE (2000) The use of rhBMP-2 in interbody fusion cages. Definitive evidence of osteoinduction in humans: a preliminary report. Spine (Phila Pa 1976) 25: 376–381.
9. Kanayama M, Hashimoto T, Shigenobu K, Yamane S, Bauer TW et al. (2006) A prospective randomized study of posterolateral lumbar fusion using osteogenic protein-1 (OP-1) versus local autograft with ceramic bone substitute: emphasis of surgical exploration and histologic assessment. Spine (Phila Pa 1976) 31: 1067–1074.
10. Govender S, Csimma C, Genant HK, Valentin-Opran A, Amit Y et al. (2002) Recombinant human bone morphogenetic protein-2 for treatment of open tibial fractures: a prospective, controlled, randomized study of four hundred and fifty patients. J Bone Joint Surg Am 84: 2123–2134.
11. Cahill KS, Chi JH, Day A, Claus EB (2009) Prevalence, complications, and hospital charges associated with use of bone-morphogenetic proteins in spinal fusion procedures. JAMA 302: 58–66.
12. Shields LB, Raque GH, Glassman SD, Campbell M, Vitaz T et al. (2006) Adverse effects associated with high-dose recombinant human bone morphogenetic protein-2 use in anterior cervical spine fusion. Spine (Phila Pa 1976) 31: 542–547.
13. Wong DA, Kumar A, Jatana S, Ghiselli G, Wong K (2008) Neurologic impairment from ectopic bone in the lumbar canal: a potential complication of off-label PLIF/TLIF use of bone morphogenetic protein-2 (BMP-2). Spine J 8: 1011–1018.
14. Carragee EJ, Mitsunaga KA, Hurwitz EL, Scuderi GJ (2011) Retrograde ejaculation after anterior lumbar interbody fusion using rhBMP-2: a cohort controlled study. Spine J 11: 511–516.
15. Carragee EJ, Hurwitz EL, Weiner BK (2011) A critical review of recombinant human bone morphogenetic protein-2 trials in spinal surgery: emerging safety concerns and lessons learned. Spine J 11: 471–491.
16. Liu Y, de Groot K, Hunziker EB (2005) BMP-2 liberated from biomimetic implant coatings induces and sustains direct ossification in an ectopic rat model. Bone 36: 745–757.
17. Liu Y, Enggist L, Kuffer AF, Buser D, Hunziker EB (2007) The influence of BMP-2 and its mode of delivery on the osteoconductivity of implant surfaces during the early phase of osseointegration. Biomaterials 28: 2677–2686.
18. Saito A, Suzuki Y, Ogata S, Ohtsuki C, Tanihara M (2003) Activation of osteo-progenitor cells by a novel synthetic peptide derived from the bone morphogenetic protein-2 knuckle epitope. Biochim Biophys Acta 1651: 60–67.
19. Saito A, Suzuki Y, Kitamura M, Ogata S, Yoshihara Y et al. (2006) Repair of 20-mm long rabbit radial bone defects using BMP-derived peptide combined with an alpha-tricalcium phosphate scaffold. J Biomed Mater Res A 77: 700–706.
20. Lee JS, Lee JS, Wagoner-Johnson A, Murphy WL (2009) Modular peptide growth factors for substrate-mediated stem cell differentiation. Angew Chem Int Ed Engl 48: 6266–6269.
21. Lee JS, Lee JS, Murphy WL (2010) Modular peptides promote human mesenchymal stem cell differentiation on biomaterial surfaces. Acta Biomater 6: 21–28.
22. Elmengaard B, Bechtold JE, Soballe K (2005) In vivo effects of RGD-coated titanium implants inserted in two bone-gap models. J Biomed Mater Res A 75: 249–255.
23. Faria ML, Lu Y, Heaney K, Uthamanthil RK, Muir P et al. (2007) Recombinant human bone morphogenetic protein-2 in absorbable collagen sponge enhances bone healing of tibial osteotomies in dogs. Vet Surg 36: 122–131.
24. Lu Y, Markel MD, Nemke B, Lee JS, Graf BK et al. (2009) Influence of hydroxyapatite-coated and growth factor-releasing interference screws on tendon-bone healing in an ovine model. Arthroscopy 25: 1427–1434.
25. Shields LB, Raque GH, Glassman SD, Campbell M, Vitaz T et al. (2006) Adverse effects associated with high-dose recombinant human bone morphogenetic protein-2 use in anterior cervical spine fusion. Spine 31: 542–547.
26. Campbell AW, Bain WE, McRae AF, Broad TE, Johnstone PD et al. (2003) Bone density in sheep: genetic variation and quantitative trait loci localisation. Bone 33: 540–548.
27. Fini M, Giavaresi G, Greggi T, Martini L, Aldini NN et al. (2003) Biological assessment of the bone-screw interface after insertion of uncoated and hydroxyapatite-coated pedicular screws in the osteopenic sheep. J Biomed Mater Res A 66: 176–183.
28. Lu Y, Nemke B, Lorang DM, Trip R, Kobayashi H et al. (2009) Comparison of a new braid fixation system to an interlocking intramedullary nail for tibial osteotomy repair in an ovine model. Vet Surg 38: 467–476.
29. Rammelt S, Heck C, Bernhardt R, Bierbaum S, Scharnweber D et al. (2007) In vivo effects of coating loaded and unloaded Ti implants with collagen, chondroitin sulfate, and hydroxyapatite in the sheep tibia. J Orthop Res 25: 1052–1061.
30. Elmengaard B, Bechtold JE, Soballe K (2005) In vivo study of the effect of RGD treatment on bone ongrowth on press-fit titanium alloy implants. Biomaterials 26: 3521–3526.
31. Kessler S, Mayr-Wohlfart U, Ignatius A, Puhl W, Claes L et al. (2003) [The impact of bone morphogenetic protein-2 (BMP-2), vascular endothelial growth factor (VEGF) and basic fibroblast growth factor (b-FGF) on osseointegration, degradation and biomechanical properties of a synthetic bone substitute]. Z Orthop Ihre Grenzgeb 141: 472–480.
32. Suarez-Gonzalez D, Barnhart K, Migneco F, Flanagan C, Hollister SJ et al. (2012) Controllable mineral coatings on PCL scaffolds as carriers for growth factor release. Biomaterials 33: 713–721.
33. Lee JS, Wagoner Johnson AJ, Murphy WL (2010) A modular, hydroxyapatite-binding version of vascular endothelial growth factor. Adv Mater 22: 5494–5498.

Determinants of Microdamage in Elderly Human Vertebral Trabecular Bone

Hélène Follet[1,2]*, Delphine Farlay[1,2], Yohann Bala[1,2], Stéphanie Viguet-Carrin[1,2], Evelyne Gineyts[1,2], Brigitte Burt-Pichat[1,2], Julien Wegrzyn[1,2,3], Pierre Delmas[1,2], Georges Boivin[1,2], Roland Chapurlat[1,2]

1 INSERM, UMR 1033, Lyon, France, **2** Université de Lyon, UMR 1033, Lyon, France, **3** Département de Chirurgie Orthopédique, Pavillon T, Hôpital Edouard Herriot, Lyon, France

Abstract

Previous studies have shown that microdamage accumulates in bone as a result of physiological loading and occurs naturally in human trabecular bone. The purpose of this study was to determine the factors associated with pre-existing microdamage in human vertebral trabecular bone, namely age, architecture, hardness, mineral and organic matrix. Trabecular bone cores were collected from human L2 vertebrae (n = 53) from donors 54–95 years of age (22 men and 30 women, 1 unknown) and previous cited parameters were evaluated. Collagen cross-link content (PYD, DPD, PEN and % of collagen) was measured on surrounding trabecular bone. We found that determinants of microdamage were mostly the age of donors, architecture, mineral characteristics and mature enzymatic cross-links. Moreover, linear microcracks were mostly associated with the bone matrix characteristics whereas diffuse damage was associated with architecture. We conclude that linear and diffuse types of microdamage seemed to have different determinants, with age being critical for both types.

Editor: Ryan K. Roeder, University of Notre Dame, United States of America

Funding: This study was supported in part by an unrestricted educational grant from Eli Lilly to INSERM. No additional external funding received for this study. The funders had no role in study design, data collection and analysis, decision to publish, or preparation of the manuscript.

Competing Interests: This study was supported in part by an unrestricted educational grant from Eli Lilly to INSERM.

* E-mail: Helene.Follet@inserm.fr

Introduction

Fatigue microdamage accumulates in bone as a result of physiological loading. [1,2,3,4] Several studies have reported microdamage in human trabecular bone occurring naturally. [5,6,7,8,9,10] Increased microdamage is associated with decreased bone strength in vitro, and thus may play a role in fragility fractures. [11] Whereas microdamage appears to increase with age [6,12] and decreased with trabecular bone volume [13], few studies have examined whether bone microarchitecture and/or characteristics of the bone matrix, such as the degree of mineralization, mineral maturity, and collagen crosslink profile are associated with the accumulation of microdamage in human trabecular bone [14,15].

In cortical bone, microcracks are observed within the interstitial bone or in interstitial bone intersecting with osteonal cement lines, and are arrested by osteons. [12,16,17] In cortical bone, microdamage appears to initiate within highly mineralized regions in cortical bone, [18] which is consistent with the linear elastic fracture mechanics theory [19,20].

Nucleation of mineral occurs in the 'hole' regions of the collagen arrays and apatite crystals develop in length along the collagen long axes and in width along channels within the collagen sheets. In such a two-phase structure, a microcrack would most likely be a break or fissure not only in the mineral matrix, but also in organic matrix. [21,22]. Thus, regarding mineral matrix, the degree of mineralization, cement lines or crystal size [23] may have a specific role in the initiation of microdamage, as they are mainly located in old interstitial regions which are more mineralized. [16,17] Indeed, changes in the morphology of the mineral crystal itself may affect the bone mechanical properties and microdamage accumulation. [24,25] For example, in human femur, crystallinity explained up to 48% of the variation in monotonic mechanical properties, and up to 64% in fatigue properties. [26] In addition to the mineral phase, the type and amount of collagen cross-links by impacting strength and stability between collagen fibers may be also associated with changes in microdamage. [27,28] Recent studies showed that the extent of advanced glycation endproducts (AGEs) were negatively associated not only with mechanical parameters [29,30,31] and microarchitecture [32] but also with microdamage. [33,34] In contrast, mature enzymatic cross-links seemed to be associated with less microdamage [33].

Altogether, the relationships between *in vivo* microdamage and the intrinsic properties of human trabecular bone remain ill-defined. In particular, little is known about what factors are specifically associated with linear and/or diffuse microdamage. Thus, the primary aims of the present study were to determine whether the degree and heterogeneity of mineralization, the mineral and organic characteristics, the microhardness and the collagen cross-links are related to the amount and type of pre-existing microdamage (ie: no damage created for this study) independently of age and trabecular bone volume in human vertebral trabecular bone from older donors.

Materials and Methods

Ethics Statement

Human bone samples were obtained from French body donation to science program (Laboratory of Anatomy, Faculty of Medicine Lyon Est, University of Lyon, France).

Specimen Preparation

L2 vertebrae were taken from 53, recently deceased Caucasians donors (22 men, 30 women), mean age of 78.3±9.9 years, with a range 54–95 years of age. The sex of one subject and the age of two subjects were not known. Bone samples were wrapped in gauze soaked with saline to keep them wet, then stored at −20°C. Vertebrae were screened using medial-lateral and anterior-posterior high-definition X-rays (Faxitron X-Ray, Lincolnshire IL, USA) to exclude prevalent fracture and significant bone diseases (e.g., metastasis, Paget's disease, osteochondritis). No additional information regarding donor disease status or medication history was available. Each vertebra was sectioned in half using an Isomet Buehler 4000 microsaw (Buehler GmbH, Düsseldorf, Germany). One hemi vertebra was dedicated to mechanical tests and the bone surrounding the cores was collected for collagen cross-links quantification by HPLC [10]; the second hemi vertebra was dedicated to the detection of pre-existing microdamage and mineral analysis. The hemi vertebrae for microdamage evaluation were bulk stained for 11 days at room temperature in 0.005 M xylenol orange (Sigma-Aldrich Corp., St. Louis, MO, USA) based in 70% ethanol. In each hemi vertebrae, a cylindrical trabecular specimen (8.25 mm diameter, 25 mm length) was removed in the supero-inferior direction from the anterior quadrant using a diamond tipped coring tool. The end plate of each vertebra was removed, as previously described. [10,35] Trabecular bone volume (BV/TV, %), trabecular thickness (Tb.Th, μm), trabecular number (Tb.N, 1/mm), trabecular separation (Tb.Sp, μm), connectivity density (Conn.D, 1/mm^3), degree of anisotropy (DA), and structure model index (SMI), which reflects the rod- versus plate-like nature of the structure, of the excised cores were assessed by microcomputed tomography, using an isotropic voxel size of 20 microns, energy (70 kVp), current (177 μA), integration time (200 ms) and a threshold corresponding to a mineral density around 0.35 g.cm^3 (μCT40, Scanco Medical AG, Brüttisellen, Switzerland). Structural indices of trabecular bone analysis were calculated using distance transformation (filling structure with spheres) without assuming anything about the shape of the bone (i.e. without plate model assumption). BV/TV was based on counting voxels.

Microdamage analysis

Trabecular cores for detection of microdamage were embedded in methylmethacrylate and cut parallel to the long axis to obtain at least three non-contiguous, parallel, 100±5 μm-thick sections for microdamage evaluation, as previously described. [35,36] Specimen were bulk stained with xylenol orange and general non-specific staining, morphologically different from microcracks, were easily identifiable. Three sections per specimen were measured using fluorescence (excitation/emission wavelength of 440–570/610 nm) microscopy at ×200 magnification and morphometry software (Bone Morpho; Explora Nova, La Rochelle, France). Microdamage appeared in orange under fluorescence light. [35,36] Microdamage was categorized and quantified as linear microcracks or diffuse damage (only few cross-hatching, which were counted as diffuse damage, Figure 1). Outcome assessments included the linear crack density, defined as the number of linear microcracks (Cr.N, #) per bone area (Cr.Dn, #/mm^2), and the diffuse damage density, defined as the number of diffuse damage regions per bone area (Dx.Dn, #/mm^2). Length was expressed as mean linear crack length (Cr.Le, μm)[1], whereas length and area density were expressed as linear length density (Cr.Le.Dn, μm/mm^2)[2] and diffuse damage area density defined as diffuse damage area per bone area (Dx.Ar.Dn, %).

NB: 1- Mean linear crack length is the mean of total length of linear cracks measured on three sections divided by the total number of linear cracks.

2- Crack length density is the mean crack length divided by the bone volume (BV) measured, by histomorphometry, on the same three sections: Cr.Le.Dn = Cr.Le/BV.

Mineralization Measurements

The mean degree of mineralization and heterogeneity of mineralization were assessed using quantitative microradiography on 100±1 μm thick sections, as previously described. [37,38,39] Outcomes included the mean degree of mineralization of bone (DMB, g/cm^3) and the heterogeneity index expressed as the mean of the widths at half-maximum height (HI, g/cm^3) measured on the individual DMB curves.

Hardness Analysis

Microhardness (Hv, kg/mm^2) was measured on polished remaining embedded blocks using a Vickers indenter with a 25 μg load for 10 seconds, as previously described [38].

Mineral at Crystal Level, and Organic Matrix Analysis by FTIRM

Each infrared spectra spectrum (Figure 2), performed on 2-μm-thick sections, was collected from an area of 30×100 μm^2 at a spectral resolution of 4 cm^{-1} and 50 scans were performed by spectrum. [40] Twenty spectra were analyzed per sample. The following variables were determined:

The mineral crystallinity index (CI) corresponds to both crystal size and perfection [40], the mineralization index (MI) is the area ratio of the bands of mineral matrix over organic matrix [41], mineral maturity (MM) was calculated as the area ratio of the apatitic phosphate over non apatitic phosphate reflecting also the age of mineral [40], carbonation was calculated as integrated area ratios ν_2CO_3 (862–894 cm^{-1}) over $\nu_1\nu_3PO_4$ (910–1184 cm^{-1}), representing the quantity of carbonates incorporated into the bone mineral, and collagen maturity (CM) was calculated as the ratio of organic matrix bands (1660/1690 cm^{-1} area ratio) [42] reflecting the evolution of the secondary structure of collagen with the mineralization [43].

Collagen Cross-links Analysis

The central part of the vertebral body around the core, containing exclusively trabecular bone, was retained for biochemical analysis. Cross-links measurements were carried out as previously described. [32,44] We assessed the content of both enzymatic nonreducible mature cross-links PYD and DPD, and the PEN induced by non-enzymatic induced, normalized to the total amount of collagen.

Statistical Analysis

Data are reported as mean values, standard deviations, ranges, median and interquartile range. As some variables were not normally distributed even after transformation, we used non-parametric tests. No significant differences between men and women were observed, consequently men and women were pooled for correlation analyses. The relationships between parameters

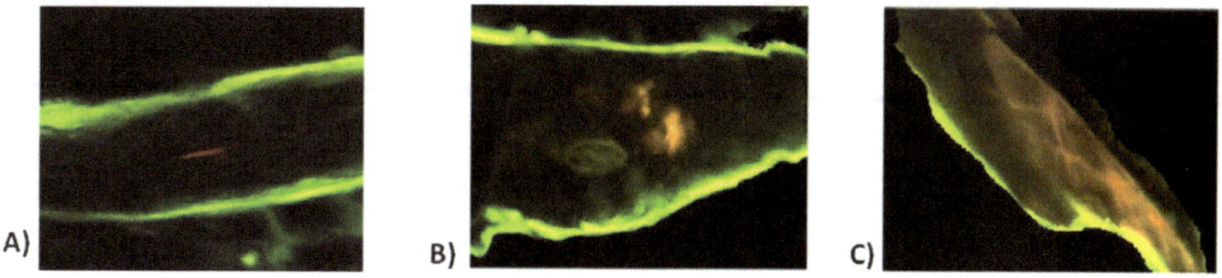

Figure 1. Pictures obtained under fluorescent light of microdamage in orange: A) Linear microcrack, B) Diffuse damage, C) Few cross-hatching microdamage were found.

were assessed by Spearman correlation coefficient (r). We used partial spearman correlation to test whether associations between parameters were significant after accounting for the contribution of BV/TV or age. All tests were two-tailed, and significance defined as $p \leq 0.05$. All statistical analyses were performed using statistical analyses software (R & SPSS 16).

Results

Association between Age, Microdamage and its Determinants

Descriptive statistics are found in Table 1. Microdamage (crack density – Figure 3a, crack length density, and diffuse damage area density), Tb.Sp, SMI, the ratio PYD/DPD and crystallinity index increased with age, whereas carbonation, BV/TV, Tb.N and DA decreased with age (Table 2). Except the ratio PYD/DPD, collagen cross-link characteristics, mineralization parameters and microhardness were not related to age (Table 3).

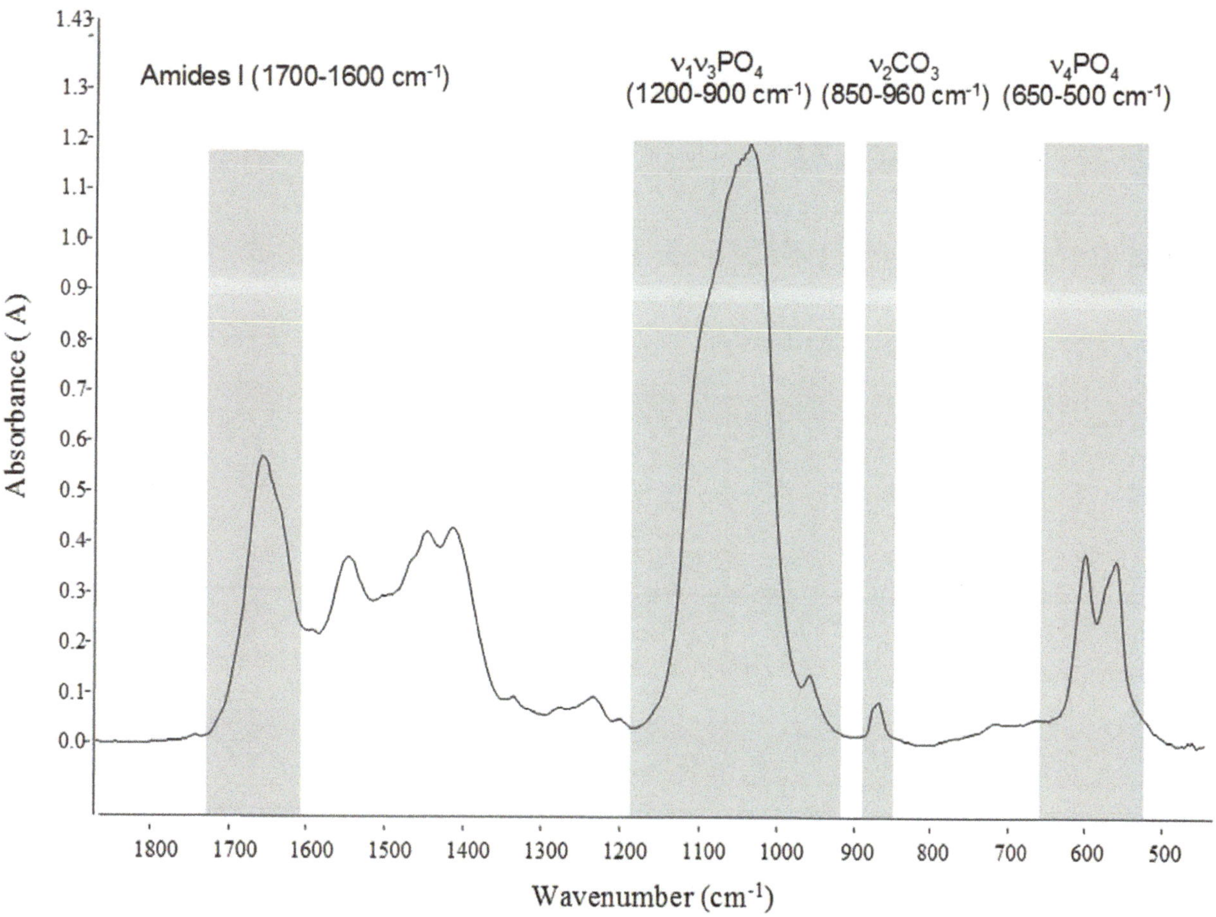

Figure 2. Infrared spectrum obtained from vertebral trabecular bone (man, 79 year-old). Spectrum is expressed as wave number (cm^{-1}) which represent the vibration modes (amide I, phosphate, carbonate).

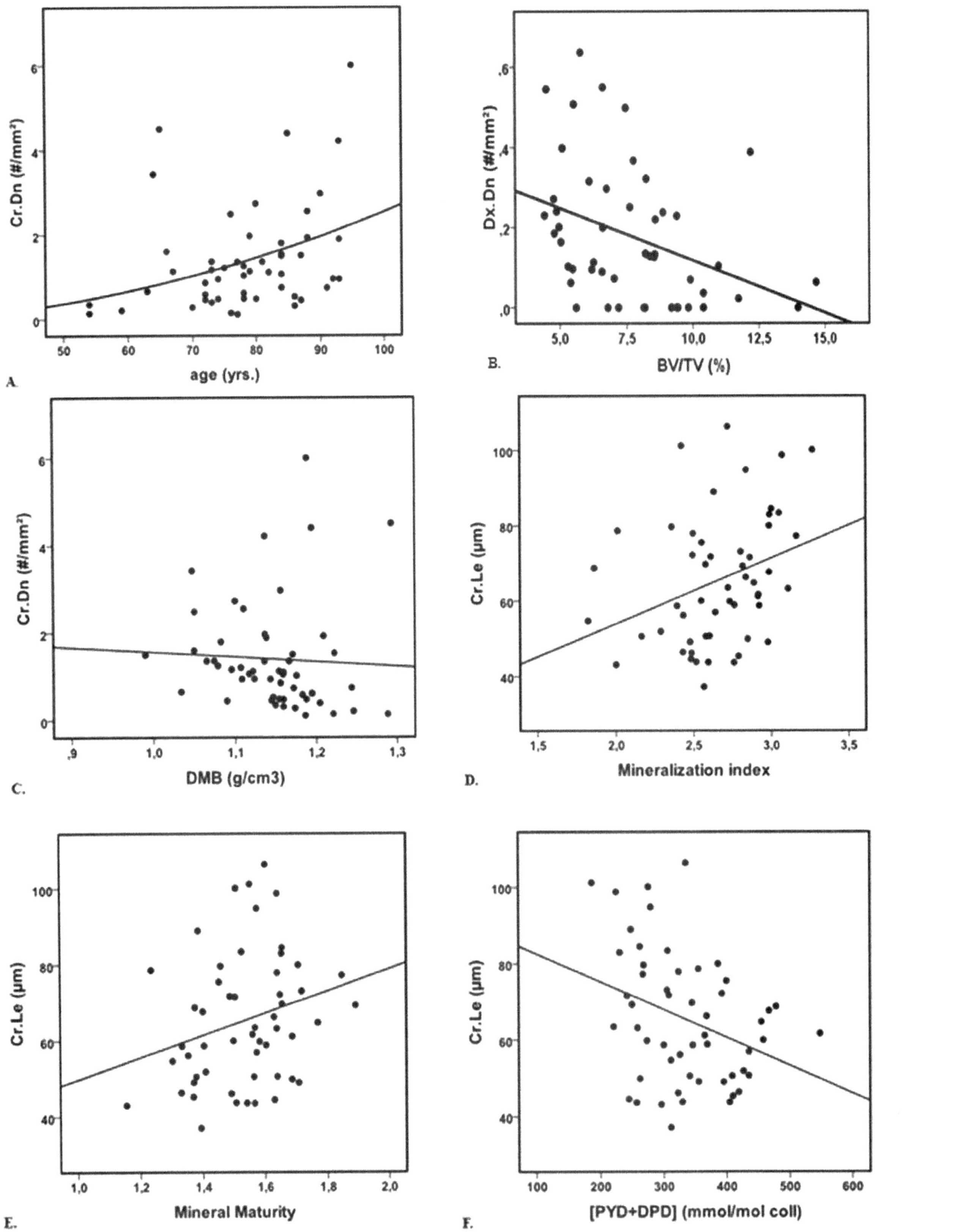

Figure 3. Bivariate Scattergrams. A) Age of donor vs Crack density – $r = 0.36$, $p = 0.010$, B) BV/TV vs Diffuse damage density, $r = -0.42$, $p = 0.003$, C) Degree of mineralization vs crack density, $r = -0.31$, $p = 0.02$, D) Mineralization index vs Crack length, $r = 0.36$, $p = 0.008$, E) Mineral maturity vs Crack length, $r = 0.30$, $p = 0.03$, F) Mature cross-links vs Crack length, $r = -0.30$, $p = 0.03$.

Table 1. Descriptive statistics, mean ± SD, range, median and interquartile range (IQR).

	n	Mean±SD	Range		Median	IQR
Age (yrs)	51	78.3±9.9	54	95	78	12.8
-FTIRM parameters	53					
Mineralization Index		2.66±0.32	1.82	3.27	2.64	0.411
Mineral Maturity		1.54±0.15	1.16	1.89	1.56	0.24
Carbonation		0.007±0.001	0.006	0.009	0.007	0.001
Collagen Maturity		4.03±0.46	2.91	5.30	3.98	0.57
Crystallinity Index		25.23±0.81	23.39	27.28	25.31	1.14
-Architecture	51					
BV/TV (%)		7.68±2.42	4.43	14.66	7.33	3.59
Tb.Th (μm)		137±18	102	187	133	28.3
Tb.Sp (μm)		1161±189	878	1932	1125	222
Tb.N (1/mm)		0.84±0.12	0.51	1.11	0.84	0.16
Connectivity density		2.03±0.80	0.74	4.32	1.87	1.14
SMI		1.77±0.49	0.33	2.52	1.80	0.74
DA		1.68±0.20	1.28	2.36	1.64	0.21
-Mineralization	53					
DMB (g/cm^3)		1.147±0.061	0.99	1.293	1.155	0.076
HI (g/cm^3)		0.287±0.087	0.122	0.525	0.274	0.111
-Hardness	53					
Hv (Kg/cm^2)		45.97±1.65	42.37	48.91	45.74	2.83
-Microdamage	53					
Cr.N (#)		22±24	1	109	15	20.3
Dx.N (#)		2.54±2.7	0	11	2.0	2.5
Cr.Dn ($\#/mm^2$)		1.408±1.24	0.114	6.012	1.109	1.132
Dx.Dn ($\#/mm^2$)		0.172±0.168	0	0.637	0.128	0.216
Cr.Le (μm)		65.37±17.15	37.1	106.37	63.24	26.79
Cr.Le.Dn ($\mu m/mm^2$)		93.1±92.8	7.68	456.3	69.35	68.0
Dx.Ar.Dn (%)		0.034±0.065	0	0.344	0.013	0.024
-Collagen X-Links	53					
PYD (mmol/mol coll)		232.1±61	126	406	225	91
DPD (mmol/mol coll)		103.6±25.9	61	192	103	32
PYD/DPD		2.30±0.65	1.398	5.65	2.184	0.635
PYD+DPD(mmol/mol coll)		335.7±78	187	548	128	91
PEN (mmol/mol coll)		20.85±9.41	6.19	54.5	18.4	11.71
Collagen (%)		22.77±2.49	15.30	28.74	23.27	3.197

After adjustment for BV/TV, crack length density, PYD/DPD, carbonation, mineral maturity and crystallinity index remained significantly correlated with age (Table 4).

Association between Bone Volume Fraction, Microarchitecture and Microdamage

Linear crack density was not associated with BV/TV. Linear crack length was positively associated with trabecular thickness (Tb.Th) and the degree of anisotropy (DA) (Table 2), even after adjusting for age (Table 3). After adjusting for BV/TV, Cr.Le remained strongly associated with Tb.Th (Table 4). In comparison, diffuse damage density was negatively correlated with BV/TV (Figure 3b), connectivity density and Tb.N, and positively correlated with Tb.Sp. After adjusting for age, diffuse damage density remained associated with BV/TV, Tb.Sp, Tb.N and connectivity, and association appeared with DA. After adjusting for BV/TV, all these associations disappeared, except for DA, which was positively correlated with damage density (Table 4). Diffuse damage area density was negatively correlated with BV/TV and Tb.N, and positively with Tb.Sp. (Table 2). After adjusting for BV/TV or age, all these associations disappeared (Table 3, Table 4).

Association between Mineral Traits and Microdamage

Crack length was positively correlated with mineralization index, mineral maturity and DMB, whereas crack density was negatively correlated with DMB (Table 2, Figure 3c). After adjusting for age, these correlations remained significant (Table 3). After adjusting for BV/TV, only mineralization index and mineral maturity remained significantly associated with crack length (Table 4, Figure 3d,e) even if it was borderline for DMB ($p = 0.056$). Carbonation and crystallinity index were not correlated to microdamage, neither before nor after adjusting for age or BV/TV. Neither heterogeneity index (HI) nor the microhardness (Hv) was associated with microdamage in vertebral trabecular bone.

Association between Collagen Cross-links, Organic Matrix Properties, and Microdamage

Crack density was positively correlated with PYD, (PYD/DPD), and tended to decrease with the percentage of collagen. Crack length was also negatively associated with PYD, DPD and (PYD+DPD), (Table 2, Figure 3f). After adjusting for age, only the relations between PYD, DPD, (PYD+DPD) and crack length remained significant (Table 3), whereas after adjusting for BV/TV, only the PYD/DPD ratio remained significantly associated to crack density and crack length density (Table 4). Crack length density was only correlated with the PYD/DPD ratio. Collagen maturity was not correlated with microdamage, even after adjusting for age or BV/TV. The non-enzymatic glycation product, PEN, was not associated with any parameters of microdamage.

Discussion

In this study, we found that microdamage in human vertebral trabecular bone was associated with age, microarchitecture, mineral characteristics and mature enzymatic cross-links, with different factors associated with linear versus diffuse damage.

Determinants of Linear Microcracks

Our finding that microdamage increases with age is in agreement with prior data reporting that linear microcracks (Cr.Dn, Cr.Le and Cr.Le.Dn) in trabecular bone from the femoral head, [11,13] the neck, [6] and vertebrae [9,35] increase exponentially with the age of the donors. [6,7,9,11,12,13,35,45] In contrast with our previous study in only 23 vertebrae, [35] but similarly to work of Fazzalari et al [6], in the current study, microarchitecture was not associated with linear crack density. Compared to Arlot et al [35], statistical difference is found in the crack density (same age, BV/TV, crack length), the measurement of damage area (in the current study, when no damage was found, a value of "zero" was indicated contrary to previous study where a "none" value was indicated) and the number of samples (23 compared to 53 presently). But the main difference is found in the architectural measurement of trabecular bone. In the previous study [35], structural parameters (BV/TV, Tb.Th, Tb.Sp, Tb.N)

Table 2. Bivariate spearman coefficient correlation (r_{sp}) between microdamage, age, architecture, mineralization degree, microhardness, mineral at crystal level, organic matrix and collagen cross-links.

	Age	Cr.Dn	Dx.Dn	Cr.Le	Cr.Le.Dn	Dx.Ar.Dn
	r_{sp}	r_{sp}	r_{sp}	r_{sp}	r_{sp}	r_{sp}
Age		**0.357***	0.232	0.02	**0.353***	**0.345***
-FTIRM parameters						
Mineralization	0.223	−0.106	−0.043	**0.358****	0.021	−0.007
Mineral Maturity	0.144	0.018	−0.11	**0.298***	0.109	−0.091
Carbonation	**−0.353***	0.053	0.082	−0.079	−0.002	−0.009
Collagen Maturity	0.045	0.025	0.034	−0.039	0.006	−0.045
Crystallinity Index	**0.336***	0.074	−0.093	0.22	0.152	−0.049
-Architecture						
BV/TV	**−0.574****	−0.20	**−0.417****	0.160	−0.151	**−0.379****
Tb.Th	0.10	0.025	0.032	**0.456****	0.157	0.034
Tb.Sp	**0.36***	−0.20	**0.424****	−0.052	0.005	**0.321***
Tb.N	**−0.34***	0.005	**−0.431****	−0.070	−0.018	**−0.317***
Conn density	−0.199	−0.187	**−0.356***	−0.102	−0.195	−0.194
SMI	**0.513****	0.085	0.213	−0.057	0.086	0.237
DA	**−0.348***	−0.043	0.216	**0.277***	0.008	0.064
-Mineralization						
DMB	0.030	**−0.314***	−0.172	**0.319***	−0.237	−0.108
HI	−0.033	−0.058	−0.075	−0.071	−0.097	−0.033
-Hardness						
Hv	0.136	−0.035	−0.087	0.233	0.024	−0.100
-Collagen X-Links						
PYD	0.272	**0.326***	0.164	**−0.30***	0.229	0.101
DPD	0.119	0.057	0.197	**−0.275***	−0.032	0.213
PYD/DPD	**0.307***	**0.326***	−0.011	−0.12	**0.279***	−0.005
PYD+DPD	0.222	0.269	0.21	**−0.296***	0.170	0.134
PEN	0.071	0.001	−0.063	0.074	0.036	−0.065
Collagen	−0.131	−0.261	−0.040	0.122	−0.180	0.008

*$p<0.05$,
**$p<0.01$.

were based on triangularization[1] of surface (ie: one more interpolation step in comparison to VOX, based on counting voxels). In present study, we used the called "Direct" measurement (DT)[2], based on distance transformation, which is more accurate. In prior study, Cr.Dn was linked with respectively TRI-BV/TV ($r=-0.51$, $p=0.017$), TRI-Tb.N ($r=-0.54$, $p=0.012$) and TRI-Tb.Sp ($r=0.53$, $p=0.013$). Using the direct measurement (DT), as in the current study, (for the same subset of samples), those previous associations does not remain, except for BV/TV: Cr.Dn and, respectively, Vox-BV/TV ($r=-0.51$, $p=0.018$), indeed, DT-Tb.N ($r=-0.31$, $p=0.17$) and DT-Tb.Sp ($r=0.32$, $p=0.15$). Furthermore, if the direct measurement was used for the previous study, crack length was also associated to the direct trabecular thickness.

NB: 1- Triangularization or TRI corresponds to traditional 2D histomorphometry, but this plate-model assumption leads to a bias in most cases. Scanco® recommends to use DT-Tb.N, DT-Tb,Sp for truly 3D results.

2- Direct measurement or DT indices are calculated using distance transformation (filling structure with spheres) without assuming anything about the shape of the bone (i.e. without plate model assumption).

The way of analysis the data is also essential. Indeed, depending of the analytical model used, Yeni et al., [46] who also studied human vertebral trabecular bone, found two different trends. A power law relationship between Cr. Dn and BV/TV was significant ($r^2=0.14$, $p=0.025$). However, a three-parameter exponential fit was not significant for the relationship between Cr. Dn and BV/TV ($p>0.07$). [46] There are too few papers on damaged aged human vertebrae to accurately compare with literature.

Average length of linear microcracks was associated with mineralization index, degree of mineralization and mineral maturity. The more mature the mineral, the longer the cracks. However, the crystallinity index was not associated with crack length. Linear microcrack density was not associated with any of the variables measured by FTIRM, suggesting that mineral maturity and/or mineralization does not influence microdamage accumulation in trabecular bone. [47] However, the degree of mineralization was inversely associated with Cr.Dn, and positively

Table 3. Spearman partial coefficient after adjustment for age; dependent variables shown along the top and independent variables along the side of the table.

	Cr.Dn	Dx.Dn	Cr.Le	Cr.Le.Dn	Dx.Ar.Dn
	r	r	r	r	r
-FTIRM parameters					
Mineralization Index	−0.197	−0.092	**0.352****	−0.071	−0.087
Mineral Maturity	−0.043	−0.179	**0.292***	0.054	−0.165
Carbonation	0.195	0.141	−0.04	0.153	0.120
Collagen Maturity	−0.005	−0.024	−0.067	−0.009	−0.087
Crystallinity Index	−0.054	−0.191	0.212	0.034	−0.195
-Architecture					
BV/TV	−0.011	**−0.389****	0.246	0.064	−0.254
Tb.Th	−0.005	0.04	**0.451****	0.114	0.031
Tb.Sp	−0.165	**0.393****	0.025	−0.159	0.232
Tb.N	0.139	**−0.398****	−0.043	0.131	−0.230
Conn density	−0.123	**−0.316***	−0.09	−0.119	−0.127
SMI	−0.093	0.173	−0.07	−0.108	0.109
DA	0.074	**0.297***	**0.328***	0.147	0.199
-Mineralization					
DMB	**−0.355****	−0.194	**0.327***	−0.270	−0.124
HI	−0.056	−0.077	−0.090	−0.095	−0.019
-Hardness					
Hv	−0.096	−0.128	0.243	−0.032	−0.165
-Collagen X-Links					
PYD	0.242	0.061	**−0.315***	0.151	−0.017
DPD	0.0012	0.130	**−0.281***	−0.082	0.160
PYD/DPD	0.24	−0.12	−0.10	0.21	−0.14
PYD+DPD	0.197	0.120	**−0.309***	0.104	0.038
PEN	−0.04	−0.094	0.09	0.005	−0.111
Collagen	−0.224	0.034	0.090	−0.166	0.079

*$p<0.05$,
**$p<0.01$.

associated with Cr.Le, meaning the more mineralized the bone was, the fewer but longer the cracks were, consistently with the positive association between elastic modulus and crack length. [10] The ensuing discrepancy between the mineralization index and DMB might be explained. Indeed, while quantitative microradiography provides results reflecting the entire bone surface of the sample, FTIRM reflects a smallest proportion of analyzed area. Therefore, the number of measurements in trabecular bone did not cover the entire bone surface, explaining the discrepancy obtained between DMB and mineralization index. It has been suggested that the more bone was mineralized, the lower the plastic deformation was and more cracks were initiated. [48] The level of mineralization might be an important factor influencing the cracks morphology. [48] Degree of mineralization and mineral maturity do not influence number or length the cracks in the same way. This finding leads to the conclusion that mineral quantity rather than mineral characteristics (maturity or crystallinity) should be used to explain cracks number.

Recent *in vitro* [49] and *ex vivo* studies [33,34] show that AGEs altered the extent of accumulated microdamage in bone tissue. Nevertheless, no association was found between PEN content and microdamage parameters, but an unexpected relationship between mature enzymatic cross-links and crack density was noted. Indeed, we found the same association between mature enzymatic cross-links and cracks density already than Saito et al [34] in cortical rib from dogs treated for 3 years with bisphosphonate. These discrepancies may be explained by the fact that microdamage may be site specific. Also, the collagen characteristic is bulk assessment (<10 mg of bone) compared to microdamage, a very localized process (thin sections). However an interesting association between mature enzymatic cross-link content and crack length was found suggesting that these cross-links, by providing strength and stability between collagen fibers, may avoid crack propagation in bone tissue. This result confirms that enzymatic cross-linking in bone is a favorable process. Lastly, collagen maturity, measured by FTIRM, was not related to microdamage whereas the collagen content, measured by HPLC, showed a negative trend with linear cracks density. This suggested that lower collagen content may be associated with numerous microcracks. Nevertheless, the orientation of the collagen fiber [50], the sacrificial bonds [51] may also participate to the propagation of microdamage and alter bone quality.

Determinants of Diffuse Damage

We found that diffuse damage in human vertebral trabecular bone was associated with age, and microarchitecture. The surface density of diffuse damage was positively associated with age, conversely to Vashishth et al. [8] who found that age did not influence the accumulation of diffuse damage in men or women. [8] However, this is partly explained by the mean age of their female population (56 years-olds) near the onset of menopause, and associated with high turnover rates. In our study, diffuse damage was only associated with microarchitecture, but not a with either characteristics of the mineral matrix nor the variables measured by FTIRM [47].

Relationship between Microcracks and Local Mechanical Properties Linked to Mineral Phase

Wang et al. showed that nanoindentation hardness was a very good predictor of bone tissue elastic modulus for both normal and osteoporotic bone tissues. [52] In another study, the same authors discussed the fact that postfailure properties of hard tissue had strong effects on bone microdamage morphology and the rate of change in apparent mechanical properties. [53] In our study, no relationship was found between hardness and microdamage, or between DMB and collagen maturity. Those hardness measurements were done at the tissue level (global level), and not at the local level of the microdamage itself. Thus, more precise measurements of hardness should be done around the microcracks to better understand the association between contact hardness and microdamage [54].

Our study has some limitations. An important limitation to the discussion of our results is that we have no information regarding medical history of persons, and therefore we cannot rule out the presence of diseases or medications that may have influenced our outcome variables. However, the anatomical specimens were radiographed to exclude bone diseases or tumors, and bone histology allowed to exclude specimens with osteomalacia. We acknowledge that many of our study subjects were old so our results are only representative of an elderly population. This

Table 4. Spearman partial coefficient after adjustment for BV/TV; dependent variables shown along the top and independent variables along the side of the table.

	Age	Cr.Dn	Dx.Dn	Cr.Le	Cr.Le.Dn	Dx.Ar.Dn
	r	r	r	r	r	r
Age		0.268	−0.056	0.194	**0.311***	0.132
-FTIRM parameters						
Mineralization	0.240	−0.151	−0.089	**0.418****	−0.008	−0.028
Mineral Maturity	**0.333***	0.021	−0.084	**0.334***	0.110	−0.062
Carbonation	**−0.326***	−0.018	0.195	−0.149	0.060	0.080
Collagen Maturity	0.106	−0.0176	0.047	0.001	−0.043	−0.072
Crystallinity Index	**0.350***	0.0286	−0.160	0.256	0.117	−0.122
-Architecture						
Tb.Th	0.240	0.045	0.129	**0.452*****	0.167	0.111
Tb.Sp	0.046	−0.169	0.242	0.216	−0.103	0.165
Tb.N	−0.037	0.140	−0.262	−0.222	0.079	−0.168
Conn density	0.084	−0.146	−0.213	−0.214	−0.168	−0.060
SMI	0.217	−0.067	−0.165	0.115	−0.010	−0.024
DA	−0.161	0.042	**0.431***	0.232	0.078	0.249
-Mineralization						
DMB	0.205	−0.269 BL	−0.049	0.258	−0.204	−0.011
HI	−0.121	−0.083	−0.157	−0.035	−0.118	−0.094
-Hardness						
Hv	0.093	−0.046	−0.154	0.246	0.028	−0.133
-Collagen X-Links						
PYD	0.1648	0.266 BL	0.045	−0.235	0.180	−0.026
DPD	0.003	−0.011	0.116	−0.223	−0.095	0.135
PYD/DPD	**0.301***	**0.327***	−0.064	−0.103	**0.285***	−0.60
PYD+DPD	0.109	0.207	0.109	−0.233	0.116	0.020
PEN	0.129	0.026	−0.002	0.030	0.050	−0.060
Collagen	−0.011	−0.229	0.025	0.110	−0.137	0.122

*$p<0.05$,
**$p<0.01$.
***$p<0.001$.

group, however, is most susceptible to fragility fractures. We are conscious that some donors may have received an osteoporosis therapy (i.e. estrogen or bisphosphonate) which may alter the relationships with microdamage. For example, bisphosphonate has an effect on the crystal characteristics as shown in BSUs of similar DMB and mineral maturity, the crystallinity was decreased in patients long-term treated with alendronate. [55] This was also shown for zoledronate, when crystallinity was measured between tetracycline labels (same chronology in both groups), it was lower in patients treated for 3 years once yearly. Moreover, another bisphosphonate (risedronate) has been associated with changes in collagen maturity assessed by FTIRM. [56] Furthermore, we did not quantify the reducible cross-links which may contribute to skeletal fragility and we only analyzed pentosidine, which explained 40% of the variance in bulk fluorescent AGE and comprise only a portion of total fluorescent AGEs that accumulate with tissue age in bone [33].

Our study also has a number of strengths. First, we have analyzed a relatively large number of sample, and only one sample per donor (compared to other studies using cadaveric tissues) comprising old donors whose age distribution reflected the population in which the majority of fragility fractures occur. Furthermore, this is among the few studies to assess mineral characteristics, collagen cross-links, and microdamage analyses on the same vertebral body.

In conclusion, trabecular microdamage increases with age, but this association is driven, at least in part, by declining BV/TV. We also found that linear and diffuse damage have different determinants. Linear microcracks are mostly influenced by the bone matrix quality whereas diffuse damage seems to be influenced by bone microarchitecture. The second finding is that, within the linear microcracks, there are also different factors that influence the density and the length of cracks.

Acknowledgments

The authors thank C. Bertholon, INSERM U1033, for her technical help for collagen crosslink analysis and J-P. Roux, INSERM U1033, for his help during the dissection of the vertebral blocs.

The authors also thank Dr. M. Arlot, INSERM U1033, for her contribution to microdamage analysis, and Dr M.L. Bouxsein, Orthopedic Biomechanics Laboratory, Beth Israel Deaconess Medical Center and

Harvard Medical School, Boston, MA, USA for her contribution in this study.

Author Contributions

Conceived and designed the experiments: HF PD. Performed the experiments: HF DF YB SVC EG BBP. Analyzed the data: HF DF YB SVC EG. Contributed reagents/materials/analysis tools: HF JW PD. Wrote the paper: HF DF YB SVC GB RC.

References

1. Donahue SW, Galley SA (2006) Microdamage in bone: implications for fracture, repair, remodeling, and adaptation. Crit Rev Biomed Eng 34: 215–271.
2. Burr DB, Turner CH, Naick P, Forwood MR, Ambrosius W, et al. (1998) Does microdamage accumulation affect the mechanical properties of bone? J Biomech 31: 337–345.
3. Luo Q, Leng H, Acuna R, Neil Dong X, Rong Q, et al. (2010) Constitutive relationship of tissue behavior with damage accumulation of human cortical bone. J Biomech 43: 2356–2361.
4. Taylor D, Hazenberg JG, Lee TC (2007) Living with cracks: damage and repair in human bone. Nat Mater 6: 263–268.
5. Fazzalari NL, Forwood MR, Manthey BA, Smith K, Kolesik P (1998) Three-dimensional confocal images of microdamage in cancellous bone. Bone 23: 373–378.
6. Fazzalari NL, Forwood MR, Smith K, Manthey BA, Herreen P (1998) Assessment of cancellous bone quality in severe osteoarthrosis: bone mineral density, mechanics, and microdamage. Bone 22: 381–388.
7. Fazzalari NL, Kuliwaba JS, Forwood MR (2002) Cancellous bone microdamage in the proximal femur: influence of age and osteoarthritis on damage morphology and regional distribution. Bone 31: 697–702.
8. Vashishth D, Koontz J, Qiu SJ, Lundin-Cannon D, Yeni YN, et al. (2000) In vivo diffuse damage in human vertebral trabecular bone. Bone 26: 147–152.
9. Wenzel TE, Schaffler MB, Fyhrie DP (1996) In vivo trabecular microcracks in human vertebral bone. Bone 19: 89–95.
10. Follet H, Viguet-Carrin S, Burt-Pichat B, Depalle B, Bala Y, et al. (2010) Effects of preexisting microdamage, collagen cross-links, degree of mineralization, age, and architecture on compressive mechanical properties of elderly human vertebral trabecular bone. J Orthop Res: Doi:10.1002/jor.21275.
11. Burr DB, Forwood MR, Fyhrie DP, Martin RB, Schaffler MB, et al. (1997) Bone microdamage and skeletal fragility in osteoporotic and stress fractures. J Bone Miner Res 12: 6–15.
12. Schaffler MB, Choi K, Milgrom C (1995) Aging and matrix microdamage accumulation in human compact bone. Bone 17: 521–525.
13. Mori S, Harruff R, Ambrosius W, Burr DB (1997) Trabecular bone volume and microdamage accumulation in the femoral heads of women with and without femoral neck fractures. Bone 21: 521–526.
14. Shi X, Liu XS, Wang X, Guo XE, Niebur GL (2010) Effects of trabecular type and orientation on microdamage susceptibility in trabecular bone. Bone 46: 1260–1266.
15. Hernandez CJ, Tang SY, Baumbach BM, Hwu PB, Sakkee AN, et al. (2005) Trabecular microfracture and the influence of pyridinium and non-enzymatic glycation-mediated collagen cross-links. Bone 37: 825–832.
16. Norman TL, Wang Z (1997) Microdamage of human cortical bone: incidence and morphology in long bones. Bone 20: 375–379.
17. Martin RB, Burr DB (1982) A hypothetical mechanism for the stimulation of osteonal remodelling by fatigue damage. J Biomech 15: 137–139.
18. Wasserman N, Yerramshetty J, Akkus O (2005) Microcracks colocalize within highly mineralized regions of cortical bone tissue. Eur J Morphol 42: 43–51.
19. Najafi AR, Arshi AR, Eslami MR, Fariborz S, Moeinzadeh MH (2007) Micromechanics fracture in osteonal cortical bone: a study of the interactions between microcrack propagation, microstructure and the material properties. J Biomech 40: 2788–2795.
20. Vashishth D, Behiri JC, Bonfield W (1997) Crack growth resistance in cortical bone: concept of microcrack toughening. J Biomech 30: 763–769.
21. Landis WJ (1995) The strength of a calcified tissue depends in part on the molecular structure and organization of its constituent mineral crystals in their organic matrix. Bone 16: 533–544.
22. Lee TC, Mohsin S, Taylor D, Parkesh R, Gunnlaugsson T, et al. (2003) Detecting microdamage in bone. J Anat 203: 161–172.
23. Augat P, Schorlemmer S (2006) The role of cortical bone and its microstructure in bone strength. Age Ageing 35 Suppl 2: ii27–ii31.
24. Burr DB (2002) Bone material properties and mineral matrix contributions to fracture risk or age in women and men. J Musculoskelet Neuronal Interact 2: 201–204.
25. Mongiorgi R, Romagnoli R, Olmi R, Moroni A (1983) Mineral alterations in senile osteoporosis. Biomaterials 4: 192–196.
26. Yerramshetty JS, Akkus O (2008) The associations between mineral crystallinity and the mechanical properties of human cortical bone. Bone 42: 476–482.
27. Fantner GE, Birkedal H, Kindt JH, Hassenkam T, Weaver JC, et al. (2004) Influence of the degradation of the organic matrix on the microscopic fracture behavior of trabecular bone. Bone 35: 1013–1022.
28. Fantner GE, Rabinovych O, Schitter G, Thurner P, Kindt JH, et al. (2006) Hierarchical interconnections in the nano-composite material bone: Fibrillar cross-links resist fracture on several length scales. Composites Science and Technology 66: 1205–1211.
29. Viguet-Carrin S, Roux JP, Arlot ME, Merabet Z, Leeming DJ, et al. (2006) Contribution of the advanced glycation end product pentosidine and of maturation of type I collagen to compressive biomechanical properties of human lumbar vertebrae. Bone 39: 1073–1079.
30. Tang SY, Zeenath U, Vashishth D (2007) Effects of non-enzymatic glycation on cancellous bone fragility. Bone 40: 1144–1151.
31. Wang X, Shen X, Li X, Agrawal CM (2002) Age-related changes in the collagen network and toughness of bone. Bone 31: 1–7.
32. Viguet-Carrin S, Follet H, Gineyts E, Roux JP, Munoz F, et al. (2010) Association between collagen cross-links and trabecular microarchitecture properties of human vertebral bone. Bone 46: 342–347.
33. Karim L, Vashishth D (2012) Heterogeneous glycation of cancellous bone and its association with bone quality and fragility. PLoS One 7: e35047.
34. Saito M, Mori S, Mashiba T, Komatsubara S, Marumo K (2008) Collagen maturity, glycation induced-pentosidine, and mineralization are increased following 3-year treatment with incadronate in dogs. Osteoporos Int 19: 1343–1354.
35. Arlot ME, Burt-Pichat B, Roux JP, Vashishth D, Bouxsein ML, et al. (2008) Microarchitecture influences microdamage accumulation in human vertebral trabecular bone. J Bone Miner Res 23: 1613–1618.
36. Burt-Pichat B, Follet H, Toulemonde G, Arlot M, Delmas P, et al. (2011) Methodological approach for the detection of both microdamage and fluorochrome labels in ewe bone and human trabecular bone. J Bone Miner Metab 29: 756–764.
37. Bala Y, Farlay D, Delmas PD, Meunier PJ, Boivin G (2010) Time sequence of secondary mineralization and microhardness in cortical and cancellous bone from ewes. Bone 46: 1204–1212.
38. Boivin G, Bala Y, Doublier A, Farlay D, Ste-Marie LG, et al. (2008) The role of mineralization and organic matrix in the microhardness of bone tissue from controls and osteoporotic patients. Bone 43: 532–538.
39. Boivin G, Meunier PJ (2002) The degree of mineralization of bone tissue measured by computerized quantitative contact microradiography. Calcif Tissue Int 70: 503–511.
40. Farlay D, Panczer G, Rey C, Delmas PD, Boivin G (2010) Mineral maturity and crystallinity index are distinct characteristics of bone mineral. J Bone Miner Metab 28: 433–445.
41. Paschalis EP, DiCarlo E, Betts F, Sherman P, Mendelsohn R, et al. (1996) FTIR microspectroscopic analysis of human osteonal bone. Calcified Tissue International 59: 480–487.
42. Paschalis EP, Verdelis K, Doty S, Boskey A, Mendelsohn R, et al. (2001) Spectroscopic characterization of collagen cross-links in bone. J Bone Miner Res 16: 1821–1828.
43. Farlay D, Duclos M-E, Gineyts E, Bertholon C, Viguet-Carrin S, et al. (2011) The ratio 1660/1690 cm-1 measured by Infrared Microspectroscopy is not specific of enzymatic collagen cross-links in bone tissue. PLoS ONE 6: e28736.
44. Viguet-Carrin S, Gineyts E, Bertholon C, Delmas PD (2009) Simple and sensitive method for quantification of fluorescent enzymatic mature and senescent crosslinks of collagen in bone hydrolysate using single-column high performance liquid chromatography. J Chromatogr B Analyt Technol Biomed Life Sci Jan 1: 1–7.
45. Kuliwaba JS, Tsangari H, Davies R, Fazzalari NL (2009) Bone microdamage accumulates in the central region of the human lumbar vertebra. Bone 44: S151–S151.
46. Yeni YN, Hou FJ, Ciarelli T, Vashishth D, Fyhrie DP (2003) Trabecular shear stresses predict in vivo linear microcrack density but not diffuse damage in human vertebral cancellous bone. Ann Biomed Eng 31: 726–732.
47. Soicher MA, Wang X, Zauel RR, Fyhrie DP (2011) Damage initiation sites in osteoporotic and normal human cancellous bone. Bone 48: 663–666.
48. Allen MR, Burr D (2007) Mineralization, Microdamage, and Matrix: How Bisphosphonates Influence Material Properties of Bone. BoneKEy-Osteovision 2007 February; 4(2): 49–60.
49. Tang SY, Vashishth D (2010) Non-enzymatic glycation alters microdamage formation in human cancellous bone. Bone 46: 148–154.
50. Peterlik H, Roschger P, Klaushofer K, Fratzl P (2006) From brittle to ductile fracture of bone. Nat Mater 5: 52–55.
51. Yeni YN, Kim DG, Dong XN, Turner AS, Les CM, et al. (2006) Do sacrificial bonds affect the viscoelastic and fracture properties of bone? Clin Orthop Relat Res 443: 101–108.
52. Wang X, Sudhaker Rao D, Ajdelsztajn L, Ciarelli TE, Lavernia EJ, et al. (2008) Human iliac crest cancellous bone elastic modulus and hardness differ with bone formation rate per bone surface but not by existence of prevalent vertebral fracture. J Biomed Mater Res B Appl Biomater 85: 68–77.

53. Wang X, Zauel RR, Fyhrie DP (2008) Postfailure modulus strongly affects microcracking and mechanical property change in human iliac cancellous bone: a study using a 2D nonlinear finite element method. J Biomech 41: 2654–2658.
54. Bala Y, Depalle B, Douillard T, Meille S, Clément P, et al. (2011) Respective roles of organic and mineral components of human cortical bone matrix in micromechanical behavior: an instrumented indentation study. J Mech Behav Biomed Mater 4: 1473–1482.
55. Bala Y, Depalle B, Farlay D, Douillard T, Meille S, et al. (2012) Bone micromechanical properties are compromised during long-term alendronate therapy independently of mineralization. J Bone Miner Res 27: 825–834.
56. Durchschlag E, Paschalis EP, Zoehrer R, Roschger P, Fratzl P, et al. (2006) Bone material properties in trabecular bone from human iliac crest biopsies after 3- and 5-year treatment with risedronate. J Bone Miner Res 21: 1581–1590.

22

Generic Rules of Mechano-Regulation Combined with Subject Specific Loading Conditions Can Explain Bone Adaptation after THA

Tomasz D. Szwedowski[¶]**, William R. Taylor***[¶]**, Markus O. Heller**[¶]**, Carsten Perka, Michael Müller, Georg N. Duda**

Julius Wolff Institute (JWI), Center for Musculoskeletal Surgery (CMSC), Center for Sports Science and Sports Medicine Berlin (CSSB), Charité – Universitätsmedizin Berlin, Berlin, Germany

Abstract

Bone adaptation after total hip arthroplasty is associated with the change in internal load environment, and can result in compromised bone stock, which presents a considerable challenge should a revision procedure be required. Under the assumption of a generic mechano-regulatory algorithm for governing bone adaptation, the aim of this study was to understand the contribution of subject specific loading conditions towards explaining the local periprosthetic remodelling variations in patients. CT scans of 3 consecutive THA patients were obtained and used for the construction of subject specific finite element models using verified musculoskeletal loading and physiological boundary conditions. Using either strain energy density or equivalent strain as mechano-transduction signals, predictions of bone adaptation were compared to DEXA derived BMD changes from 7 days to 12 months post-implantation. Individual changes in BMD of up to 33.6% were observed within the 12 month follow-up period, together with considerable inter-patient variability of up to 26%. Estimates of bone adaptation using equivalent strain and balanced loading conditions led to the best agreement with *in vivo* measured BMD, with RMS errors of only 3.9%, 7.3% and 7.3% for the individual subjects, compared to errors of over 10% when the loading conditions were simplified. This study provides evidence that subject specific loading conditions and physiological boundary constraints are essential for explaining inter-patient variations in bone adaptation patterns. This improved knowledge of the rules governing the adaptation of bone following THA helps towards understanding the interplay between mechanics and biology for better identifying patients at risk of excessive or problematic periprosthetic bone atrophy.

Editor: Ryan Keith Roeder, University of Notre Dame, United States of America

Funding: This work was financially supported by Zimmer Orthopaedics Inc. (Warsaw, Indiana, United States of America) and the Deutsche Forschungsgemeinschaft DFG SFB 760. The funders had no role in study design, data collection and analysis, decision to publish, or preparation of the manuscript.

Competing Interests: The authors have the following conflicts: The study was partially funded by Zimmer GmbH.

* E-mail: bill.taylor@charite.de

¶ These authors contributed equally to this work.

Introduction

Periprosthetic bone loss continues to be a burden after total hip arthroplasty (THA) and exhibits substantial inter-patient variability in clinical radiographic measures [1–5]. Periprosthetic bone mineral density (BMD) changes are associated with the internal load distribution, where the local bone is thought to adapt to the requirements of loading and function [5–8]. Abrupt changes to the internal loading environment, such as after the implantation of a joint endoprosthesis, lead to a short term adaptation of the bone, resulting in periprosthetic bone atrophy in regions that become unloaded. Such bone loss is believed to influence THA longevity by undermining implant fixation and contributing to the risk of aseptic loosening [9,10]. The resulting compromised bone stock presents a considerable challenge should a revision procedure be required [11–13].

Although the mechanisms dictating individual patterns of bone adaptation are thought to be mechanically driven, the rules governing these processes remains unclear. To establish these rules of tissue adaptation, a number of computational models have been developed that aim to predict the changes in periprosthetic bone [14–24]. Such predictions of bone adaptation generally rely on models of the interplay between mechanics and biology [25], in which an increase in local loading leads to net bone deposition, while decreased loading results in bone loss, in order to return to customary physiological load levels within the tissue. Previous investigations have predominantly used changes in strain energy density (SED) following THA [9,14,22,26,27] as a remodelling signal to induce bone mineral changes. The choice of strain energy density was reasoned as being an indirect measure that represents a simplified index for bone gain or bone loss [14,15]. However, an investigation comparing the adaptation driven by different mechanical remodelling signals did not show strain energy density to be superior against the outcome of animal experiments *in vivo* [17].

In addition to animal experiments, determination of the accuracy and validity of remodelling algorithms in clinical THA cohorts has relied upon comparisons against averaged longitudinal measurements [22,23]. Such generic comparisons have partially achieved good agreement with RMS errors of approximately 5% [23] against cohort averaged DEXA measurements. However, these comparisons could not account for excessive trochanteric resorption [22] and predictions of less net resorption than occurred *in vivo* was observed in Gruen zones 1 and 2 [23]. Whilst the rules of mechanically regulated bone remodelling in such models have therefore been able to describe the general patterns of periprosthetic adaptation, they fail to explain the mechano-biological aetiology of the individual variations. Such discrepancies are generally thought to be guided by biological adaptive capacity, where it has been widely considered that the genome, proteome and secretome drive the patient specific response. In this study, we want to analyse to what degree mechanical specificity alone can explain the patient specific variations observed. If such individual adaptation is indeed related to subject specific musculoskeletal loading conditions, then next to genetic pre-disposition and molecular biological pathways, the patient specific intrinsic physical constraints [28–30] have to be taken into account if biological adaptation processes are to be successfully characterised.

Currently, the mechanisms of tissue adaptation following e.g. an abrupt change to the loading conditions after THA, are not well understood. Under the assumption of a generic mechano-regulatory algorithm for governing bone adaptation, the aim of this study was to understand the contribution of subject specific loading conditions towards explaining the local periprosthetic remodelling variations in patients.

Methods

Subjects and DEXA acquisition

Finite element models for predictions of bone adaptation were constructed for 3 consecutive patients who underwent a primary elective total hip arthroplasty, receiving an uncemented Zimmer Alloclassic® stem and Allofit® Pressfit- cup (Zimmer®, Warsaw, IN, USA) from the identical surgical team. The study was approved by the local ethics committee, and after providing written informed consent to participate, each of the three patients (2 female, 1 male, aged 68.7±2.3) received a three joint CT scan (hip, knee, ankle) that included the entire femur, both pre- and post-operatively (GE Centricity, 0.5 mm pixel size, slice thickness of 1 and 5 mm respectively). In addition, radiographic (DEXA) measurements were performed on each patient at 7 days and 12 months after surgery, and changes in BMD were determined within each Gruen zone.

Finite element models

Pre-operative femoral bone geometry was reconstructed using automated statistical shape modelling techniques (ZIB Amira, Zuse Institute Berlin) [31] with manual correction if necessary. Post-operative femoral geometry, specifically including the location of the resection plane and implant position, was determined from the post-operative CT scan. The triangulated surface reconstructions (intact, post-operative and implant) were converted into NURBS surface representations and anatomic landmarks were determined using the methods of Heller and co-workers (2001) (Geomagic Studio 10, Geomagic Inc., Triangle Park, NC). Virtual implantation and resection of the intact femoral head was performed using Boolean operations on the parametric representations of the femur, implant and resection plane (NX 3.0, Siemens PLN, Köln, DE).

The post-operative femur and implant assembly, that inherently included the anatomy of the intact femur, was then meshed using parabolic tetrahedral finite elements (MSC Patran 2008, MSC Software Corp., Santa Ana, CA) using a global mesh seed of 3.5 mm with a local refinement in areas of high detail (Figure 1). The mesh contained all solids required to construct both the intact and implanted models from the single assembly, allowing mesh congruency in regions common to the intact and implanted femurs, thus facilitating direct mapping of mechanical signals between the models. All models accounted for non-linear geometric effects (Abaqus 6.7-1, Dassault Systèmes, France).

Material Properties

A calibration phantom (Model #13002 Mindways Software, Inc., CA, USA) was placed under the thigh during all pre-operative CT scans, which allowed transformation of the CT values (in Hounsfeld units) into an apparent bone density. These average local densities were geometrically mapped onto each finite element of the femur model. Elastic modulus was then determined for each element by scaling the apparent density according to an established empirical relationship: $E = 15.1\ \rho^{2.25}$ [32]. All materials were modelled as linear elastic isotropic assuming a Poisson's ratio of 0.3.

Individual Loading and Mechanical Boundary Conditions

Two sets of different musculoskeletal loading conditions were applied to each patient model and were classified as either simplified or complex. In the simplified loading scenario a reduced set of musculoskeletal loads (Figure 2). was applied to both the pre- and post-operative models according to published data from Heller and co-workers [33]. The musculoskeletal forces were

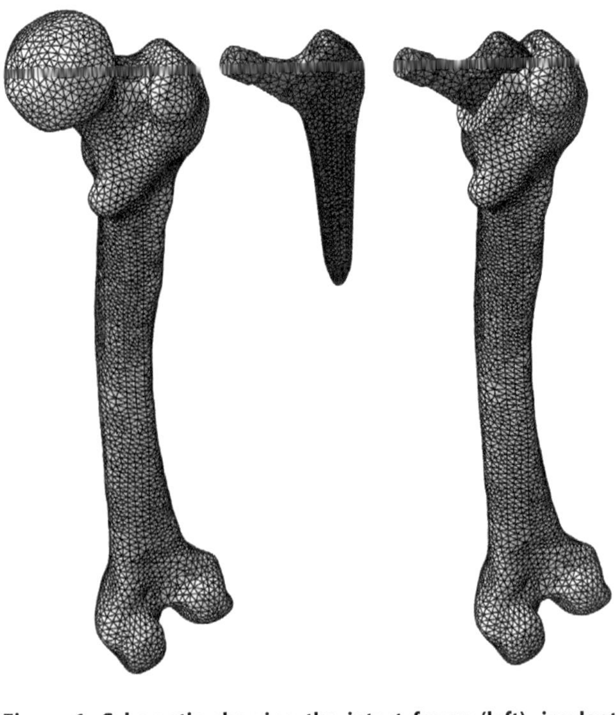

Figure 1. Schematic showing the intact femur (left), implant (centre) and implanted femur (right) meshes, consisting of approximately 80,000 second order tetrahedral elements.

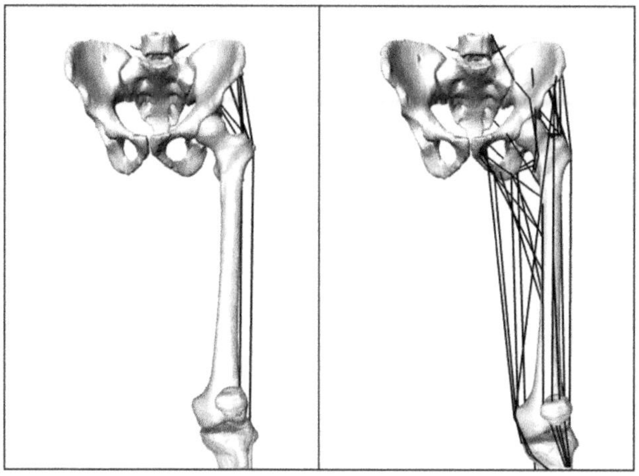

Figure 2. Simplified (left) and complex (right) musculoskeletal models used in the determination of subject specific muscle and joint loading. The simplified loading employs only the musculature that acts over the trochanteric region.

scaled to each patient's body weight and the femur was fully constrained at the mid-diaphysis.

For the complex loading scenario, the intact and implanted hip, knee and ankle centres, femoral neck axis and femoral shaft axis were determined and used to transform all reconstructions into a local femoral coordinate system. Musculoskeletal loading was determined for each patient for both the intact anatomy and the implanted femur configurations using a previously validated musculoskeletal model [34,35]. This analysis accounted for subject specific anatomy/implantation (femoral antetorsion, caput-collum-diaphyseal angle (CCD) angle, neck length, limb length, limb alignment), as well as muscle origins and insertions (Figure 2). The forces corresponding to maximum joint loading (20% gait cycle) for the intact and implanted anatomies were then applied to the respective models.

Bone Remodelling Algorithms

Bone remodelling was governed according to a tri-linear curve [9] that possessed a 'lazy zone' in which net bone apposition and deposition rates remained in equilibrium, while increased loads stimulated local bone deposition and unloading resulted in local bone resorption (Figure 3). In a first step, the equivalent strain $\varepsilon_{\mathrm{equivalent}} = \sqrt{\varepsilon_{ij}\varepsilon_{ij}}$ was employed as the mechanical remodelling signal for establishing the reference (intact pre-operative) loading conditions. This signal for the implanted model was then compared with the intact model and the course of remodelling simulated using an iterative adaptive bone remodelling algorithm. The lazy zone (S_1 & S_2) was specified as ± 100 με relative to the intact element-specific equivalent strain [16]. Remodelling proceeded in an iterative fashion, where a reduction in mechanical remodelling signal relative to the intact situation stimulated a decrease in element density and vice versa with a maximum change per iteration (saturation level) when the signal difference was 2000 με or more. Mechanical remodelling signal deviations of between 100 ($S_{sat,res}$) and 2000 με ($S_{sat,dep}$) from the reference signal resulted in a linear change in remodelling to a maximum rate or (saturation) of density change. A parametric study was performed to identify the remodelling rate (saturation) for which 25 iterations successfully reached remodelling equilibrium (all elements $< 15\%$ of max remodelling). To compare remodelling signals, a similar

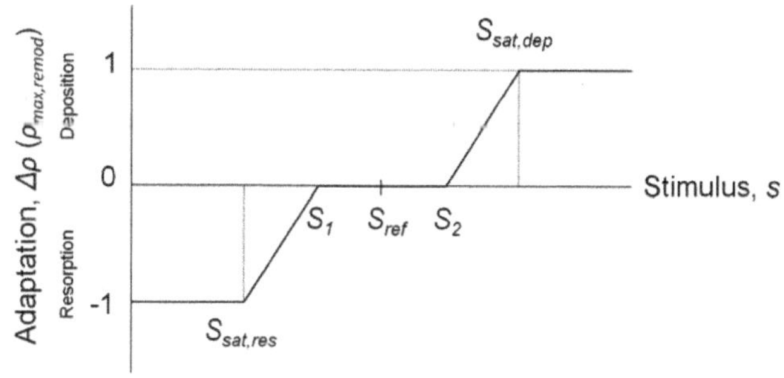

Figure 3. Mechanostat remodelling scheme. Change in the local density of bone for each time step, $\Delta\rho$, was governed by the local stimulus (s) according to the following rules:

$$\text{If } s \le S_{sat,dep} \quad \Delta\rho = -\rho_{\max,re\,\mathrm{mod}}$$

$$\text{If } S_1 \ge s > S_{sat,res} \quad \Delta\rho = \frac{-(S_1 - s)}{(S_1 - S_{sat,res})}$$

$$\text{If } S_1 \ge s \ge S_2 \quad \Delta\rho = 0$$

$$\text{If } S_{sat,dep} > s \ge S_2 \quad \Delta\rho = \frac{(s - S_2)}{(S_{sat,dep} - S_2)}$$

$$\text{If } s \ge S_{sat,dep} \quad \Delta\rho = \rho_{\max,re\,\mathrm{mod}}$$

where $S_{sat,dep}$ and $S_{sat,res}$ were the stimuli at which deposition and resorption saturation occurred respectively, and S_1 and S_2 defined the limits of the lazy zone. $\rho_{\max,re\,\mathrm{mod}}$ was the maximum rate of change of density for each of the remodelling steps.

iterative model was investigated using strain energy density (SED) to drive the adaptive changes.

Post-processing

For comparison against DEXA measurements, the bone mineral densities for each finite element were sampled onto a regular grid and projected to simulate a 2D DEXA image. The bone mineral content contained within each Gruen Zone was then computed and normalized against the projected area (area BMD) that included only bone and excluded regions coincident with the implant. The ability of the various models to predict the clinical changes in BMD due to adaptation from the post-op to the 1 year follow-up time point was determined by evaluating the RMS error between the predicted and measured BMD changes for each Gruen zone.

Results

Over the course of the investigation, none of the patients experienced postoperative complications. The 3 patients exhibited periprosthetic bone atrophy of -8.1, -18.4 and -16.9% 12 months postoperatively, as measured using DEXA and averaged over 7 Gruen zones. All three patients exhibited atrophy in the most proximal regions (Gruen zones 1 and 7), ranging from -9.2 to -17.2% and -15.9 to -33.6% respectively (Figure 4).

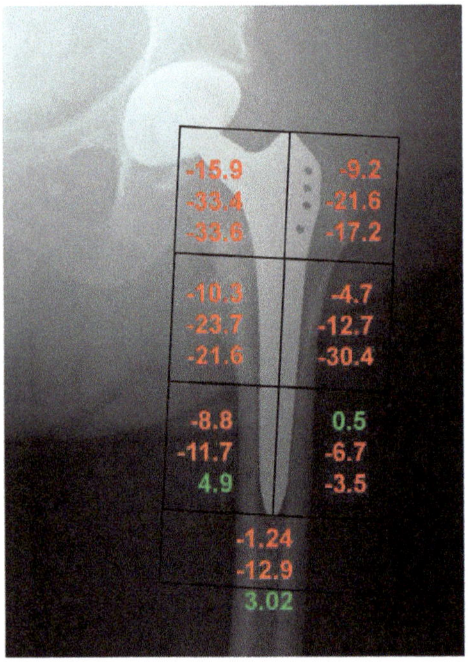

Figure 4. Summary of clinically measured changes in BMD from 7 days to 12 months after surgery. Values are presented for each patient as the percentage change relative to the 7 days postoperative BMD.

The corresponding FE models demonstrated average BMD changes (from 7 days to 12 months after implantation) of −7.5, −18.1 and −15.5% relative to the immediate postoperative BMD for the 3 patients respectively. Individual Gruen zone specific changes measured using DEXA were then compared to the subject specific FEA predictions, and exhibited considerable variation across patients and also as a consequence of loading conditions and mechano-regulation were observed (Figure 5).

For all three subjects, FEA predictions of the bone adaptation within each Gruen Zone demonstrated that mechano-regulation based on equivalent strain and that incorporated the complex musculoskeletal loading conditions (including physiological boundary constraints) resulted in the best agreement with the clinical DEXA measurements (Figure 5). The mean RMS error for the 3 patients was 6.2% while the patient specific RMS errors were 3.9%, 7.3% and 7.3% (Table 1). Adaptation based on equivalent strain with simplified loading conditions, rather than loading conditions that included the full anatomical complexity, reduced the levels of agreement with DEXA measurements to 10.7% overall. The overall best and worst case predictions on a patient and Gruen zone level were: equivalent strain and complex loading (best: 0.4%, worst: 16.0%), equivalent strain with simplified loading (0.4%, 28.1%), SED with complex loading (0.9%, 42.3%), and SED with simplified loading (0.3%, 84.4%) (Figure 5).

SED based predictions with complex loading had an average RMS error of 20%, which increased to 23.4% under simplified loading conditions. Individually (Table 1): subject 1 exhibited little change in agreement (complex loading; 12.3%, simplified loading; 12.6%), subject 2 showed an overall improvement of 21.1%, while subject 3 exhibited a reduction in agreement with complex loading (−11.6%).

In general, the three patient models exhibited unloading in the lower trochanteric region (Gruen zones 1 and 2), and a localized increase in loading directly adjacent to the implant in the proximal lateral region (Gruen zone 1). These patterns correspond to atrophy and bone densification respectively in the trabecular region (Figure 6). Additionally, patterns of unloading of the calcar region (Gruen zone 7) and an increase in loading at the tip of the implant (Gruen zone 4) corresponded to regions of atrophy and densification respectively. Regions of net bone atrophy and deposition exhibited similarities between the two signal types in the complex loading environment, but the application of simplified loading conditions led to more locally varied adaptation patterns.

Discussion

Bone loss following THA is well documented and frequently associated with changes in the mechanical environment. A detailed understanding of the rules that governing bone adaptation as well as the influence of subject specific factors is, however, lacking. In this study, we assumed that generic mechano-regulatory rules govern bone adaptation and then evaluated the contribution of subject specific anatomy and loading conditions towards explaining the local periprosthetic remodelling variations in 3 patients. The results of this study suggest that while generic rules of mechano-regulation can indeed estimate the broad patterns of periprosthetic bone adaptation observed *in vivo*, knowledge of the subject specific anatomy and loading conditions is indeed required before local variations in bone mineral changes can be discriminated.

This study has demonstrated that considerations regarding balanced musculoskeletal loading conditions [36] that enforce physiological deformation patterns [29,36] play a critical role for accurate predictions of periprosthetic bone adaptation. It is known that subtle changes to a subject's anatomy can play a critical role the internal loading conditions [37]. It therefore becomes apparent that simplified loading assumptions that have been predominantly employed in periprosthetic femoral remodelling studies, may not capture the complex balanced, subject specific loading conditions [36], and therefore enforce non-physiological deformation constraints [29]. Simplified loading conditions therefore seem limited in their ability to contribute towards understanding the underlying mechanisms that control the subject specific maintenance of bone stock [21].

In our study, 3 patients were observed over 12 months, resulting in average *in vivo* Gruen zone BMD changes of approximately −14.5%, with an RMS error of 6.2%. These results demonstrated that by considering detailed, subject specific loading conditions, the highly variable *in vivo* BMD outcomes of our three patients were all well predicted using our techniques (Figure 4). Importantly, the patient group displayed variations in periprosthetic bone adaptation patterns with average BMD changes ranging between −8.1 and −18.0%, with considerable inter-patient variation between the Gruen zones, and these variations could be explained in the models. Here, the equivalent strain based predictions and complex musculoskeletal loading conditions derived from subject specific analyses were accurate to within the magnitude of error observed in longitudinal DEXA measurements [38]. Although the study by Turner and co-workers [23] has suggested good agreement (5% RMS error) between longitudinal BMD changes and remodelling predictions based on equivalent strain, these predictions were assessed against cohort averaged values of bone remodelling, where local variations between and within individuals become obscured.

This study was able to compare the outcome of equivalent strain or SED mechano-regulation, and specifically how abrupt changes in the stimulus that result from implantation dictate predictions of

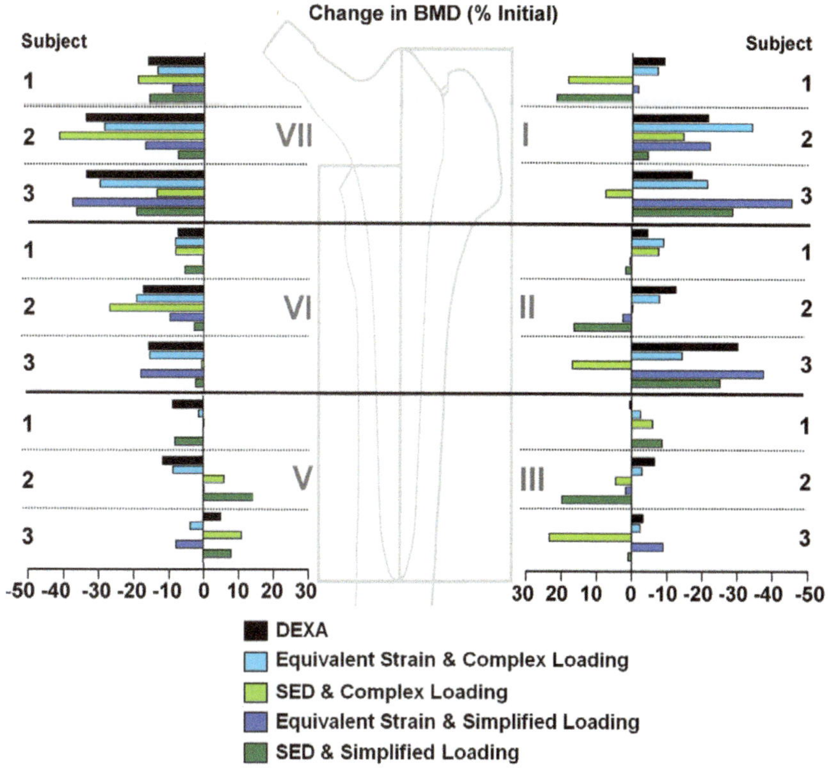

Figure 5. Comparison of change in BMD (% from initial) measured using DEXA against the adaptation signal based predictions of BMD. Also shown is the effect of simplified versus complex musculoskeletal loads depicted as the total change in the BMD of individual Gruen Zones.

periprosthetic bone remodelling (Figure 6). The changes in the signals (Figure 5) indicated that an unloading occurred most prominently in: 1. the calcar region (Gruen zone 7) and 2. the proximal lateral regions (Gruen zones 1 and 2), with localized increases adjacent to the implant. These changes were associated with decreases in BMD in the same general locations, reflecting clinical observations [3,38] with the notable exception in some cases that densification adjacent to the implant occurred in Gruen zone 1. Since these local phenomena appear to be due to boundary effects at the bone-implant interface, more detailed models that incorporate such interactions may be required before a more complete understanding of the local load transfer mechanisms across this interface can be reliably achieved.

The results of this study have demonstrated a better agreement between longitudinal clinical radiographic measurements and computational bone remodelling predictions based on equivalent strain than those based on SED [9,14,26,39] as the mechano-regulatory signal. This result is supported by previous work predicting experimentally observed adaptation patterns in a turkey ulna model [16] that did not find SED to be superior to other mechanical signals. Although these studies have contributed towards instilling confidence in the 'mechanostat' model of bone adaptation [40,41], individual specific patterns and their dependence on musculoskeletal forces, including implantation, have never been demonstrated. Equivalent strain as an alternative to SED was first used by Taylor an co-workers [17] and Turner and co-workers [23] based on work by Stülpner and co-workers [42] and derived from Mikic and Carter [43]. The rationale was that although bone adaptation stimuli could be based on stress or strain, strain was a parameter most likely detectable by bone. Furthermore, in the study of Kerner and co-workers [22], the SED mechanical signal was suggested to be responsible for resorption of the lesser trochanteric region, a result deemed clinically unrealistic. The results presented in this current study indicate that SED consistently invokes a proportionally larger change after implantation and exhibits larger local signal gradients than equivalent strain (Figure 6). This is likely related to the fact that SED is proportional to the square of the strain and therefore more sensitive to the changes in pre- to post-op signal.

For the first time this work considered the effect of physiological boundary conditions that enforce realistic femoral deformation

Table 1. The root mean square (RMS) error (%) values for subject specific comparisons between the 12 month *in vivo* DEXA measurement and model variations that include equivalent strain and strain energy density based remodelling and their combinations with simplified and complete balanced musculoskeletal loading conditions.

RMS error (%)	Subject			
	1	2	3	Mean
Equivalent Strain & Simplified Loading	6.6	13.1	12.4	10.7
Equivalent Strain & Complex Loading	3.9	7.3	7.3	6.2
SED & Simplified Loading	12.6	39.8	17.8	23.4
SED & Complex Loading	12.3	18.7	29.4	20.2

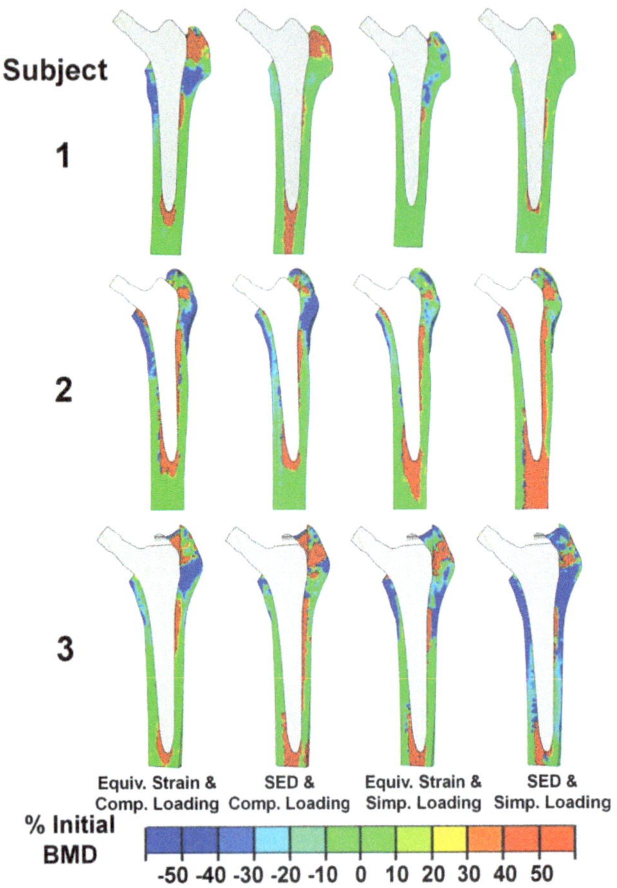

Figure 6. Percentage change in BMD distribution due to adaptation predicted using equivalent strain and strain energy density signals, as well as due to loading conditions, from the implanted to 12 months post-op situation.

patterns [29] and therefore internal loading conditions on predictions of bone adaptation. Additionally, in this study, the muscle and joint contact forces were taken from a musculoskeletal model [33,35] that had previously been validated against forces measured *in vivo* using instrumented telemetric hip implants [44]. Musculoskeletal loading in this study was adapted to the patients' geometry, where the musculoskeletal force predictions took into account the hip joint anatomy both before and after implantation. Patient specific gait patterns, however, were not included in this study, where kinematics were assumed to be the same both before and after implantation. The role of including subject specific gait patterns and external ground reaction forces might alter the characteristics of load estimations. Although not available in this study, one elegant approach for differentiating the impact of periprosthetic stress-shielding from global changes in limb loading, could be to normalise the proximal BMD to a reference BMD taken at a location well distal to the stem tip (sufficiently below Gruen Zone IV) pre- and post-operatively [45].

This investigation was able to achieve good agreement with DEXA BMD measurements despite certain limitations. DEXA can only produce a two dimensional projection that inherently reduces the amount of information available regarding the distribution of BMD. The third dimension is partially preserved in the operation of planar summation, but the spatial distribution is partially obscured. DEXA measurements also obscure information in regions that are coincident with the implant, and simplification into individual Gruen zone values further reduces the local specificity. However, in this study, DEXA allowed a quantitative and reproducible comparison for determining the adaptation of bone at multiple locations for longitudinal assessment of BMD in these subjects.

In summary, this study has demonstrated in three THA patients that under the assumption of generic bone adaptation rules, the variability in bone remodelling patterns between individuals can only be predicted when subject specific anatomy and loading conditions are taken into consideration. Additionally, this study has shown that mechano-regulation driven by an equivalent strain signal can produce good estimations of bone tissue adaptation. Here, the high level of agreement against clinical measurements using these techniques establishes a foundation for examining the variation in individual BMD adaptation patterns. This improved knowledge of the rules governing the adaptation of bone following the abrupt mechanical changes that occur due to the implantation of a prosthesis helps towards understanding the interplay between mechanics and biology for better identification of patients at risk of excessive or problematic periprosthetic bone atrophy.

Acknowledgments

The authors would like to thank Andrew Speirs and Adam Henderson for their contribution to the modelling techniques, as well as Annette Bowitz and Anne Zergiebel for the clinical administrative support.

Author Contributions

Conceived and designed the experiments: MH WT GD CP MM. Performed the experiments: MM TS. Analyzed the data: TS WT MH. Contributed reagents/materials/analysis tools: TS WT MH. Wrote the paper: GD WT MH TS CP.

References

1. Engh CA, McGovern TF, Schmidt LM (1993) Roentgenographic densitometry of bone adjacent to a femoral prosthesis. Clin Orthop Relat Res. pp 177–190.
2. Smart RC, Barbagallo S, Slater GL, Kuo RS, Butler SP, et al. (1996) Measurement of periprosthetic bone density in hip arthroplasty using dual-energy x-ray absorptiometry. Reproducibility of measurements. J Arthroplasty 11: 445–452.
3. Kiratli BJ, Heiner JP, McBeath AA, Wilson MA (1992) Determination of bone mineral density by dual x-ray absorptiometry in patients with uncemented total hip arthroplasty. J Orthop Res 10: 836–844.
4. Kiratli BJ, Checovich MM, McBeath AA, Wilson MA, Heiner JP (1996) Measurement of bone mineral density by dual-energy x-ray absorptiometry in patients with the Wisconsin hip, an uncemented femoral stem. J Arthroplasty 11: 184–193.
5. Perka C, Heller M, Wilke K, Taylor WR, Haas NP, et al. (2005) Surgical approach influences periprosthetic femoral bone density. Clin Orthop Relat Res 432: 153–159.
6. Rubin CT, Lanyon LE (1987) Kappa Delta Award paper. Osteoregulatory nature of mechanical stimuli: function as a determinant for adaptive remodeling in bone. J Orthop Res 5: 300–310.
7. Wolff J (2010) The classic: on the theory of fracture healing. 1873. Clin Orthop Relat Res 468: 1052–1055.
8. Wolff J (2010) The classic: on the inner architecture of bones and its importance for bone growth. 1870. Clin Orthop Relat Res 468: 1056–1065.
9. Huiskes R (1993) Stress shielding and bone resorption in THA: clinical versus computer-simulation studies. Acta Orthop Belg 59 Suppl 1: 118–129.
10. Sumner DR, Galante JO (1992) Determinants of stress shielding: design versus materials versus interface. Clin Orthop Relat Res. pp 202–212.
11. Dunbar MJ, Blackley HR, Bourne RB (2001) Osteolysis of the femur: principles of management. Instr Course Lect 50: 197–209.
12. Rosenbaum TG, Bloebaum RD, Ashrafi S, Lester DK (2006) Ambulatory activities maintain cortical bone after total hip arthroplasty. Clin Orthop Relat Res 450: 129–137.

13. Wilkinson JM, Hamer AJ, Rogers A, Stockley I, Eastell R (2003) Bone mineral density and biochemical markers of bone turnover in aseptic loosening after total hip arthroplasty. J Orthop Res 21: 691–696.
14. Huiskes R (1987) Finite element analysis of acetabular reconstruction. Noncemented threaded cups. Acta Orthop Scand 58: 620–625.
15. Schmitz MJ, Clift SE, Taylor WR, Hertig D, Warner MD, et al. (2004) Investigating the effect of remodelling signal type on the finite element based predictions of bone remodelling around the thrust plate prosthesis: a patient-specific comparison. Proc Inst Mech Eng H 218: 417–424.
16. Taylor WR, Ploeg H, Hertig D, Warner MD, Clift SE (2004) Bone remodelling of a proximal femur with the thrust plate prosthesis: an in vitro case. Comput Methods Biomech Biomed Engin 7: 131–137.
17. Taylor WR, Warner MD, Clift SE (2003) Finite element prediction of endosteal and periosteal bone remodelling in the turkey ulna: effect of remodelling signal and dead-zone definition. Proc Inst Mech Eng H 217: 349–356.
18. Weinans H, Huiskes R, van Rietbergen B, Sumner DR, Turner TM, et al. (1993) Adaptive bone remodeling around bonded noncemented total hip arthroplasty: a comparison between animal experiments and computer simulation. J Orthop Res 11: 500–513.
19. Van Rietbergen B, Huiskes R, Weinans H, Sumner DR, Turner TM, et al. (1993) ESB Research Award 1992. The mechanism of bone remodeling and resorption around press-fitted THA stems. J Biomech 26: 369–382.
20. Huiskes R, van Rietbergen B (1995) Preclinical testing of total hip stems. The effects of coating placement. Clin Orthop Relat Res. pp 64–76.
21. Bitsakos C, Kerner J, Fisher I, Amis AA (2005) The effect of muscle loading on the simulation of bone remodelling in the proximal femur. J Biomech 38: 133–139.
22. Kerner J, Huiskes R, van Lenthe GH, Weinans H, van Rietbergen B, et al. (1999) Correlation between pre-operative periprosthetic bone density and post-operative bone loss in THA can be explained by strain-adaptive remodelling. J Biomech 32: 695–703.
23. Turner AW, Gillies RM, Sekel R, Morris P, Bruce W, et al. (2005) Computational bone remodelling simulations and comparisons with DEXA results. J Orthop Res 23: 705–712.
24. Scannell PT, Prendergast PJ (2009) Cortical and interfacial bone changes around a non-cemented hip implant: simulations using a combined strain/damage remodelling algorithm. Med Eng Phys 31: 477–488.
25. Epari DR, Taylor WR, Heller MO, Duda GN (2006) Mechanical conditions in the initial phase of bone healing. Clin Biomech (Bristol, Avon) 21: 646–655.
26. Huiskes R, Weinans H, Dalstra M (1989) Adaptive bone remodeling and biomechanical design considerations for noncemented total hip arthroplasty. Orthopedics 12: 1255–1267.
27. Huiskes R, Weinans H, Grootenboer HJ, Dalstra M, Fudala B, et al. (1987) Adaptive bone-remodeling theory applied to prosthetic-design analysis. J Biomech 20: 1135–1150.
28. Kleemann RU, Heller MO, Stoeckle U, Taylor WR, Duda GN (2003) THA loading arising from increased femoral anteversion and offset may lead to critical cement stresses. J Orthop Res 21: 767–774.
29. Speirs AD, Heller MO, Duda GN, Taylor WR (2007) Physiologically based boundary conditions in finite element modelling. J Biomech 40: 2318–2323.
30. Speirs AD, Heller MO, Taylor WR, Duda GN, Perka C (2007) Influence of changes in stem positioning on femoral loading after THR using a short-stemmed hip implant. Clin Biomech (Bristol, Avon) 22: 431–439.
31. Kainmueller D, Lamecker H, Zachow S, Hege HC (2009) An articulated statistical shape model for accurate hip joint segmentation. Conf Proc IEEE Eng Med Biol Soc 2009: 6345–6351.
32. Les CM, Keyak JH, Stover SM, Taylor KT, Kaneps AJ (1994) Estimation of material properties in the equine metacarpus with use of quantitative computed tomography. J Orthop Res 12: 822–833.
33. Heller MO, Bergmann G, Kassi JP, Claes L, Haas NP, et al. (2005) Determination of muscle loading at the hip joint for use in pre-clinical testing. J Biomech 38: 1155–1163.
34. Heller MO, Bergmann G, Deuretzbacher G, Durselen L, Pohl M, et al. (2001) Musculo-skeletal loading conditions at the hip during walking and stair climbing. J Biomech 34: 883–893.
35. Taylor WR, Heller MO, Bergmann G, Duda GN (2004) Tibio-femoral loading during human gait and stair climbing. J Orthop Res 22: 625–632.
36. Duda GN, Heller M, Albinger J, Schulz O, Schneider E, et al. (1998) Influence of muscle forces on femoral strain distribution. J Biomech 31: 841–846.
37. Heller MO, Taylor WR, Perka C, Duda GN (2003) The influence of alignment on the musculo-skeletal loading conditions at the knee. Langenbecks Arch Surg 388: 291–297.
38. Kilgus DJ, Shimaoka EE, Tipton JS, Eberle RW (1993) Dual-energy X-ray absorptiometry measurement of bone mineral density around porous-coated cementless femoral implants. Methods and preliminary results. J Bone Joint Surg Br 75: 279–287.
39. Huiskes R, Weinans H, van Rietbergen B (1992) The relationship between stress shielding and bone resorption around total hip stems and the effects of flexible materials. Clin Orthop Relat Res. pp 124–134.
40. Frost HM (1987) Bone "mass" and the "mechanostat": a proposal. Anat Rec 219: 1–9.
41. Frost HM (2003) Bone's mechanostat: a 2003 update. Anat Rec A Discov Mol Cell Evol Biol 275: 1081–1101.
42. Stulpner MA, Reddy BD, Starke GR, Spirakis A (1997) A three-dimensional finite analysis of adaptive remodelling in the proximal femur. J Biomech 30: 1063–1066.
43. Mikic B, Carter DR (1995) Bone strain gage data and theoretical models of functional adaptation. J Biomech 28: 465–469.
44. Bergmann G, Deuretzbacher G, Heller M, Graichen F, Rohlmann A, et al. (2001) Hip contact forces and gait patterns from routine activities. J Biomech 34: 859–871.
45. Bryan JM, Sumner DR, Hurwitz DE, Tompkins GS, Andriacchi TP, et al. (1996) Altered load history affects periprosthetic bone loss following cementless total hip arthroplasty. J Orthop Res 14: 762–768.

Impaired Angiogenesis during Fracture Healing in GPCR Kinase 2 Interacting Protein-1 (GIT1) Knock Out Mice

Guoyong Yin[1,3], Tzong-Jen Sheu[2], Prashanthi Menon[1], Jinjiang Pang[1], Hsin-Chiu Ho[2], Shanshan Shi[2], Chao Xie[2], Elaine Smolock[1], Chen Yan[1], Michael J. Zuscik[2], Bradford C. Berk[1]*

1 Aab Cardiovascular Research Institute and the Department of Medicine, University of Rochester Medical Center, Rochester, New York, United States of America, **2** Center for Musculoskeletal Research and the Department of Orthopaedics and Rehabilitation, University of Rochester Medical Center, Rochester, New York, United States of America, **3** Orthopaedic Department, The First Affiliated Hospital of Nanjing Medical University, Jiangsu, China

Abstract

G protein coupled receptor kinase 2 (GRK2) interacting protein-1 (GIT1), is a scaffold protein that plays an important role in angiogenesis and osteoclast activity. We have previously demonstrated that GIT1 knockout (GIT1 KO) mice have impaired angiogenesis and dysregulated osteoclast podosome formation leading to a reduction in the bone resorbing ability of these cells. Since both angiogenesis and osteoclast-mediated bone remodeling are involved in the fracture healing process, we hypothesized that GIT1 participates in the normal progression of repair following bone injury. In the present study, comparison of fracture healing in wild type (WT) and GIT1 KO mice revealed altered healing in mice with loss of GIT1 function. Alcian blue staining of fracture callus indicated a persistence of cartilagenous matrix in day 21 callus samples from GIT1 KO mice which was temporally correlated with increased type 2 collagen immunostaining. GIT1 KO mice also showed a decrease in chondrocyte proliferation and apoptosis at days 7 and 14, as determined by PCNA and TUNEL staining. Vascular microcomputed tomography analysis of callus samples at days 7, 14 and 21 revealed decreased blood vessel volume, number, and connection density in GIT1 KO mice compared to WT controls. Correlating with this, VEGF-A, phospho-VEGFR2 and PECAM1 (CD31) were decreased in GIT1 KO mice, indicating reduced angiogenesis with loss of GIT1. Finally, calluses from GIT1 KO mice displayed a reduced number of tartrate resistant acid phosphatase-positive osteoclasts at days 14 and 21. Collectively, these results indicate that GIT1 is an important signaling participant in fracture healing, with gene ablation leading to reduced callus vascularity and reduced osteoclast number in the healing callus.

Editor: Luc Malaval, INSERM U1059/LBTO, Université Jean Monnet, France

Funding: This work was supported by NIH/NHLBI R01 HL063462 (to BCB), National Natural Science Foundation of China Grant #81271988 (to GY), NIH/NIAMS P50 AR054041-5471 (to MJZ) and NIH/NIAMS P30 AR061307. The funders had no role in study design, data collection and analysis, decision to publish, or preparation of the manuscript.

Competing Interests: The authors have declared that no competing interests exist.

* E-mail: brad_berk@urmc.rochester.edu

These authors contributed equally to this work.

Introduction

Fracture healing is a complex process involving an early inflammatory phase, recruitment, expansion and differentiation of mesenchymal cells, and production of cartilage and bone matrix in a temporally regulated manner [1–3]. After fracture, the repair process begins with hematoma formation and an inflammatory response [2]. In this early inflammatory phase, lack of blood vessels causes a regional hypoxic environment leading to the formation of a cartilagenous template that initiates a process of differentiation that recapitulates endochondral ossification [4]. Included are the proliferation and differentiation of mesenchymal progenitor cells into chondrocytes [1,5] which facilitate deposition of extracellular matrix components at the fracture site resulting in the formation of the transient soft callus [4]. In an initial remodeling phase, the avascular cartilagenous callus is converted into a vascularized and mineralized tissue that is remodeled by osteoclasts during an initial cartilage resorption phase [6], and then later in a bone remodeling phase that sculpts the healed skeletal element into the anatomically appropriate shape [7–9]. The importance of vascular invasion during endochondral bone formation has been established, with defects in bone vasculature having been reported in osteoporosis and rickets [10]. Thus, not surprisingly, during skeletal repair, neoangiogenesis driven by vascular endothelial growth factor (VEGF) is required to support nutrient and oxygen transport, with tissue oxygenation being required for osteogenic differentiation [11–16]. Further suggesting the need for this angiogenic cascade of events in the repair process, pharmacologic inhibition of angiogenesis has been shown to impair fracture healing by reducing/delaying callus mineralization [17].

G protein coupled receptor kinase 2 (GRK2) interacting protein 1 (GIT1) was originally identified by its binding to GRK2 and its effects on adrenergic receptor endocytosis [18]. GIT1 has five functional domains, including a zinc finger domain responsible for ARF-GAP activity, three ankyrin repeats, a Spa2 homology domain (SHD), a synaptic localization domain (SLD), and a conserved carboxyl-terminal region that interacts with paxillin (PBS) [19]. Through these domains, GIT1 interacts with diverse proteins including ARF6, MEK, phospholipase C-γ (PLCγ), p21-activated kinase (PAK)-interacting exchange factor (PIX) and paxillin [20,21]. GIT1 has diverse biological functions, which we have shown to include a critical role in pulmonary vascular development by regulating VEGF induced PLCγ and ERK1/2 activation [22]. GIT1 is also upregulated in atherosclerotic plaques and regulates endothelial cell and vascular smooth muscle cell migration [23]. Recently, we identified an important role of GIT1 in bone physiology based on its regulation of osteoclast sealing zone formation, a critical step required for the function of this cell [24]. Based on the observations that GIT1 plays an important role in angiogenesis and osteoclast function, both of which are critical for bone repair, we hypothesized that GIT1 is an important molecular player in the bone healing process.

In the present study, we established that loss of GIT1 alters the fracture healing process. Homozygous GIT1 knockout (GIT1 KO) mice display a persistence of cartilagenous callus evidenced by preservation of Alcian Blue staining and type 2 collagen content. Chondrocyte differentiation was impacted by loss of GIT1, with PCNA and TUNEL staining revealing decreased proliferation and apoptosis of chondrocytes. We used microcomputed tomography (microCT) to investigate overall callus volume and vascular parameters and discovered that GIT1 KO mice have reduced vessel volume and vessel number, which correlated with decreased expression of VEGF-A and VEGFR2. We also examined osteoclst numbers in the callus, and document a reduced number of TRAP-stained cells during the remodeling phases of healing in mice with loss of GIT1 function. Overall, findings documented in this report establish that GIT1 is important for the normal progression of the bone healing program via effects on callus vascularization and osteoclast number, improtant determinants for callus mineralization and remodeling respectively.

Materials and Methods

Ethics Statement

To ensure the humane treatment of mice in this study, all experiments involving mice were performed with the approval and supervision of the University Committee on Animal Resources, the AALAC-, OLAW- and USDA-approved IACUC at the University of Rochester Medical Center.

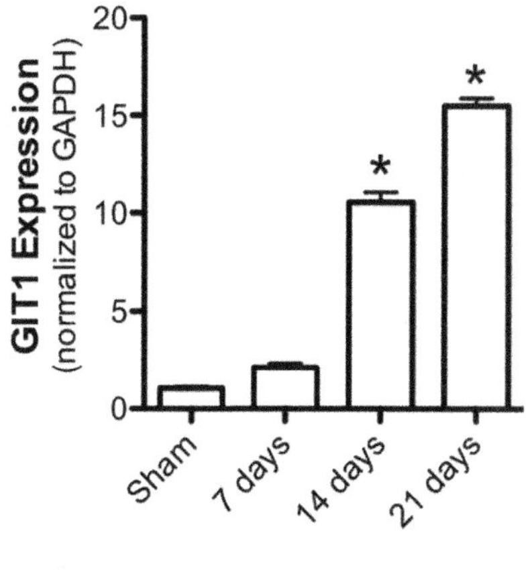

Figure 1. GIT1 mRNA is expressed during fracture healing. WT mice were administered femur fractures and fractured femora were harvested for isolation of mRNA from the callus at 7, 14, and 21 days post-injury. qPCR was performed to examine the profile of GIT1 expression. Bars represent mean GIT1 expression level relative to GAPDH +/− SEM (N = 4, *p<0.05).

Animals

Homozygous GIT1 knockout (GIT1 KO) mice were generated on the C57/BL6 background as described in Pang et al [22]. Chimeric mice generated were backcrossed for more than 7 generations. GIT1 KO mice at age of 10–12 weeks were used for femoral fracture with WT littermates used as controls. It is important to note that because of the high rate of perinatal lethality in GIT1 KO mice due to a pulmonary defect [22] and because of sensitivity to anesthesia, we were limited to an experimental strategy that included only 3 KO mice at each of 3 harvest time points post-fracture: 7, 14 and 21 days.

Mouse Femur Fracture Model

Femur fractures in mice were performed as described in Xie et al [25]. Briefly, mice were anesthetized using a mixture of ketamine and xylazine delivered via intraperitoneal injection. The skin and the underlying tissues over the left knee were incised. A 25-gauge needle was inserted through the patellar tendon and into the medullary canal of the femur. A mid-diaphyseal fracture was created via three-point bending using an Einhorn device [1]. After fracture, 0.5 mg/kg buprenorphine (Abbott labs, North Chicago, Illinois) was administered subcutaneously to each mouse daily for 3 days to control pain. Radiographs were obtained on 7, 14, and 21 days under anesthesia using a Faxitron X-ray system (Faxitron X-ray, Wheeling, Illinois).

Quantitative Real Time PCR (qPCR)

Fracture calluses from WT mice (n = 4) per time point (7, 14, 21 days) were carefully excised from the lower limb. The soft tissue surrounding the calluses was removed and the samples were flash-frozen in liquid N_2. Frozen samples were placed in a Tissuelyser (Qiagen, Venlo, Netherlands) along with 1 mL of TRIzol (Invitrogen, Carlesbad, CA). Homogenization was performed using a frequency of 30 Hz for a time of 3 minutes. The samples were checked for adequate disruption and the mRNA was purified according to the TRIzol System protocol. The concentration of stock mRNA was determined in triplicate using a Nanodrop photospectrometer. The mRNA was diluted in RNase-free water and aliquoted into working dilutions of 0.5 µg/µL. A cDNA library was synthesized using 0.5 µg of callus mRNA by a commercially available reverse transcription kit (Invitrogen, Carlesbad, CA). qPCR analyses were performed using murine-specific primers for *GIT1* and *GAPDH*. The qPCR reactions were performed using SyberGreen (ABgene, Rochester, NY) in a RotorGene real time PCR machine (Corbett Research, Carlsbad, CA). GIT1 expression was normalized using GAPDH expression as an internal control.

Microcomputed Tomography Imaging

Microcomputed tomography imaging (microCT) was performed to assess mineralized callus volume and vascularity as we have previously described [25–28]. Vascular networks at the cortical bone junction and around the fractures were examined using microCT analysis combined with perfusion of a lead chromate based contrast agent [29]. Briefly, Microfil MV-122 (Flow Tech, Inc., Carver, Massachusetts) contrast media, a radiopaque silicone rubber compound containing lead chromate, was perfused via the heart along with 4% paraformaldehyde following an initial vascular flush with heparinized saline. After perfusion, the fractured femur was removed and scanned using a microCT imaging system (VivaCT 40; Scanco Medical AG, Basserdorf, Switzerland) at resolution of 10.5 µm to image bone and vasculature. The samples were subsequently decalcified for 21 days using a 10% EDTA solution. After complete decalcification, the samples were scanned again to image only vascularization within the callus. By registering the 2-D slices before and after decalcification, contour lines were drawn to define a VOI that only included the vasculature in or immediately adjacent to the fracture callus itself. The reconstructed scan images were globally thresholded based on intensity values to render 3-D images of the vasculature in new bone callus, excluding the vessels in the surrounding tissues. Three-dimensional morphometric analysis, based on direct distance transform methods, was subsequently performed on the 3-D images using algorithms that are commonly used to model trabecular bone morphology. This facilitated quantification and analysis of vascular network morphology including vessel volume, number, spacing, and connection density. It should be noted that all measurements of the vascular network were constrained by the limit of resolution of the scanner (10 μm) and the permeability of the networks to the viscous Microfil. Careful heparinization and consistent application of perfusion conditions were established to ensure comparability between mice.

Histology and Histomorphometry

Fractured femora harvested for microCT analysis were processed for histology as previously described [30]. Briefly, femora were disarticulated at the knee and hip, denuded of soft tissue, and fixed at RT in 10% NBF for 72 hours. After three washes in phosphate buffered saline (PBS), fixed femora were decalcified in 10% EDTA for 7 to 14 days. Tissues were then processed using a Tissue-Tek VIP 6 tissue processor (Sakura Finetek USA, Inc., Torrance, CA, USA) and embedded in paraffin. Serial 3 μm thick sagittal sections were obtained from a 60 μm region spanning the center of the fracture callus. Three sections, each separated by approximately 25 to 50 μm, were stained with Alcian Blue Hematoxylin/Orange G and histomorphometric analysis was performed using a point counting method as described previously [31]. Briefly, blinded sections were analyzed using a standardized eyepiece grid under the 10× objective to determine the percent of total callus area composed of cartilage and woven bone. Cartilage was defined as tissue with positive Alcian Blue stain. Woven bone was counted whenever a trabecular structure was observed, regardless of staining. Cortical bone and internal (i.e. intramedullary) callus were not included in these analyses. At each intersection of a horizontal and vertical grid line, the identity of the underlying tissue was determined, with the outcomes for every intersection documented and counted. Based on the number of counted intersections on each slide, the relative area of each tissue type as a percentage of the callus area (i.e. grid intersections that fell within the callus domain) was calculated.

Immunohistochemistry

Previosly published methods were employed for immunohistochemical analysis of PCNA and VEGFR2 expression [32] and type 2 collagen expression [33]. Briefly, for either antigen, sections were incubated at 60°C for 30 minutes, followed by deparaffinization in xylene and hydration in gradient ethanol. Sections were permeabilized in PBS containing 0.2% Triton X-100 (Sigma, St. Louis, MO) for 10 min, washed in PBS, blocked with 3% H_2O_2 in methanol for 30 minutes, and 3% goat serum in PBS for 30 minutes. Sections were then incubated with primary antibodies overnight at 4°C. The next day, sections were washed with PBS and incubated with biotinylated secondary antibodies (Vector Laboratories, Burlingame, CA) in blocking buffer for 30 minutes. After washing with PBS, ABC reagent (Vector Laboratories) was added for 30 minutes and sections were washed again before detection with AEC reagent (Vector Laboratories). Negative controls were performed on adjacent sections by omitting primary antibodies. All sections were analyzed using an Olympus VS120 Whole Slide Imager and quantification was performed using the automated Visiopharm Integrator System (Visiopharm, Hoersholm, Denmark) and its associated software.

Immunofluorescence

Slides from WT and GIT1 KO femure fractures were deparaffinized in xylene, rehydrated in graded ethanol, and rinsed in distilled, deionized H_2O as described above. For PECAM1 (CD31) detection, slides were boiled for 15 minutes in citrate buffer (Zymed Laboratories, San Francisco, CA), cooled for 20 minutes, and washed in PBS for 5 minutes. Slides were then blocked with normal goat serum containing 5% BSA in PBS for 30–60 minutes and incubated overnight with primary antibodies diluted 1:100 in blocking buffer. After two rinses with PBS, the sections were incubated in the dark for 1 hour at 37°C with rabbit secondary antibody diluted 1:500 in normal rabbit serum. Slides were rinsed in PBS before the addition of Topro3 nuclear stain (Invitrogen, Grand Island, NY) and then mounted with Prolong Gold mounting media (Invitrogen). Confocal images were captured using Zeiss LSM 510 Axioskop 2 microscope (Zeiss Microimaging, Thornwood, NY) and analyzed with Zen 2007 software (Zeiss, San Diego, CA).

Osteoclast Quantification

Three sections per callus were stained for tartrate-resistant acid phosphatase (TRAP) using a previously described method [34]. Briefly, after deparaffinization and rehydration with distilled water, sections were incubated at 37°C for 25 minutes in a solution of anhydrous sodium acetate (Sigma), L-(+) tartaric acid (Sigma), glacial acetic acid, fast red violet LB salt (Sigma), naphthol AS-MX phosphate (Sigma), ethylene glycol monoethyl ether (Sigma), and distilled water. Sections were rinsed in distilled water, counterstained with hematoxylin for 10 seconds and then placed in ammonia water for 5 seconds. Quantification was completed using the 10× objective and Osteomeasure software (Osteo-Metrics, Inc., Decatur, GA) to contour bone perimeter within the callus and identify osteoclast number as a percentage of covered bone surface perimeter and as a number of cells per mm of bone surface. Osteoclasts were defined as multi-nucleated, TRAP-positive cells seated on a bone surface.

Statistical Analysis

All values are expressed as mean +/− SEM. Statistical differences between groups were detected using either ANOVA (when >2 experimental groups were compared) or two-tailed unpaired Student's t tests (when only 2 experimental groups were compared). A p-value less than 0.05 ($p<0.05$) was considered significant.

Results

GIT1 is Expressed during Fracture Healing

To establish that GIT1 is expressed and regulated during the fracture healing process, qPCR was performed on mRNA isolated from the healing callus of WT mice at days 7, 14 and 21 post-fracture. Consistent with previously published work identifying GIT1 function in vascular tissue and osteoclasts, GIT1 is upregulated significantly by day 14 and remains highly-expressed at day 21 (Fig. 1). These timepoints correspond to callus revascularization, cartilage remodeling and woven bone remodeling in the temporal progression of healing. These results set the

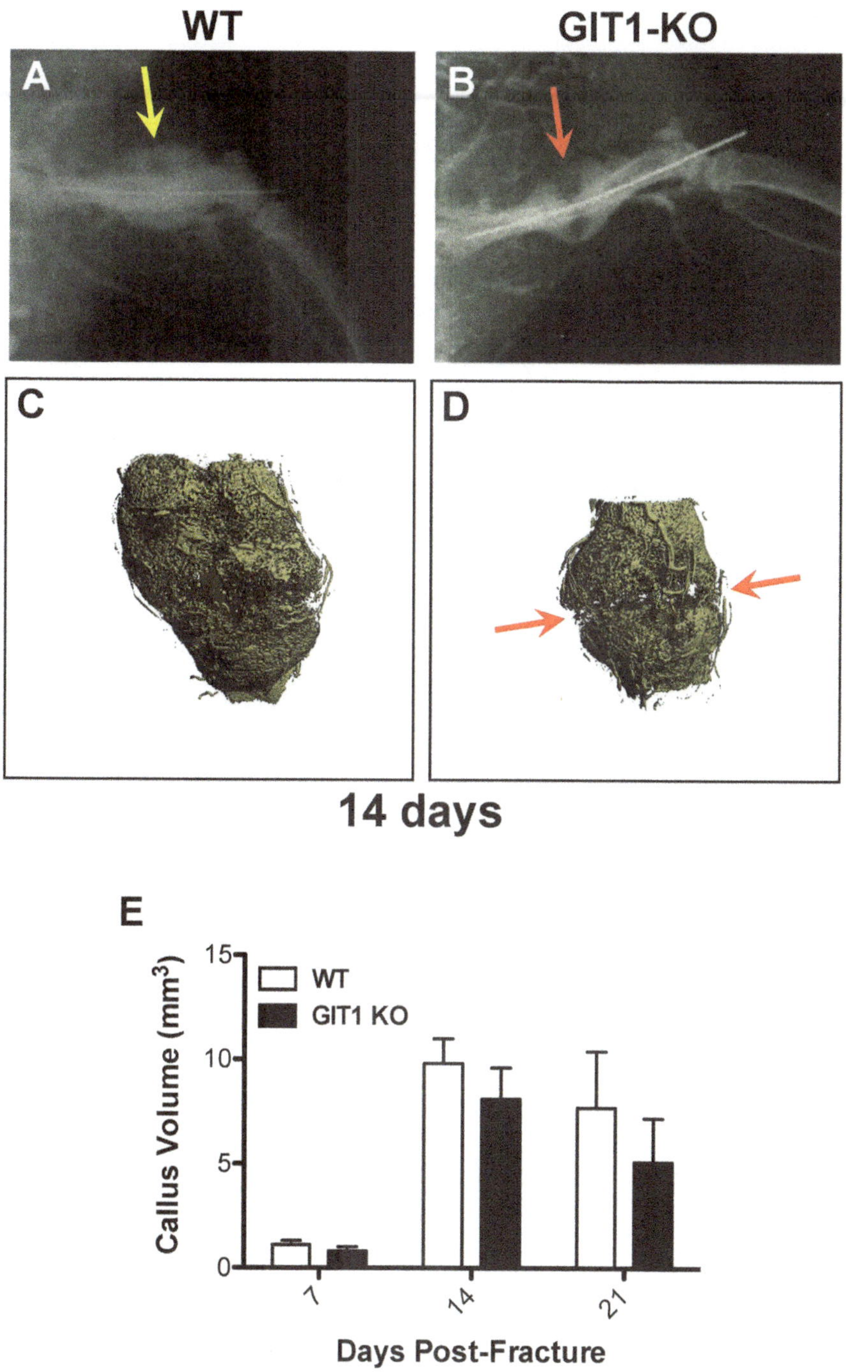

Figure 2. Disjunction persists at 14 days post-fracture in GIT1 KO mice. Femur fractures were induced in 10-week-old WT and GIT1 KO mice. Fractured femora were harvested for analysis at 7, 14, and 21 days post-injury. Radiographs obtained at the 14 day time point consistently revealed radiolucency in GIT1 KO calluses (B, red arrow) compared with calluses from WT mice (A, yellow arrow). This was supported by microCT analysis, which revealed lack of bridging mineral in GIT1 KOs (D, red arrows) compared to a connected shell of mineral in WT controls (C). Further quantification of callus geometry via microCT indicated that there were no differences in mineralized callus volume between WT and GIT1 KO mice (E). Bars represent mean callus volume (mm^3) +/− SEM (N = 3, *$p<0.05$).

stage for study of bone healing in mice in the context of GIT1 loss-of-function.

Fracture Healing is Impaired in GIT1 KO Mice

To begin investigating the role of GIT1 in the fracture healing process, we induced femoral fractures in WT and GIT1 KO mice and assessed the healing process by radiographical evaluation and microCT analysis of mineralized callus volume. At day 14, loss of radiolucency at the fracture site in WT mice suggested the normal pacing of repair (Fig. 2A), while the healing process was delayed in GIT1 KO mice (Fig. 2B, red arrow). Representative microCT reconstructions confirm persistence of disjunction in GIT1 KO

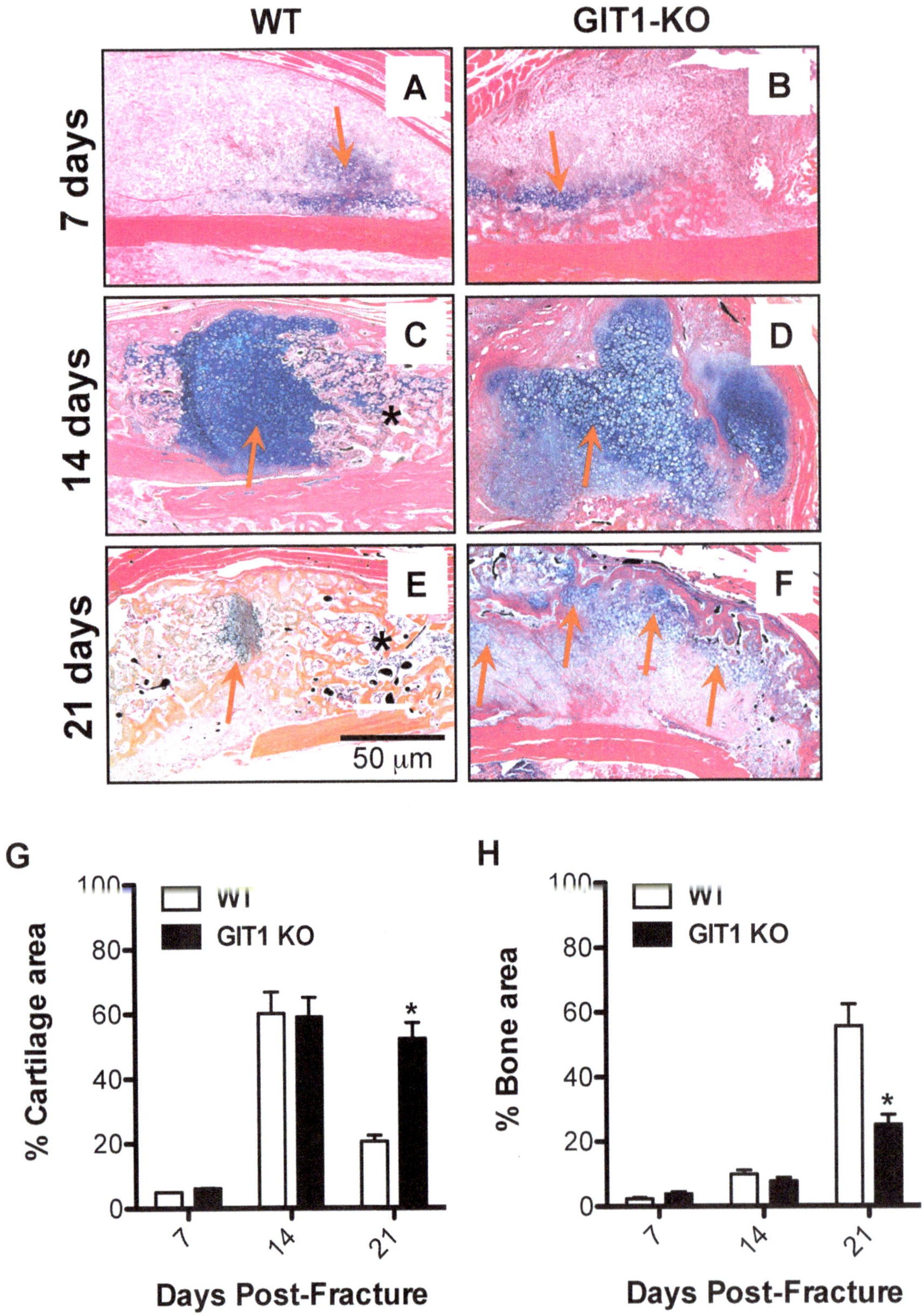

Figure 3. Cartilage persists and woven bone callus is delayed in GIT1 KO mice. Histological analysis of fracture callus cartilage content was performed via Alcian Blue Hematoxylin/Orange G staining. Representative stains of calluses from WT and GIT1 KO mice at 1, 2 and 3 weeks post-fracture are displayed (A–F). Red arrows denote Alcian Blue-stained cartilagenous matrix and asterisks denote mineralized woven bone. Histomorphometry was performed on triplicate sections from multiple mice, with % Cartilage Area (G) and % Bone Area (H) quantified. Bars represent % Area (cartilage or bone) +/− SEM (*$p<0.05$, $N=3$).

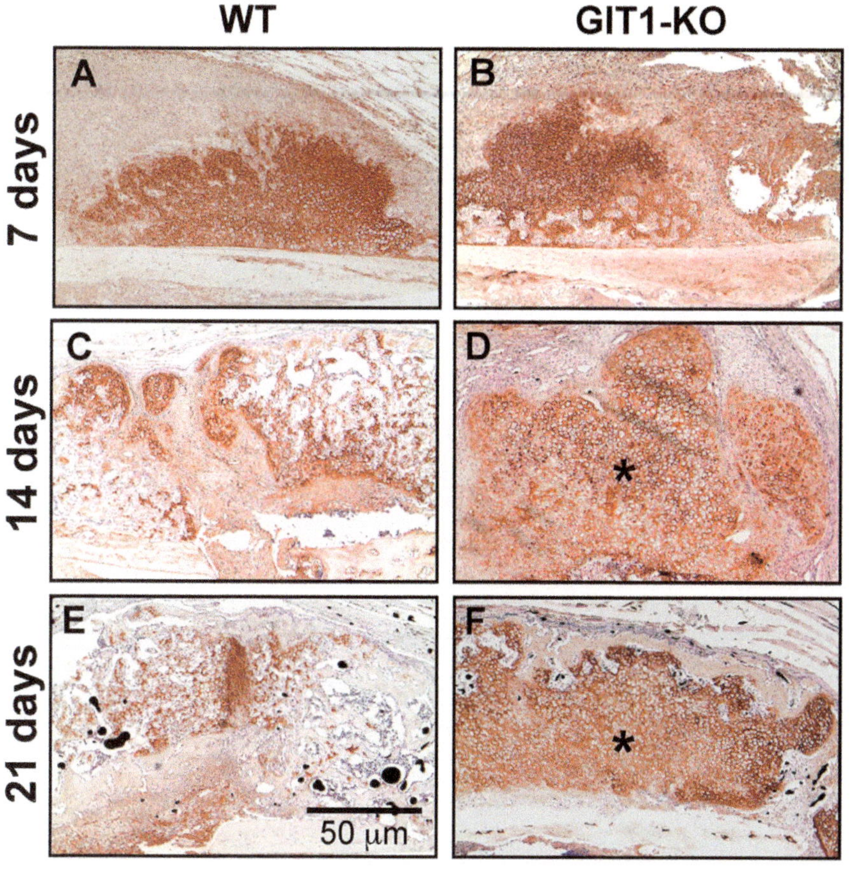

Figure 4. Type 2 collagen-containing matrix persists in GIT1 KO mice. Tissue sections cut from WT and GIT1 KO mice were analyzed for COL2A1 content using an immunohistochemistry approach. Representative stains at 7, 14 and 21 days post-fracture are depicted, with asterisks denoting areas within the callus at 2 and 3 weeks post-fracture in GIT1 KO mice (D and F respectively) that have more robust/persistent staining.

mice (Fig. 2D, red arrows indicating disjunction) compared to WT mice (Fig. 2C) at 14 days post-fracture, although quantification of mineralized callus volume in cohorts of animals failed to achieve significance at any timepoint, only revealing a trend toward a decrease (Fig. 2E).

Chondrocyte Maturation is Delayed in Fracture Callus of GIT1 KO Mice

Alcian Blue was used to stain extracellular matrix surrounding chondrocytes within the fracture callus, with representative sections depicted (Fig. 3A–F). At days 7 and 14 post-fracture, cartilage matrix content in WT mice (Fig. 3A and 3C) was similar to that in GIT1 KO mice (Fig. 3B and 3D). However, unlike in WT mice (Fig. 3E), cartilaginous callus in GIT1 KO mice was still present at day 21 (red arrows, Fig. 3F). Histomorphometric quantification of callus cartilage and bone content confirmed that at 21 days post-fracture, GIT1 KO mice had persistent cartilage (Fig. 3G) that was at the expense of woven bone (Fig. 3H).

To further examine the cartilage phenotype, we performed COL2A1 immunohistochemistry in WT and GIT1 KO mice at 7, 14 and 21 days post-fracture. Representative stained sections are displayed in Fig. 4, with GIT1 KO mice trending toward persistence of COL2A1 at 14 and 21 days (Fig. 4D and 4F) compared to matched sections from WT mice (Fig. 4C and 4E). These results suggest that cartilage persists in the fracture callus of GIT1 KO mice at the expense of woven bone formation.

Chondrocyte Proliferation and Apoptosis is Reduced in Fracture Callus of GIT1 KO Mice

To explore the possible association between persistent cartilagenous callus and changes in chondrocyte proliferation and apoptosis, we performed PCNA immunostaining and TUNEL immunofluorescence respectively. At days 7 and 14, PCNA-positive cells were more abundant in the cartilaginous soft callus of WT mice (Fig. 5A and 5C) relative to calluses from GIT1 KO mice (Fig. 5B and 5D). Histomorphometry confirmed this, establishing that GIT1 KO chondrocytes were less proliferative at 7 and 14 days post fracture (Fig. 5E). Regarding apoptosis, representative TUNEL-stained sections reveal that the percentage of TUNEL-positive cells (relative to DAPI) was reduced in GIT1 KO chondrocytes at both day 14 and 21 post-fracture (Fig. 6A–H). Again, this was confirmed quantitatively (Fig. 6I), indicating that GIT1 KO chondrocytes are less apoptotic during the time period of healing that normally involves remodeling of the cartilagenous callus (i.e. conversion to bone) and associated programmed death of chondrocytes. While GIT1 appears to have a role in modulating proliferation and death of chondrocytes, it is not clear how these combined phenotypes (reduced mitosis and death in the GIT1 KO group) account for the net persistence of the cartilagenous callus and the delay in its conversion to woven bone.

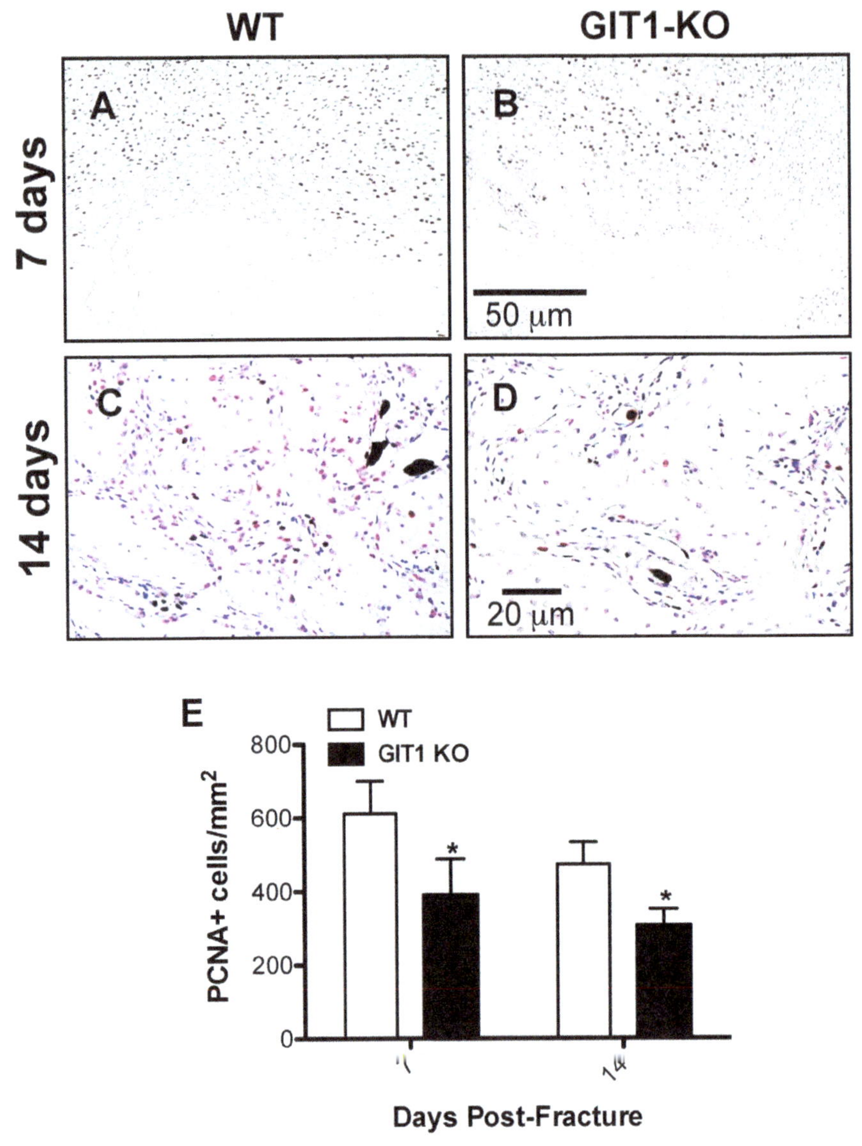

Figure 5. Chondrocyte proliferation is reduced in GIT1 KO mice. Representative PCNA staining is shown at 7 and 14 days post-fracture in WT mice (A and C) and at 7 (B) and 14 days (D) post-fracture in GIT1 KO mice (B and D respectively). Histomorphometry was performed on triplicate sections from multiple mice to quantify the number of PCNA-positive cells per unit callus area (E). The data is presented as mean of the number of PCNA positive cells/mm^2+/− SEM (*$p<0.05$, N = 3).

Blood Vessel Volume and Number are Decreased in Fracture Callus of GIT1 KO Mice

Based on our previously published results demonstrating a pulmonary vascular deficit in GIT1 KO mice, we hypothesized that delayed bone repair in these animals could be due to impaired angiogenesis in the fracture callus. Therefore, we performed quantitative vascular microCT analyses to evaluate neovascularization at day 7, 14, and 21 post-fracture in WT and GIT1 KO mice. Representative reconstructions indicated reduced callus vascularity in KO mice compared to the WT cohort, with GIT1 KO mice displaying a marked reduction in vessel volume, number, and connectivity (Fig. 7A–F). These apparent changes were supported by quantifation of various vascular parameters, substantiating that compared to the WT cohort, GIT KO mice had reduced vessel volume (Fig. 7G), reduced vessel number (Fig. 7H), increased spacing between vessels (Fig. 7I) and reduced connection density (Fig. 7J). It should be noted that the quantification of reduced vessel connectivity (i.e. connection density) is influenced by the efficiency of vessel perfusion with contrast agent, and there may not be adequate filling in vascular beds with smaller vessel diameters, reducing the accuracy of the connectivity algorithm and conclusions that are drawn from it.

Neovascularization is Impaired in the Fracture Callus of GIT1 KO Mice

To further evaluate angiogenesis, we analyzed vessel number using an antibody against PECAM1 (CD31), an endothelial cell marker. A strong signal was observed in vessels of the callus from WT mice at days 7 and 14 (Fig. 8A and 8C). In contrast, the number of PECAM1$^+$ vessels was dramatically reduced in GIT1 KO mice (Fig. 8B and 8D). Quantification of the number of blood vessels revealed a 60% reduction in GIT1 KO mice (Fig. 8E) at

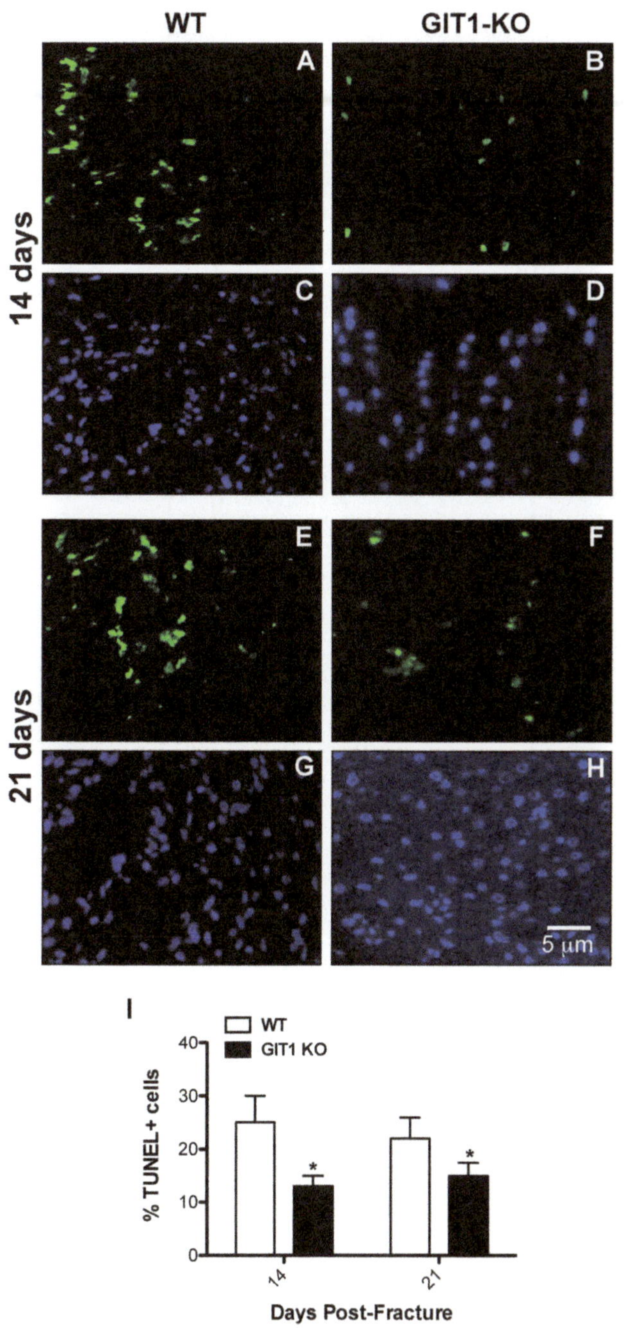

Figure 6. Chondrocyte TUNEL staining is reduced in GIT1 KO mice. Chondrocyte apoptosis was assessed in WT and GIT1 KO mice at 14 and 21 days post-fracture. Representative TUNEL immunofluorescence and DAPI staining at both time points is presented in WT mice (A/C and E/G respectively) and in GIT1 KO mice (B/D and F/H respectively). Quantitative histomorphometric analyses of the number of TUNEL-positive cells per unit area in triplicate sections from three WT and GIT1 KO mice at 14 and 21 days post-fracture are presented (I). Bars represent the percent of TUNEL positive cells/mm^2+/− SEM (*$p<0.05$, N = 3).

both 7 and 14 days post-fracture. In order to examine why vessel parameters (from the vascular microCT findings, Fig. 7) and vessel density (PECAM1) were lower in GIT1 KO mice, we first analyzed the amount of phospho-VEGFR2 expressed in the callus. Compared to WT mice, the phospho-VEGFR2 positivity was reduced in GIT1 KO mice at 14 and 21 days post-fracture (Fig. 9A–D). Quantification in multiple mice from each cohort supported this, revealing a 50% reduction in GIT1 KO mice at days 14 and 21 (Fig. 9E). Since the active form of VEGF receptor was significantly decreased at 14 and 21 days, we next examined VEGF expression levels. Representative immunohistochemistry at 14 days post-fracture depicts reduced VEGF expression in GIT1 KO callus compared to WT controls (Fig. 9F–G). Taken together, these findings indicate that GIT1 is critical for VEGF induced microvessel sprouting in fracture callus, and GIT1 deficiency impairs neoangiogenesis in response to injury.

Osteoclast Number is Reduced in GIT1 KO Fracture Callus

As mentioned, alterations in callus chondrocyte proliferation and apoptosis cannot explain the healing phenotype seen in GIT1 KO mice. Since we have previously established that osteoclast differentiation and activity is impaired in GIT1 KO mice [24], we therefore focused on assessing osteoclast numbers. To assess osteoclast number, histology-based quantification of the number of TRAP-positive cells was performed in callus samples from both WT and GIT1 KO mice at days 7, 14 and 21 post-fracture. Although there was no difference in the number of the TRAP positive cells and the amount of cartilaginous callus (Alcian blue) between WT (Fig. 10A and 10C) and GIT1 KO mice (Fig. 10B and 10D) mice at day 7, differences were observed at days 14 and 21. The increased percentage of cartilaginous callus in GIT1 KO mice compared to WT mice at day 21 (Fig. 3) was concordant with what appeared to be a marginally decreased TRAP positivity in the GIT1 KO cohort at day 14 (Fig. 10C, 10D, 10G and 10H), and a significant decrease in TRAP staining at day 21 (Fig. 10E, 10F, 10G and 10H). This net reduction in osteoclast number in GIT1 KO mice could account for the larger amount/persistence of cartilage callus in these animals that we have observed via Alcian Blue staining (seen in both Fig. 10 and Fig. 3).

Discussion

Delayed and/or failed fracture repair are major public health issues that impact populations in the United States and throughout the world. Musculoskeletal deficits that result from delayed healing post-injury and post-surgery limits the performance of normal daily activities, compromises the function of various organ systems, and has a debilitating impact on psychological health and social function [35–41]. Given the scope of this public health crisis, it is the goal of researchers in the field to further understand the molecular basis for normal and pathologic healing with the aim of developing novel therapeutic strategies.

Endochondral-based healing, which predominates in the repair of long bones, requires the correct temporospatial coordination of a series of molecular and cellular events [42]. From a tissue architecture perspective, these events are organized into four overlapping phases – (1) inflammation, (2) soft (cartilaginous) callus formation, (3) resorption of cartilage and hard (woven bone) callus formation, and (4) woven bone remodeling. Mesenchymal stem cells (MSCs) and chondro−/osteo-progenitor populations that primarily reside in the periosteum are essential throughout fracture repair [43,44]. The transition from soft to hard callus requires angiogenesis, because increased tissue oxygen concentration is necessary for osteoprogenitors to mineralize the matrix. Additionally, functional osteoclasts are needed to remove the cartilage matrix during woven bone formation and to remodel the woven bone callus to ultimately recapitulate the normal structure of the injured element.

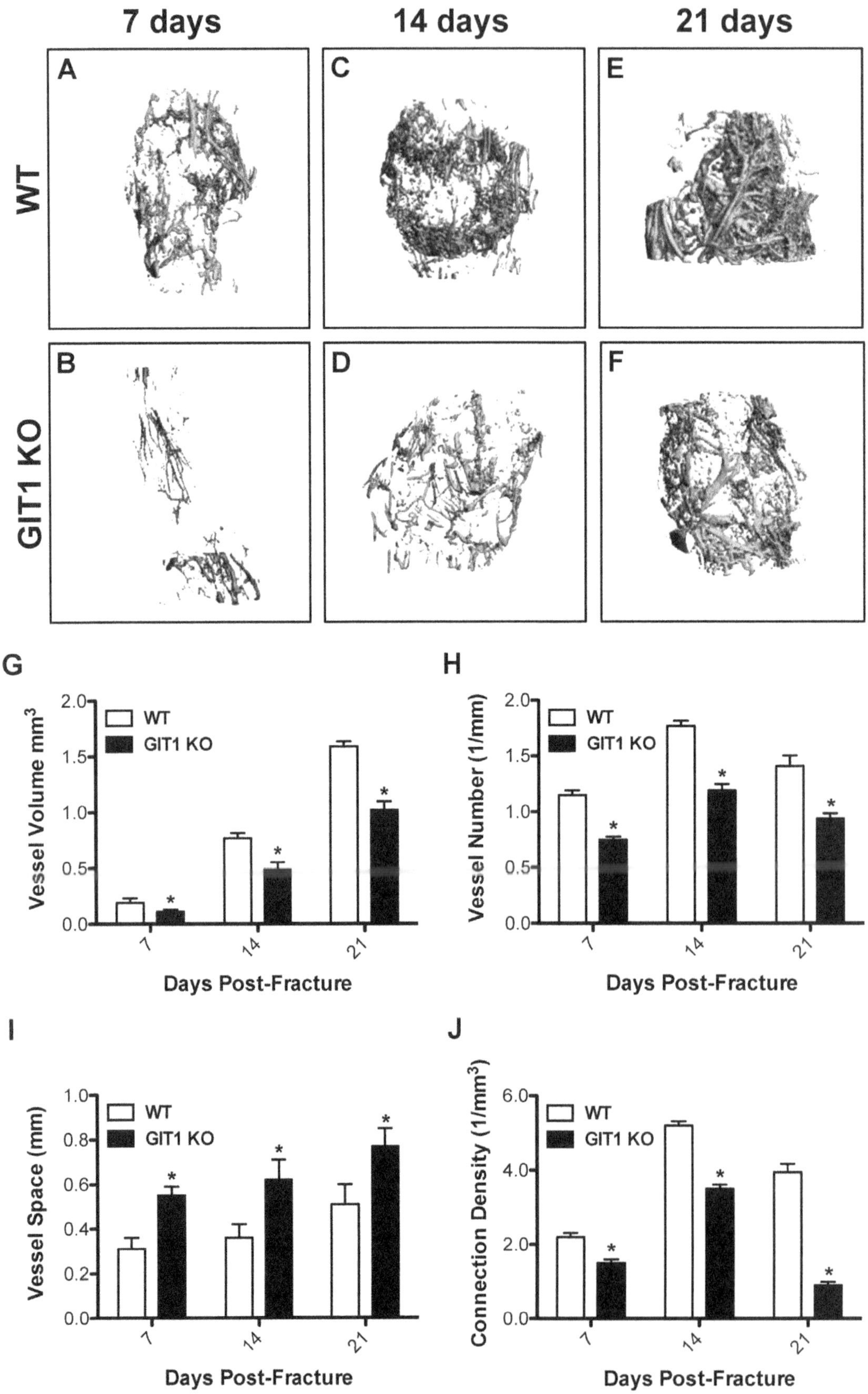

Figure 7. Fracture callus vascularity is reduced in GIT1 KO mice. To visualize and quantify callus vascularity, WT and GIT1 KO mice were perfused with lead chromate microfilm perfusion reagent. Harvested femora were decalcified and representative vascular microCT reconstructions

from each experimental group at 7, 14 and 21 days post-fracture are presented. Reduced vascularity in GIT1 KO mice (A, C, E) compared to WT control mice (B, D, F) was evident at all time points. Quantification of callus vascular parameters, including Vessel Volume (G), Vessel Number (H), Vessel Spacing (I) and Connection Density (J) supported these findings, with GIT1 KO mice possessing reduced callus vessel volume, vessel number and connection density and increased space between vessels compared to callus from WT mice. Bars represent mean for each value +/− SEM (N = 3, $*p < 0.05$).

Our group has recently documented a critical role for GIT1 in pulmonary vascular development [22] and in the formation of functional osteoclasts via regulation of sealing zone formation [24]. Given these unique roles for GIT1, both critical for normal tissue morphogenesis in fracture repair, we became interested in the function of this protein during the bone healing process. Based on

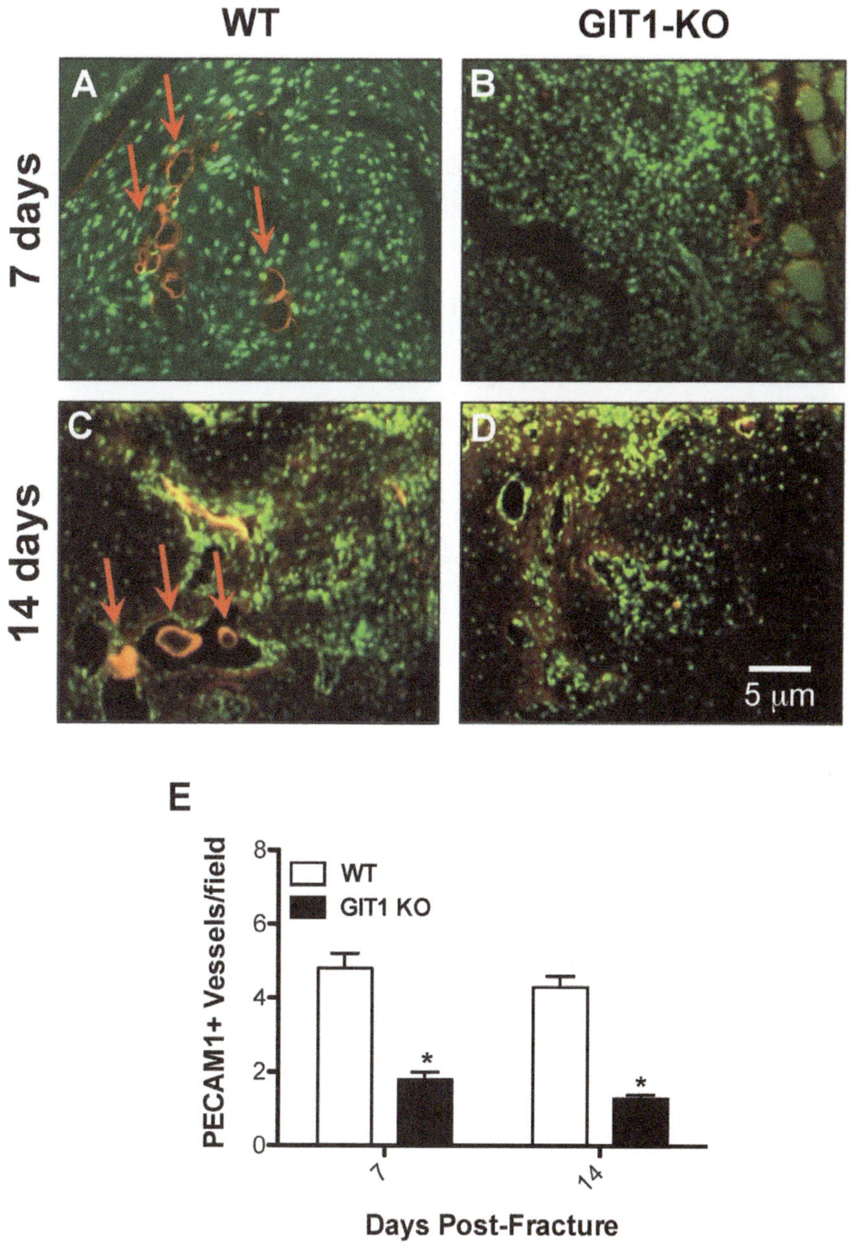

Figure 8. PECAM1$^+$ blood vessel number is reduced in GIT1 KO mice. Representative PECAM1 immunofluorescence is presented at 7 and 14 days post-fracture in WT mice (A and C) and GIT1$^{-/-}$ mice (B and D). Histomorphometry was performed to quantify the average number of positively-stained blood vessels present in each field of view on each section analyzed. Three sections (from 3 levels within each callus, 25–50 μm apart) were viewed using the 10× objective, with counts being collected from 3 fields of view in each section. All counts from each callus (9 fields total) were averaged. Vessel counting using this approach confirmed the immunofluorescence in panels A–D, with WT calluses possessing between 2 and 3-fold more PECAM1$^+$ vessels than GIT1 KO calluses at both time points (E). Bars represent mean number of PECAM1$^+$ vessels/field +/− SEM ($*p<0.01$, N = 3).

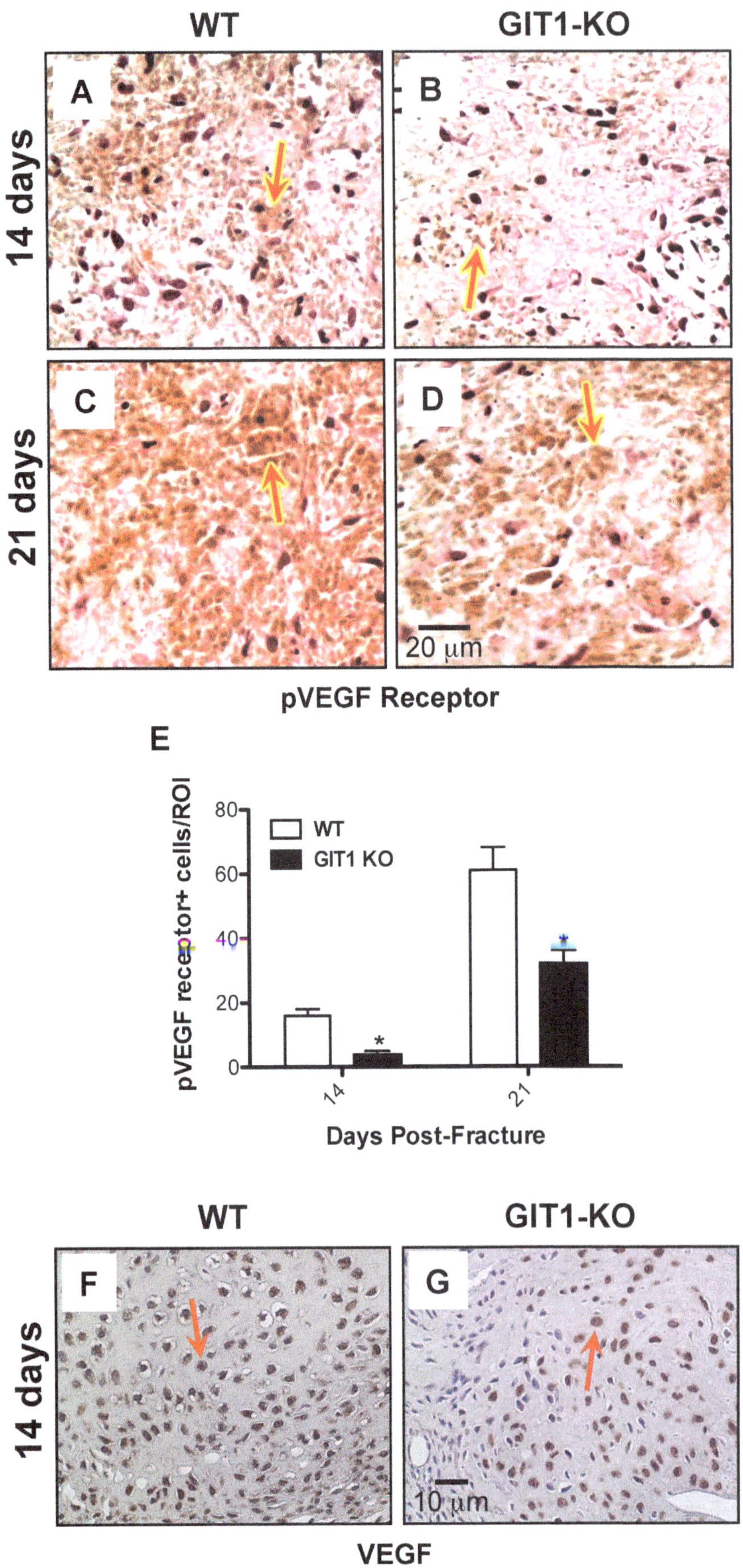
WT
GIT1-KO
14 days
21 days
A
B
C
D
20 µm
pVEGF Receptor
E
pVEGF receptor+ cells/ROI
80
60
40
20
0
WT
GIT1 KO
*
14
21
Days Post-Fracture
WT
GIT1-KO
14 days
F
G
10 µm
VEGF

Figure 9. VEGF signaling is reduced in GIT1 KO mice. Phospho-VEGF receptor immunostaining was performed on fracture calluses from WT and GIT1 KO mice at 2 and 3 weeks post-fracture. Panels A-D depict representative staining profiles, with Phospho-VEGF receptor-positive cells staining red as indicated by red arrows. Histomorphometry was performed to quantify the number of Phospho-VEGF receptor-positive cells per unit callus area (E). Data is presented as the mean number of positive cells per unit area (i.e. region of interest) +/− SEM (*$p<0.01$, $N=3$). Additionally, immunohistochemistry was performed of assess VEGF levels in fracture calluses from WT (F) and GIT1 KO mice (G). Representative histological sections of calluses at 2 weeks post-fracture are presented, depicting reduced expression in KO mice. VEGF positive cells are stained reddish-brown as indicated by red arrows.

our previous work, we hypothesized that loss of GIT1 function will lead to delayed healing in a mouse model of femur fracture due to i) impaired neovascularization of the callus and ii) inhibited cartilage and woven bone remodeling due to reduced osteoclast number and/or function. Supporting this hypothesis, our results indicate that GIT1 deficiency leads to a fracture healing defect that is driven by two primary effects: altered neovascularization of the callus in early-mid stage healing, and reduced osteoclast number during primary and secondary callus remodeling.

Regarding blood vessels in the callus, successful bone repair requires the revascularization of injured tissues to provide oxygen, facilitate metabolic waste management, and deliver a population of circulating precursor cells that may contribute to healing either directly or in a paracrine manner. Angiogenesis during the repair process is thought to be modulated by VEGFs and their cognate receptors VEGFR1 and VEGFR2. It has been demonstrated that delivery of VEGF during mouse femur fracture healing enhances vascular ingrowth into the callus and accelerates repair by promoting bony bridging [45]. This has been confirmed in allograft bone healing, where VEGF gene therapy accelerates the healing process [26]. Conversely, inhibition of new blood vessel formation by injecting TNP-470, an endostatin-like anti-angiogenesis agent [46], prevented fracture healing in a rodent fracture model [17]. Here, we show for the first time that GIT1 may be an important regulator of angiogenesis during fracture repair, thus having a direct impact of the progression of the healing process. Previously we demonstrated that GIT1 is required for activation of PLC-γ and ERK1/2 in endothelial cells and osteoblasts, leading to the regulation of VEGF expression in osteoblasts through the GIT1-ERK1/2 signaling axis [47]. In the present study, we demonstrate that loss of GIT1 results in reduced VEGF expression and phospho-VEGFR2 (active form) in the fracture callus. We also found that GIT1 deficiency significantly decreased small vessel connectivity density and PECAM1 expression in the fracture callus. Correlated with this, vascular microCT analyses revealed reduced overall vessel volume, number and connection density coupled with increased spacing between vessels. These results suggest that the impaired fracture healing process in GIT1 KO mice is at least in part related to impaired VEGF-induced angiogenesis, implicating GIT1 as central regulator of angiogenesis in the context of bone healing.

In addition to the resulting vascular defect described above, the loss of GIT1 function likely also contributes to impaired fracture healing due to altered primary and secondary remodeling because of a defect in osteoclast formation and/or function. We have previously published that GIT1 is required for appropriate osteoclast function via its role in regulating cytoskeletal-related ruffled border and sealing zone formation [24]. Following the formation of the cartilagenous callus, an initial phase of osteoclast-driven remodeling removes the cartilage template, which is then replaced by mineralized woven bone matrix. This occurs in response to macrophage colony-stimulating factor (M-CSF), RANK ligand (RANKL) and osteoprotegerin (OPG) [6]. This initial woven bone matrix is subsequently replaced by organized lamellar bone through a second remodeling process that is the final step in achieving an anatomically correct skeletal element. This second remodeling process is also governed by osteoclasts, which become dominant in this final stage due to the induction of IL-1 and TNF-α and the subsequent expansion of the functional osteoclast population [7,8] via RANKL in the remodeling callus [9]. In this report, histomorphometric analysis revealed persistent cartilaginous callus that could be the result of delayed cartilage matrix removal due to reduced osteoclast number (and possibly activity) in GIT1 deficient mice that was seen at day 14 and 21 (i.e. during primary and secondary callus remodeling). This phenotype could be related to both the reduced number of osteoclasts observed in the callus area as well as reduced formation of resorbing zones (ruffled border), a known phenotype following loss of GIT1 [24]. Overall, these findings suggest that osteoclast-dependent callus remodeling is likely at least partially impaired in GIT1 KO mice. The molecular basis of this effect may involve several mechanisms including altered RANKL and OPG expression, or cytoskeletal defects that alter osteoclast function, a subject requiring further study.

In addition to these central defects in fracture healing seen in GIT1 KO mice, we also observed an alteration in normal chondrogenic differentiation and cartilage persistence. While expression of Sox9, the master inducer of chondrogenesis, was not altered (data not shown), there was reduced chondrocyte proliferation and apoptosis (Fig. 7 and 8). This was in conjunction with enhanced Alcian Blue staining and cartilage persistence coupled with delayed woven bone formation (Fig. 5) and type 2 collagen immunoreactivity (Fig. 6). Since it is not known if there is a direct role for GIT1 in normal chondrocyte physiology, we postulate that these defects could be indirect and downstream of impaired neovascularization of the callus and/or reduced osteoclast formation and function. Further effort is required to determine any potential direct effects of GIT1 deficiency on chondrocyte differentiation.

In conclusion, data is presented in this report that supports a previously unappreciated role for GIT1 as a regulator of bone fracture healing. GIT1 deficiency leads to decreased revascularization of the fracture callus, decreased chondrocyte proliferation and apoptosis, and reduced osteoclast number. Since the fragility of the GIT1 KO model severely limited the completion of a full evaluation of healing including a higher N for histologic and microCT analyses, mRNA profiling of the callus to further establish molecular mechanism, and performance of biomechanical testing, further study into the role of GIT1 in fracture repair is required. The development of a floxed GIT1 KO model allowing temporal and tissue-specific gene ablation would facilitate the next step in the study of mechanism that would alleviate the high rate of mortality leading to the low number of mice available to populate the experimental groups included in this study. Despite this shortcoming, the results presented clearly define GIT1 as a contributor to bone repair. We speculate that agents targeting activation of GIT1 could be exploited to i) improve callus vascularization in the early phases of healing, and ii) accelerate osteoclast-driven remodeling steps, in particular the resorption of cartilagenous callus that is required to clear the path for deposition of woven bone and stabilization of the fracture site.

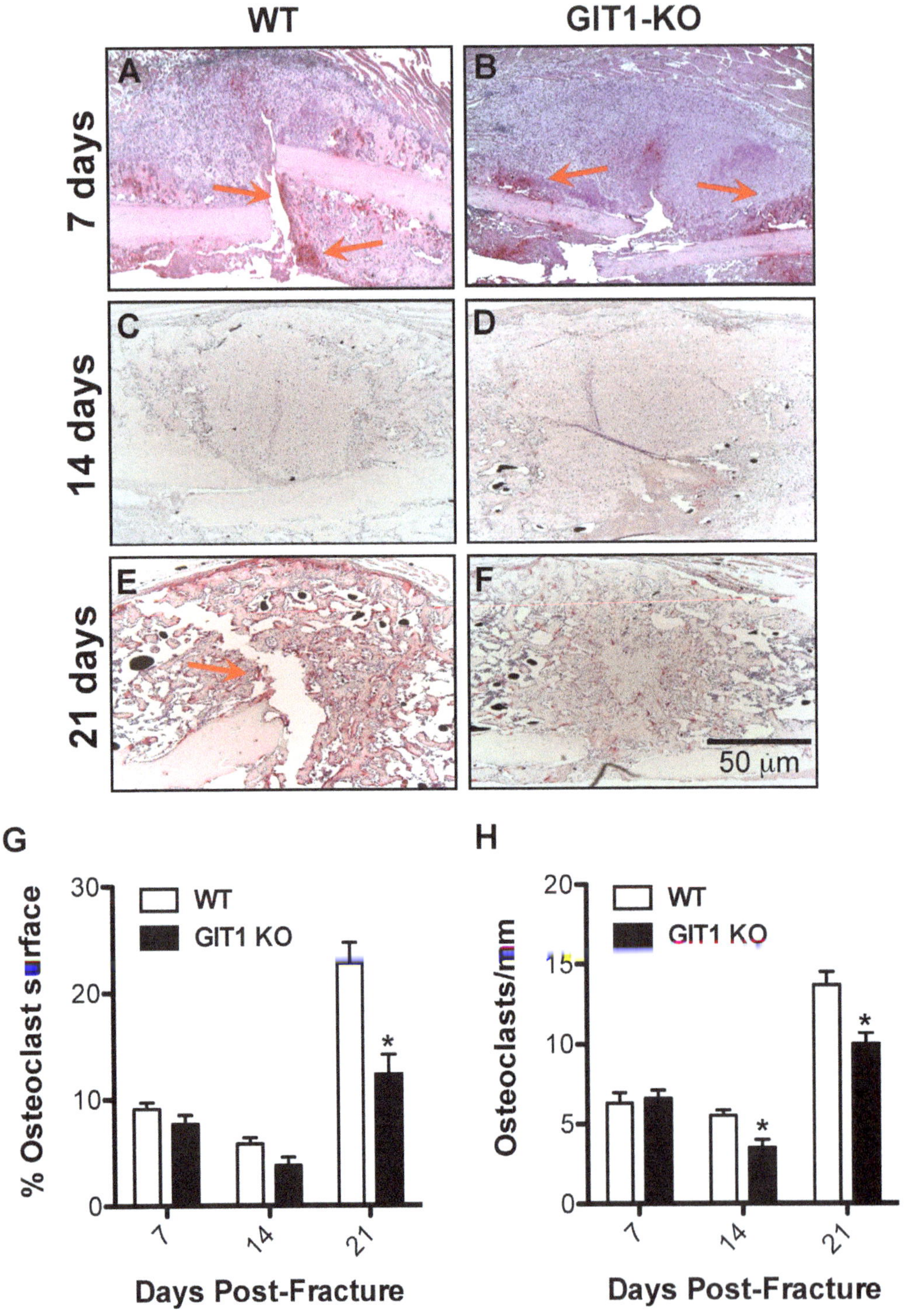

Figure 10. Osteoclast number is reduced in GIT1 KO mice. The presence of osteoclasts in the fracture callus of WT and GIT1 KO mice was assessed at 7 (A and B respectively), 14 (C and D respectively) and 21 days (E and F respectively) post-fracture via TRAP staining. Histomorphometry to quantify percentage of osteoclast surface (G) and osteoclast number per unit bone surface (H) was also performed on triplicate sections from multiple mice, with bars representing the mean for each parameter +/− SEM (*$p<0.05$, $N=3$).

Acknowledgments

We thank Dr. Tianfang Li and Dr. Yufeng Dong for helpful suggestions and thoughtful discussion of data, and we thank Michael Thullen for assistance with all microCT analysis of mineralized and vascular tissues.

Author Contributions

Conceived and designed the experiments: GY TJS MJZ BCB. Performed the experiments: GY TJS. Analyzed the data: GY TJS PM JP HH SS CX ES CY MJZ BCB. Contributed reagents/materials/analysis tools: GY TJS ES MJZ BCB. Wrote the paper: GY TJS.

References

1. Einhorn TA (1998) The cell and molecular biology of fracture healing. ClinOrthop: S7–21.
2. Gerstenfeld LC, Cullinane DM, Barnes GL, Graves DT, Einhorn TA (2003) Fracture healing as a post-natal developmental process: molecular, spatial, and temporal aspects of its regulation. JCell Biochem 88: 873–884.
3. Marsell R, Einhorn TA (2011) The biology of fracture healing. Injury 42: 551–555.
4. Thompson Z, Miclau T, Hu D, Helms JA (2002) A model for intramembranous ossification during fracture healing. Journal of Orthopaedic Research 20: 1091–1098.
5. Li G, White G, Connolly C, Marsh D (2002) Cell proliferation and apoptosis during fracture healing. J Bone Miner Res 17: 791–799.
6. Kon T, Cho TJ, Aizawa T, Yamazaki M, Nooh N, et al. (2001) Expression of osteoprotegerin, receptor activator of NF-kappaB ligand (osteoprotegerin ligand) and related proinflammatory cytokines during fracture healing. Journal of Bone and Mineral Research 16: 1004–1014.
7. Mountziaris PM, Mikos AG (2008) Modulation of the inflammatory response for enhanced bone tissue regeneration. Tissue Eng Part B Rev 14: 179–186.
8. Ai-Aql ZS, Alagl AS, Graves DT, Gerstenfeld LC, Einhorn TA (2008) Molecular mechanisms controlling bone formation during fracture healing and distraction osteogenesis. J Dent Res 87: 107–118.
9. Gerstenfeld LC, Sacks DJ, Pelis M, Mason ZD, Graves DT, et al. (2009) Comparison of effects of the bisphosphonate alendronate versus the RANKL inhibitor denosumab on murine fracture healing. J Bone Miner Res 24: 196–208.
10. Maes C, Kobayashi T, Selig MK, Torrekens S, Roth SI, et al. (2010) Osteoblast precursors, but not mature osteoblasts, move into developing and fractured bones along with invading blood vessels. Dev Cell 19: 329–344.
11. Pufe T, Wildemann B, Petersen W, Mentlein R, Raschke M, et al. (2002) Quantitative measurement of the splice variants 120 and 164 of the angiogenic peptide vascular endothelial growth factor in the time flow of fracture healing: a study in the rat. Cell Tissue Res 309: 387–392.
12. Eckardt H, Bundgaard KG, Christensen KS, Lind M, Hansen ES, et al. (2003) Effects of locally applied vascular endothelial growth factor (VEGF) and VEGF-inhibitor to the rabbit tibia during distraction osteogenesis. J Orthop Res 21: 335–340.
13. Ferguson C, Alpern E, Miclau T, Helms JA (1999) Does adult fracture repair recapitulate embryonic skeletal formation? Mechanisms of Development 87: 57–66.
14. Glowacki J (1998) Angiogenesis in fracture repair. Clin Orthop Relat Res: S82–89.
15. Gerber HP, Vu TH, Ryan AM, Kowalski J, Werb Z, et al. (1999) VEGF couples hypertrophic cartilage remodeling, ossification and angiogenesis during endochondral bone formation. NatMed 5: 623–628.
16. Athanasopoulos AN, Schneider D, Keiper T, Alt V, Pendurthi UR, et al. (2007) Vascular endothelial growth factor (VEGF)-induced up-regulation of CCN1 in osteoblasts mediates proangiogenic activities in endothelial cells and promotes fracture healing. Journal of Biological Chemistry 282: 26746–26753.
17. Hausman MR, Schaffler MB, Majeska RJ (2001) Prevention of fracture healing in rats by an inhibitor of angiogenesis. Bone 29: 560–564.
18. Premont RT, Claing A, Vitale N, Freeman JL, Pitcher JA, et al. (1998) beta2-Adrenergic receptor regulation by GIT1, a G protein-coupled receptor kinase-associated ADP ribosylation factor GTPase-activating protein. Proc Natl Acad Sci U S A 95: 14082–14087.
19. Natarajan K, Yin G, Berk BC (2004) Scaffolds direct Src-specific signaling in response to angiotensin II: new roles for Cas and GIT1. Mol Pharmacol 65: 822–825.
20. Haendeler J, Yin G, Hojo Y, Saito Y, Melaragno M, et al. (2003) GIT1 mediates Src-dependent activation of phospholipase Cgamma by angiotensin II and epidermal growth factor. J Biol Chem 278: 49936–49944.
21. Yin G, Haendeler J, Yan C, Berk BC (2004) GIT1 functions as a scaffold for MEK1-extracellular signal-regulated kinase 1 and 2 activation by angiotensin II and epidermal growth factor. Mol Cell Biol 24: 875–885.
22. Pang J, Hoefen R, Pryhuber GS, Wang J, Yin G, et al. (2009) G-protein-coupled receptor kinase interacting protein-1 is required for pulmonary vascular development. Circulation 119: 1524–1532.
23. Wang J, Taba Y, Pang J, Yin G, Yan C, et al. (2009) GIT1 mediates VEGF-induced podosome formation in endothelial cells: critical role for PLCgamma. Arterioscler Thromb Vasc Biol 29: 202–208.
24. Menon P, Yin G, Smolock EM, Zuscik MJ, Yan C, et al. (2010) GPCR kinase 2 interacting protein 1 (GIT1) regulates osteoclast function and bone mass. J Cell Physiol 225: 777–785.
25. Xie C, Liang B, Xue M, Lin AS, Loiselle A, et al. (2009) Rescue of impaired fracture healing in COX-2−/− mice via activation of prostaglandin E2 receptor subtype 4. AmJPathol 175: 772–785.
26. Ito H, Koefoed M, Tiyapatanaputi P, Gromov K, Goater JJ, et al. (2005) Remodeling of cortical bone allografts mediated by adherent rAAV-RANKL and VEGF gene therapy. NatMed 11: 291–297.
27. Zhang X, Xie C, Lin AS, Ito H, Awad H, et al. (2005) Periosteal progenitor cell fate in segmental cortical bone graft transplantations: implications for functional tissue engineering. Journal of Bone and Mineral Research 20: 2124–2137.
28. Dhillon RS, Xie C, Tyler W, Calvi LM, Awad HA, et al. (2013) PTH-enhanced structural allograft healing is associated with decreased angiopoietin-2-mediated arteriogenesis, mast cell accumulation, and fibrosis. J Bone Miner Res 28: 586–597.
29. Duvall CL, Taylor WR, Weiss D, Guldberg RE (2004) Quantitative microcomputed tomography analysis of collateral vessel development after ischemic injury. Am J Physiol Heart Circ Physiol 287: H302–310.
30. Zhang X, Schwarz EM, Young DA, Puzas JE, Rosier RN, et al. (2002) Cyclooxygenase-2 regulates mesenchymal cell differentiation into the osteoblast lineage and is critically involved in bone repair. JClinInvest 109: 1405–1415.
31. Naik AA, Xie C, Zuscik MJ, Kingsley P, Schwarz EM, et al. (2009) Reduced COX-2 expression in aged mice is associated with impaired fracture healing. Journal of Bone and Mineral Research 24: 251–264.
32. Konishi H, Wu J, Cooke JP (2010) Chronic exposure to nicotine impairs cholinergic angiogenesis. Vasc Med 15: 47–54.
33. Arasapam G, Scherer M, Cool JC, Foster BK, Xian CJ (2006) Roles of COX-2 and iNOS in the bony repair of the injured growth plate cartilage. J Cell Biochem 99: 450–461.
34. Boyce BF, Xing L (2008) Functions of RANKL/RANK/OPG in bone modeling and remodeling. Arch Biochem Biophys 473: 139–146.
35. Alarcon T, Gonzalez-Montalvo JI, Gotor P, Madero R, Otero A (2011) Activities of daily living after hip fracture: profile and rate of recovery during 2 years of follow-up. Osteoporos Int 22: 1609–1613.
36. Brenneman SK, Barrett-Connor E, Sajjan S, Markson LE, Siris ES (2006) Impact of recent fracture on health-related quality of life in postmenopausal women. J Bone Miner Res 21: 809–816.
37. Ding R, McCarthy ML, Houseknecht E, Ziegfeld S, Knight VM, et al. (2006) The health-related quality of life of children with an extremity fracture: a one-year follow-up study. J Pediatr Orthop 26: 157–163.
38. Giannoudis PV, Harwood PJ, Kontakis G, Allami M, Macdonald D, et al. (2009) Long-term quality of life in trauma patients following the full spectrum of tibial injury (fasciotomy, closed fracture, grade IIIB/IIIC open fracture and amputation). Injury 40: 213–219.
39. Lonnroos E, Kautiainen H, Sund R, Karppi P, Hartikainen S, et al. (2009) Utilization of inpatient care before and after hip fracture: a population-based study. Osteoporos Int 20: 879–886.
40. Olerud P, Ahrengart L, Soderqvist A, Saving J, Tidermark J (2010) Quality of life and functional outcome after a 2-part proximal humeral fracture: a prospective cohort study on 50 patients treated with a locking plate. J Shoulder Elbow Surg 19: 814–822.
41. Silverman SL, Shen W, Minshall ME, Xie S, Moses KH (2007) Prevalence of depressive symptoms in postmenopausal women with low bone mineral density and/or prevalent vertebral fracture: results from the Multiple Outcomes of Raloxifene Evaluation (MORE) study. J Rheumatol 34: 140–144.
42. Schindeler A, McDonald MM, Bokko P, Little DG (2008) Bone remodeling during fracture repair: The cellular picture. Semin Cell Dev Biol 19: 459–466.
43. Zhang X, Naik A, Xie C, Reynolds D, Palmer J, et al. (2005) Periosteal stem cells are essential for bone revitalization and repair. JMusculoskeletNeuronalInteract 5: 360–362.
44. Zuscik MJ, O'Keefe RJ (2009) Skeletal Healing. In: Rosen CJ, editor. Primer on the Metabolic Bone Diseases and Disorders of Mineral Metabolism: American Society of Bone and Mineral Research. 61–65.
45. Street J, Bao M, deGuzman L, Bunting S, Peale FV Jr, et al. (2002) Vascular endothelial growth factor stimulates bone repair by promoting angiogenesis and bone turnover. ProcNatlAcadSciUSA 99: 9656–9661.
46. Moulton KS, Heller E, Konerding MA, Flynn E, Palinski W, et al. (1999) Angiogenesis inhibitors endostatin or TNP-470 reduce intimal neovascularization and plaque growth in apolipoprotein E-deficient mice. Circulation 99: 1726–1732.
47. Rui Z, Li X, Fan J, Ren Y, Yuan Y, et al. (2012) GIT1Y321 phosphorylation is required for ERK1/2- and PDGF-dependent VEGF secretion from osteoblasts to promote angiogenesis and bone healing. Int J Mol Med 30: 819–825.

Permissions

All chapters in this book were first published in PLOS ONE, by The Public Library of Science; hereby published with permission under the Creative Commons Attribution License or equivalent. Every chapter published in this book has been scrutinized by our experts. Their significance has been extensively debated. The topics covered herein carry significant findings which will fuel the growth of the discipline. They may even be implemented as practical applications or may be referred to as a beginning point for another development.

The contributors of this book come from diverse backgrounds, making this book a truly international effort. This book will bring forth new frontiers with its revolutionizing research information and detailed analysis of the nascent developments around the world.

We would like to thank all the contributing authors for lending their expertise to make the book truly unique. They have played a crucial role in the development of this book. Without their invaluable contributions this book wouldn't have been possible. They have made vital efforts to compile up to date information on the varied aspects of this subject to make this book a valuable addition to the collection of many professionals and students.

This book was conceptualized with the vision of imparting up-to-date information and advanced data in this field. To ensure the same, a matchless editorial board was set up. Every individual on the board went through rigorous rounds of assessment to prove their worth. After which they invested a large part of their time researching and compiling the most relevant data for our readers.

The editorial board has been involved in producing this book since its inception. They have spent rigorous hours researching and exploring the diverse topics which have resulted in the successful publishing of this book. They have passed on their knowledge of decades through this book. To expedite this challenging task, the publisher supported the team at every step. A small team of assistant editors was also appointed to further simplify the editing procedure and attain best results for the readers.

Apart from the editorial board, the designing team has also invested a significant amount of their time in understanding the subject and creating the most relevant covers. They scrutinized every image to scout for the most suitable representation of the subject and create an appropriate cover for the book.

The publishing team has been an ardent support to the editorial, designing and production team. Their endless efforts to recruit the best for this project, has resulted in the accomplishment of this book. They are a veteran in the field of academics and their pool of knowledge is as vast as their experience in printing. Their expertise and guidance has proved useful at every step. Their uncompromising quality standards have made this book an exceptional effort. Their encouragement from time to time has been an inspiration for everyone.

The publisher and the editorial board hope that this book will prove to be a valuable piece of knowledge for researchers, students, practitioners and scholars across the globe.

List of Contributors

Christin Habig and Ottmar Distl
Institute for Animal Breeding and Genetics, University of Veterinary Medicine Hannover (Foundation), Hannover, Germany

Robert Geffers
Department of Cell Biology, Helmholtz Centre for Infection Research, Braunschweig, Germany

Hana Chang and Shannon R. Moore
Department of Biomedical Engineering, Case Western Reserve University, Cleveland, Ohio, United States of America

Melissa L. Knothe Tate
Department of Biomedical Engineering, Case Western Reserve University, Cleveland, Ohio, United States of America
Department of Mechanical & Aerospace Engineering, Case Western Reserve University, Cleveland, Ohio, United States of America

Ulf R. Knothe
Department of Orthopaedic Surgery, Cleveland Clinic, Cleveland, Ohio, United States of America

Nigel A. Morrison, Alexandre A. Stephens, Nicolette Fozzard and James D. Doecke
School of Medical Sciences, Griffith University, Southport, Australia

Motomi Osato
Institute of Molecular and Cell Biology, Singapore, Singapore

Patsie Polly and Timothy C. Tan
Department of Pathology and Inflammation and Infection Research Centre, School of Medical Sciences, University of New South Wales, Sydney, Australia

Namiko Yamashita
Cancer Science Institute of Singapore, National University of Singapore, Singapore, Singapore

Julie Pasco
School of Medicine, Deakin University, Geelong, Australia

Graeme Jones
The Menzies Institute, Hobart, Australia

Stuart H. Ralston
Centre for Molecular Medicine, The University of Edinburgh, Edinburgh, Scotland

Philip N. Sambrook
Royal North Shore Hospital, The University of Sydney, Sydney, Australia

Richard L. Prince
Western Australian Institute of Medical Research and the Department of Endocrinology and Diabetes, Sir Charles Gairdner Hospital, Perth, Australia

Geoff C. Nicholson
Rural Clinical School, School of Medicine, The University of Queensland, Toowoomba, Australia

Andrew J. Burghardt and Sharmila Majumdar
Musculoskeletal Quantitative Imaging Research Group, Department of Radiology, University of California San Francisco, San Francisco, California, United States of America

Björn Jobke
Musculoskeletal Quantitative Imaging Research Group, Department of Radiology, University of California San Francisco, San Francisco, California, United States of America
Institute of Radiology, Helios Klinikum Berlin-Buch, Berlin, Germany

Burkhard Muche and Jutta Semler
Department of Bone Metabolism and Osteology, Immanuel Hospital Berlin-Wannsee, Berlin, Germany

Michael Hahn and Michael Amling
Department of Osteology & Biomechanics, University Medical Center Hamburg-Eppendorf, Hamburg, Germany

Björn Busse
Department of Osteology & Biomechanics, University Medical Center Hamburg-Eppendorf, Hamburg, Germany

Materials Sciences Division, Lawrence Berkeley National Laboratory, University of California, Berkeley, California, United States of America

Song Yao, Lara E. Sucheston, Warren Davis and Christine B. Ambrosone
Department of Cancer Prevention and Control, Roswell Park Cancer Institute, Buffalo, New York, United States of America

Shannon L. Smiley, Philip L. McCarthy Jr. and Theresa Hahn
Department of Medicine, Roswell Park Cancer Institute, Buffalo, New York, United States of America

Jeffrey M. Conroy
Department of Cancer Genetics, Roswell Park Cancer Institute, Buffalo, New York, United States of America

Norma J. Nowak
Department of Cancer Genetics, Roswell Park Cancer Institute, Buffalo, New York, United States of America
Department of Biochemistry, University at Buffalo, Buffalo, New York, United States of America

Christopher L. Newman and Matthew R. Allen
Department of Anatomy and Cell Biology, Indiana University School of Medicine, Indianapolis, Indiana, United States of America

Neal X. Chen
Division of Nephrology, Department of Medicine, Indiana University School of Medicine, Indianapolis, Indiana, United States of America

Sharon M. Moe
Division of Nephrology, Department of Medicine, Indiana University School of Medicine, Indianapolis, Indiana, United States of America
Roudebush VA Medical Center, Indianapolis, Indiana, United States of America

Max A. Hammond
Weldon School of Biomedical Engineering, Purdue University, West Lafayette, Indiana, United States of America

Joseph M. Wallace
Weldon School of Biomedical Engineering, Purdue University, West Lafayette, Indiana, United States of America
Department of Biomedical Engineering, Indiana University—Purdue University, Indianapolis, Indiana, United States of America

Jeffry S. Nyman
Department of Orthopaedic Surgery and Rehabilitation and Vanderbilt Center for Bone Biology, Vanderbilt University Medical Center, Nashville, Tennessee, United States of America
Department of Veterans Affairs, Tennessee Valley Healthcare System, Nashville, Tennessee, United States of America

Keiyo Takubo, Ayako Nakamura-Ishizu and Toshio Suda
Department of Cell Differentiation, The Sakaguchi Laboratory of Developmental Biology, Keio University School of Medicine, Tokyo, Japan

Hirono Iriuchishima
Department of Cell Differentiation, The Sakaguchi Laboratory of Developmental Biology, Keio University School of Medicine, Tokyo, Japan
Department of Medicine and Clinical Science, Gunma University Graduate School of Medicine, Maebashi, Gunma, Japan

Yoshitaka Miyakawa
Division of Hematology, Department of Internal Medicine, Keio University School of Medicine, Tokyo, Japan

Yoshiteru Miyauchi, Nobuyuki Fujita, Kana Miyamoto and Takeshi Miyamoto
Department of Orthopedic Surgery, Keio University School of Medicine, Tokyo, Japan

Eiji Ikeda
Department of Pathology, Yamaguchi University Graduate School of Medicine, Ube, Yamaguchi, Japan

Masahiro Kizaki
Division of Hematology, Department of Internal Medicine, Keio University School of Medicine, Tokyo, Japan
Department of Hematology, Saitama Medical Center, Saitama Medical University, Saitama, Japan

Yoshihisa Nojima
Department of Medicine and Clinical Science, Gunma University Graduate School of Medicine, Maebashi, Gunma, Japan

Yongzheng He, Yaling Liu, Xiaohua Wu, Karl Staser, Su-Jung Park, Jin Yuan, Xianlin Yang, Xiaohong Li, Li Jiang and Shi Chen
Departments of Pediatrics, Indiana University School of Medicine, Indianapolis, Indiana, United States of America
Herman B Wells Center for Pediatric Research, Indiana University School of Medicine, Indianapolis, Indiana, United States of America

Steven D. Rhodes
Herman B Wells Center for Pediatric Research, Indiana University School of Medicine, Indianapolis, Indiana, United States of America
Anatomy and Cell Biology, Indiana University School of Medicine, Indianapolis, Indiana, United States of America

Feng-Chun Yang
Departments of Pediatrics, Indiana University School of Medicine, Indianapolis, Indiana, United States of America
Herman B Wells Center for Pediatric Research, Indiana University School of Medicine, Indianapolis, Indiana, United States of America
Anatomy and Cell Biology, Indiana University School of Medicine, Indianapolis, Indiana, United States of America

Thomas Funck-Brentano, Hilène Lin, Eric Hay, Marie-Dominique Ah Kioon, Corinne Schiltz, Frédéric Lioté, Marie-Christine de Vernejoul and Martine Esther Cohen-Solal
INSERM U606, Centre Viggo Petersen and Université Paris-Diderot Paris 7, Hôpital Lariboisière, Paris, France
Didier Hannouche and Rémy Nizard
Department of Orthopedics, Centre Viggo Petersen and Université Paris-Diderot Paris 7, Hôpital Lariboisière, Paris, France

Orcel
Department of Rheumatology, Centre Viggo Petersen and Universite´ Paris-Diderot Paris 7, Hôpital
Lariboisière, Paris, France

Hiroaki Kimura, Haruhiko Akiyama and Takashi Nakamura
Department of Orthopaedics, Kyoto University, Kyoto, Japan

Zhaoping Zhang, Jian Min Deng, Richard R. Behringer and Benoit de Crombrugghe
Department of Molecular Genetics, The University of Texas M. D. Anderson Cancer Center, Houston, Texas, United States of America

Kin Ming Kwan
Department of Molecular Genetics, The University of Texas M. D. Anderson Cancer Center, Houston, Texas, United States of America
Department of Biology, The Chinese University of Hong Kong, Shatin, Hong Kong SAR, China

Bryant G. Darnay
Department of Experimental Therapeutics, The University of Texas M. D. Anderson Cancer Center, Houston, Texas, United States of America

Han, Huan Zhao, Li Ni, Jiajun Han, Yun Zhou, Yannan Gu, Xuesong Zhu, Huilin Yang and Qin Shi
Orthopedic Department, the First Affiliated Hospital of Soochow University, Suzhou, P.R. China

Wen Zhang
Orthopedic Institute of Soochow University, Suzhou, P.R. China

Jun Gu
Orthopedic Department, the Second Affiliated Hospital of Soochow University, Suzhou, P.R. China

Jie Sun
Division of Nanobiomedicine, Suzhou Institute of Nano-Tech and Nano-Bionics, Chinese Academy of Sciences, Suzhou, P.R. China

Xianglin Hou and Jianwu Dai
State Key Laboratory of Molecular Developmental Biology, Institute of Genetics and Developmental Biology, Chinese Academy of Sciences, Beijing, P.R. China

Natalia Mejía-Gaviria
Department of Pediatrics, University of Oviedo, Oviedo, Spain

Óscar Álvarez-García
Department of Pediatrics, University of Oviedo, Oviedo, Spain
Laboratory of Growth and Cancer, Instituto Universitario de Oncología del Principado de Asturias, Oviedo, Asturias, Spain

Enrique García-López, Vanessa Loredo, Helena Gil-Peña and Flor Á. Ordóñez
Department of Pediatrics, Hospital Universitario Central de Asturias, Oviedo, Spain

Julián Rodríguez-Suárez
Department of Pediatrics, University of Oviedo, Oviedo, Spain
Department of Pediatrics, Hospital Universitario Central de Asturias, Oviedo, Spain

Fernando Santos
Department of Pediatrics, University of Oviedo, Oviedo, Spain
Laboratory of Growth and Cancer, Instituto Universitario de Oncología del Principado de Asturias,
Oviedo, Asturias, Spain
Department of Pediatrics, Hospital Universitario Central de Asturias, Oviedo, Spain

Kathryn J. Swoboda, Sandra P. Reyna, Bernard LaSalle, Susan L. Sorenson, Janine Wood, Mark B. Bromberg and Gary M. Chan,
Departments of Neurology, Pediatrics, Neonatology and General Clinical Research Center, University of Utah School of Medicine, Salt Lake City, Utah, United States of America

Charles B. Scott
CBS Squared, Inc, Fort Washington, Pennsylvania, United States of America

Thomas W. Prior, Bakri Elsheikh and John T. Kissel
Departments of Molecular Pathology and Neurology, Ohio State University Medical Center, Columbus, Ohio, United States of America

Gyula Acsadi
Departments of Neurology and Pediatrics, Wayne State University School of Medicine, Detroit, Michigan, United States of America

Thomas O. Crawford
Departments of Neurology and Pediatrics, Johns Hopkins University School of Medicine, Baltimore, Maryland, United States of America

Kristin J. Krosschell
Department of Physical Therapy and Human Movement Sciences, Feinberg School of Medicine, Northwestern University, Chicago, Illinois, United States of America

Guy D'Anjou
Division of Pediatric Neurology, Hôpital Sainte-Justine Montréal, Montréal, Québec, Canada

Mary K. Schroth
Department of Pediatrics, University of Wisconsin School of Medicine, Madison, Wisconsin, United States of America

Louise R. Simard
Department of Biochemistry and Medical Genetics, University of Manitoba, Winnipeg, Manitoba, Canada

Wei Yi
Department of Mechanics, Huazhong University of Science and Technology, Wuhan, Hubei, China

Qing Tian
Tongji Medical College, Huazhong University of Science and Technology, Wuhan, Hubei, China

Zhipeng Dai
Tongji Medical College, Huazhong University of Science and Technology, Wuhan, Hubei, China

Xiaohu Liu
Department of Mechanics, Huazhong University of Science and Technology, Wuhan, Hubei, China

Romain Dacquin, Chantal Domenget, Pierre Jurdic and Irma Machuca-Gayet
Institut de Génomique Fonctionnelle de Lyon, Universitéde Lyon, CNRS, Ecole Normale Supérieure de Lyon, Lyon, France

Atsushi Kumanogoh and Hitoshi Kikutani
Department of Immunopathology, Research Institute for Microbial Diseases, Osaka University, Suita, Osaka, Japan

Tyler J. O'Neill and Laura Rivera
Dalla Lana School of Public Health, University of Toronto, Toronto, Ontario, Canada

Vladi Struchkov
Dalla Lana School of Public Health, University of Toronto, Toronto, Ontario, Canada
Faculty of Medicine, University of Toronto, Toronto, Ontario, Canada

Hla-Hla Thein
Dalla Lana School of Public Health, University of Toronto, Toronto, Ontario, Canada

Ontario Institute for Cancer Research/Cancer Care Ontario, Toronto, Ontario, Canada

Ahmad Zaheen
Faculty of Medicine, University of Toronto, Toronto, Ontario, Canada

Chun-Chun Cheng, Felix Shih-Hsiang Hsiao and Shau-Ping Lin
Institute of Biotechnology, National Taiwan University, Taipei, Taiwan

Shinn-Chih Wu
Institute of Biotechnology, National Taiwan University, Taipei, Taiwan
Department of Animal Science and Technology, National Taiwan University, Taipei, Taiwan

Wei-Shiung Lian and Ching-Feng Cheng
Department of Medical Research, Tzu Chi General Hospital and Department of Pediatrics, Tzu Chi University, Hualien, Taiwan
Institute of Biomedical Sciences, Academia Sinica, Taipei, Taiwan

Yen-Hua Lee, Chia-Chun Chang, Guan-Yu Xiao and Hsin-Yi Huang
Department of Animal Science and Technology, National Taiwan University, Taipei, Taiwan

I-Hsuan Liu
Department of Animal Science and Technology, National Taiwan University, Taipei, Taiwan
Research Center for Developmental Biology and Regenerative Medicine, National Taiwan University, Taipei, Taiwan

Teng-Kuei Cheng
Department of Animal Science and Technology, National Taiwan University, Taipei, Taiwan
Department of Animal Science and Biotechnology, Tunghai University, Taichung, Taiwan

Jin-Kang Zhang, Liu Yang, Guo-Lin Meng, Zhi Yuan, Jing Fan, Dan Li, Tian-Hui-Min Hu, Bo-Yuan Wei, Zhuo-Jing Luo and Jian Liu
Institute of Orthopedic Surgery, Xijing Hospital, Fourth Military Medical University, Xi9an, People's Republic of China

Jian-Zong Chen
Research Center of Traditional Chinese Medicine, Xijing Hospital, Fourth Military Medical University, Xi'an, People's Republic of China

Yao Shi
Department of Pharmacology, School of Pharmacy, Fourth Military Medical University, Xi'an, People's Republic of China

Eugenia Negredo, Anna Bonjoch, Carla Estany and Jordi Puig
Lluita contra la SIDA Foundation, Hospital Universitari Germans Trias i Pujol, Universitat Autònoma de Barcelona, Barcelona, Spain

Moisés Gómez-Mateu and Guadalupe Gómez
Statistics and Operations Research Department, Universitat Politècnica de Catalunya, Barcelona, Spain

Nuria Perez-Alvarez
Lluita contra la SIDA Foundation, Hospital Universitari Germans Trias i Pujol, Universitat Autònoma de Barcelona, Barcelona, Spain
Statistics and Operations Research Department, Universitat Politècnica de Catalunya, Barcelona, Spain

Bonaventura Clotet
Lluita contra la SIDA Foundation, Hospital Universitari Germans Trias i Pujol, Universitat Autònoma de Barcelona, Barcelona, Spain
Irsicaixa Foundation, Barcelona, Spain

Joaquin Rosales, Silvana di Gregorio and Luis del Rio
CETIR Centre Mèdic, Barcelona, Spain

Brett Nemke
Comparative Orthopaedic Research Laboratory, School of Veterinary Medicine, University of Wisconsin-Madison, Madison, Wisconson, United States of America

Yan Lu
Comparative Orthopaedic Research Laboratory, School of Veterinary Medicine, University of Wisconsin-Madison, Madison, Wisconson, United States of America
Orthopedics and Rehabilitation, University of Wisconsin, Madison, Wisconson, United States of America

Jae Sung Lee, Ray Vanderby Jr. and Kevin Royalty
Departments of Biomedical Engineering, University of Wisconsin, Madison, Wisconson, United States of America

Ben K. Graf and Richard Illgen III
Orthopedics and Rehabilitation, University of Wisconsin, Madison, Wisconson, United States of America

Mark D. Markel
Comparative Orthopaedic Research Laboratory, School of Veterinary Medicine, University of Wisconsin-Madison, Madison, Wisconson, United States of America
Orthopedics and Rehabilitation, University of Wisconsin, Madison, Wisconson, United States of America

William L. Murphy
Departments of Biomedical Engineering, University of Wisconsin, Madison, Wisconson, United States of America
Pharmacology, University of Wisconsin, Madison, Wisconson, United States of America
Orthopedics and Rehabilitation, University of Wisconsin, Madison, Wisconson, United States of America

Hélène Follet, Delphine Farlay, Yohann Bala, Stéphanie Viguet-Carrin, Evelyne Gineyts, Brigitte Burt-Pichat, Pierre Delmas, Georges Boivin and Roland Chapurlat
INSERM, UMR 1033, Lyon, France
Université de Lyon, UMR 1033, Lyon, France

Julien Wegrzyn
INSERM, UMR 1033, Lyon, France
Université de Lyon, UMR 1033, Lyon, France
Département de Chirurgie Orthopédique, Pavillon T, Hôpital Edouard Herriot, Lyon, France

Tomasz D. Szwedowski, William R. Taylor, Markus O. Heller, Carsten Perka, Michael Müller and Georg N. Duda
Julius Wolff Institute (JWI), Center for Musculoskeletal Surgery (CMSC), Center for Sports Science and Sports Medicine Berlin (CSSB), Charite´ - Universita¨tsmedizin Berlin, Berlin, Germany

Prashanthi Menon, Jinjiang Pang, Elaine Smolock, Chen Yan and Bradford C. Berk
Aab Cardiovascular Research Institute and the Department of Medicine, University of Rochester Medical Center, Rochester, New York, United States of America

Tzong-Jen Sheu, Hsin-Chiu Ho, Shanshan Shi, Chao Xie and Michael J. Zuscik
Center for Musculoskeletal Research and the Department of Orthopaedics and Rehabilitation, University of Rochester Medical Center, Rochester, New York, United States of America

Guoyong Yin
Aab Cardiovascular Research Institute and the Department of Medicine, University of Rochester Medical Center, Rochester, New York, United States of America
Orthopaedic Department, The First Affiliated Hospital of Nanjing Medical University, Jiangsu, China

Index

A

Anti-mm Therapies, 55, 64

Antiproliferative, 85, 103, 108

Atomic Force Microscopy, 47, 54

B

Bi-layered Membrane, 9-10

Biological Process, 1-2, 6-7

Bisphosphonate, 29-32, 36-37, 45-46, 81-82, 183, 199-200, 223

Bone Adaptation, 203-204, 206-208

Bone Biopsies, 29-31, 36-37

Bone Marrow Cross Transplantation, 130

Bone Marrow Mononuclear Cells, 67, 75, 138

Bone Mass, 27, 29, 35-36, 46-47, 49-50, 53, 72, 85-88, 91, 93, 123-125, 130-131, 134-138, 140-141, 167, 170, 175-176, 223

Bone Metabolism, 29, 39-40, 44-45, 75, 185

Bone Mineral Density, 1-2, 18, 27-28, 31-32, 34-37, 39, 41-42, 44-46, 54, 67-68, 72, 74, 77, 82, 94, 96, 100, 112-113, 115, 117, 120, 129-130, 139, 141-143, 148, 150-151, 167, 169, 175, 177, 179, 181, 185, 208-209, 223

Bone Morphogenetic, 85, 93-95, 102, 186-187, 192

Bone Morphogenetic Protein-2, 85, 94-95, 102, 192

Bone Regeneration, 16-17, 94-95, 101-102

Bone Resorption, 30, 36-37, 55, 68-71, 77-79, 81, 83-86, 88, 90-91, 130-131, 133-134, 136-138, 140, 147-148, 167, 172, 176, 185, 208-209

Bone-implant Gap, 186-187, 189-191

Bone-resorbing Mediators, 167

Broadband Ultrasound Attenuation, 18-19, 22-23

C

Cardio-facio-cutaneous Syndrome, 67, 72

Cartilage Metabolism, 77, 81

Catechol-o-methyltransferase, 2, 4, 7-8

Cell Proliferation, 14, 55, 75, 90, 92, 103, 107-108, 152, 154, 156, 158-159, 164, 223

Chemoresistance, 55, 63

Chicken Genome, 1, 6

Chondrocyte Proliferation, 104, 106, 210, 215-217, 221

Chronic Kidney Disease, 47, 53-54, 147

Cleidocranial Displaysia, 18

Collagen Binding Domain, 94-95, 100-102

Collagen Morphology, 47-49, 51, 53

Colony-forming Unit, 68, 85, 87, 171

Cortical Bone, 11, 15-17, 31, 47, 49, 52-54, 69, 90, 93, 169, 193, 201-202, 208, 211, 223

Crystallinity Index, 194-195, 197-198, 200-201

Cycle Energy Dissipation, 47-49, 51

D

Dxa Scan, 40, 45, 177-178, 180, 183

E

Elastomer Membrane, 9, 11, 14

F

Femoral Head Support Device, 121-122, 124-125, 129

Femoral Neck Bmd, 18, 20, 22-23, 28

Fracture Healing Process, 161, 210-212, 221

G

Gene Expression, 1-3, 6-7, 28, 41-42, 67, 83, 120, 139, 155, 157, 163, 169

Genetic Variants, 28, 39-40, 45

Glutamine, 18-20, 25, 27-28, 162

Growth Hormone, 103-104, 111

Growth Retardation, 103-104, 111

H

Hematopoietic Cell

Transplantation, 39, 41-42, 44-45

Hematopoietic Cells, 45, 67-68, 72, 152-154

Hepatitis C Virus, 141, 143, 146, 148-150

Hip Arthroplasty, 176, 203-204, 208-209

Hiv-hepatitis, 141

Human Runx2, 18-20

Hybridization, 1, 6-7, 57, 65, 85-86, 91-93, 104, 106-107, 110-111

Hydrogen Peroxide, 167-168, 176

I

Iliac Crest Biopsies, 29-31, 52, 202

Immune Responsiveness, 1, 3

Immunoglobulin, 3-4, 55

J

Joint Endoprosthesis, 203

L

Lb Laying Hens, 1-2

Lohmann Selected Leghorn, 1, 3-5, 7
Lumbar Spine, 19, 21-22, 31, 40, 44, 95, 102, 144, 147, 178

M
Membrane Controls, 9, 14-15
Membranes Incorporating, 9-10, 13
Mesenchymal Cell, 18, 223
Mesenchymal Stem Cells, 152, 154, 161, 164-166, 192
Micro-computed Tomograph, 15
Micro-computed Tomography, 9, 13-14, 16-17, 30, 37, 72, 94, 169, 174
Monoclonal Antibody, 39, 83
Multiple Myeloma, 55-56, 65-66
Myeloma Cells, 55-60, 63

N
Neuronal Cells, 1, 165
Neutralizing Antibody, 77, 79, 82-83
Nitrogen Mustard, 55
Nuclear Localization, 23-24, 27

O
Osteoarthritis, 77, 83-84, 201
Osteoclasts, 29-31, 36, 44, 49, 55, 57-59, 61, 67-73, 75-76, 80, 85-86, 90, 93, 107, 130-140, 167, 170-172, 210, 212, 217, 219, 221-222
Osteoporosis, 17-19, 21-22, 27-31, 35-37, 39-40, 44-47, 54, 74-75, 81, 83-85, 88, 90-91, 93, 121-122, 125, 127, 129-130, 141-142, 144, 148-151, 167-168, 170-172, 174-178, 180-183, 185, 200-201, 210
Osteoprotegerin, 75, 77, 83-84, 172, 221, 223
Ovarian Function, 130-131, 135-138
Oxidative Stress, 1-2, 167-168, 170-171, 173-176

P
Periosteal Transplant Strips, 9, 12, 14
Periosteum, 9-17, 86, 165, 217
Plasmids, 20
Pluripotent Cells, 9, 15, 17
Polyglutamine, 18-19, 28
Preosteoblasts, 15, 85, 93

R
Raman Spectroscopy, 47-49, 52
Rapamycin, 103-111

S
Salidroside, 167-176
Single Nucleotide
Polymorphisms, 39, 45
Spinal Muscular Atrophy, 112, 119-120
Spine Fusion Model, 95
Strain Energy Density, 203, 207
Strontium Ranelate, 29-30, 32, 34-37
Strontium Ranelate Treatment, 29, 32, 35-37

T
Tissue Generation, 9, 13, 16
Tumor Resection, 10
Tunneling Resorption, 29, 35

U
Ultrasound Attenuation, 18-19, 22-23, 26

V
Valproic Acid, 112-113, 120
Vitamin D Receptor, 24, 26, 28, 40